Annual Update in Intensive Care and Emergency Medicine 2019

The series *Annual Update in Intensive Care and Emergency Medicine* is the continuation of the series entitled *Yearbook of Intensive Care and Emergency Medicine* in Europe and *Intensive Care Medicine: Annual Update* in the United States.

Jean-Louis Vincent
Editor

Annual Update in Intensive Care and Emergency Medicine 2019

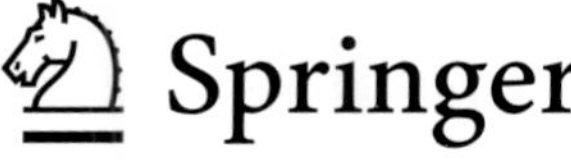

Editor
Prof. Jean-Louis Vincent
Dept. of Intensive Care
Erasme Hospital
Université libre de Bruxelles
Brussels, Belgium
jlvincent@intensive.org

ISSN 2191-5709 ISSN 2191-5717 (electronic)
Annual Update in Intensive Care and Emergency Medicine
ISBN 978-3-030-06066-4 ISBN 978-3-030-06067-1 (eBook)
https://doi.org/10.1007/978-3-030-06067-1

Library of Congress Control Number: 2019931833

Cover design: WMXDesign GmbH, Heidelberg

This Springer imprint is published by the registered company Springer Nature Switzerland AG
The registered company address is: Gewerbestrasse 11, 6330 Cham, Switzerland

Contents

Part IV Cardiac Arrest

Part V Cardiac Function

Part VI Shock

Part VII Hemodynamic and Respiratory Monitoring

Abbreviations

AKI	Acute kidney injury
ARDS	Acute respiratory distress syndrome
CAP	Community-acquired pneumonia
COPD	Chronic obstructive pulmonary disease
CPR	Cardiopulmonary resuscitation
CRRT	Continuous renal replacement therapy
CT	Computed tomography
CVP	Central venous pressure
ECMO	Extracorporeal membrane oxygenation
EEG	Electroencephalogram
GFR	Glomerular filtration rate
ICU	Intensive care unit
IL	Interleukin
LPS	Lipopolysaccharide
MAP	Mean arterial pressure
NO	Nitric oxide
NOS	Nitric oxide synthase
PAC	Pulmonary artery catheter
PAOP	Pulmonary artery occlusion pressure
PEEP	Positive end-expiratory pressure
PPV	Pulse pressure variation
RBC	Red blood cell
RCT	Randomized controlled trial
ROS	Reactive oxygen species
RRT	Renal replacement therapy
RV	Right ventricular
$ScvO_2$	Central venous oxygen saturation
SvO_2	Mixed venous oxygen saturation
TBI	Traumatic brain injury
TNF	Tumor necrosis factor
VAP	Ventilator-associated pneumonia
VILI	Ventilator-induced lung injury

Part I

Precision Medicine

Precision Medicine in the Intensive Care Unit: Identifying Opportunities and Overcoming Barriers

1

T. L. Palmieri and N. K. Tran

1.1 Introduction

Is precision medicine really precise? Precision in medicine can only be achieved with precision diagnostics. Unfortunately, barriers, such as access to clean electronic medical data, accurate and precise laboratory tests, and a propensity to over simplify complex pathophysiology, hinder this transformation to achieve the 'four Ps' of precision medicine: Personalized, Preventive, Predictive, and Participatory.

The rapid evolution of intensive care medicine has resulted in advancements for integration of technology with disease pathophysiology. The result: improved therapeutics and reduced patient mortality and morbidity. However, current medical practice is predicated on the Cnidarian School of Medicine, a three-tiered approach consisting of: (1) patient evaluation and disease diagnosis; (2) comparison and matching to a similar patient population via databases or data sets; and (3) initiation and monitoring of treatment [1]. As such, treatment is reactive and compartmentalized; intensivists initiate therapy for a specific organ system after disease identification. The ultimate success of treatment, however, relies on the interaction between the individual, the disease and the treatment. For example, infection is diagnosed by obtaining a sample of the infectious source, identifying an inciting organism, and choosing an antibiotic based on culture results in a petri dish. The efficacy of that treatment is dependent on the patient, the organism, the therapy, and the interaction among the three. Current paradigms tend to underestimate the variability and complexity of the system.

T. L. Palmieri (✉)
Firefighters Burn Institute, Burn Center at the University of California, Davis, CA, USA

Burns Department, Shriners Hospitals for Children Northern California, Sacramento, CA, USA
e-mail: tlpalmieri@ucdavis.edu

N. K. Tran
Department of Pathology and Laboratory Medicine, UC Davis School of Medicine, Davis, CA, USA

J.-L. Vincent (ed.), *Annual Update in Intensive Care and Emergency Medicine 2019*, Annual Update in Intensive Care and Emergency Medicine,
https://doi.org/10.1007/978-3-030-06067-1_1

The four pillars of precision medicine allow healthcare to be proactive and predictive, enabling clinicians to address the patient-disease-therapy triad by developing targeted patient and disease-specific therapies [2]. Initial precision medicine endeavors focused on oncology, an arena in which genetic biomarkers transformed therapeutic interventions [3]. Molecular oncology has created a better understanding of malignancies and identified exploitable targets, such as human epidermal growth factor receptor 2 (HER2), for therapy. However, application in intensive care, which represents a significant health burden, has been far slower. This is due to multiple factors, including the complex nature of critical illness in an intensive care unit (ICU), poor characterization of patient populations (generalized definitions), lack of informatics that integrate physiologic data with laboratory and genetic data, timeliness of usable data analysis, and appropriate clinical trial platforms that can capture discreet patient populations [4]. However, the ICU, housing patients with the greatest severity of illness, also has the greatest opportunity for benefit for improving both patient survival and quality of life while also containing cost. The purpose of this chapter is to present a framework for application of precision medicine in the ICU and introduce potential current challenges and future areas of conflict that may arise.

1.2 Definitions

Clarity in definitions is essential to any discussion of medical treatment paradigms. Perhaps the greatest example is the definition of the 'critically ill' patient by the United States (US) Food and Drug Administration (FDA)—it does not exist! How can a disease be studied or targeted if it is not well defined? Further exacerbating the challenges faced by intensivists in defining the 'critically ill' population is the variation of the definition between institutions. In 2015, US hospitals were faced with a dilemma involving the intended use of point-of-care blood glucose monitoring systems. At the time, no blood glucose monitoring device was approved by the FDA for use in critically ill patients, and point-of-care glucose monitoring in these patients was considered off label use. Due to the lack of a definition of critical illness, hospitals were stymied in trying to conform to the regulations and risked citation by regulatory agencies including the Centers for Medicare and Medicaid Services (CMS).

Another definition challenge has been the transformation of the term individualized medicine, to personalized medicine, to now, precision medicine. Although personalized medicine has many overlapping features with precision medicine, personalized medicine and precision medicine are distinct concepts. The concept of personalized medicine, introduced in the early 2000s, was partially developed in response to the completion of the human genome project. As such, personalized medicine emphasizes specific analyses for unique treatments for each individual patient [5]. Essentially, the personalized medicine model is an N-of-1: individuals receive customized treatment designed specifically for them. Precision medicine, on the other hand, is characterized by tailoring medical treatment to patient characteristics, i.e., classifying individuals into subpopulations with different susceptibilities, disease biology and/or prognosis, or response to treatment. Hence, the model is 1-of-N [6]. Accurate identification of subgroups, likely by genomic, metabolomic, proteomic, and immunologic data, will be essential for the success of the precision medicine model.

Due to the complexity of critical care and the multifaceted nature of the ICU environment, it is important to distinguish populations based on prognosis versus prediction. Prognostic patient selection involves the selection of patients with a greater chance of a disease-related event, such as mortality, whereas predictive selection involves selection of patients more likely to respond to an intervention based on biological mechanisms associated with a disease [7]. Prognostic precision medicine examples predominate in sepsis [8]. Predictive precision medicine is advancing rapidly with the advent of pharmacogenomics, allowing for the more targeted use of antibiotics in sepsis [9]. Both forms will be needed in the ICU setting. The most logical approach is to first define patient subpopulations followed by the use of targeted therapies designed for that population.

1.3 Diagnosis

One of the more exciting aspects of precision medicine in the ICU is its potential to identify subgroups with similar disease states or outcomes based on biomarkers. A range of critical illnesses are defined by syndromes or clinical signs which may or may not be caused by a single underlying disease, including acute respiratory syndrome (ARDS), sepsis, acute kidney injury (AKI) and delirium [10]. Sepsis trials, in particular, have suffered from this syndromic issue. Unfortunately, although biomarkers have been proposed to define a host of clinical conditions ranging from sepsis [11] to AKI [12], all have lacked the specificity necessary to define study populations.

Additional challenges with diagnosis include significant variation within laboratory testing methodology. Modern medicine has often taken for granted what is being tested. For example, a serum lactate cut-off of 2 or 4 mmol/L has often been used as part of sepsis protocols. However, the lack of standardization of lactate as a test is an underappreciated limitation. Ridenour et al. reported that many lactate tests differ significantly as values approach 4 mmol/L [13].

Even cardiac troponin (cTn), a very common biomarker of myocardial injury, is not standardized. Differences between cTnI and cTnT are well known, but, the reference materials (National Institute of Standards and Technology Standard Reference Material 2921) for manufacturers are native cTn-ICT ternary complexes [14]. However, biologically, cTn could exist as dimers, trimers, and monomers—each with a different epitope targeted by various assays. Thus, cTnI between different manufacturers are different as illustrated by their 99th percentile cut offs. In summary, to achieve precision medicine, we must also achieve precision laboratory testing. Table 1.1 shows the intrinsic differences between different common critical care tests based on the assay used to perform the test.

Table 1.1 Variation between common critical care tests

Purpose	Biomarker (standard)	Manufacturer	Platform	Format	Methodology	Challenges
Cardiac injury	Troponin I (SRM 2921)	Abbott	Architect	Mainframe	Chemiluminescent immunoassay	Biologically released troponin can be monomeric, dimeric, and/or trimeric with differing epitopes detected by each immunoassay. Different troponin I assays cannot be compared, nor can I against T assays [15, 16]
		Beckman Coulter	DxI	Mainframe	Chemiluminescent immunoassay	
		Siemens	Centaur	Mainframe	Chemiluminescent immunoassay	
	Troponin T (SRM 2921)	Roche Diagnostics	Elecsys	Mainframe	Electro-chemiluminescent immunoassay	
Coagulation	PT/INR (multiple, recombinant or rabbit thromboplastin)	Abbott	i-STAT	POCT	Electrochemical	Multiple standards exist for PT/INR tests. Some assays use rabbit thromboplastin, others use recombinant human thromboplastin. Recent reformulations resulted in significant differences between POCT and lab [17]
		Instrumentation Laboratories	ACL TOPS	Mainframe	Spectrophotometric	
		Roche Diagnostics	CoaguChek XS	POCT	Electrochemical	
Glycemic control	Glucose (SRM 965b, IDMS)	Abbott	i-STAT	POCT	Enzymatic (GO)	Previous studies show statistically significant differences across POCT and laboratory platforms using paired specimens despite efforts to standardize [18]
		Beckman Coulter	DxC	Mainframe	Enzymatic (GO)	
			AU	Mainframe	Enzymatic (HK)	
		Nova Biomedical	StatSensor	POCT	Enzymatic (GO)	
		Radiometer	ABL90	POCT	Enzymatic (GO)	
		Roche Diagnostics	c702	Mainframe	Enzymatic (HK)	
		Siemens	epoc	POCT	Enzymatic (GO)	

Liver function	ALP, ALT, AST, GGT (None)	Abbott	Piccolo	POCT	Enzyme activity	Since 1971, it has been established that it is not feasible to determine the true accuracy of enzyme activity assays [19]
		Beckman Coulter	DxC	Mainframe	Enzyme activity	
		Roche Diagnostics	c701	Mainframe	Enzyme activity	
Perfusion	Lactate (None)	Abbott	i-STAT	POCT	Electrochemical	Lactate is not standardized, with several studies showing significant discordance as values approach 4 mmol/L and beyond [20]
		Beckman Coulter	DxC	Mainframe	Electrochemical	
		Nova Biomedical	StatStrip	POCT	Electrochemical	
		Radiometer	ABL90	POCT	Electrochemical	
		Roche Diagnostics	c702	Mainframe	Electrochemical	
		Siemens	epoc	POCT	Electrochemical	
Renal function	Creatinine (SRM 967, IDMS)	Abbott	i-STAT	POCT	Electrochemical	Although creatinine was standardized to SRM 967 by IDMS, variations in methods and the significant biological variability of the biomarker causes substantial discordance between platforms [21]
		Beckman Coulter	DxC Cartridge	Mainframe	Electrochemical	
			DxC Jaffe	Mainframe	Jaffe Reaction	
		Nova Biomedical	StatSensor	POCT	Enzymatic	
		Radiometer	ABL90	POCT	Enzymatic	
		Roche Diagnostics	c702	Mainframe	Enzymatic	
		Siemens	epoc	POCT	Enzymatic	

ALP alkaline phosphatase, *ALT* alanine transferase, *AST* aspartate aminotranasferase, *GGT* gamma glutamyl transferase, *IDMS* isotope dilution mass spectrometry, *INR* international normalized ratio, *POCT* point-of-care testing, *PT* prothrombin time, *SRM* standardized reference method, *GO* glucose oxidase, *HK* hexokinase

1.4 Treatment

Several studies have used biomarker data to identify predictive cohorts that would respond to a therapeutic intervention. For example, several groups have analyzed biomarkers in ARDS to predict responsiveness to positive end-expiratory pressure (PEEP) and fluid management [22, 23]. However, the more precise identification of subtypes may make prospective trial conduct problematic, as the number of patients eligible for a study will diminish. Trials will require a greater number of participating centers, more advanced screening methods, longer conduct times, and different trial methodologies to achieve statistical significance.

1.5 Potential Conflicts/Weaknesses

Why has the adoption of precision medicine in the ICU been slower than in oncology? Perhaps the most intuitive argument is the lack of a clear well-defined target (disease process and subpopulation). Oncologists can target a cancer molecular signature in a specific organ or system. Patients in an ICU are admitted for diverse problems ranging from sepsis to cardiac failure, traumatic or burn injury to postoperative cardiac care. As such, ICU patients often have multiple potential targets. For example, a patient admitted with a closed head injury has frequently sustained other injuries (such as hemorrhagic trauma or burns) and/or has multiple organ system dysfunction, which could lead to conflicts in treatment. Should a patient with a closed head injury and major burn be treated with massive fluid resuscitation to address the burn injury or with fluid restriction to minimize intracranial edema? Precise treatment of one disease may have no effect or may even adversely impact morbidity and mortality from another medical issue. Precision medicine may assist in formulating an answer to such questions, but the answers will be late in coming, as the precise treatment of the index injuries or diseases must occur prior to determining the best treatment for combined problems. Although clinicians have made tremendous progress in the identification of pathophysiology of illness, the understanding of the complex interplay among multiple medical issues remains elusive in many medical conditions commonly encountered in the ICU.

In addition, one therapy may alter the efficacy of another. Perhaps the best example of this occurred at the end of the twentieth century. Two landmark studies, the TRICC (Transfusion Requirements in Critical Care), which reported that stable ICU patients could be maintained at a hemoglobin of 7 g/dL as opposed to the traditional 10 g/dL [24], and Van den Berghe's intensive insulin therapy study [25], which suggested that tight glycemic control improved outcomes in critically ill patients, were published. As a result, many critically ill patients were treated with both a restrictive transfusion policy and tight glycemic control. However, clinical practice combining the two strategies had a different outcome. Tight glycemic control did not yield the benefits that were reported in the randomized trial. The subsequent NICE SUGAR study suggested harm using tight glycemic control [26]. Why? First, there was a distinct difference in the types of patients enrolled. The Van den Berghe study enrolled a very specific subpopulation, whereas the NICE-SUGAR trial had much broader enrollment criteria. Second, and equally important, the methodology for glycemic control (i.e., point-of-care glucose testing) used by most clinicians for glucose monitoring in NICE-SUGAR differed from that used in the Van den Berghe trial (serum glucose). Unbeknownst to the NICE-SUGAR investigators at that time, point-of-care glucose monitoring overestimated serum glucose levels by as much as 20% in anemic patients, likely creating unrecognized hypoglycemia in the cohort [27]. The application of the TRICC trial restrictive transfusion policy, in which ICU patients have sustained anemia, may have influenced the outcomes for patients also treated with tight glycemic control. Independently both strategies worked. Together they did not. Is tight glycemic control beneficial? The answer will require an in-depth understanding of the metabolomics of various forms of critical illness and subsequent application of targeted strategies to address the clinical variations. The application of precision medicine to the ICU will need to carefully consider the potential conflicts inherent in treating multiple different medical issues simultaneously.

The intersection of the TRICC trial and the glycemic trial also illustrate another important concept: precision medicine in the ICU will require standardization of sample collection, storage, testing and reporting; assurance of quality and reproducibility of test results; timely reporting of clinically applicable results; and clear delineation of test results in a format that clinicians can understand and apply. Recent reports from the precision method Surgical Critical Care Initiative (SC2i) have attributed data quality as the largest hurdle to the development of a comprehensive precision medicine program [28]. Even today, clinicians are bombarded with test results that need to be integrated to treat patients. Yet key elements remain unstandardized. Lactate is but one example. Lactate is currently measured using different platforms. However, no reference method or traceable material exists for lactate, resulting in non-standardized testing [13]. This is compounded by the influence of pre-analytic factors, such as testing delays and interfering substances, which can falsely elevate lactate levels. As a result, lactate measurements may vary by as much as 1.5 mmol/L for values >2 mmol/L [29]. The use of lactate in clinical trials should carefully evaluate the platforms used as well as the timing of sample analysis to assure comparable results between centers and platforms. Knowledge of how samples are analyzed and what they mean will be essential if precision medicine is to be 'precise'. Standard operating procedures, use of certified clinical laboratories, specimen storage protocols and quality assurance for every step of the laboratory analytic process will need to be employed not just for clinical samples, but for metabolomics, genomics, biomarkers, and other testing methodologies.

1.6 Pharmacokinetics

One of the core principles of precision medicine is delivery of the right treatment at the right dose at the right time. Understanding pharmacokinetics, pharmacogenomics, and pharmacokinetic variability among critically ill patients will help guide appropriate medication administration in the critical care setting. Changes in pharmacokinetics are both drug-specific and time sensitive and are often influenced by other treatment modalities. For example, hypothermia reduces phase I cytochrome P450 metabolism, thus increasing concentration of drugs (such as fentanyl, midazolam) that are metabolized using this system [30]. In contrast, the metabolic rate of severe burn patients is more than doubled, resulting in augmented renal clearance of many agents [31]. Effective dosing of antimicrobial agents as well as narcotics requires drug doses far exceeding the 'normal' standards. Drug interactions may also influence pharmacokinetics of a given agent. Concomitant administration of medications may increase, decrease or offset the effect of any given agent. This can be particularly problematic in the ICU, as patients receive multiple different agents. Critically ill burn patients, for example, receive, on average, more than 40 agents, many of which interact with each other [32]. Pharmacogenomics, which evaluates the influence of patient genomic makeup on pharmacokinetics and pharmacodynamics, will likely play a major role in future ICU precision medicine practice.

1.7 Data Collection and Analysis

Regardless of the type of patient being studied, the data acquired in precision medicine efforts will include not just patient physiologic and 'routine' laboratory analyses (such as electrolytes, blood counts) but also genomic, proteomic, metabolomic and transcriptome data; biomarkers; and data from other sources. Current electronic health records are fraught with inconsistent and inaccurate data due to both machine and human limitations. Data recording, integration, and interpretation will require quality assurance prior, during, and after data integration into a centralized data repository. New data management and analytic techniques (including machine learning) will be required to integrate the data sources and develop valid, clinically meaningful, and actionable data with which to treat patients. One of the keys to successful implementation of precision medicine in ICU patients is consistency in data acquisition, storage and reporting. This will require a level of collaboration far beyond what has occurred in medicine to date. In addition, how data are analyzed will need to be standardized. Study results can also vary depending upon how informatics is used.

Precision medicine will require fundamental changes in the conduct of clinical trials. Specific requirements will include development of trial methodologies that streamline collaboration to generate sufficient data for studies of smaller, better defined patient cohorts; additional time allotted to complete patient enrollment, and different trial platforms employing computer-based learning to maximize output from any given trial. One promising methodology, the registry-based randomized controlled trial (RRCT) uses data collected for other reasons, such as registry data, to identify appropriate targets for trial enrollment [33]. The RRCT can be used to identify patients who already meet pre-specified enrollment criteria (with their associated built-in screening, data capture and outcomes measurements), thus identifying new subjects for consent. This type of methodology is designed to optimize patient enrollment and increase collaborations among centers. In essence, the RRCT can use prognostic precision medicine to assign patients to different predictive therapeutic options. Another potential new trial design is the platform trial, which uses response-adaptive randomization to test multiple treatments in a pre-specified patient group. The system uses Bayesian analysis to identify effective treatments for specific patient subgroups [34]. Ineffective treatments are eventually discarded, as are patient groups that do not benefit from a given treatment. Essentially, the platform trial system is an example of computer learning applied to clinical trials.

1.8 The Future

The key to successful implementation of precision medicine in the ICU is collaboration. Different disease processes are in different stages of precision medicine development, particularly with respect to subgroup identification and delineation. For example, oncology has identified subgroups based on genomic markers; sepsis uses broad-based physiologic definitions; trauma and burn patients are categorized on the basis of injury characteristics. Each has unique cohort identification requirements and will require a different strategy to develop meaningful subgroup analysis. Informed groups consisting of clinicians, biostatisticians, basic scientists, epidemiologists and pharmacologists need to gather for the major disease processes to delineate the current state of the disease process, identify the key steps needed to identify subpopulations for prognostic marker testing, and map out the initial course to define prognostic markers. Concurrently, biomarker development at both the bench and clinical level should continue to validate subgroup selection and study conduct for the given subgroup, as biomarker development requires time for development, testing and implementation.

Just as disease states need to be defined, so do data capture and processing. Consistent and coherent data analysis will rely heavily on the development of a universal critical care ontology that can accommodate specialty-specific topics so that data gathered are all based on the same foundation [35]. Currently different hospitals use different electronic health records, each with a unique structure. Harnessing the power of the electronic health record to gather physiologic data requires either all programs to use the same data capture system (unlikely) or the development of algorithm-based programs that can extract common data elements from multiple different data sources and collate data into a consistent, analyzable database. These data will then need to be combined with biomarker data, including genomic, metabolomic and proteomic data. Database development teams consisting of informaticists, biostatisticians, scientists and clinicians will need to unite to complete this challenging process, which will be essential to the development of precision medicine.

1.9 Conclusion

The vision for precision medicine in the ICU has been articulated. The goal is visible on the horizon. However, the road leading to the vision is unpaved, the ground is rocky, the path crooked and the construction team has not yet been assembled.

Success will depend on collaboration, strategic resource utilization, funding availability, flexibility and patience. New technologies and trial designs will need to be created. Collaborations will need to be extended. The traditional medical paradigm will need to change. The ICU team has the dedication and capability necessary to complete the journey. We just need to take the first step.

References

1. Sugeir S, Naylor S. Critical care and personalized or precision medicine: who needs whom? J Crit Care. 2018;43:401–5.
2. Naylor S. What's in a name? The evolution of "P-medicine". J Precision Med. 2015;2:15–29.
3. Collins FS, Varmus H. A new initiative on precision medicine. N Engl J Med. 2015;372:793–5.
4. Vincent J. The coming era of precision medicine for intensive care. Crit Care. 2017;21(Suppl 3):314.
5. Redekop WK, Madsi D. The faces of personalized medicine: a framework for understanding its meaning and scope. Value Health. 2013;16:S4–9.
6. Zhang XD. Precision medicine, personalized medicine, omics, and big data: concepts and relationships. J Pharmacogenomics Pharmacoproteomics. 2015;6:e14.
7. Wong HR. Intensive care medicine in 2050: precision medicine. Intensive Care Med. 2017;43:1507–9.
8. Langley RJ, Tsalik EL, van Velkinburgh JC, et al. An integrated clinic-metabolomic model improves prediction of death in sepsis. Sci Transl Med. 2013;5:195ra95.
9. Aung AK, Haas DW, Hulgan T, Phillips EJ. Pharmacogenomics of antimicrobial agents. Pharmacogenomics. 2014;15:1903–30.
10. Sweeney TE, Khatri P. Generalizable biomarkers in critical care: toward precision medicine. Crit Care Med. 2017;45:934–9.
11. Pierrakos C, Vincent JL. Sepsis biomarkers: a review. Crit Care. 2010;14:R15.
12. McMahon BA, Koyner JL. Risk stratification for acute kidney injury: are biomarkers enough? Adv Chronic Kidney Dis. 2016;23:167–78.
13. Ridenour RV, Gada RP, Brost BC, Karon BS. Comparison of lactate values between point-of-care and central laboratory analyzers. Am J Clin Pathol. 2007;128:168–71.
14. Apple FS. Counterpoint: standardization of cardiac troponin I assays will not occur in my lifetime. Clin Chem. 2011;58:169–71.
15. Christenson RH, Bunk DM, Schimmel H, et al. Point; Put simply, standardization of cardiac troponin I is complicated. Clin Chem. 2012;58:165–8.
16. Gaze DC, Collinson PO. Multiple molecular forms of circulating cardiac troponin: analytical and clinical significance. Ann Clin Biochem. 2008;45:349–55.
17. Kost GJ, Tran NK, Louie RF, et al. Assessing the performance of handheld glucose testing for critical care. Diabetes Technol Ther. 2008;10:445–51.
18. Moss DW, Baron DN, Walker PG, et al. Standardization of clinical enzyme assays. J Clin Pathol. 1971;24:740–3.
19. Pieroini L, Bargnoux AS, Cristl JP, et al. Did creatinine standardization give benefits to the evaluation of glomerular filtration rate. EJIFCC. 2017;28:251–7.
20. Poller L. International normalized ratios (INR): the first 20 years. J Thromb Haemost. 2004;2:849–60.
21. Tolan NV, Wockenfus AM, Koch CD, et al. Analytical performance of three whole blood point-of-care lactate devices compared to plasma lactate comparison methods sand a flow-injection mass spectrometry method. Clin Biochem. 2017;50:168–73.
22. Calfee CS, Delucchi K, Parsons PE, Thompson BT, Ware LB, Matthay MA. Subphenotypes in acute respiratory distress syndrome: latent class analysis of data from two randomized controlled trial. Lancet Respir Med. 2014;2:611–20.

23. Famous KR, Delucchi K, Ware LB, et al. ARDS subphenotypes respond differently to randomized fluid management strategy. Am J Respir Crit Care Med. 2016;195:331–8.
24. Hebert PC, Wells G, Blajchman MA, et al. A multicenter, randomized, controlled clinical trial of transfusion requirements in critical care. N Engl J Med. 1999;340:409–17.
25. Van den Berghe G, Wouters P, Weekers F, et al. Intensive insulin therapy in critically ill patients. N Engl J Med. 2001;345:1359–67.
26. Investigators TNICE-SUGARS. Intensive versus conventional glucose control in critically ill patients. N Engl J Med. 2009;360:1283–97.
27. Ceriotti F, Kaczmarek E, Guerra E, et al. Comparative performance assessment of point-of-care testing devices for measuring glucose and ketones at the patient bedside. J Diabetes Sci Technol. 2015;9:268–77.
28. Belard A, Buchman T, Dente CJ, Potter BK, Kirk A, Elster E. The Uniformed Services University's Surgical critical Care Initiative (SC2I): bringing precision medicine to the critically ill. Mil Med. 2018;183:487–95.
29. Lima K, Caynak R, Tran NK. Lactate monitoring for severe sepsis and septic shock: are all lactate measurements the same? Crit Care Med. 2016;44:443.
30. Empey PE, Miller TM, Philbrick AH, et al. Mild hypothermia decreases fentanyl and midazolam steady-state clearance in a rat model of cardiac arrest. Crit Care Med. 2012;40:1221–8.
31. Udy AA, Roberts JA, Lipman J, Blot S. The effects of major burn related pathophysiological changes on the pharmacokinetics and pharmacodynamics of drug use: an appraisal utilizing antibiotics. Adv Drug Deliv Rev. 2017;123:65–74.
32. Godwin Z, Lima K, Greenhalgh D, Palmieri T, Sen S, Tran NK. A retrospective analysis of clinical laboratory interferences caused by frequently administered medications in burn patients. J Burn Care Res. 2016;37:10–7.
33. Lauer MS, D'Agostina RB. The randomized registry trial-the next disruptive technology in clinical research? N Engl J Med. 2013;369:1579–81.
34. Maslove DM, Lamontagne F, Marshall JC, Heyland KD. A path to precision in the ICU. Crit Care. 2017;21:79–88.
35. Noy NF, Shah NH, Whetzel PL, et al. BioPortal: ontologies and integrated data resources at the click of a mouse. Nucleic Acids Res. 2009;37:170–3.

Precision Delivery in Critical Care: Balancing Prediction and Personalization

2

V. X. Liu and H. C. Prescott

2.1 Introduction

Recent developments in healthcare data availability, advanced analytic algorithms, and high-performance computing have produced incredible enthusiasm about a new age of data-driven healthcare [1–8]. When it comes to clinical care specifically, 'precision delivery' is an emerging term to describe the "routine use of patients' electronic health record (EHR) data to predict risk and personalize care to substantially improve value" (Table 2.1) [7, 9, 10]. While clinical risk prediction tools have a long history in critical care, novel machine learning applications can offer improved predictive performance by maximally leveraging large-scale, complex EHR and other data [5]. Perhaps, even more importantly, these approaches may help overcome the problem of heterogeneity, which is routinely noted to be a hallmark of critical illness as well as a major barrier to improved treatment [11–13]. In this chapter, we discuss the overarching concept of 'precision delivery', the important balance between clinical risk prediction and personalization, and the future challenges and applications of data-driven critical care delivery.

V. X. Liu (✉)
Kaiser Permanente Division of Research, Oakland, CA, USA
e-mail: Vincent.x.liu@kp.org

H. C. Prescott
Department of Medicine and Institute for Social Research, University of Michigan and VA Center for Clinical Management Research, VA Ann Arbor Healthcare System, Ann Arbor, MI, USA

J.-L. Vincent (ed.), *Annual Update in Intensive Care and Emergency Medicine 2019*, Annual Update in Intensive Care and Emergency Medicine,
https://doi.org/10.1007/978-3-030-06067-1_2

Table 2.1 Key domains and concepts underlying the potential of precision delivery in critical care

Key domains	Concepts
Electronic health record (EHR) data	Granular EHR data are becoming increasingly ubiquitous in healthcare and these data can now be used routinely to inform data-driven approaches to clinical care delivery
Risk prediction	Machine learning algorithms can facilitate the use of complex, multi-faceted EHR data to improve the performance and capability of risk prediction models across many adverse outcomes of interest
Personalization	Machine learning can also be used to identify underlying subgroups within a heterogeneous cohort of at-risk patients allowing for treatments to be maximally targeted towards responsive subgroups
Improved value	When embedded within well-defined clinical pathways and delivered at the right moment, targeted care can improve outcomes while also reducing unnecessary resource utilization across large populations of patients

2.2 A Changing Landscape: The Fourth Industrial Revolution

In God we trust; all others must bring data. (frequently attributed to W. Edwards Deming)

Klaus Schwab, the founder of the World Economic Forum, notes that we are in the midst of a rapid societal upheaval driven by technological advances that are evolving at an exponential, rather than linear, scale [14, 15]. Prior industrial revolutions were marked by incredible achievements yielding the steam engine, the light bulb, the telephone, the internal combustion engine, the personal computer, and the internet. Today, the Fourth Industrial Revolution is heralded by advances in data availability, mobile computing, machine learning and artificial intelligence, robotics and autonomous vehicles, energy innovation, and nano- and bio-technology. Given the pace and complexity of change driven by these technological advances, it remains unclear how this revolution will impact societies and individuals. However, we are already bearing witness to rapid disruptions of existing industries and norms driven by expanded uses of data to risk stratify individuals and tailor actions to suit their needs.

Familiar examples of these disruptions outside of healthcare include the Amazon recommender system which uses item-based collaborative filtering algorithms when a customer is preparing to purchase a specific item to identify other 'related' items that are likely to be of interest [16]. This and other innovations have already altered the landscape of consumer purchases. Similar systems are also in place at Netflix, whose suite of algorithms seek to deliver the 'Netflix experience' by combining prediction and recommender systems that leverage personal interests, prior viewed content, and temporal trends in activity [17]. This approach has allowed Netflix to target content development to highly-specific subgroups and vastly increase the viewable or 'effective' size of their library even within narrow genres. Similar algorithmic approaches are used in applications like advertisement targeting software to surface the most relevant marketing content based on prediction algorithms using background browsing data.

2.3 Precision Delivery in Healthcare

In healthcare today, precision delivery describes a similar process for leveraging data-driven predictive approaches to improve the value of clinical care [9]. Rapid expansions in the availability of health data driven primarily through the increasing ubiquity of EHRs and other key emerging data sources (e.g., sensors, -omics), along with advances in machine learning algorithms have improved the performance and capability of contemporary risk stratification models. Machine learning algorithms can rapidly sift through voluminous and complex data to find clinically-relevant risk strata by applying computationally-intensive statistical modeling at scale [18, 19]. These risk models can then be used to improve the personalization of patient care by identifying patient subgroups in whom specific interventions can have the maximum impact, or those in whom specific interventions are unlikely to offer any benefit. Precision delivery is based on using this prediction-personalization approach, deployed at precisely the right moment in clinical treatment, to drive improved clinical outcomes [10]. At the same time, given the rapid rise in healthcare expenditures in the United States and in many other nations, the hope is that the precision delivery model can control or even reduce healthcare costs through improved patient targeting.

2.4 Critical Care: A Risk-Based Specialty

It is important to note that risk prognostication is not a new concept in medicine and has long been used to identify patient groups who might benefit from specific, targeted interventions [20]. Indeed, one could argue that the field of critical care arose as a byproduct of risk prognostication: a system in which patients with key observable criteria portending a high risk of imminent death (e.g., vital signs, traumatic injury, organ failure) were identified and triaged to a setting of increased monitoring and clinician staffing [21].

Given this history, it comes as no surprise then that the field of critical care has also been a leader in the development of clinical risk stratification models [22–24]. Highly robust mortality models developed decades ago, prior to the routine use of personal computers, continue to be widely used today. For example, the Acute Physiology and Chronic Health Evaluation II (APACHE II) scoring system, published in 1985 and based on 12 routine physiologic measurements [25], remains a common risk stratification system used even for contemporary, high-profile randomized controlled trials. Similarly, the Sepsis-related/Sequential Organ Failure Assessment (SOFA) score from 1996 [26, 27], continues to play a key role in severity of illness assessment as well as in the definition of sepsis [28].

2.5 Novel Capabilities with Improved Data and Computation

Critical care already has a robust history of risk prognostication, but recent innovations in data and computation provide several new opportunities (Table 2.2). First, the breadth of data available for incorporation into prediction algorithms has

Table 2.2 Potential capabilities available through improved platforms for data collection, analysis, and computation

Domain	Improvements
Electronic health record (EHR) data	Increasing routine collection of health data within the EHR fosters a vastly increased breadth of data available for incorporation into clinical risk prediction models. In general, models developed with expanded data have shown improved predictive performance
Variable subset selection or dimensionality reduction	With a vastly increased set of variables, or 'feature space', the risk of identifying random associations increases. Machine learning algorithms can be used to statistically identify the most relevant variables to a specific problem of interest
Non-parametric modeling	Traditional risk prediction algorithms largely depended on linear modeling, which places potential limitations on interactions between complex data elements. Improved computation platforms allow for more flexible modeling approaches to maximally leverage EHR data. However, they may also decrease the interpretability of prediction models
Real-time predictive modeling	As greater numbers of risk prediction models are incorporated within EHR systems, the incremental costs of additional calculations are small (when compared with the costs of manual calculation). This allows for multiple models to be calculated for each patient, as well as multiple time points for model updating (e.g., every minute, hour, or day).
User-friendly systems	Alarm fatigue and distractions already plague clinicians working in high-acuity settings. By tuning model parameters at the development and deployment stages, models can be embedded within clinical workflows to enhance, rather than distract, clinical care

expanded tremendously, owing to the transition from pen and paper recording of data into automated EHR-based data collection. Thus, while simpler hand-calculated models continue to be calculated and used even in modern EHR systems (e.g., the Model for End-Stage Liver Disease [MELD] score), most newer prediction models now incorporate a considerably larger set of variables or 'features'. In general, these models show improved predictive capability, at least when measured by standard quantitative performance metrics like test error rates, area under the receiver operating characteristic (AUC) curves, or positive predictive values [1, 2, 5].

However, the expansion of variables available for model inclusion, or the 'feature space', brings with it new challenges related to finding robust data signals within the noise. This is an area in which machine learning excels, because algorithms can be used to empirically identify the most relevant subset of variables in a model (i.e., dimensionality reduction) as well as to apply non-parametric modeling approaches to complex data that account for non-linear relationships between variables [18, 19]. For example, gradient boosted trees, which iteratively combine many individual weaker decision trees based on random subsets of data to improve classification, have shown robust performance across many different types of clinical risk prediction challenges.

This use of machine learning algorithms does not come without cost. Computationally-intensive platforms are often needed to implement advanced modeling strategies, particularly in large databases. However, the cost of these platforms has decreased tremendously while their availability has also increased rapidly, largely offsetting these concerns in all but the most complex scenarios. There is also an important trade-off between the ease of model development or scoring and the ability to interpret and apply the risk predictions themselves [19]. While some methods, like decision tree-based models, offer moderate degrees of intelligibility (i.e., the ability to understand which variables are driving predictions), others, like the deep learning neural networks recently used by Google [29], are considerably more challenging to interpret. Traditional linear models, including logistic regression, have generally shown weaker predictive performance in recent comparisons but offer the advantage of allowing for high degrees of intelligibility and potentially easier technical implementation. In some cases, extensions of linear models, like penalized logistic regression models—designed to identify the subset of variables which maximally contribute to prediction—have shown similar performance to other non-parametric approaches [18].

In addition to the advantages afforded by an expanded universe of potential variables and more flexible modeling approaches, the widespread uptake of EHRs and mobile computing has facilitated the deployment of real-time risk scoring and display without requiring significant additional manual effort. Thus, the incremental operating costs associated with using an EHR-based system to simultaneously calculate and display 100 risk models compared with only a single model may be relatively modest. This would certainly not be the case for individuals who might have to manually calculate and record 100 risk scores for each patient every hour.

This flexibility offers further opportunities to deploy risk models that are more user-centric and aligned with the so-called "5 rights of clinical decision support" [30]: providing the right information, to the right people, in the right format, through the right channels, and at the right time. Given that all clinicians, and in particular those operating in high-acuity environments like the intensive care unit (ICU), are already vulnerable to alarm fatigue and distractions, few would be excited about using an EHR system that simultaneously displayed 100 risk scores for each patient [31]. Instead, a more sustainable approach would be to allow risk prediction scoring to occur silently in the background, with specific alerts only surfacing when a key alert threshold has been crossed or users actively seek out the information. A car dashboard offers a familiar example outside of healthcare of a data display that has remained remarkably focused over many decades, despite the tremendous increase in the number of onboard computers constantly surveilling specific automotive functions.

2.6 Current Risk Prediction Applications in Critical Care

As described above, critical care already has numerous models designed to predict hospital mortality [22, 23]. Recent machine learning-based models incorporate a variety of newer elements including variable transformations, time-series data, and unstructured data from clinical documentation (Table 2.3). While these have contributed to some improvement in predictive performance, in many cases, the incremental gains have been modest and of uncertain benefit for clinical practice [32–34]. The capabilities available through natural language processing (NLP), a field that leverages computational approaches for understanding text-based, unstructured

Table 2.3 Balancing prediction and personalization in precision delivery by leveraging supervised and unsupervised machine learning approaches

	Prediction	Personalization
Goal	Precisely quantify the risk of experiencing an adverse outcome, while minimizing the false-positive rate associated with a given risk alert threshold	Identify subgroups of patients from a diverse at-risk group who would respond to specific targeted treatments
Machine learning approach	Supervised learning approaches fit a set of model variables to a pre-defined outcome of interest	Unsupervised learning approaches surface latent subgroups based on identifying underlying patterns and associations
Examples	ICU mortality Early warning scores Sepsis 'sniffers'	Subgroups responsive to statin therapy in acute respiratory distress syndrome; steroids in pediatric septic shock

documents like clinical notes or pathology reports, are now in wide use outside healthcare. However, the advantages of NLP in predictive models for patients who already have 'high-density' structured data available during hospitalization (i.e., frequent physiologic, laboratory, and treatment data) remain unclear [35].

Another active area of risk prediction relevant to critical care includes risk models designed to identify ward patients with a high likelihood of imminent deterioration [36, 37]. Again, many simpler scores (e.g., the Modified Early Warning Score [MEWS]; National Early Warning Score [NEWS]) have already seen widespread use within routine clinical workflows. Broadly speaking, more advanced scores (e.g., Advance Alert Monitor [AAM]; electronic Cardiac Arrest Risk Triage [eCART]; Rothman Index) demonstrate modest to moderate levels of improvement compared to existing models [38–42]. Where they are likely to excel is in their ability to reduce the number of false positives that trigger the need for clinical workup when compared to simpler models. Given the clinical burden imposed by the need to workup false positive alerts to find a single 'true positive' case, favorable reductions in the 'workup-to-detection ratio' or the 'number needed to screen' could have considerable downstream benefits on clinician sustainability and uptake.

Other areas of active focus include risk prediction models designed to accelerate the identification, triage or treatment of sepsis patients [43–50]. Although several reports suggest that use of risk prediction models has contributed to large reductions in sepsis-related mortality, it is unclear whether the described benefits actually accrue from the quantitative risk stratification (i.e., the relative improvement in the discrimination and performance of the model itself versus other screening criteria) or from the increased attention to sepsis and the clinical workflow alignment that becomes essential when an alerting system is turned on (i.e., the creation of a team-based standardized process for screening, identification, treatment, escalation and hand-off). Even prior to the advent of real-time predictive models, similar reductions in sepsis adverse outcomes were previously reported as part of system-wide quality improvement efforts.

In addition to these focus areas, a growing number of models are targeted towards increasingly prominent problems facing patients with acute and critical illness including the development of brain dysfunction or delirium [51–54], acute kidney injury (AKI) or organ failure [55–63], respiratory failure or acute respiratory distress syndrome (ARDS) [60–63], extended length of stay and post-ICU sequelae of severe illness [33, 64–66], and specific infectious types or complications (e.g., *Clostridium difficile*) [66–69]. Over the coming years, we will almost certainly see extensive growth in the development, reporting and testing of numerous predictive models incorporating EHR data with machine learning techniques to predict non-mortality outcomes.

2.7 Heterogeneity: The Hallmark of Severe and Critical Illness

Given the fundamental role that risk stratification has played in the birth and growth of the critical care specialty, the field is naturally suited to develop and deploy diverse risk models. However, while implementing broad risk prognostication tools to trigger protocolized care approaches has improved outcomes, our ability to further improve outcomes is pushing up against substantial limitations [11, 13]. In particular, the failures of numerous randomized controlled trials intended to identify novel pharmaceutical treatments for key ICU conditions like sepsis and ARDS has been particularly vexing.

There has been growing recognition that underlying heterogeneity in critical care patients represents a major barrier to the identification of specific treatments that can be targeted to responsive subgroups. Thus, while intense focus is currently placed on developing risk prediction models (i.e., a scale that quantifies each patient's risk for some adverse outcome like mortality, readmission, unexpected ICU transfer or chronic critical illness), the emerging frontier must focus on risk personalization models (i.e., models which predict the likelihood that a patient subgroup will respond to a specific therapy). To contextualize this concept within the framework of precision delivery, much more attention now needs to be shifted to the latter half of the prediction-personalization paradigm.

2.8 Unsupervised Machine Learning Approaches and Personalization

Fortunately, this is another area in which machine learning has shown excellent promise [18]. The development of standard risk prediction models focuses on using supervised learning methods in which model input variables are fit to a known outcome variable in a training dataset and then subsequently to a test dataset. However, to uncover potentially actionable subgroups within a high-risk cohort, unsupervised learning approaches—in which input variables are known but there is no corresponding pre-defined outcome variable—can be used to identify subgroups based on a variety of similarity or association metrics (Table 2.3).

For example, although mortality risk models are widely used in critical care to identify the sickest patients, they do not necessarily identify the patients most likely to benefit from a specific therapy. For example, even if a model perfectly predicts a cohort of patients as having a mortality risk of 32%, it could easily fail to distinguish patients who would be harmed or helped by liberal fluid administration. Similarly, even if early warning scores perfectly predicted impending adverse outcomes, they do not offer any insight into whether individual deteriorating patients would benefit most from improved respiratory support, vasopressor use or infection control.

Because unsupervised machine learning approaches can be used to identify or unmask underlying subgroups within a diverse sample, they have tremendous potential to help characterize the heterogeneity that is currently seen as a barrier to both identifying new treatments and applying treatments to individual patients. By leveraging high-dimensional statistical associations and pattern recognition they offer promise for effectively uncovering latent groupings that might be amenable to targeted treatment. However, because even the number of potential subgroups partitioned can vary wildly based on the unsupervised modeling approach and their specific parameters, it can be challenging to definitively establish the validity of the output. Emerging research is now demonstrating the power of using unsupervised approaches within existing clinical trial data to confirm that latent groups surfaced through statistical approaches differ in their responsiveness to specific treatments [70, 71]. It is likely that these unsupervised approaches will hold particular utility when they are paired with granular prospectively collected data where specific treatments are assigned through randomization and where machine learning methods can be used to evaluate heterogeneity in treatment effects.

2.9 Considerations: Assessing the Value of Increasing Model Performance

While there is great enthusiasm about the routine use of risk prediction models in healthcare, the incremental value of building and deploying ever higher-performing models remains unclear. As it stands today, there are very few clinical decisions, particularly in the inpatient setting, that are strictly based on precisely-defined, narrow risk thresholds—for example, a theoretical situation in which a highly accurate model predicting a risk of kidney injury of 23% would always prompt a different action than a risk of 29%. In most clinical situations, decisions are typically made across broader strata (e.g., mild, moderate or high risk categories), in part, because we often have only a limited menu of interventions available. Thus, investments allocated to achieving a model with an additional 1–2% in discriminative performance might instead be better spent on improving local calibration, personalization, technical implementation, workflow alignment or new model development. However, the tradeoff between increases in model predictive performance and their translation into improved personalized care or outcomes remains poorly characterized.

2.10 Considerations: Moving Beyond Clinical Data

In this chapter, we have focused primarily on clinical data available through the EHR; however, heterogeneity in critical illness arises from diverse sources including temporal trajectories of illness, genetic predisposition, immune status and mechanisms of disease. A growing set of technologies (e.g., sensors, gene expression, immune profiling, biomarkers, -omics, nanotechnology) are improving our ability to precisely and dynamically characterize patients along these axes of heterogeneity. As these tools become increasingly available outside research settings, they are likely to drastically improve the performance of risk prediction models and, more importantly, personalization approaches. At the same time, early-stage clinical risk prediction models are likely to continue to serve an important gatekeeper role in deciding which high-risk patients would benefit most from additional more focused, and likely more costly, testing.

2.11 Considerations: Risk Prediction Model Fatigue

In some instances, real-time risk prediction models have already been shut down because they are perceived to be contributing to alert and documentation fatigue without improving clinical care. For example, sepsis models designed to accelerate early identification in the emergency department may result in alerts that arrive after clinicians have already begun treatment for sepsis. Similarly, a model designed to target delirium, which frequently alerts after clinicians have already initiated treatment or prevention measures, may be viewed as overly burdensome or frankly useless. Thus, careful collaboration between end-users, model designers and technical implementation teams is needed to ensure that risk models improve value for clinicians, while minimizing burdens. In the model development phase, risk prediction models should be tuned to minimize false positive rates. Once the models have begun deployment, they can be initially set to alarm at high specificity risk thresholds while clinicians are gaining experience with their predictions, with gradual decreases in specificity once confidence and familiarity have been established.

2.12 Considerations: Workforce Development and Artificial Intelligence

The current precision delivery framework demands clinicians who can contextualize risk prediction alerts and personalize a patient's care at a precise moment in their illness. While clinicians receive general training in biostatistics, they often fail to understand how concepts like specificity or false positive rates actually translate into clinical decision-making. Thus, as risk models become as routine in clinical practice as laboratory tests, ongoing workforce education and training remain essential to ensuring that risk predictions are used correctly. Into the future, the inevitable progression towards artificial intelligence agents—computing systems which continuously improve and learn while also having autonomy over their actions and interventions—will continue and is likely to fundamentally alter health-care delivery.

2.13 Conclusion

The foundation of critical care is a risk stratification approach to identify patients with the highest risk of imminent mortality who require enhanced triage and treatment. Although critical care practitioners have long contributed to the development of robust risk prediction models, emerging advances in data availability and machine learning offer new potential for improvement. Precision delivery describes a paradigm that incorporates a prediction-personalization approach to clinical care, facilitating the delivery of targeted interventions at the precise moment. Although much attention is currently focused on building risk prediction models, there is an urgent need to employ machine learning approaches to understand heterogeneity among critically ill patients. Unsupervised learning approaches can be used to unpack heterogeneity and improve targeted treatment for responsive subgroups. When embedded within careful workflows that minimize burdensome alerting, precision delivery holds the potential to greatly improve the value of healthcare into the future.

References

1. Obermeyer Z, Emanuel EJ. Predicting the future—big data, machine learning, and clinical medicine. N Engl J Med. 2016;375:1216–9.
2. Murdoch TB, Detsky AS. The inevitable application of big data to health care. JAMA. 2013;309:1351–2.
3. Celi LA, Mark RG, Stone DJ, Montgomery RA. "Big data" in the intensive care unit. Closing the data loop. Am J Respir Crit Care Med. 2013;187:1157–60.
4. Naylor CD. On the prospects for a (deep) learning health care system. JAMA. 2018;320:1099–100.
5. Hinton G. Deep learning—a technology with the potential to transform health care. JAMA. 2018;320:1101–2.
6. Darcy AM, Louie AK, Roberts LW. Machine learning and the profession of medicine. JAMA. 2016;315:551–2.
7. Bates DW, Saria S, Ohno-Machado L, Shah A, Escobar G. Big data in health care: using analytics to identify and manage high-risk and high-cost patients. Health Aff (Millwood). 2014;33:1123–31.
8. Liu VX. Toward the "plateau of productivity": enhancing the value of machine learning in critical care. Crit Care Med. 2018;46:1196–7.
9. Parikh RB, Kakad M, Bates DW. Integrating predictive analytics into high-value care: the dawn of precision delivery. JAMA. 2016;315:651–2.

10. Parikh RB, Schwartz JS, Navathe AS. Beyond genes and molecules—a precision delivery initiative for precision medicine. N Engl J Med. 2017;376:1609–12.
11. Cohen J, Vincent JL, Adhikari NK, et al. Sepsis: a roadmap for future research. Lancet Infect Dis. 2015;15:581–614.
12. Seymour CW, Coopersmith CM, Deutschman CS, et al. Application of a framework to assess the usefulness of alternative sepsis criteria. Crit Care Med. 2016;44:e122–30.
13. Prescott HC, Calfee CS, Thompson BT, Angus DC, Liu VX. Toward smarter lumping and smarter splitting: rethinking strategies for sepsis and acute respiratory distress syndrome clinical trial design. Am J Respir Crit Care Med. 2016;194:147–55.
14. National Academies of Sciences, Engineering, and Medicine. The fourth industrial revolution: proceedings of a workshop-in brief. Washington: National Academies Press; 2017.
15. Schwab K. The fourth industrial revolution. New York: Crown Publishing Group; 2017.
16. Smith B, Linden G. Two decades of recommender systems at Amazon.com. IEEE Internet Comput. 2017;21:12–8.
17. Gomez-Uribe CA, Hunt N. The Netflix recommender system: algorithms, business value, and innovation. ACM Trans Manage Inf Syst. 2016;6:1–19.
18. Hastie T, Tibshirani R, Friedman JH. The elements of statistical learning. New York: Springer Science+Business Media; 2017.
19. Kuhn M, Johnson K. Applied predictive modeling. New York: Springer; 2016.
20. Vincent JL. The future of critical care medicine: integration and personalization. Crit Care Med. 2016;44:386–9.
21. Vincent JL. Critical care—where have we been and where are we going? Crit Care. 2013;17(Suppl 1):S2.
22. Vincent JL, Moreno R. Clinical review: scoring systems in the critically ill. Crit Care. 2010;14:207.
23. Liu V. Keeping score of severity scores: taking the next step. Crit Care Med. 2016;44:639–40.
24. Castella X, Artigas A, Bion J, Kari A. A comparison of severity of illness scoring systems for intensive care unit patients: results of a multicenter, multinational study. The European/North American Severity Study Group. Crit Care Med. 1995;23:1327–35.
25. Knaus WA, Draper EA, Wagner DP, Zimmerman JE. APACHE II: a severity of disease classification system. Crit Care Med. 1985;13:818–29.
26. Vincent JL, de Mendonca A, Cantraine F, et al. Use of the SOFA score to assess the incidence of organ dysfunction/failure in intensive care units: results of a multicenter, prospective study. Working group on "sepsis-related problems" of the European Society of Intensive Care Medicine. Crit Care Med. 1998;26:1793–800.
27. Ferreira FL, Bota DP, Bross A, Melot C, Vincent JL. Serial evaluation of the SOFA score to predict outcome in critically ill patients. JAMA. 2001;286:1754–8.
28. Singer M, Deutschman CS, Seymour CW, et al. The third international consensus definitions for sepsis and septic shock (Sepsis-3). JAMA. 2016;315:801–10.
29. Rajkomar A, Oren E, Chen K, Dai AM, Hajaj N. Scalable and accurate deep learning for electronic health records. NPJ Digital Med. 2018;18:1–10.
30. Osheroff J, Teich JM, Levick D, et al. Improving outomes with clinical decision support: an implementer's guide. Chicago: HIMSS Publishing; 2012.
31. Sendelbach S, Funk M. Alarm fatigue: a patient safety concern. AACN Adv Crit Care. 2013;24:378–86.
32. Badawi O, Liu X, Hassan E, Amelung PJ, Swami S. Evaluation of ICU risk models adapted for use as continuous markers of severity of illness throughout the ICU stay. Crit Care Med. 2018;46:361–7.
33. Weissman GE, Hubbard RA, Ungar LH, et al. Inclusion of unstructured clinical text improves early prediction of death or prolonged ICU stay. Crit Care Med. 2018;46:1125–32.
34. Lee J, Maslove DM, Dubin JA. Personalized mortality prediction driven by electronic medical data and a patient similarity metric. PLoS One. 2015;10:e0127428.
35. Sjoding MW, Liu VX. Can you read me now? Unlocking narrative data with natural language processing. Ann Am Thorac Soc. 2016;13:1443–5.

36. Alam N, Hobbelink EL, van Tienhoven AJ, van de Ven PM, Jansma EP, Nanayakkara PW. The impact of the use of the early warning score (EWS) on patient outcomes: a systematic review. Resuscitation. 2014;85:587–94.
37. McGaughey J, Alderdice F, Fowler R, Kapila A, Mayhew A, Moutray M. Outreach and Early Warning Systems (EWS) for the prevention of intensive care admission and death of critically ill adult patients on general hospital wards. Cochrane Database Syst Rev. 2007;Issue 3:CD005529.
38. Escobar GJ, LaGuardia JC, Turk BJ, Ragins A, Kipnis P, Draper D. Early detection of impending physiologic deterioration among patients who are not in intensive care: development of predictive models using data from an automated electronic medical record. J Hosp Med. 2012;7:388–95.
39. Kipnis P, Turk BJ, Wulf DA, et al. Development and validation of an electronic medical record-based alert score for detection of inpatient deterioration outside the ICU. J Biomed Inform. 2016;64:10–9.
40. Green M, Lander H, Snyder A, Hudson P, Churpek M, Edelson D. Comparison of the between the flags calling criteria to the MEWS, NEWS and the electronic Cardiac Arrest Risk Triage (eCART) score for the identification of deteriorating ward patients. Resuscitation. 2018;123:86–91.
41. Churpek MM, Yuen TC, Winslow C, et al. Multicenter development and validation of a risk stratification tool for ward patients. Am J Respir Crit Care Med. 2014;190:649–55.
42. Finlay GD, Rothman MJ, Smith RA. Measuring the modified early warning score and the Rothman index: advantages of utilizing the electronic medical record in an early warning system. J Hosp Med. 2014;9:116–9.
43. Olenick EM, Zimbro KS, D'Lima GM, Ver Schneider P, Jones D. Predicting Sepsis risk using the "sniffer" algorithm in the electronic medical record. J Nurs Care Qual. 2017;32:25–31.
44. Harrison AM, Thongprayoon C, Kashyap R, et al. Developing the surveillance algorithm for detection of failure to recognize and treat severe sepsis. Mayo Clin Proc. 2015;90:166–75.
45. Alsolamy S, Al Salamah M, Al Thagafi M, et al. Diagnostic accuracy of a screening electronic alert tool for severe sepsis and septic shock in the emergency department. BMC Med Inform Decis Mak. 2014;14:105.
46. Rolnick J, Downing NL, Shepard J, et al. Validation of test performance and clinical time zero for an electronic health record embedded severe sepsis alert. Appl Clin Inform. 2016;7:560–72.
47. Herasevich V, Pieper MS, Pulido J, Gajic O. Enrollment into a time sensitive clinical study in the critical care setting: results from computerized septic shock sniffer implementation. J Am Med Inform Assoc. 2011;18:639–44.
48. Despins LA. Automated detection of sepsis using electronic medical record data: a systematic review. J Healthc Qual. 2017;39:322–33.
49. Manaktala S, Claypool SR. Evaluating the impact of a computerized surveillance algorithm and decision support system on sepsis mortality. J Am Med Inform Assoc. 2017;24:88–95.
50. Henry KE, Hager DN, Pronovost PJ, Saria S. A targeted real-time early warning score (TREWScore) for septic shock. Sci Transl Med. 2015;7:299ra122.
51. Wassenaar A, Schoonhoven L, Devlin JW, et al. Delirium prediction in the intensive care unit: comparison of two delirium prediction models. Crit Care. 2018;22:114.
52. Lindroth H, Bratzke L, Purvis S, et al. Systematic review of prediction models for delirium in the older adult inpatient. BMJ Open. 2018;8:e019223.
53. Marra A, Pandharipande PP, Shotwell MS, et al. Acute brain dysfunction: development and validation of a daily prediction model. Chest. 2018;154:293–301.
54. Mestres Gonzalvo C, de Wit H, van Oijen BPC, et al. Validation of an automated delirium prediction model (DElirium MOdel (DEMO)): an observational study. BMJ Open. 2017;7:e016654.
55. Hodgson LE, Roderick PJ, Venn RM, Yao GL, Dimitrov BD, Forni LG. Correction: the ICE-AKI study: impact analysis of a clinical prediction rule and electronic AKI alert in general medical patients. PLoS One. 2018;13:e0203183.

56. Mohamadlou H, Lynn-Palevsky A, Barton C, et al. Prediction of acute kidney injury with a machine learning algorithm using electronic health record data. Can J Kidney Health Dis. 2018;5:1–9.
57. Klein SJ, Brandtner AK, Lehner GF, et al. Biomarkers for prediction of renal replacement therapy in acute kidney injury: a systematic review and meta-analysis. Intensive Care Med. 2018;44:323–36.
58. Haines RW, Lin SP, Hewson R, et al. Acute kidney injury in trauma patients admitted to critical care: development and validation of a diagnostic prediction model. Sci Rep. 2018;8:3665.
59. Koyner JL, Adhikari R, Edelson DP, Churpek MM. Development of a multicenter ward-based AKI prediction model. Clin J Am Soc Nephrol. 2016;11:1935–43.
60. Bauman ZM, Gassner MY, Coughlin MA, Mahan M, Watras J. Lung injury prediction score is useful in predicting acute respiratory distress syndrome and mortality in surgical critical care patients. Crit Care Res Pract. 2015;2015:157408.
61. Beitler JR, Schoenfeld DA, Thompson BT. Preventing ARDS: progress, promise, and pitfalls. Chest. 2014;146:1102–13.
62. Levitt JE, Calfee CS, Goldstein BA, Vojnik R, Matthay MA. Early acute lung injury: criteria for identifying lung injury prior to the need for positive pressure ventilation. Crit Care Med. 2013;41:1929–37.
63. Levitt JE, Bedi H, Calfee CS, Gould MK, Matthay MA. Identification of early acute lung injury at initial evaluation in an acute care setting prior to the onset of respiratory failure. Chest. 2009;135:936–43.
64. LaFaro RJ, Pothula S, Kubal KP, et al. Neural network prediction of ICU length of stay following cardiac surgery based on pre-incision variables. PLoS One. 2015;10:e0145395.
65. Verburg IW, Atashi A, Eslami S, et al. Which models can I use to predict adult ICU length of stay? A systematic review. Crit Care Med. 2017;45:e222–31.
66. Escobar GJ, Baker JM, Kipnis P, et al. Prediction of recurrent Clostridium difficile infection using comprehensive electronic medical records in an integrated healthcare delivery system. Infect Control Hosp Epidemiol. 2017;38:1196–203.
67. Zilberberg MD, Reske K, Olsen M, Yan Y, Dubberke ER. Development and validation of a recurrent Clostridium difficile risk-prediction model. J Hosp Med. 2014;9:418–23.
68. Reveles KR, Mortensen EM, Koeller JM, et al. Derivation and validation of a Clostridium difficile infection recurrence prediction rule in a national cohort of veterans. Pharmacotherapy. 2018;38:349–56.
69. Oh J, Makar M, Fusco C, et al. A generalizable, data-driven approach to predict daily risk of Clostridium difficile infection at two large academic health centers. Infect Control Hosp Epidemiol. 2018;39:425–33.
70. Delucchi K, Famous KR, Ware LB, et al. Stability of ARDS subphenotypes over time in two randomised controlled trials. Thorax. 2018;73:439–45.
71. Wong HR, Sweeney TE, Hart KW, Khatri P, Lindsell CJ. Pediatric sepsis endotypes among adults with sepsis. Crit Care Med. 2017;45:e1289–91.

Part II

Acute Respiratory Failure and ARDS

Acute Respiratory Failure in the Oncologic Patient: New Era, New Issues

3

B. L. Ferreyro and L. Munshi

3.1 Introduction

Recent decades have seen an increase in the number of patients living with cancer. This trend has resulted in an increase in intensive care unit (ICU) utilization across this population [1]. Acute respiratory failure is the most frequent medical complication leading to critical illness in oncologic patients [2–4]. Historically, there has been a reluctance to admit cancer patients to the ICU given their poor outcomes, particularly in the setting of hematologic malignancy and invasive mechanical ventilation [5]. ICU treatment limitations or refusal of admission was advocated [6]. Major advances in oncologic care, critical care and more meticulous attention to where the conditions overlap, have resulted in marked improvement in short-term survival in this population [1, 7, 8]. Despite these major advances, acute respiratory failure in this population remains complex with unique challenges surrounding diagnosis and management compared to the general ICU population. This chapter provides a comprehensive overview of acute respiratory failure in the oncologic population and highlights specific considerations for the intensivist. We will focus on the important differences between the immunocompromised oncologic patient and general intensive care population, the spectrum of causes of acute respiratory failure with a specific focus on toxicities related to newer cancer therapies, diagnostic approach, management and an up-to-date overview of prognosis.

B. L. Ferreyro
Interdepartmental Division of Critical Care Medicine, Department of Medicine, Mount Sinai Hospital/University Health Network, University of Toronto, Toronto, ON, Canada

Internal Medicine Department, Hospital Italiano de Buenos Aires, Buenos Aires, Argentina

L. Munshi (✉)
Interdepartmental Division of Critical Care Medicine, Department of Medicine, Mount Sinai Hospital/University Health Network, University of Toronto, Toronto, ON, Canada
e-mail: Laveena.munshi@sinaihealthsystem.ca

J.-L. Vincent (ed.), *Annual Update in Intensive Care and Emergency Medicine 2019*, Annual Update in Intensive Care and Emergency Medicine,
https://doi.org/10.1007/978-3-030-06067-1_3

Table 3.1 Advances in oncologic care and the implications for critical care

Advance	New critical care challenges
Earlier detection of disease	Increased number of patients with cancer Earlier treatment with potential toxicities causing acute respiratory failure
Novel and more effective treatment options	Known/unknown toxicities causing acute respiratory failure with uncertainty in optimal management (example pulmonary toxicity due to immune check point inhibitions)
Treatments with reduced toxicities for advanced age	Older patients with more comorbidities receiving treatment and admitted to ICU
Sustained cancer control	Shift from an acute to a chronic disease model

3.2 The Evolution of Oncologic Critical Care over Time

Historically, candidacy for oncologic treatment was reserved for early stage disease across functional patients with minimal comorbid conditions. Recent advances in oncologic care have resulted in (1) earlier detection of malignancies; (2) a broader range of available therapies across different stages of disease; (3) gentler therapeutic options for the aging population living long enough to be diagnosed with cancer; (4) precision medicine/targeted therapies; and, most recently, (5) engineered T cells that have the ability to re-program the immune system to recognize and attack cancer cells [8–10]. This paradigm shift in cancer care has not been free of new challenges for the medical community. With these advances comes a higher rate of critical illness. While most oncologic admissions to the ICU are planned post-surgical admissions, the profile of those being admitted for medical indications is changing. Infectious acute respiratory failure and sepsis remain the leading causes of medical-oncologic ICU admissions; however, we are seeing a surge in elderly patients presenting with disease- or treatment-associated critical illness and unique toxicities associated with newer therapies. As oncologic care is becoming more complex with intensive regimens, newer therapies and higher volumes, certain centers are developing specialized ICUs for the management of cancer patients, recognizing a need for critical care support and expansion of oncologic critical care knowledge. Table 3.1 highlights some of the recent advances in oncology and the critical care implications of these changes.

3.3 Differences Between Oncologic and Non-oncologic Patients

While trying to define the characteristics and outcomes of acute respiratory failure in the oncologic population it is important to consider why this patient population is different to a non-oncologic ICU group. We feel the key differences are associated with (1) their immunocompromised state; (2) higher risk of non-infectious causes of acute respiratory failure; and (3) potential greater risk of frailty at the time of critical illness. Oncologic patients are usually considered to be immunocompromised. This can be a result of the underlying disease (e.g., acute leukemia with functional neutropenia) or secondary to the treatment (e.g., patient with solid tumor after chemotherapy). Although the mechanisms leading to immunosuppression are different across all oncologic patients, these patients all share an increased vulnerability to develop common community-acquired and opportunistic infections. Furthermore, the underlying cause of acute respiratory failure in this population can also be non-infectious (direct involvement by the tumor or treatment-related toxicity), making the differential diagnosis even more challenging particularly when infectious/non-infectious causes occur concurrently.

Oncologic patients often exhibit frailty because of their complex trajectory through their disease, exposure to recurrent hospitalizations, risk of nutrition interruption or impairment, and possible exposure to corticosteroids. This state could put them at higher risk in the face of invasive procedures.

It is important to note that the characteristics and outcomes of critically ill oncologic patients differ in those with hematologic malignancies and those with solid tumors. Patients with hematologic malignancies are more frequently admitted with higher acuity conditions, whereas patients with solid tumors are more frequently admitted perioperatively [4]. In the subset of solid tumor patients admitted with medical-induced critical illness, their characteristics and outcomes mirror the general ICU population to a greater degree than those with hematologic malignancies [1]. This difference is attributable to the more profound and prolonged nature of immunosuppression across the hematologic malignancies, making such patients more vulnerable to bacterial, viral and invasive fungal respiratory infections. Furthermore, patients with hematologic malignancies also face a higher risk of non-infectious respiratory complications than those with solid tumors given the heightened doses of cytoreductive/myeloablative therapies, and a higher risk of immune reconstitution reactions.

3.4 Causes of Acute Respiratory Failure in Oncologic Patients

Acute respiratory failure in the oncologic population can be broadly classified as infectious and non-infectious. The latter can further be categorized into disease-related or treatment-related. The clinician needs to keep a broad differential and always consider the coexistence of more than one cause as is seen in 15–20% of cases [4]. Table 3.2 outlines the differential diagnoses to consider in the oncologic population.

3.4.1 Infectious

Oncologic patients face an increased risk of community-acquired and opportunistic infections, which can be secondary to bacteria, virus and fungi. The lung is a

Table 3.2 Classification of respiratory failure in oncology patients

Predominant site of involvement	Infectious	Non-infectious	
		Disease-related	Treatment-related
Airway		Extrinsic upper airway obstruction Bronchial invasion Bronchial obstruction	Anaphylactic reactions to chemotherapy or targeted therapies
Lung parenchyma	Bacterial, fungal, viral infections	Direct lung invasion by the tumor Leukostasis	Cardiogenic pulmonary edema Immune checkpoint Inhibitor toxicity/other medication-associated pneumonitis CAR T-cell induced lung injury
	Acute respiratory distress syndrome Pulmonary hemorrhage (secondary to infection/ necrotizing pneumonia)	Pulmonary hemorrhage (secondary to direct tumor invasion)	Acute respiratory distress syndrome Alveolar hemorrhage
Vascular disorders	Angioinvasive aspergillosis	Thromboembolic disease Carcinomatous lymphangitis	
Pleura and chest wall	Empyema	Malignant effusions Chest wall tumors Malignant ascites or bowel obstructions	
Nervous system		Paraneoplastic neuropathy/myopathy Spinal cord involvement	Chemotherapy associated polyneuropathy

CAR chimeric antigen receptor

frequent site of infection in patients with cancer. The underlying predominant deficit in the immune system can help narrow the differential of potential pathogens. It is important to note that the clinical presentation of pulmonary infections in this population frequently presents atypical features.

Neutropenic patients face a higher risk of infections caused by staphylococcus species, Gram-negative bacilli and fungal agents, mainly if neutropenia persists. *Aspergillus* species are the most frequent fungal etiology of pneumonia in neutropenic patients, followed by *Zygomycetes* and *Fusarium*.

In patients with impaired cell-mediated immunity, the spectrum of pulmonary infections is different. Intracellular bacteria, such as *Listeria*, *Nocardia* and *Legionella* species, should be considered in this setting. Mycobacterial infectious are also common in patients with cellular immune dysfunction.

Beyond community-acquired viral pathogens, pulmonary viral infections specific to this group include cytomegalovirus (CMV). CMV usually presents diagnostic challenges due to the potential colonization of the airway without established infection. *Pneumocystis jirovecii* pneumonia is a common opportunistic infection in patients with cell-mediated immune dysfunction. Originally described in patients with human immunodeficiency virus (HIV) infection, it has been increasingly recognized as a common pathogen in patients with hematologic malignancies and solid tumors. Recently, Azoulay and colleagues reported the results of a multivariable risk prediction model to assist with the early recognition of *P. jirovecii* pneumonia in patients with hematologic malignancies. The variables in this score included age, lymphoprolipherative disorder, *P. jirovecii* pneumonia prophylaxis, timing of symptoms and ICU admission, the presence of shock and radiological findings [11].

3.4.2 Non-infectious: Disease-Related

Disease-induced acute respiratory failure can arise from multiple mechanisms and accounts for approximately 10% of cases [4]. Direct tumor invasion or extrinsic compression by tumor cells can be seen in carcinomatous lymphangitis, leukostasis, malignant pleural effusions, bulky mediastinal malignancies and tumor cell embolism [2]. Furthermore, pulmonary embolism should always be suspected when assessing the causes of acute respiratory failure in an oncologic patient, particularly in the absence of radiographic evidence of infiltrates.

3.4.3 Non-infectious: Treatment-Related

There is a wide range of treatment-associated pulmonary complications. The incidence of treatment-associated lung toxicity across studies evaluating acute respiratory failure in immunocompromised patients is 3.4–10% [12, 13]. The predominant mechanism of lung injury stems from an exaggerated inflammatory cytokine release as a consequence of the drug, its impact on the tumor cell, or an appropriate 'on target' but 'off tumor' effect of targeted treatment [9].

3.4.3.1 Non-infectious: Treatment-Related—Novel Treatments

Immune checkpoint inhibitors (ICIs) are a new group of drugs that have revolutionized the treatment of cancer. They work by reprogramming T cells to generate an anti-tumor response [14–16]. However, they are also associated with inflammatory adverse effects which may range from mild endocrine, dermatologic, and gastrointestinal complications to more severe neurologic or pulmonary toxicity. The incidence of severe lung toxicity associated with ICIs is 2% [14, 15, 17]. Pneumonitis is considered one of the most common causes of ICI-related death [15]. Pulmonary-related toxicity usually presents as pneumonitis at a median time of 3 months post-treatment initiation [18]. Earlier and later time periods have been reported [15]. Obtaining sputum samples for microbiologic assessment or performing bronchoscopy with bronchoalveolar lavage (BAL) can help to exclude concomitant infection. Treatment includes corticosteroids. Immunosuppressants, such as infliximab, cyclophosphamide and mycophenolate, are recommended by some experts in non-respondent patients although this has not been evaluated extensively [14, 15].

Chimeric antigen receptor-T cell therapy consists of modified T cells infused into patients to recognize tumor antigens and initiate an immune attack of cancer cells [9, 16]. Outcomes across Chimeric antigen receptor-T cell therapy intervention trials have been promising for select hematologic malignancies and are projected to revolutionize cancer treatment [10]. Unfortunately, this treatment is associated with cytokine release syndrome, seen in greater than 60% of cases [9]. Its most severe forms (grade 3–4 toxicity), reported in approximately 15% of cases, may be associated with acute respiratory failure and acute respiratory distress syndrome (ARDS) [9].

3.4.3.2 Non-infectious: Treatment-Related—Tumor Lysis Syndrome

Tumor lysis syndrome is an acute life-threatening condition resulting from massive release of cell products into the blood [19, 20]. It is usually associated with rapid cell death after treatment initiation, but it can also occur spontaneously [20]. It is characterized by electrolyte abnormalities (hyperkalemia, hyperphosphatemia, hyperuricemia, hypocalcemia) leading to acute kidney injury, cardiac arrhythmias and potentially multiorgan failure [19]. Life-threatening acute respiratory failure and ARDS associated with tumor lysis syndrome have been described [21, 22].

3.4.3.3 Non-infectious: Treatment-Related—Radiation

Radiation-induced lung injury can present as acute radiation pneumonitis (usually between 1 and 3 months after irradiation) or as pulmonary fibrosis. The acute form usually is self-limiting and responds to corticosteroids whereas the fibrotic form responds poorly to treatment.

3.4.3.4 Non-infectious: Treatment-Related—Immune Reconstitution

Immune recovery or immune reconstitution can lead to acute respiratory failure and is due to an exaggerated inflammatory response as the immune system recovers from a period of prolonged neutropenia. This has been described after neutrophil recovery in hematology malignancy patients or peri-engraftment following autologous/allogeneic stem cell transplant. It is theorized that it may be more common in the setting of an infectious precipitant as is seen in the HIV setting. Treatment includes consideration for corticosteroids depending upon its severity. A series of other inflammatory conditions exist that can cause acute respiratory failure and ARDS, such as inflammation induced by the underlying condition (hemophagocytic lymphohistiocytosis) or treatment (differentiation syndrome from all-trans retinoic acid for acute promyelocytic leukemia) [23]. The allogeneic stem cell transplant patient has a series of unique treatment-associated conditions that can induce acute respiratory failure and severe ARDS. These conditions, range from pre-engraftment diffuse alveolar hemorrhage, to peri-engraftment syndrome and idiopathic pneumonia syndrome [24–26]. While these occur at different phases of the post-stem cell trajectory, the consistent features associated with these conditions include their association with preconditioning regimens and their high mortality in the setting of severe respiratory failure and need for invasive mechanical ventilation.

3.5 Diagnostic Work-Up and Undiagnosed Acute Respiratory Failure

An accurate diagnosis is key to guide early prognostication, institution of appropriate therapy, and initiation of necessary supportive care. Recognizing and projecting the reversibility of the underlying cause is an important factor in deciding the need for monitoring, transfer for ICU admission and eventually the decision for intubation. This also needs to take into consideration the oncologic diagnosis, pending treatments and underlying prognosis. A wide spectrum of differential diagnosis should be kept in consideration, including infectious and non-infectious causes and the possibility of dual infections or concomitant infections/non-infectious etiologies. In patients with pulmonary infiltrates, laboratory studies need to be considered in light of the type and degree of immunosuppression. The work-up may include a series of non-invasive serum and sputum microbiologic tests (sputum cultures, induced sputum for *P. jirovecii*, CMV serum evaluation, serum galactomannan, nasopharyngeal swab for viral polymerase chain reaction, etc.); imaging modalities (computed tomography [CT] thorax, echocardiography if cardiogenic pulmonary edema is considered) and possible BAL for further microbiologic evaluation if no diagnosis has been yielded. The routine and upfront use of BAL in hypoxic oncologic immunocompromised patients with undetermined lung infiltrates is controversial. Conflicting evidence exists surrounding its safety in patients with high oxygen requirements (potentially precipitating endotracheal intubation) [27, 28]; however, evidence has demonstrated that given the debatable diagnostic yield, a strategy of first pursuing non-invasive tests may be warranted in the appropriate population [27]. There may exist a subset of patients for whom the need for BAL as an initial diagnostic strategy is warranted at an earlier time point (e.g., to rule out extrinsic compression or pulmonary hemorrhage, or to rule out infections with potentially toxic treatment profiles). Figure 3.1 outlines an approach to diagnosis.

Finally, despite an extensive diagnostic work up, approximately 13–40% of oncologic patients have undiagnosed acute respiratory failure [4, 29]. Undiagnosed acute respiratory failure is associated with a worse prognosis. It remains unclear whether it is a disease entity within itself or occult infectious/non-infectious etiology not appropriately identified. The role of lung biopsy has been considered in this population in the setting of acute respiratory failure or ARDS, but, given the immunosuppressed state, frequent thrombocytopenia, risk of bronchopleural fistula in light of positive pressure ventilation, and morbidity and mortality with the procedure; it is not pursued frequently [30].

3.6 Management

The mainstays of management of the oncologic patient with acute respiratory failure remain rapid identification of etiology and institution of appropriate therapy. This therapy may range from antimicrobial coverage for possible infections, chemotherapy/radiation therapy for disease-induced acute respiratory failure (e.g., leukostasis

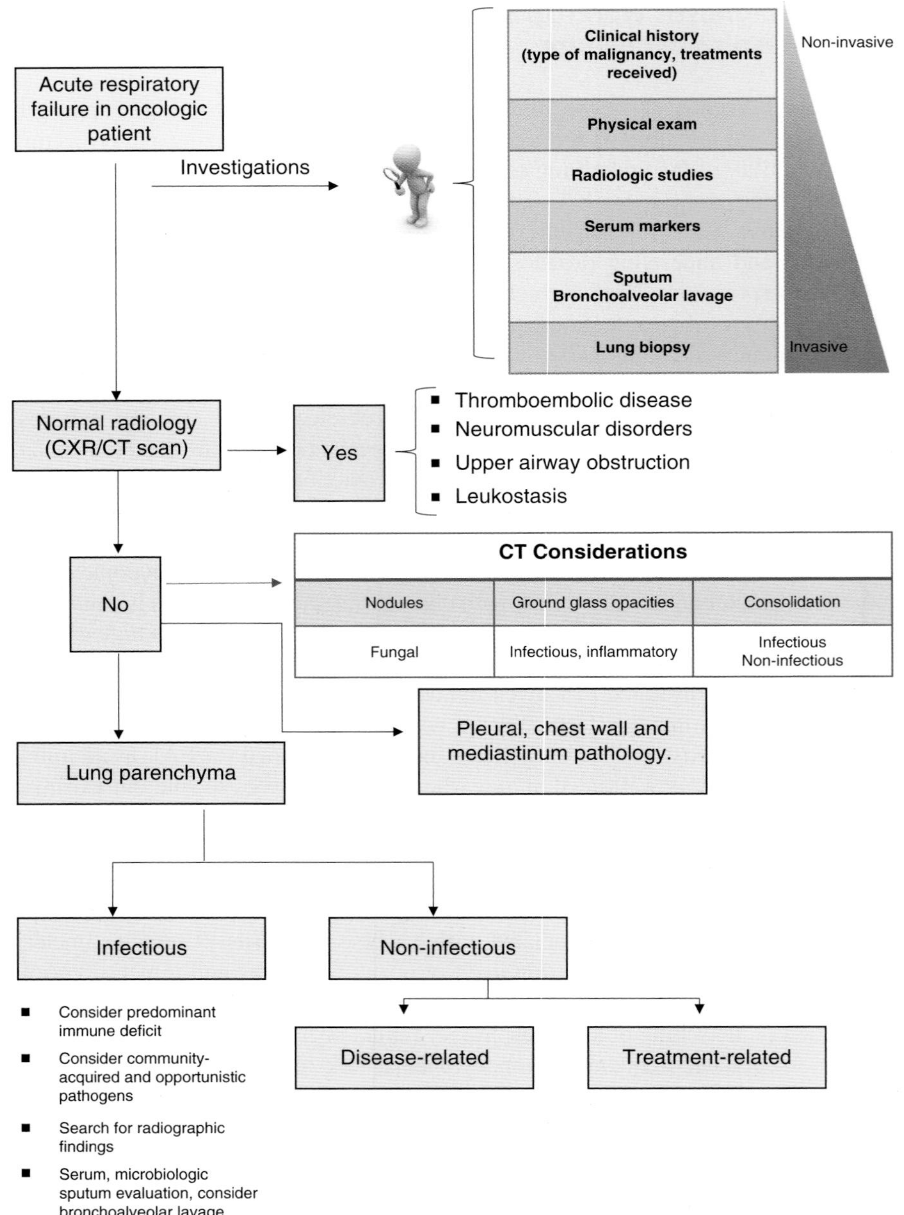

Fig. 3.1 Diagnostic considerations in acute respiratory failure among oncologic patients

or airway compression from lymphoma), or corticosteroid/anti-interleukin-6 (IL-6) therapy to blunt inflammation related to possible drug toxicities. Of utmost importance is the rapid identification of cause and initiation of treatment early in the course of acute respiratory failure in order to prevent the development of ARDS or need for invasive mechanical ventilation. For disease-associated complications, such as leukostasis or tumor infiltration, historic reservations to initiate chemotherapy in the ICU have been dispelled by more recent data demonstrating its feasibility and lack of association with increased mortality [31]. While mortality rates across acute respiratory failure in this population have decreased (40–70%) [3, 7, 32], there is a subset that continue to have an unacceptably high mortality, particularly in the setting of invasive mechanical ventilation [32, 33]. The high mortality in the face of mechanical ventilation is likely attributable to (1) more aggressive infectious organisms with a higher risk of drug resistance; (2) adverse events of appropriate antimicrobial treatments; (3) an immunocompromised state that delays eradication of the infection; (4) difficulty or delays in diagnosis; and (5) a higher risk of frailty—which may subject these patients to a higher risk of respiratory muscle weakness prolonging their recovery from critical illness. It remains unclear whether these patients are more susceptible to ventilator-associated lung injury or the harms associated with ventilator-associated lung injury. Given an increased mortality in the setting of invasive mechanical ventilation compared to the general ICU population, a subset of literature has focused on optimal strategies of non-invasive oxygen therapy to prevent intubation.

3.6.1 Supportive Care During Early Acute Hypoxemic Respiratory Failure

Three non-invasive oxygen strategies have been evaluated in immunocompromised and oncologic acute respiratory failure: continuous oxygen therapy, non-invasive ventilation, and high-flow nasal cannula (HFNC)—each with unique physiologic properties. They are often applied in the setting of severe hypoxemic acute respiratory failure in an attempt to prevent the need for invasive mechanical ventilation.

Continuous low-flow oxygen therapy via face mask is the most common mechanism of oxygen delivery in the setting of acute hypoxemic respiratory failure. Its greatest limitation remains the limited inspired flow rate (up to 15 L/min). When hypoxia is combined with a high work of breathing, entrainment of ambient air (which could be liters) from around the mask may result in a dilution of the inspired oxygen to the alveoli. This results in insufficient delivery of the intended oxygen concentrations to the alveoli. Inability to provide alveolar recruitment and the risk of local oxygen toxicity (tracheobronchitis/mucociliary disturbance) are also limitations to this non-invasive strategy.

Non-invasive ventilation (NIV) has the ability to provide continuous positive airway pressure and assist each breath with augmented pressure. The seal generated by the NIV interface (via facemask or helmet) permits alveolar recruitment. Two historic trials in immunocompromised patients established biologic plausibility for the benefit of NIV compared to continuous oxygen therapy in patients with acute respiratory failure [34, 35]. These trials demonstrated that, in early acute respiratory failure, the application of NIV instead of continuous oxygen therapy was associated with a decreased need for invasive mechanical ventilation and mortality. Given the limited generalizability of those historic trials to the populations we manage today, a more recent trial by Lemiale and colleagues re-evaluated this question and demonstrated no difference in outcomes between NIV and continuous oxygen therapy [36].

Humidified HFNC is a novel device for oxygen delivery that allows for higher flow oxygen delivery via large bore nasal cannula (40–60 L/min of flow). Theoretic mechanisms of benefit include higher flow of inspired oxygen delivery outstripping any ambient air that could be entrained, dead space washout, a small amount of positive end-expiratory pressure (PEEP) generated and humidification to enhance mucociliary clearance. The Florali trial by Frat and colleagues demonstrated reduced 90-day mortality with HFNC compared to NIV and continuous oxygen therapy across the general ICU population with acute respiratory failure [37]. In a *post hoc* analysis focusing on immunocompromised patients (excluding severe neutropenia), there were no differences with HFNC compared to continuous oxygen on rates of intubation but a persistent benefit of HFNC compared to NIV [38]. These results are intriguing as it is theorized that it may not be the HFNC *per se* resulting in a beneficial impact, but potentially harm induced by NIV. The median tidal volumes in the NIV arm were 9 mL/kg thus leading the authors to hypothesize that ventilator-associated lung injury could be contributing to the increased harm noted. The authors, in a subsequent study, found that a PaO_2/FiO_2 <200 mmHg or tidal volumes ≥9 mL/kg were associated with NIV failure [39].

Finally, in a systematic review by Sklar and colleagues evaluating non-invasive oxygen strategies in immunocompromised patients, the majority of whom had an oncologic diagnosis, seven studies (randomized controlled trials [RCTs] or observational studies with propensity score matching) were evaluated comparing HFNC to conventional oxygen or NIV. Mortality was found to be lower in the HFNC arms compared to the pooled oxygen control arms (continuous oxygen therapy or NIV). This study was exploratory but warrants further investigation [40].

3.6.2 Supportive Care During ARDS

A secondary analysis of the LUNG SAFE database, an international, multicenter observational study of patients with ARDS, was conducted focusing on an immunocompromised cohort [29]. Across this cohort, 20% of patients with ARDS underwent NIV as their first line supportive management instead of invasive mechanical ventilation. Focusing on observational studies of ARDS across oncology patients, 40–50% underwent NIV as first-line [32, 33]. While the original studies evaluating the utility of NIV in immunocompromised patients focused on early acute respiratory failure and the role of NIV in preventing the need for intubation, these initial promising data has led to NIV creep into more severe subgroups of ARDS [29, 32, 33]. In an observational study by Azoulay and colleagues evaluating management and outcomes of oncologic patients with ARDS, 70% of those who underwent initial NIV, eventually failed and required invasive mechanical ventilation [32]. However, high failure rates are not consistently reported, as the failure rate noted by Rathi and colleagues was 40% [33]. Across these two studies—amongst the largest to evaluate ARDS in the oncology population—NIV failure was an independent risk factor for mortality with mortality rates higher than in patients managed with an initial strategy of invasive mechanical ventilation. Given the observational nature of these data, it remains unclear whether this increased mortality is due to unmeasured confounders, such as higher severity of illness not captured in the multivariable analysis, physician reservation to intubate based upon subtle patient factors (e.g., frailty) or whether the use of NIV was associated with higher tidal volumes resulting in greater lung injury and increased mortality in this population. On the contrary, of the 60% who did not require invasive mechanical ventilation after NIV in the study by Rathi and colleagues, their ICU mortality rates were the lowest (29%) compared to cohorts with an initial strategy of invasive mechanical ventilation (61%) and NIV failure (71%). Given the retrospective nature of these studies, future, research should focus on delineating how to identify which patient populations, if any, may benefit from a time-limited trial of NIV in the setting of ARDS. Until further research, we propose the following management algorithm to consider in oncologic patients in the setting of acute respiratory failure and ARDS (Fig. 3.2).

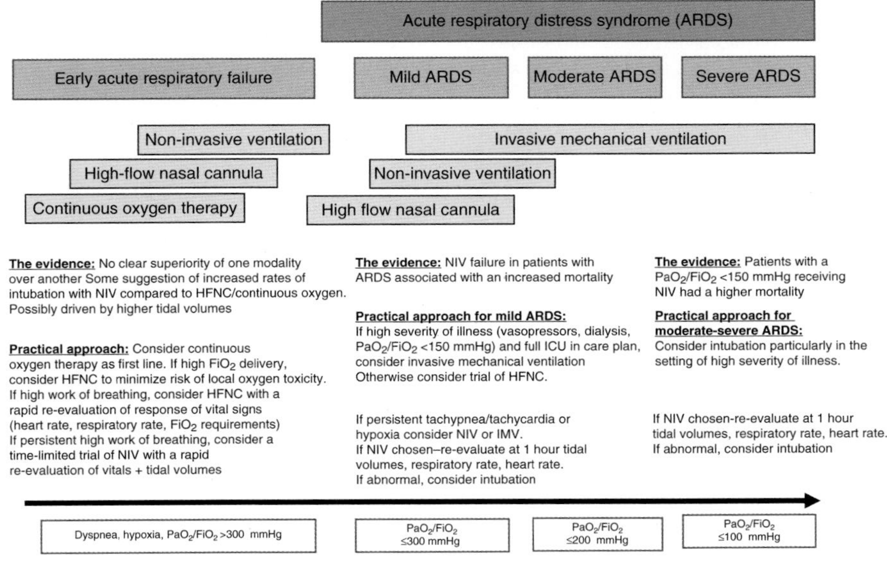

Fig. 3.2 Invasive and non-invasive oxygenation strategies for oncology patients with acute hypoxemic respiratory failure. *NIV* non-invasive ventilation, *HFNC* high-flow nasal cannula; *IMV* invasive mechanical ventilation

3.7 Prognosis and Future Research Considerations

Historic hospital mortality rates across patients with hematologic malignancy developing critical illness were >80% [41]. More recent up-to-date data demonstrate more favorable short-term prognoses ranging from <10% in the post-surgical oncologic patient, 30–50% in the solid or hematologic malignancy patient, to upwards of 60% across allogeneic stem cell transplant patient requiring invasive mechanical ventilation [42–45]. Improved outcomes are likely attributable to better patient selection for oncologic and intensive care, advances in antimicrobial prophylaxis, infection control and antimicrobial management, earlier identification and a better understanding of the causes of acute respiratory failure and better overall supportive care with more specialized centers/units and subspecialists managing these patients. Factors consistently found to be associated with high mortality in the oncologic critically ill population include age and comorbid conditions, poor functional and frailty status, treatment refractory graft-vs-host disease in allogeneic stem cell transplant patients, NIV failure in the setting of ARDS, invasive fungal infections requiring invasive mechanical ventilation and number of organs failed evaluated after 3–5 days of ICU admission and mechanical ventilation. Early and routine discussions with the oncologist and patient/substitute decision makers in guiding ongoing care decisions is imperative to ensuring that the resources dedicated to the care of this patient is bridging them to a meaningful recovery or candidacy for ongoing oncologic treatment if indicated [46].

Future research should focus on advancing diagnostic strategies to delineate more precisely and rapidly the etiology of acute respiratory failure, strategies to blunt pulmonary and systemic inflammation that can result as a consequence of otherwise effective cancer therapies, the role of biomarkers in predicting the onset of acute respiratory failure, clarifying optimal non-invasive oxygen strategies and the role of NIV and finally long-term outcomes across survivors of acute respiratory failure.

3.8 Conclusion

With the paradigm shift in cancer care comes a unique host of critical care conditions and challenges for the intensivist. Acute respiratory failure in the oncologic host has a very broad infectious and non-infectious differential. Early recognition of acute respiratory failure and a thorough evaluation for the etiology is critical to preventing progression to ARDS and need for invasive mechanical ventilation. Optimal non-invasive oxygen strategies remain unclear. Adherence to pressure- and volume-limited strategies remains imperative in this population. Future research must focus on better identification of 'undiagnosed' acute respiratory failure, optimal initial supportive care strategies for mild ARDS and long-term outcomes.

References

1. Taccone F, Artigas A, Sprung C, et al. Characteristics and outcomes of cancer patients in European ICUs. Crit Care. 2009;13:R15.
2. Pastores SM. Acute respiratory failure in critically ill patients with cancer. Diagnosis and management. Crit Care Clin. 2001;17:623–46.
3. Mokart D, Etienne A, Esterni B, et al. Critically ill cancer patients in the intensive care unit: short-term outcome and 1-year mortality. Acta Anaesthesiol Scand. 2011;56:178–89.
4. Azoulay E, Pickkers P, Soares M, et al. Acute hypoxemic respiratory failure in immunocompromised patients: the Efraim multinational prospective cohort study. Intensive Care Med. 2017;316:1–12.
5. Kress JP, Christenson J, Pohlman AS, et al. Outcomes of critically ill cancer patients in a university hospital setting. Am J Respir Crit Care Med. 1999;160:1957–61.
6. Task Force of the American College of Critical Care Medicine, Society of Critical Care Medicine. Guidelines for intensive care unit admission, discharge and triage. Crit Care Med. 1999;27:633–8.
7. Azoulay E, Mokart D, Pène F, et al. Outcomes of critically ill patients with hematologic malignancies: prospective multicenter data from France and Belgium—a groupe de recherche respiratoire en réanimation onco-hématologique study. J Clin Oncol. 2013;31:2810–22.
8. Schellongowski P, Sperr W, Wohlfarth P, et al. Critically ill patients with cancer: chances and limitations of intensive care medicine—a narrative review. ESMO Open. 2016;201:1.
9. Gutierrez C, McEvoy C, Mead E, et al. Management of the critically ill adult chimeric antigen receptor-t cell therapy patient. Crit Care Med. 2018;46:1402–10.
10. June CH, Sadelain M. Chimeric antigen receptor therapy. N Engl J Med. 2018;379:64–73.
11. Azoulay E, Roux A, Vincent F, et al. A multivariable prediction model for Pneumocystis jirovecii pneumonia in hematology patients with acute respiratory failure. Am J Respir Crit Care Med. 2018;198:1519–26.
12. Dhokarh R, Li G, Schmickl CN, et al. Drug-associated acute lung injury. Chest. 2012;142:845–50.
13. Reinert T, Baldotto CS, Nunes FAP, et al. Bleomycin induced lung injury. J Cancer Res. 2013;2013:1–9.
14. Wills B, Brahmer JR, Naidoo J. Treatment of complications from immune checkpoint inhibition in patients with lung cancer. Curr Treat Options Oncol. 2018;19:1–21.
15. Brahmer JR, Lacchetti C, Schneider BJ, et al. Management of immune-related adverse events in patients treated with immune checkpoint inhibitor therapy: American Society of Clinical Oncology Clinical Practice Guideline. J Clin Oncol. 2018;36:1714–68.
16. Neelapu SS, Tummala S, Kebriaei P, et al. Chimeric antigen receptor T-cell therapy—assessment and management of toxicities. Nat Rev Clin Oncol. 2018;15:47–62.
17. Nishino M, Giobbie-Hurder A, Hatabu H, Ramaiya NH, Hodi FS. Incidence of programmed cell death 1 inhibitor-related pneumonitis in patients with advanced cancer: a systematic review and meta-analysis. JAMA Oncol. 2016;2:1607–16.
18. Postow M, Sidlow R, Hellmann D. Immune related adverse events associated with immune checkpoint blockade. N Engl J Med. 2018;378:158–68.
19. Mirrakhimov AE, Voore P, Khan M, et al. Tumor lysis syndrome: a clinical review. World J Crit Care Med. 2015;4:130–8.
20. Howard SC, Jones DP, Pui CH. The tumor lysis syndrome. N Engl J Med. 2011;364:1844–54.
21. Macaluso A, Genova S, Maringhini S, et al. Acute respiratory distress syndrome associated with tumor lysis syndrome in a child with acute lymphoblastic leukemia. Pediatr Rep. 2015;7:5760–2.
22. Bell CM, Stewart TE. Acute respiratory distress syndrome associated with tumour lysis syndrome in leukemia. Can Respir J. 1997;4:48–51.
23. Seguin A, Galicier L, Boutboul D, et al. Pulmonary involvement in patients with hemophagocytic lymphohistiocytosis. Chest. 2016;149:1294–301.

24. Yadav H, Nolan ME, Bohman JK, et al. Epidemiology of acute respiratory distress syndrome following hematopoietic stem cell transplantation. Crit Care Med. 2016;44:1082–90.
25. Lucena CM, Torres A, Rovira M, et al. Pulmonary complications in hematopoietic SCT: a prospective study. Bone Marrow Transplant. 2014;49:1293–9.
26. Panoskaltsis-Mortari A, Griese M, Madtes DK, et al. An official American Thoracic Society research statement: noninfectious lung injury after hematopoietic stem cell transplantation: idiopathic pneumonia syndrome. Am J Respir Crit Care Med. 2011;183:1262–79.
27. Azoulay E, Mokart D, Lambert J, et al. Diagnostic strategy for hematology and oncology patients with acute respiratory failure. Am J Respir Crit Care Med. 2010;182:1038–46.
28. Deotare U, Merman E, Pincus D, et al. The utility and safety of flexible bronchoscopy in critically ill acute leukemia patients: a retrospective cohort study. Can J Anaesth. 2018;65:2 72–9.
29. Cortegiani A, Madotto F, Gregoretti C, et al. Immunocompromised patients with acute respiratory distress syndrome: a secondary analysis of the LUNG SAFE database. Crit Care. 2018;22:157–72.
30. Chellapandian D, Lehrnbecher T, Phillips B, et al. Bronchoalveolar lavage and lung biopsy in patients with cancer and hematopoietic stem-cell transplantation recipients: a systematic review and meta-analysis. J Clin Oncol. 2015;33:501–15.
31. Pastores S, Goldman D, Shaz D, et al. Characteristics and outcomes of patient with hematologic malignancies receiving chemotherapy in the intensive care unit. Cancer. 2018;124: 3025–36.
32. Azoulay E, Lemiale V, Mokart D, et al. Acute respiratory distress syndrome in patients with malignancies. Intensive Care Med. 2014;40:1106–14.
33. Rathi N, Haque S, Nates R, et al. Noninvasive positive pressure ventilation vs invasive mechanical ventilation as first-line therapy for acute hypoxemic respiratory failure in cancer patients. J Crit Care. 2017;39:56–62.
34. Hilbert G, Gruson D, Vargas F, et al. Noninvasive ventilation in immunosuppressed patients with pulmonary infiltrates. N Engl J Med. 2001;344:481–7.
35. Antonellli M, Conti G, Bufi M, et al. Noninvasive ventilation for treatment of acute respiratory failure in patients undergoing solid organ transplant: a randomized trial. JAMA. 2000;283:235–41.
36. Lemiale V, Mokart D, Resche-Rigon M, et al. Effect of noninvasive ventilation vs oxygen therapy on mortality among immunocompromised patients with acute respiratory failure: a randomized clinical trial. JAMA. 2015;314:1711–20.
37. Frat JP, Thille AW, Mercat A, et al. High-flow oxygen through nasal cannula in acute hypoxemic respiratory failure. N Engl J Med. 2015;372:2185–96.
38. Frat JP, Ragot S, Girault C, et al. Effect of non-invasive oxygenation strategies in immunocompromised patients with severe acute respiratory failure: a post-hoc analysis of a randomised trial. Lancet Respir Med. 2016;4:646–53.
39. Frat JP, Ragot S, Coudroy R, et al. Predictors of intubation in patients with acute hypoxemic respiratory failure treated with a noninvasive oxygenation strategy. Crit Care Med. 2018;46:208–15.
40. Sklar M, Mohamed A, Orchanian-Cheff A, et al. The impact of high flow nasal oxygen in the immunocompromised critically ill: a systematic review and meta-analysis. Respir Care. 2018; 63:1555–66.
41. Lloyd-Thomas A, Dhaliwal H, Lister T, et al. Intensive therapy for life-threatening medical complications of hematologic malignancy. Intensive Care Med. 1986;12: 317–24.
42. Bos MM, Bakhshi-Raiez F, Dekker JW, et al. Outcomes of intensive care unit admissions after elective cancer surgery. Eur J Surg Oncol. 2013;39:584–92.
43. Fisher R, Dangoisse C, Crichton S, et al. Short-term and medium-term survival of critically ill patients with solid tumors admitted to the intensive care unit: a retrospective analysis. BMJ Open. 2016;6:e011363.

44. Darmon MR, Bernal T, Borges M, et al. Ventilatory support in critically ill hematology patients with respiratory failure. Crit Care. 2012;16:R133.
45. Van Vliet M, Verburg I, Boogaard M, et al. Trends in admission prevalence, illness severity and survival of hematological patients treated in Dutch intensive care units. Intensive Care Med. 2014;40:1275–84.
46. Soares M, Bozza F, Azevedo L, et al. Effects of organizational characteristics on outcomes and resource use in patients with cancer admitted to Intensive Care Units. J Clin Oncol. 2016;34:3315–24.

Universal Low Tidal Volume: Early Initiation of Low Tidal Volume Ventilation in Patients with and without ARDS

4

J.-T. Chen and M. N. Gong

4.1 Introduction

Lung protective ventilation using 6 mL/kg of ideal body weight is the standard of practice in patients with acute respiratory distress syndrome (ARDS). The use of low tidal volume ventilation was associated with decreased morbidity and mortality in the ARMA trial [1]. The use of low tidal volume of 6 mL/kg of predicted body weight (PBW) conferred a mortality reduction of 22% [1]. A recent large epidemiologic study, LUNG SAFE, demonstrated that not only is ARDS underdiagnosed, there is also a significant delay in recognition [2]. There is growing evidence in support of the use of low tidal volume ventilation as early as possible in patients with acute respiratory failure, both with and without ARDS [3, 4]. Given that as many as half of the patients admitted to the intensive care unit (ICU) come directly from the emergency department (ED) [5], and many others come to the ICU after major surgery, it is important to understand ventilator practices for patients in the ED and operating rooms and how these practices in the early part of mechanical ventilation may be important to the later outcomes of patients.

In 2014, Sutherasan et al. reviewed the pathophysiology of ventilator-induced lung injury (VILI) and the use of protective ventilation using low tidal volume in the operating room and the ICU [6]. In this chapter, we will expand upon their review by discussing recent findings on the early initiation of low tidal volume ventilation in patients without ARDS, patients with respiratory failure in the ED and other specific clinical situations, and discuss barriers to universal application of low tidal volume ventilation.

J.-T. Chen · M. N. Gong (✉)
Department of Critical Care, Montefiore Medical Center, New York, NY, USA
e-mail: mgong@montefiore.org

J.-L. Vincent (ed.), *Annual Update in Intensive Care and Emergency Medicine 2019*, Annual Update in Intensive Care and Emergency Medicine,
https://doi.org/10.1007/978-3-030-06067-1_4

4.2 Timing of Low Tidal Ventilation in ARDS and in Non-ARDS

Mechanical ventilation can be life-saving in patients with critical illness, but it can be injurious too. Invasive mechanical ventilation is helpful if it decreases the work of breathing, secures the airway, and assists in gas exchange in acute respiratory failure. However, invasive mechanical ventilation is also known to contribute to injury of the lung. Ventilator-associated lung injuries include atelectrauma, volutrauma, barotrauma, release of reactive oxygen species (ROS) from high oxygen content, and biotrauma [7]. Since the ARMA trial demonstrated that lung protective ventilation with tidal volumes of 6 mL/kg PBW led to improved survival and more ventilator-free days, low tidal volume ventilation to target plateau pressures ≤30 cmH_2O has become the recommended standard of care in patients with ARDS [1, 8]. Nevertheless, multiple studies have shown poor recognition and limited compliance with low tidal volume ventilation in patients with ARDS (Fig. 4.1). This observation is especially discouraging, as there is growing evidence that earlier initiation of low tidal ventilation is better than later.

In patients with ARDS, early exposure to low tidal volume ventilation was associated with better survival rates than low tidal volume ventilation that was initiated later in the course of mechanical ventilation [9]. Needham et al. followed 482 patients with ARDS and monitored their tidal volumes over the duration of their mechanical ventilation. They found that for every 1 mL/kg increase in initial tidal volume beyond 6.5 mL/kg, there was an associated 23% increase in ICU mortality [9]. Furthermore, they found that in patients who were exposed to both high and low tidal volume ventilation during the course of their mechanical ventilation, the risk of ICU mortality was lower among those receiving lower tidal volume early on compared to those patients who were ventilated at higher tidal volume initially and then adjusted to lower tidal volume. This is in contrast to an earlier retrospective

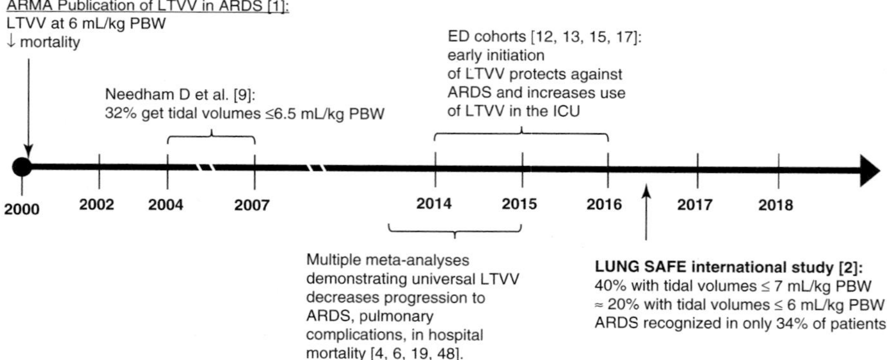

Fig. 4.1 Timeline of evolution of low tidal volume ventilation (LTVV). Despite evidence supporting the use of LTVV in 2000 [1], the LUNG SAFE study in 2016 [2] still reported low adoption of LTVV. *PBW* predicted body weight, *ARDS* acute respiratory distress syndrome, *ED* emergency department

study by Checkley et al., who found that exposure to high tidal volume for 48 h before enrollment to an ARDSNet trials was not associated with in-hospital mortality [10]. However, high plateau pressure within 48 h prior to trial enrollment was associated with in-hospital mortality, which suggests that lack of lung protective ventilation early in the course of ARDS can affect later outcomes. This study only examined patients enrolled into ARDS clinical trials and may therefore suffer from selection bias (e.g., patients who died within 48 h or whose family or physicians refused enrollment into ARDS trials were not enrolled in these studies and their tidal volumes were not measured) and may be insufficiently powered to detect an effect from early high tidal volume [11].

Low tidal volume ventilation was also protective against the development of ARDS in critically ill patients who did not have acute lung injury at initiation of invasive mechanical ventilation [12–17]. In a single center retrospective review of patients initially without ARDS who were receiving mechanical ventilation, patients with higher initial tidal volume were more likely to meet ARDS criteria within 48 h of mechanical ventilation than those with lower tidal volumes [18]. In a study in which ICU patients without ARDS were randomized to receive high versus low tidal volume ventilation at the time of mechanical ventilation, patients who were ventilated at tidal volumes of 10 mL/kg PBW were five times more likely to develop ARDS than those ventilated at 6 mL/kg PBW [16]. A meta-analysis of ICU patients without ARDS who received low (≤7 mL/kg PBW) versus high (>10 mL/kg of PBW) tidal volume demonstrated an increased incidence of pulmonary complications, such as development of ARDS or pneumonia (adjusted OR 0.72, 95% CI 0.52–0.98) [19]. There was no difference between patients receiving high and intermediate (between 7 and 10 mL/kg PBW) tidal volumes.

Finally, a retrospective analysis of highly granular electronic health record data on tidal volume found that exposure to more than 12 h of high tidal volume (>8 mL/kg PBW) was associated with increased mortality. Exposure to 8 mL/kg PBW for 12 or 24 h was associated with increased in-hospital mortality (OR 1.66 [95% CI 1.15–2.38] for 12 h, OR 1.51 [95% CI 1.08–2.11] for 24 h) [20]. Interestingly, average tidal volume was not associated with mortality.

Many of these studies are observational. However, a randomized controlled trial (RCT) recently compared low tidal volume ventilation of 4–6 mL/kg PBW with higher tidal volumes of 8–10 mL/kg PBW in patients without ARDS [21]. The primary outcome measured was ventilator-free days at day 28 after randomization. Other secondary endpoints included ICU and hospital lengths of stay, sedation and neuromuscular blockade use, ICU delirium and acquired weakness, pulmonary complications, and mortality. The study completed recruitment in 2017 [22].

4.3 Review and Update of Evidence in the Operating Room

A number of RCTs of intraoperative lung protective ventilation in patients without ARDS have been conducted, and their results are consistent with the observational studies described above. The IMPROVE trial randomized 400 patients with surgical procedures averaging 200 min to receive 10–12 mL/kg PBW without positive end-expiratory pressure (PEEP) vs. 6–8 mL/kg PBW with PEEP between 6 and 8 cmH_2O and regular recruitment maneuvers. The low tidal volume group had less post-operative pulmonary (pneumonia, need for invasive or non-invasive ventilation [NIV] for acute respiratory failure) and extrapulmonary (sepsis and shock, and death) complications [14]. One criticism of this study is that the use of 10–12 mL/kg PBW is higher than what is commonly used in the operating room [23]. Nevertheless, these results indicate that higher tidal volume for even short periods of time can result in more postoperative complications even in non-acutely injured lungs in patients undergoing surgery.

In surgical patients, tidal volume of 9 mL/kg of PBW was associated with a higher incidence of pulmonary complications and hypoxemia in a meta-analysis and review by Sutherasan et al. [6]. Higher tidal volume was an independent risk factor for multiorgan failure. In this meta-analysis of surgical ventilator practice, high tidal volume in the operating room, even for a short time, was associated with more hypoxemia, more pulmonary complications, increased time on the ventilator, increased ICU and hospital lengths of stay, and increased mortality [6]. Interestingly, there was no difference in the development of postoperative pulmonary complications in surgical patients receiving high PEEP and recruitment vs. low PEEP (≤ 2 cmH_2O), if the patients were ventilated with low tidal volume (7.2 vs. 7.1 mL/kg PBW) [24]. When 19 randomized controlled trials comparing intraoperative ventilator strategies were analyzed together in a meta-analysis, low tidal volume (5–8 mL/kg PBW vs. 8–12 mL/kg PBW) protected against lung injury and pulmonary infections, regardless of the type of surgery [25].

Despite this evidence, in an epidemiologic study the most commonly used tidal volume intraoperatively was "500 mL" [26]. This one size does not fit all patients. Using the Centers for Disease Control and Prevention (CDC) data for height in the US population, about 10% of men and up to 85% of women would be receiving a tidal volume >8 mL/kg if the tidal volume is set at 500 mL [27]. By using this commonly set tidal volume, the average woman is exposed to high tidal volumes by predicted weight intraoperatively which may explain in part why female ARDS patients were more likely to receive high tidal volume ventilation in the ICU [28, 29].

4.4 Acute Respiratory Failure in the Emergency Department

Acute respiratory failure is a common presentation to the ED. The ED was the source of 45.2% of admissions to the ICU in a large cohort study [5]. Post-intubation management, such as confirming endotracheal tube placement with a chest radiograph, oral gastric decompression, early sedation protocol, appropriate tidal volume, obtaining arterial blood gas, and end-tidal CO_2 monitoring were associated with reduced mortality [30]. However, adherence to these practices in the ED setting has been found to be sub-optimal. The prevalence of ARDS at the time of intubation in the ED is about 6.8–8% [12, 13, 31] but 14–27.5% progress to ARDS later on in the ICU [13, 15, 17, 32]. Although the ED is a major source of patients with acute respiratory failure requiring invasive mechanical ventilation, the tidal volume settings for these patients are highly variable [13, 17]. The tidal volume most commonly observed in the ED was 500 mL in a cohort of mechanically ventilated patients, suggesting a default "one size fits all" setting similar to surgical ventilator practices [13, 17, 33]. Furthermore, unlike surgical patients who would be extubated after their procedure, critically ill patients (even without ARDS) who are intubated in the ED will continue to require mechanical ventilation in the ICU, and their initial tidal volume and ventilator setting influences how they are ventilated subsequently in the ICU [5].

4.5 Therapeutic Momentum: From the ED to the ICU

There is great variability in ventilator practice in the emergency room, and lung-protective ventilation is rarely used in patients with or without ARDS [12, 13, 17]. Initial ventilator settings in the ED are usually high and highly variable in patients with or without ARDS at the time of intubation. In addition, the initial tidal volume influences subsequent practice in the ICU. In one ED cohort, only 15% of patients received the recommended tidal volume setting at initiation and 41% of patients with initially high tidal volumes never had any adjustment of their tidal volumes. An additional 44% of patients were exposed to an average of 14 h (standard deviation of 16.8 h) of high tidal volumes before the ventilator was adjusted [17]. Similarly, in another study, only 10% of the patients initially without ARDS in the ED had their tidal volume settings adjusted in a cohort of patients intubated for sepsis who later developed ARDS [12]. In a different single center cohort characterizing mechanical ventilation practice in the ED, there was a significant correlation between ED and ICU ventilator settings [13]. About 42% of patients received the same ventilator setting in the ICU as their last ED setting, and up to 28% of them had that same tidal volume for the following 24 h. Transition between tidal volumes in the ICU was infrequent and high initial tidal volume and admission from the ED was independently associated with longer exposure to high tidal volume [20]. Given that Sjording et al. reported that exposure to tidal volume >8 mL/kg PBW for 12 h or more was associated with increased mortality, this would suggest that the majority of patients intubated in the ED may be exposed to potentially injurious tidal volume that is associated with higher mortality [20]. Careful consideration of ventilator settings in the ED can improve compliance with low tidal volume ventilation in the ICU.

In fact, there is evidence suggesting that even pre-hospital tidal volume influences ultimate ICU ventilator settings. Stoltze et al. showed that the use of low tidal volume ventilation was rare in a cohort of patients intubated and transferred to the study hospital [34]. Although rare, the use of low tidal volume ventilation in transfers was associated with a 7.06-times increased likelihood of receiving low tidal volumes during hospitalization. However, there was no difference in tidal volume received between patients who subsequently developed ARDS and those who did not, as both groups received relatively high tidal volumes (between 8 and 9 mL/kg PBW).

The Lung-Protective Ventilation Initiated in the ED (LOV-ED) investigators tested the feasibility of using a universal lung protective ventilation protocol in the ED to reduce the development of ARDS and ventilator associated conditions [15]. They performed a systematic implementation of low tidal volume ventilation using the ARDSnet protocol, limiting plateau pressure, setting PEEP ≥5 cmH_2O and increasing PEEP if body mass index (BMI) was high, initiating FiO_2 at 0.3–0.4 instead of 1.0, adjusting respiratory rate between 20 and 30 breaths per minute, and keeping the head of the bed elevated. Not only were they able to reduce the tidal volume used in the ED, but patients were five times more likely to receive low tidal volume ventilation in the ICU after implementation. Using propensity score analysis, there was an absolute risk reduction in ARDS and ventilator associated conditions of 7.1% (adjusted OR 0.47, 95% CI 0.31–0.71) and mortality reduction of 14.5% (adjusted OR 14.5%, 95% CI 0.35–0.63). Lung protective ventilation in the ED was also associated with increased ventilator-free days and shorter ICU and hospital lengths of stay. Importantly, there was significant correlation between low tidal volume use in the ED and ICU. This study highlights that early implementation of best care in acute respiratory failure and critical illness in the ED can influence subsequent critical care practices in the ICU and affect later outcomes. One of the limitations of this study was that it was a before and after comparison. However, time series analysis suggests that there were no systemic temporal changes to explain the differences.

4.6 Lung Protective Ventilation After Cardiac Arrest

Cardiopulmonary resuscitation (CPR) with effective chest compression can lead to pulmonary injuries, such as lung contusion, atelectasis, aspiration and pulmonary edema [35], which are associated with prolonged mechanical ventilation, length of stay and higher mortality [35, 36].

Ventilator practices for these patients have evolved in the ICU. The average tidal volume has decreased significantly from 9.04 mL/kg PBW to 7.95 mL/kg of PBW in these patients [36]. While hypoxemia (PaO_2 <60 mmHg) is associated with 28-day mortality, high tidal volume and plateau pressure or lower PEEP are also associated with ICU-acquired pneumonia or ARDS. A more recent secondary analysis in 2018 to characterize ventilator practices in the targeted temperature management trial cohort found that non-survivors were more hypoxic and had higher respiratory rates and higher driving pressures [37]. Survivors and non-survivors of cardiac arrests had similar tidal volumes (median 7.7 [IQR 6.4–8.7] mL/kg of PBW), with more than 60% of the cohort receiving tidal volumes greater than or equal to 8 mL/kg.

Keeping patients within normoxemia (PaO_2 70–100 mmHg, SpO_2 92–97%) and normocarbia/hypercarbia ($PaCO_2$ 40–50 mmHg) ranges is recommended for favorable neurologic outcomes. As these post-cardiac arrest patients are at risk of developing ARDS and pulmonary complications given pulmonary injury and the overall dysregulated state, lung protective ventilation with low tidal volume is also recommended [38]. Beitler et al. reported that survivors of out-of-hospital cardiac arrest who received tidal volumes ≤8 mL/kg PBW had cerebral performance category (CPC) scores of 1 or 2, indicating minor neurocognitive deficit to moderate disability, compared with a CPC score >3 indicating severe disability, coma/vegetative state, or death in those receiving tidal volumes >8 mL/kg PBW [39]. Again, although cardiac arrest patients are placed on mechanical ventilation for reasons other than primarily pulmonary injuries, they are likely to develop pulmonary complications that can lead to worse outcomes.

4.7 Lung Protective Ventilation in Patients with Increased Intracranial Pressure or Traumatic Brain Injury

There are data to suggest that low tidal volume ventilation may also be beneficial in patients with increased intracranial pressures, especially if you can avoid hyper- and hypo-ventilation. Hyperventilation causes cerebral vasoconstriction and reduced cerebral blood volume leading to decreased intracranial pressure [40]. Inappropriate hyperventilation post-traumatic brain injury (TBI) can cause secondary ischemia during the decreased global cerebral blood flow after the first day of traumatic injury. Hyperventilation and hypoventilation ($PaCO_2$ <35 and $PaCO_2$ >45 mmHg) on arterial blood gas within 20 min of arrival to the hospital is associated with a 14-times increased risk of in-hospital mortality. Furthermore, high tidal volume ventilation is associated with the development of ARDS after severe brain injury [41], and ARDS in patients with TBI is associated with a three-fold increased risk of persistent vegetative state and death [42]. High tidal volume ventilation for the purpose of hyperventilation is unlikely to be beneficial to patients with TBI.

Some may be reluctant to use low tidal volume ventilation in patients with elevated intracranial pressure, because of concerns for hypoventilation which can increase intracranial pressure. However, hypoventilation can often be avoided by increasing the respiratory rate when you lower the tidal volume. In an observational study, patients with TBI and ARDS tolerated low tidal volume ventilation (between 6 and 7 mL/kg PBW) and 5–15 cmH_2O of PEEP could be achieved without increases in $PaCO_2$ just by adjusting the respiratory rate [43]. There was no significant change in intracranial pressure or cerebral perfusion pressure. In fact, both systemic and brain tissue oxygenation improved with this strategy.

4.8 Perceived Barriers to Low Tidal Volume Ventilation in ARDS and Non-ARDS

Despite the evidence supporting low tidal volume ventilation in acute respiratory failure with and without ARDS, the application of low tidal volume is not widespread (Fig. 4.1). In the LUNG SAFE study, 35% of ARDS patients received tidal volumes >8 mL/kg. Patients with recognized ARDS received on average 7.5 mL/kg PBW, only slightly less than those with unrecognized ARDS (mean 7.7 mL/kg PBW) [2]. Similarly, adoption of lung-protective ventilation is also low in the non-ARDS population. Approximately 40% of the intubated patients in four academic EDs received tidal volume >8 mL/kg PBW [33]. The barriers to using low tidal volume ventilation in ARDS and non-ARDS include under-recognition of ARDS, inappropriate use of body weight and height, concern for hypercarbia/respiratory acidosis and increased sedation requirements [2, 17, 44, 45].

4.9 Under-Recognition of ARDS and Reluctance to Use Low Tidal Volume Ventilation in At-Risk Patients with Acute Respiratory Failure

A perceived barrier to adapting low tidal volume ventilation is that the patient has not met criteria for ARDS on initial endotracheal intubation. Some clinicians may feel that low tidal volume ventilation is not indicated in these patients even if they are at risk of developing ARDS. This factor, coupled with a lack of recognition of when the patient does meet ARDS criteria, can result in under-utilization of low tidal volume ventilation in patients with, and at-risk for, ARDS. This is especially notable because the initial tidal volume and ventilator practice after intubation can affect later outcomes, and the initial practice often persists beyond the ED into the ICU for a large proportion of the patient's duration of mechanical ventilation. Fuller et al. suggested making the default setting for tidal volume 6–8 mL/kg PBW in the ED for all comers with acute respiratory failure [15]. Clinicians can still adjust the tidal volume upwards if they think it is clinically indicated, but that becomes their conscious decision. By setting low tidal volume ventilation as the default initial setting, it can serve as a "nudge" for the clinician to use the appropriate ventilator setting in most patients [46].

4.10 Calculation of Predicted Body Weight

The LOV-ED study demonstrated that successful implementation of low tidal volume ventilation in the ED setting is possible. In the observational trials on mechanical ventilator practices in the ED and surgery, average tidal volume was approximately 500 mL regardless of patient height and/or sex [13, 17, 33]. This suggests that existing practice uses an empiric ventilator setting, without calculation of the PBW of the patients. Calculation of PBW can be facilitated by obtaining the actual height from the patients or surrogates whenever possible, otherwise by measuring the patient using a measuring tape to obtain proper height. Calculation of PBW can be automated within electronic health records and displayed whenever mechanical ventilator parameters are entered into the system. Although height may be more commonly measured before surgery and for patients in the ICU, this is rarely done for patients in the ED. Arming respiratory therapists with tape measures and tidal volume calculator apps on their phones may be one strategy to bring consistent ventilator practices to patients in different areas of the hospital.

4.11 Concern About Sedation

One argument against the use of low tidal volume ventilation is that patients ventilated with low tidal volumes will need more sedation which goes against the current best practice to minimize sedation in patients on mechanical ventilation. In a secondary analysis of the ARMA cohort within a single institution, there was no significant difference between the choice of sedative, dose or duration of sedation between ARDS patients receiving ventilation with tidal volumes of 6 mL/kg or 12 mL/kg PBW [47]. Furthermore, multiple meta-analyses indicate that low tidal volume ventilation is not associated with increased sedation requirements [19, 48]. Serpa Neto et al. evaluated sedation practices using a meta-analysis of non-ARDS patients in the ICU receiving low (≤6 mL/kg PBW), intermediate (6–10 mL/kg PBW), and high (≥10 mL/kg PBW) tidal volumes. There was no difference in duration of sedation or the type and dose of medication required for sedation [48].

4.12 Concern About Respiratory Acidosis

Some clinicians are reluctant to decrease tidal volume out of a concern about possible respiratory acidosis [44]. Alveolar ventilation is dependent on respiratory rate and tidal volume. Although decreasing tidal volume may affect ventilation, appropriate adjustment of respiratory rate can match the required minute ventilation and avoid respiratory acidosis. In situations such as intracranial conditions, where hypercarbia should be avoided, adjusting the respiratory rate can match the needed minute ventilation [43]. Low tidal volume ventilation in non-ARDS patients in the ED was associated with no clinically significant difference in pH and $PaCO_2$ when adequate ventilation by respiratory rate adjustment was applied [15].

4.13 Conclusion

Early initiation of low tidal volume ventilation in patients without ARDS decreased the risk of developing ARDS, led to shorter lengths of stay, and decreased mortality. We advocate the routine use of PBW obtained by height measurement to set the initial tidal volume at 6–8 mL/kg PBW with PEEP ≥5 cmH_2O on the ventilator for patients at risk of ARDS. Furthermore, oxygenation monitoring is necessary, because the clinical presentation can progress to hypoxemia. Early recognition of ARDS allows prompt adjustment of tidal volume to ≤6 mL/kg PBW. Implementing low tidal volumes in the ED prior to the patient arriving on the ICU is feasible and improves compliance with lung protective ventilation in the ICU.

References

1. Bower RG, Matthay MA, Morris A, et al. Ventilation with lower tidal volumes as compared with traditional tidal volumes for acute lung injury and the acute respiratory distress syndrome. The Acute Respiratory Distress Syndrome Network. N Engl J Med. 2000;342:1301–8.
2. Bellani G, Laffey JG, Pham T, et al. Epidemiology, patterns of care, and mortality for patients with acute respiratory distress syndrome in intensive care units in 50 countries. JAMA. 2016;315:788–800.
3. Fuller BM, Mohr NM, Drewry AM, et al. Lower tidal volume at initiation of mechanical ventilation may reduce progression to acute respiratory distress syndrome: a systematic review. Crit Care. 2013;17:R11.
4. Serpa Neto A, Cardoso SO, Manetta JA, et al. Association between use of lung-protective ventilation with lower tidal volumes and clinical outcomes among patients without acute respiratory distress syndrome: a meta-analysis. JAMA. 2012;308:1651–9.
5. Lilly CM, Zuckerman IH, Badawi O, et al. Benchmark data from more than 240,000 adults that reflect the current practice of critical care in the United States. Chest. 2011;140:1232–42.
6. Sutherasan Y, Vargas M, Pelosi P. Protective mechanical ventilation in the non-injured lung: review and meta-analysis. Crit Care. 2014;18:211.
7. Slutsky AS, Ranieri VM. Ventilator-induced lung injury. N Engl J Med. 2013;369:2126–36.
8. Fan E, Del Sorbo L, Goligher EC, et al. An Official American Thoracic Society/European Society of Intensive Care Medicine/Society of Critical Care Medicine Clinical Practice Guideline: mechanical ventilation in adult patients with acute respiratory distress syndrome. Am J Respir Crit Care Med. 2017;195:1253–63.
9. Needham DM, Yang T, Dinglas VD, et al. Timing of low tidal volume ventilation and intensive care unit mortality in acute respiratory distress syndrome. A prospective cohort study. Am J Respir Crit Care Med. 2015;191:177–85.
10. Checkley W, Brower R, Korpak A, et al. Effects of a clinical trial on mechanical ventilation practices in patients with acute lung injury. Am J Respir Crit Care Med. 2008;177:1215–22.
11. Cornish S, Wynne R, Klim S, Kelly AM. Protective lung strategies: a cross sectional survey of nurses knowledge and use in the emergency department. Australas Emerg Nurs J. 2017;20:87–91.
12. Fuller BM, Mohr NM, Dettmer M, et al. Mechanical ventilation and acute lung injury in emergency department patients with severe sepsis and septic shock: an observational study. Acad Emerg Med. 2013;20:659–69.
13. Fuller BM, Mohr NM, Miller CN, et al. Mechanical ventilation and ARDS in the ED: a multicenter, observational, prospective, cross-sectional study. Chest. 2015;148:365–74.
14. Futier E, Constantin JM, Paugam-Burtz C, et al. A trial of intraoperative low-tidal-volume ventilation in abdominal surgery. N Engl J Med. 2013;369:428–37.
15. Fuller BM, Ferguson IT, Mohr NM, et al. Lung-protective ventilation initiated in the emergency department (LOV-ED): a quasi-experimental, before-after trial. Ann Emerg Med. 2017;70:406–18. e404
16. Determann RM, Royakkers A, Wolthuis EK, et al. Ventilation with lower tidal volumes as compared with conventional tidal volumes for patients without acute lung injury: a preventive randomized controlled trial. Crit Care. 2010;14:R1.
17. Allison MG, Scott MC, Hu KM, et al. High initial tidal volumes in emergency department patients at risk for acute respiratory distress syndrome. J Crit Care. 2015;30:341–3.
18. Gajic O, Frutos-Vivar F, Esteban A, et al. Ventilator settings as a risk factor for acute respiratory distress syndrome in mechanically ventilated patients. Intensive Care Med. 2005;31:922–6.
19. Neto AS, Simonis FD, Barbas CS, et al. Lung-protective ventilation with low tidal volumes and the occurrence of pulmonary complications in patients without acute respiratory distress syndrome: a systematic review and individual patient data analysis. Crit Care Med. 2015;43:2155–63.

20. Sjoding MW, Gong MN, Hass MLS, Iwashyna TJ. Evaluating delivery of low tidal volume ventilation in six ICUs using electronic health record data. Crit Care Med. 2019;47:56–61.
21. Simonis FD, Binnekade JM, Braber A, et al. PReVENT—protective ventilation in patients without ARDS at start of ventilation: study protocol for a randomized controlled trial. Trials. 2015;16:226.
22. Anonymous. PRotective VENTilation in Patients Without ARDS (PReVENT-NL) NCT02153294. 2014. https://clinicaltrialsgov/ct2/show/study/NCT02153294. Accessed 8 Oct 2018.
23. Wanderer JP, Blum JM, Ehrenfeld JM. Intraoperative low-tidal-volume ventilation. N Engl J Med. 2013;369:1861.
24. PROVHILO Investigators. High versus low positive end-expiratory pressure during general anaesthesia for open abdominal surgery (PROVHILO trial): a multicentre randomised controlled trial. Lancet. 2014;384:495–503.
25. Gu WJ, Wang F, Liu JC. Effect of lung-protective ventilation with lower tidal volumes on clinical outcomes among patients undergoing surgery: a meta-analysis of randomized controlled trials. CMAJ. 2015;187:E101–9.
26. Kroell W, Metzler H, Struber G, et al. Epidemiology, practice of ventilation and outcome for patients at increased risk of postoperative pulmonary complications: LAS VEGAS—an observational study in 29 countries. Eur J Anaesthesiol. 2017;34:492–507.
27. Fryar CD, Gu Q, Ogden CL, Flegal KM. Anthropometric reference data for children and adults: United States, 2011–2014. Vital Health Stat. 2016;2016:1–46.
28. Sasko B, Thiem U, Christ M, et al. Size matters: an observational study investigating estimated height as a reference size for calculating tidal volumes if low tidal volume ventilation is required. PLoS One. 2018;13:e0199917.
29. Han S, Martin GS, Maloney JP, et al. Short women with severe sepsis-related acute lung injury receive lung protective ventilation less frequently: an observational cohort study. Crit Care. 2011;15:R262.
30. Bhat R, Goyal M, Graf S, et al. Impact of post-intubation interventions on mortality in patients boarding in the emergency department. West J Emerg Med. 2014;15:708–11.
31. Goyal M, Houseman D, Johnson NJ, et al. Prevalence of acute lung injury among medical patients in the emergency department. Acad Emerg Med. 2012;19:E1011–8.
32. Kor DJ, Talmor DS, Banner-Goodspeed VM, et al. Lung Injury Prevention with Aspirin (LIPS-A): a protocol for a multicentre randomised clinical trial in medical patients at high risk of acute lung injury. BMJ Open. 2012;2:e001606.
33. Wilcox SR, Richards JB, Fisher DF, et al. Initial mechanical ventilator settings and lung protective ventilation in the ED. Am J Emerg Med. 2016;34:1446–51.
34. Stoltze AJ, Wong TS, Harland KK, et al. Prehospital tidal volume influences hospital tidal volume: a cohort study. J Crit Care. 2015;30:495–501.
35. Perbet S, Mongardon N, Dumas F, et al. Early-onset pneumonia after cardiac arrest: characteristics, risk factors and influence on prognosis. Am J Respir Crit Care Med. 2011;184:1048–54.
36. Sutherasan Y, Penuelas O, Muriel A, et al. Management and outcome of mechanically ventilated patients after cardiac arrest. Crit Care. 2015;19:215.
37. Harmon MBA, van Meenen DMP, van der Veen A, et al. Practice of mechanical ventilation in cardiac arrest patients and effects of targeted temperature management: a substudy of the targeted temperature management trial. Resuscitation. 2018;129:29–36.
38. Johnson NJ, Carlbom DJ, Gaieski DF. Ventilator management and respiratory care after cardiac arrest: oxygenation, ventilation, infection, and injury. Chest. 2018;153:1466–77.
39. Beitler JR, Ghafouri TB, Jinadasa SP, et al. Favorable neurocognitive outcome with low tidal volume ventilation after cardiac arrest. Am J Respir Crit Care Med. 2017;195:1198–206.
40. Dumont TM, Visioni AJ, Rughani AI, et al. Inappropriate prehospital ventilation in severe traumatic brain injury increases in-hospital mortality. J Neurotrauma. 2010;27:1233–41.

41. Mascia L, Zavala E, Bosma K, et al. High tidal volume is associated with the development of acute lung injury after severe brain injury: an international observational study. Crit Care Med. 2007;35:1815–20.
42. Holland MC, Mackersie RC, Morabito D, et al. The development of acute lung injury is associated with worse neurologic outcome in patients with severe traumatic brain injury. J Trauma. 2003;55:106–11.
43. Nemer SN, Caldeira JB, Santos RG, et al. Effects of positive end-expiratory pressure on brain tissue oxygen pressure of severe traumatic brain injury patients with acute respiratory distress syndrome: a pilot study. J Crit Care. 2015;30:1263–6.
44. Wright BJ, Slesinger TL. Low tidal volume should not routinely be used for emergency department patients requiring mechanical ventilation. Ann Emerg Med. 2012;60:216–7.
45. Elmer J, Huang DT. Lung-protective ventilation in the emergency department. Ann Emerg Med. 2017;70:419–20.
46. Halpern SD. Using default options and other nudges to improve critical care. Crit Care Med. 2018;46:460–4.
47. Kahn JM, Andersson L, Karir V, et al. Low tidal volume ventilation does not increase sedation use in patients with acute lung injury. Crit Care Med. 2005;33:766–71.
48. Serpa Neto A, Simonis FD, Barbas CS, et al. Association between tidal volume size, duration of ventilation, and sedation needs in patients without acute respiratory distress syndrome: an individual patient data meta-analysis. Intensive Care Med. 2014;40:950–7.

5 Recruitment Maneuvers and Higher PEEP, the So-Called Open Lung Concept, in Patients with ARDS

P. van der Zee and D. Gommers

5.1 Introduction

The acute respiratory distress syndrome (ARDS) is a hypoxemic syndrome primarily treated using supportive mechanical ventilation. Although mechanical ventilation is life-saving, it can cause ventilator-induced lung injury (VILI). Therefore, the goal of mechanical ventilation is to achieve adequate gas exchange while minimizing lung injury. Multiple mechanical ventilation strategies have been developed to limit VILI. These strategies are based on the pathophysiological concept that alveolar overdistention, shear-stress, and atelectrauma (i.e., the cyclical opening and closing of unstable alveoli) are possible mechanisms that result in VILI. Targets that might aggravate or attenuate VILI, notably tidal volume and positive end-expiratory pressure (PEEP), have become the subject of extensive research.

The ARDS Network (ARDSNet) trial aimed to reduce overdistention, if necessary at the cost of suboptimal gas exchange [1]. This trial demonstrated that a ventilation strategy with low tidal volume and limited plateau pressure (Pplat $\leq$30 cmH_2O) reduced mortality rate. Lachmann proposed to reduce atelectrauma and shear-stress by using recruitment maneuvers and subsequent use of higher PEEP: the "open lung concept" [2].

The open lung concept, combined with low tidal volume seems appealing from a pathophysiological perspective, and has been very promising in experimental ARDS models [3, 4]. However, clinical evidence is inconsistent. A meta-analysis comparing higher PEEP (13–15 cmH_2O) and low PEEP ventilation strategies reported a reduction in mortality rate, but only in a subgroup analysis of patients with moderate to severe ARDS [5]. Another meta-analysis reported a reduced mortality rate in patients with ARDS treated according to the open lung concept [6]. Amato and

P. van der Zee · D. Gommers (✉)
Department of Adult Intensive Care Medicine, Erasmus MC,
Erasmus University Rotterdam, Rotterdam, The Netherlands
e-mail: d.gommers@erasmusmc.nl

J.-L. Vincent (ed.), *Annual Update in Intensive Care and Emergency Medicine 2019*, Annual Update in Intensive Care and Emergency Medicine,
https://doi.org/10.1007/978-3-030-06067-1_5

colleagues demonstrated in a multilevel mediation analysis that an increase in PEEP reduced mortality rate in patients with ARDS, but only if this resulted in a decreased driving pressure [7].

The recent Alveolar Recruitment for ARDS Trial (ART) renewed the controversies about the efficacy of recruitment maneuvers and application of higher PEEP levels [8]. This trial reported that a recruitment maneuver combined with higher PEEP increased mortality rate in patients with moderate to severe ARDS. It was proposed that the overdistention caused by recruitment maneuvers and higher PEEP might be more harmful than the shear-stress and atelectrauma it prevents [9]. This raises the following question: should we abandon the open lung concept in our patients with ARDS?

In this chapter, we will briefly discuss the pathophysiology of ARDS and VILI, limitations and indications of the open lung concept, bedside monitoring to guide the open lung concept, and airway pressure release ventilation (APRV) as an alternative.

5.2 The Pathophysiology of ARDS and VILI

The pathophysiology of ARDS is based on the triad of alveolar-capillary membrane injury, high-permeability (alveolar) edema and inflammation [10]. Histologically this is characterized by diffuse alveolar damage [11]. The “baby lung” model describes the pathophysiological effects of ARDS, mainly edema, on lung mechanics [12]. It is based on observations that atelectasis and edema are preferentially distributed to dependent lung regions, whereas independent lung regions are relatively well-aerated. The amount of collapse and edema formation correlates with ARDS severity. Although intrinsic elasticity of the independent lung region is nearly normal, lung function is restricted by the collapsed dependent lung region. Because the ARDS lung is small and not stiff, the term “baby lung” was proposed [12].

The pathophysiological triad cannot be routinely measured in clinical practice. Therefore, arterial hypoxemia and bilateral opacities on chest imaging are used as clinical surrogates in the Berlin definition of ARDS [13]. Because the Berlin definition is not based on pathophysiological criteria, it poses several limitations in clinical research. Only half of clinically diagnosed patients with ARDS have diffuse alveolar damage at autopsy [14]. In addition, pulmonary and extrapulmonary insults may induce ARDS, both with a different response to PEEP [15]. As a consequence, ARDS is a heterogeneous syndrome.

The Berlin definition of ARDS specified disease severity according to the PaO_2/FiO_2 ratio at a PEEP level of at least 5 cmH_2O. This classification is important, as recruitability is dependent on disease severity. However, PEEP has a major effect on the PaO_2/FiO_2 ratio and application of high PEEP could mask ARDS severity. Caironi and colleagues [16] reported that 54% of patients with mild ARDS at clinical PEEP (i.e., >5 cmH_2O) were reclassified as either moderate or severe ARDS at 5 cmH_2O PEEP. In addition, the correlation between ARDS severity and lung recruitability improved significantly at 5 cmH_2O [16]. Therefore, a fixed PEEP level should be used to assess disease severity and recruitability.

Injurious mechanical ventilation in experimental models results in diffuse alveolar damage, including interstitial and alveolar edema, hyaline membrane formation, and cell infiltration [17]. Therefore, VILI cannot be distinguished from ARDS and is potentially the most important insult that sustains or aggravates ARDS. As ARDS is characterized by baby lungs, alveolar overdistention of the independent lung is considered to be a major contributor to VILI. Initially it was unclear whether high tidal volume, high airway pressure, or both resulted in VILI. Dreyfuss and colleagues distinguished tidal volume from airway pressures in a rat model [18]. Pulmonary edema formation was assessed after 20 min of mechanical ventilation according to the following protocols: (1) high pressure (45 cmH_2O) and high tidal volume (40 mL/kg); (2) high pressure (45 cmH_2O) and lower tidal volume (19 mL/kg)—lower tidal volume was achieved by a thoracoabdominal strap avoiding chest wall distention; and (3) negative inspiratory pressure (iron lung) and high tidal volume (44 mL/kg). They observed that edema increased significantly in groups 1 and 3 compared to group 2, indicating that high volume and not high pressure caused lung injury. In addition, in a fourth group they reported that 10 cmH_2O PEEP reduced edema formation.

Protti and colleagues demonstrated the beneficial effect of PEEP in combination with a reduced tidal volume [3]. In a pig model, they divided the end-inspiratory lung volume (i.e., strain) into a component generated by PEEP (static strain = PEEP volume/functional residual capacity) and a component generated by tidal volume (dynamic strain = tidal volume/functional residual capacity). Four groups were ventilated with a total strain of 2.5 (close to total lung capacity): (1) V_{PEEP} 0% and tidal volume 100%; (2) V_{PEEP} 25% and tidal volume 75%; (3) V_{PEEP} 50% and tidal volume 50%; and (4) V_{PEEP} 75% and tidal volume 25%. After 54 h, all pigs in the tidal volume 100% group had died due to massive lung edema, whereas none of the pigs in the V_{PEEP} 75% and tidal volume 25% group had died or developed pulmonary edema. At the end of the experiment, sudden removal of PEEP in the last group did not result in pulmonary edema formation, indicating that the integrity of the alveolar-capillary barrier was preserved and PEEP did not only counteract the extravasation of plasma. PEEP has a protective effect, but tidal volume should be reduced during application of high PEEP levels.

The use of higher PEEP levels is accompanied by an increase in Pplat >30 cmH_2O. Since the ARDSNet trial reported that a combination of low tidal volume and a Pplat $\leq$30 cmH_2O reduced mortality rates, physicians are cautious with the use of high airway pressures. However, Pplat is exerted over the entire respiratory system, including the lungs and chest wall. Chest wall elastance varies widely in patients with ARDS and contributes between 20 and 50% to total respiratory system elastance (E_{RS}) [19]. A Pplat of 30 cmH_2O exerted at a stiff chest wall (50% of E_{RS}) results in a transpulmonary pressure of 15 cmH_2O, whereas a similar Pplat exerted at a normal chest wall (20% of E_{RS}) results in a transpulmonary pressure of 24 cmH_2O. Therefore, Pplat provides little information about the transpulmonary pressure, i.e., the distending force on the lung.

In conclusion, there is sufficient experimental evidence that high tidal volume and not high airway pressure is important in the development of VILI. In addition, higher PEEP levels are beneficial if tidal volume is reduced in order to limit the total strain (overdistention). Thus, a combination of higher PEEP and low tidal volume should be applied to reduce the development of VILI.

5.3 The Open Lung Concept

In 1970, Mead and colleagues developed a mathematical model to estimate intrapulmonary pressures in a heterogeneously ventilated lung [20]. They stated that at the interfaces of open and collapsed lung, a transpulmonary pressure of 30 cmH_2O could result in local pressures of 140 cmH_2O. Based on these estimates, Lachmann hypothesized that shear-stress might be the major cause of structural damage and VILI [2]. In order to minimize shear-stress and atelectrauma in heterogeneously ventilated lungs, he proposed to "open up the lung and keep the lung open".

Traditionally the open lung concept consists of a recruitment maneuver to open up the collapsed lung and high PEEP to maintain alveolar stability. According to the LaPlace law ($P = 2\gamma/r$, where P is the pressure within an alveolus, γ is the surface tension of the alveolar wall, and r is the radius of the alveolus), more pressure is required to open a collapsed or deflated alveolus in comparison to an open alveolus. Surfactant impairment in severe ARDS further increases opening pressure as a result of increased surface tension. In addition, the opening pressure of collapsed alveoli has to overcome the alveolar retractive force and the compressing force on the alveolus by surrounding lung tissue. The sum of these pressures is estimated to be 45–60 cmH_2O in patients with ARDS [9].

An elegant example of opening the dependent lung, although not by using high airway pressures, is the application of prone positioning. In the supine position, the weight of the ventral lungs, heart and abdominal viscera increases pleural pressure in the dorsal lung regions. The decrease in transpulmonary pressure (airway pressure minus pleural pressure) results in a reduced distending force on the dependent lung. In addition, pulmonary edema in ARDS gradually increases lung mass. Eventually the dependent lung collapses under its own weight and ventilation is redistributed to the baby lung. Application of the prone position changes gravitational forces; the dorsal lung becomes the independent lung region and is re-aerated. Due to conformational shape matching (the anatomic tendency to overdistend ventral lung regions despite gravitational forces) and a greater lung mass on the dorsal side, aeration in the prone position is more homogeneously distributed [21]. Perfusion is also distributed more homogeneously in the prone position. As a result, ventilation-perfusion matching and oxygenation improves [22]. Early large randomized controlled trials did not confirm the theoretical advantages of prone positioning. However, a meta-analysis suggested a reduction in mortality rate in patients with severe ARDS [23]. The beneficial effects of prone positioning were confirmed by the PROSEVA trial [24]. Patients with severe ARDS (PaO_2/FiO_2 ratio <150 mmHg) assigned to the prone group had a significantly lower 28-day mortality rate (16.0%) compared to the supine group (32.8%). Therefore, opening up the lung by prone positioning is recommended in severe ARDS.

5.3.1 The Open Lung Concept in Mild to Moderate ARDS

The American Thoracic Society Clinical Practice Guideline for mechanical ventilation in adult patients with ARDS recommends limiting Pplat to 30 cmH_2O, in line with the ARDSNet trial [25]. This raises the following question: can a lung be fully open at a Pplat ≤30 cmH_2O? Cressoni and colleagues investigated whether mechanical ventilation with a Pplat of 30 cmH_2O actually recruited the lung [26]. They included 33 patients with mild to severe ARDS. Four computed tomography (CT) scans were done: one at 5 cmH_2O PEEP, and three at Pplat of 19 ± 0, 28 ± 0, and 40 ± 2 cmH_2O during a <5 s breath holding episode. Lung recruitment was defined as the amount of lung tissue (grams) that regained inflation as a result of the applied airway pressures (Fig. 5.1). They found that the amount of lung recruitment achieved with a Pplat increase from 30 to 45 cmH_2O was negligible in patients with mild to moderate ARDS. In contrast, a similar increase in Pplat in patients with severe ARDS resulted in a significant amount of lung recruitment. These results confirm that the amount of recruitable tissue increases with ARDS severity.

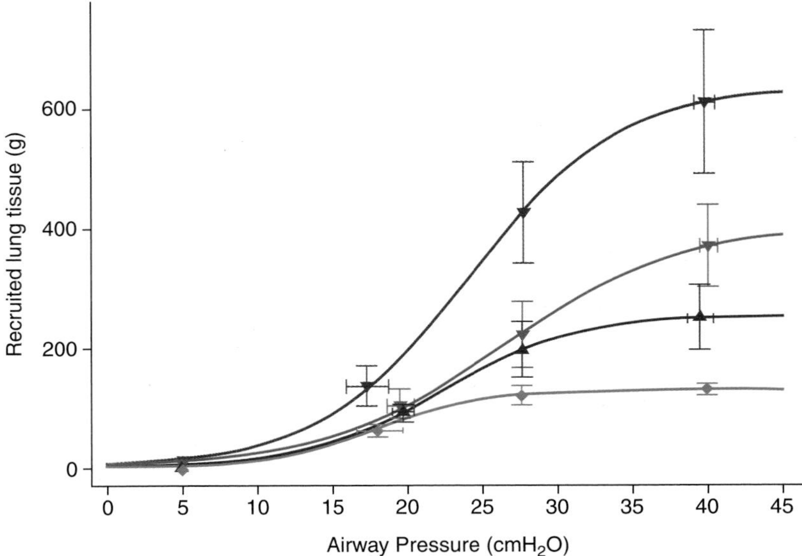

Fig. 5.1 Lung recruitment as a function of airway pressure. This figure represents the amount of lung tissue (grams) recruited as a function of applied airway pressure. Estimates were based on computed tomography (CT) images of patients with acute respiratory distress syndrome (ARDS). Green: mild ARDS, blue: moderate ARDS, red: severe ARDS, dark red: severe ARDS with veno-venous extracorporeal membrand oxygenation (VV-ECMO). From [26] with permission

Multiple clinical studies have assessed the effects of recruitment maneuvers in patients with ARDS. A recent meta-analysis included 15 randomized controlled trials (a total of 3134 patients) that compared the open lung concept with other mechanical ventilation strategies in patients with ARDS [6]. The authors reported a reduced mortality rate in the patients treated according to the open lung concept. However, this meta-analysis was performed prior to the ART trial. The multicenter ART included 1010 patients with moderate to severe ARDS [8]. The objective of the study was to compare recruitment maneuvers with PEEP titrated according to best respiratory system compliance ("High PEEP") to the ARDSNet protocol ("Low PEEP"). The initial recruitment maneuver consisted of PEEP increments up to a maximum Pplat of 60 cmH_2O. Subsequently, a decremental PEEP trial was performed and the PEEP associated with the best compliance plus 2 cmH_2O was applied. After three cases of resuscitated cardiac arrests, the recruitment maneuver was modified to a maximum Pplat of 50 cmH_2O. The high PEEP strategy resulted in an increased 28-day mortality rate (55.3% vs. 49.3%). There are two major explanations for the increased mortality rate after a recruitment maneuver. A first explanation is the included study population, as 599 of 1010 patients (59.3%) had moderate ARDS. According to Fig. 5.1, an increase of Pplat to 60 cmH_2O in moderate ARDS results in a negligible amount of recruited lung tissue at the cost of overdistention. A subgroup analysis supports this hypothesis, as the increase in mortality rate was more pronounced in patients with moderate ARDS, whereas mortality was similar in the two groups in patients with severe ARDS. Gattinoni and colleagues estimated the power delivered to the lung during the ART trial. They found that the power delivered to mild ARDS lungs was three times greater than to severe ARDS lungs (1169 Joule vs. 390 Joule) [9]. Second, the ART trial did not distinguish between responders and non-responders. A mean reduction in driving pressure of only 2 cmH_2O was found, indicating that the recruitment maneuver was inadequate to open up the lung and increase functional residual capacity in most patients. In conclusion, this study found an increased mortality rate after the application of a mild recruitment maneuver and subsequent PEEP titration based on best compliance in patients with moderate ARDS.

In addition, a trial comparing high-frequency oscillatory ventilation (HFOV) with the ARDSNet protocol in patients with moderate to severe ARDS was terminated prematurely, as a trend towards increased mortality was observed in the HFOV group [27]. In this trial, HFOV was applied in accordance with the open lung concept strategy: first a recruitment maneuver was performed by increasing the distending pressure to 40 cmH_2O. Subsequently, mean airway pressure was set at 30 cmH_2O and reduced based on target oxygenation in combination with very low tidal volume (1–2 mL/kg) and high respiratory frequency. However, as in the ART trial, a subgroup analysis demonstrated that mortality rate was not increased if HFOV was applied in patients with severe ARDS. An individual patient data meta-analysis of four HFOV trials (1552 patients with ARDS) found that HFOV might even reduce mortality rate in patients with severe ARDS, whereas mortality was increased in patients with mild ARDS

[28]. This suggests that a strategy of higher mean airway pressure results in an increased mortality rate in patients with moderate ARDS due to PEEP or distending pressure, whereas in patients with severe ARDS higher mean airway pressure might be beneficial.

5.3.2 The Open Lung Concept in Severe ARDS

In patients with severe refractory hypoxemia under the ARDSNet protocol there are three possible treatment strategies: (1) maintain ARDSNet protocol and accept hypoxemia; (2) convert to venovenous extracorporeal membrane oxygenation (VV-ECMO); or (3) initiate mechanical ventilation according to the open lung concept, thus accepting airway pressures >30 cmH_2O (Fig. 5.2). The EOLIA trial compared early application of VV-ECMO with the ARDSNet protocol in patients with very severe ARDS [29]. The authors reported that VV-ECMO did not reduce 60-day mortality rate. In addition, VV-ECMO is associated with a high complication rate (up to 40%), including intracranial hemorrhage resulting in death [30].

In a retrospective analysis of patients treated according to the open lung concept who met the EOLIA inclusion criteria, we observed a 30-day mortality rate of 25% as compared to 35–46% in the EOLIA trial [29]. This supports our hypothesis that there is an indication for the open lung concept in patients with severe ARDS. However, it is essential that recruitment maneuvers and high Pplat are guided by strict monitoring.

Inspiratory pressure is limited by transpulmonary pressure instead of Pplat. Transpulmonary pressure is estimated with an esophageal balloon catheter. An inspiratory transpulmonary pressure of <25 cmH_2O is considered to be lung protective ventilation regardless of Pplat [19]. Grasso and colleagues measured transpulmonary pressure in 14 patients with severe ARDS who were referred to their ICU

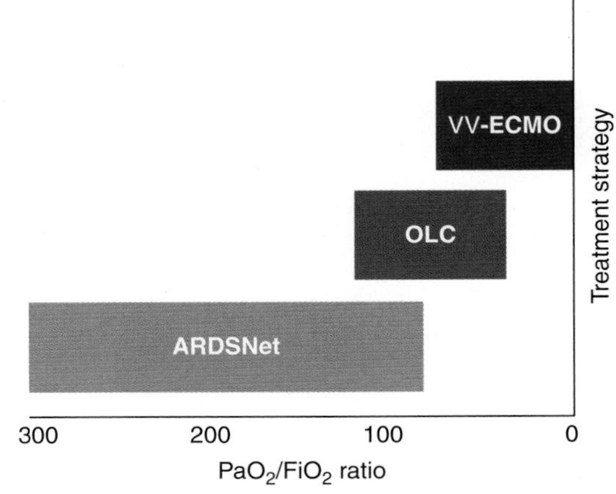

Fig. 5.2 Indication for the open lung concept (OLC) in acute respiratory distress syndrome (ARDS). This figure represents the indication for ARDSNet protocol, OLC and venovenous extracorporeal membrane oxygenation (VV-ECMO) according to the PaO_2/FiO_2 ratio

for VV-ECMO [19]. In half of the patients, transpulmonary pressure was >25 cmH_2O and in these patients VV-ECMO was initiated. In the other patients, transpulmonary pressure was <25 cmH_2O and therefore PEEP was increased from 17 to 22 cmH_2O until transpulmonary pressure was equal to 25 cmH_2O. The authors accepted airway pressures up to 38 cmH_2O. In these patients, oxygenation improved and they did not require VV-ECMO.

In order to prevent overdistention, it is important to distinguish responders to a recruitment maneuver from non-responders. Responders can be identified by an increase in oxygenation, compliance and/or a significant reduction in driving pressure. The reduction in driving pressure is a direct result of opening up the lung, thereby increasing functional residual capacity. In our experience, driving pressure is reduced rapidly after a recruitment maneuver in responders. The extent to which the driving pressure has to decrease in order to be a responder is unclear. The multilevel mediation analysis by Amato and colleagues suggests that a driving pressure of ≤ 15 cmH_2O reduces mortality rate in patients with ARDS [7]. However, in the ART trial, driving pressure was reduced from 13.5 to 11.5 cmH_2O after a recruitment maneuver and still resulted in an increased mortality rate. Although driving pressure decreased initially, an increase was observed afterwards, whereas driving pressure in the control group remained stable. This suggests that maintaining a low stable driving pressure might be more important than the absolute value of the driving pressure. In non-responders, functional residual capacity does not increase after a recruitment maneuver. Thus, PEEP should not be increased as this results in increased overdistention of the baby lung (Fig. 5.3).

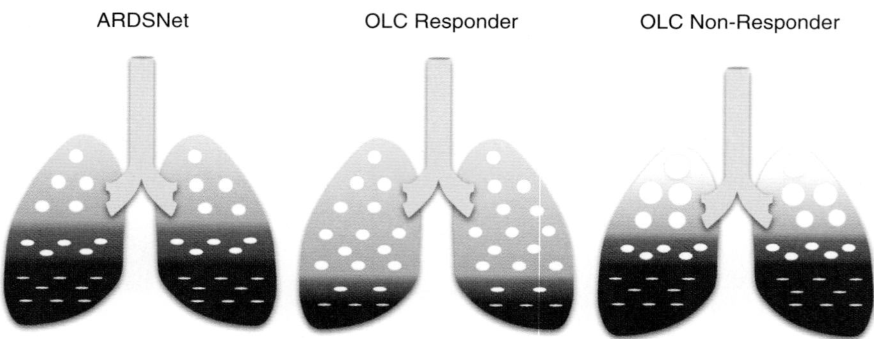

Fig. 5.3 Responders and non-responders to the open lung concept (OLC). Lung aeration at expiration is schematically depicted in the ARDSNet protocol (left) and in responders (middle) and non-responders (right) to the OLC, i.e., a recruitment maneuver and higher positive end-expiratory pressure (PEEP) levels. In responders, functional residual capacity increases in response to recruitment, resulting in reduced strain and driving pressure. In non-responders, functional residual capacity does not increase following a recruitment maneuver. Subsequent application of higher PEEP levels results in alveolar overdistention. Very light blue: overdistention; light blue: normally aerated lung tissue; dark blue: collapsed alveoli

5.4 Slow Recruitment with Airway Pressure Release Ventilation

Time is an important variable in both alveolar recruitment and stabilization, yet often overlooked. The application of 30 cmH_2O to a lung inflated at 5 cmH_2O for 2 s opens up approximately 75% of alveoli [31]. Continuation of 30 cmH_2O for 40 s gradually increases the proportion of open alveoli to 85%. In the expiratory phase, there is a delay of approximately 0.17 s before alveolar collapse commences and at 0.25 s an alveolus is collapsed [32]. Inspiration time in the ARDSNet protocol is too short to recruit the majority of alveoli and too long to prevent the alveoli from collapsing. APRV might address both problems. APRV consists of a continuous positive airway pressure (P_{high}) with a brief intermittent release phase (P_{low}) for expiration and CO_2 removal. Patients are allowed to breath spontaneously independent of ventilator cycles. P_{high} slowly recruits the lung and a short P_{low} prevents alveolar collapse. Eventually, the lung is open and stable. However, in experimental models, heterogeneity is increased if P_{low} is set too long, giving the alveoli sufficient time to collapse [33]. Zhou and colleagues compared APRV 50% with the ARDSNet protocol in patients with moderate to severe ARDS [34]. They reported a trend towards a reduced ICU mortality in the APRV group: 19.7% vs. 34.3%. The number of ventilator-free days, oxygenation and respiratory system compliance were in favor of the APRV group. In this study, the investigators aimed for a spontaneous minute ventilation of at least 30% of total minute ventilation. The contraction of the diaphragm during spontaneous breathing is more pronounced in the dorsal lung region and assists in opening up even the most dependent lung regions. In conclusion, APRV results in an open lung by slow recruitment, alveolar stabilization and contraction of the diaphragm.

5.5 Conclusion

The objective of the open lung concept is to achieve an open and homogeneously ventilated lung. From a pathophysiological perspective the open lung concept seems beneficial, because shear-stress and atelectrauma are reduced. An open and more homogeneously ventilated lung can be achieved by the application of prone position or high airway pressures. In patients with severe ARDS, prone position has been shown to reduce mortality rates.

Multiple studies using recruitment maneuvers with airway pressures up to 50–60 cmH_2O showed improved oxygenation and not reduced mortality rates. The ART trial found an increased mortality rate when a recruitment maneuver was combined with decremental PEEP titration based on best compliance in patients with moderate to severe ARDS [8]. The application of HFOV and high mean airway pressures in patients with ARDS increased mortality rate as well [27]. However, subgroup analyses of both trials showed that mortality rate increased in patients with moderate ARDS, but was similar or even reduced in patients with severe ARDS [28]. Apparently, the application of higher PEEP or distending pressures increases mortality in patients with moderate ARDS due to overdistention, despite best PEEP titration. This observation indicates that high airway pressures should not be used in patients with moderate ARDS.

We propose that the open lung concept should be applied in patients with severe ARDS with refractory hypoxemia under the ARDSNet protocol, but only if a patient is a responder to recruitment. In patients who do not respond to recruitment, PEEP should be reduced and VV-ECMO may be considered. As both the open lung concept and VV-ECMO require clinical expertise, we recommend that this strategy be applied in tertiary referral centers. The exact definition of a responder remains to be elucidated. After a recruitment maneuver, driving pressure, oxygenation, and compliance should improve, but to what extent remains unclear.

Acknowledgment We thank Nathalie Timmerman for her support in the preparation of figures.

References

1. Brower R, Matthay M, Morris A, et al. Ventilation with lower tidal volumes as compared with traditional tidal volumes for acute lung injury and the acute respiratory distress syndrome. The Acute Respiratory Distress Syndrome Network. N Engl J Med. 2000;342:1301–8.
2. Lachmann B. Open up the lung and keep the lung open. Intensive Care Med. 1992;18:319–21.
3. Protti A, Andreis DT, Monti M, et al. Lung stress and strain during mechanical ventilation: any difference between statics and dynamics? Crit Care Med. 2013;41:1046–55.
4. Jain SV, Kollisch-Singule M, Satalin J, et al. The role of high airway pressure and dynamic strain on ventilator-induced lung injury in a heterogeneous acute lung injury model. Intensive Care Med Exp. 2017;5:25.
5. Briel M, Meade M, Mercat A, et al. Higher vs lower positive end-expiratory pressure in patients with acute lung injury and acute respiratory distress syndrome: systematic review and meta-analysis. JAMA. 2010;303:865–73.
6. Lu J, Wang X, Chen M, et al. An open lung strategy in the management of acute respiratory distress syndrome: a systematic review and meta-analysis. Shock. 2017;48:43–53.
7. Amato MB, Meade MO, Slutsky AS, et al. Driving pressure and survival in the acute respiratory distress syndrome. N Engl J Med. 2015;372:747–55.
8. Cavalcanti AB, Suzumura EA, Laranjeira LN, et al. Effect of lung recruitment and titrated positive end-expiratory pressure (PEEP) vs low PEEP on mortality in patients with acute respiratory distress syndrome: a randomized clinical trial. JAMA. 2017;318:1335–45.
9. Cipulli F, Vasques F, Duscio E, Romitti F, Quintel M, Gattinoni L. Atelectrauma or volutrauma: the dilemma. J Thorac Dis. 2018;10:1258–64.
10. Thompson BT, Chambers RC, Liu KD. Acute respiratory distress syndrome. N Engl J Med. 2017;377:1904–5.
11. Tomashefski JF Jr. Pulmonary pathology of acute respiratory distress syndrome. Clin Chest Med. 2000;21:435–66.
12. Gattinoni L, Marini JJ, Pesenti A, Quintel M, Mancebo J, Brochard L. The "baby lung" became an adult. Intensive Care Med. 2016;42:663–73.
13. Ranieri VM, Rubenfeld GD, Thompson BT, et al. Acute respiratory distress syndrome: the Berlin Definition. JAMA. 2012;307:2526–33.
14. Kao KC, Hu HC, Chang CH, et al. Diffuse alveolar damage associated mortality in selected acute respiratory distress syndrome patients with open lung biopsy. Crit Care. 2015;19:228.
15. Gattinoni L, Pelosi P, Suter PM, Pedoto A, Vercesi P, Lissoni A. Acute respiratory distress syndrome caused by pulmonary and extrapulmonary disease. Different syndromes? Am J Respir Crit Care Med. 1998;158:3–11.

16. Caironi P, Carlesso E, Cressoni M, et al. Lung recruitability is better estimated according to the Berlin definition of acute respiratory distress syndrome at standard 5 cmH_2O rather than higher positive end-expiratory pressure: a retrospective cohort study. Crit Care Med. 2015;43:781–90.
17. Slutsky AS, Ranieri VM. Ventilator-induced lung injury. N Engl J Med. 2013;369:2126–36.
18. Dreyfuss D, Soler P, Basset G, Saumon G. High inflation pressure pulmonary edema. Respective effects of high airway pressure, high tidal volume, and positive end-expiratory pressure. Am Rev Respir Dis. 1988;137:1159–64.
19. Grasso S, Terragni P, Birocco A, et al. ECMO criteria for influenza A (H1N1)-associated ARDS: role of transpulmonary pressure. Intensive Care Med. 2012;38:395–403.
20. Mead J, Takishima T, Leith D. Stress distribution in lungs: a model of pulmonary elasticity. J Appl Physiol. 1970;28:596–608.
21. Gattinoni L, Taccone P, Carlesso E, Marini JJ. Prone position in acute respiratory distress syndrome. Rationale, indications, and limits. Am J Respir Crit Care Med. 2013;188:1286–93.
22. Henderson AC, Sa RC, Theilmann RJ, Buxton RB, Prisk GK, Hopkins SR. The gravitational distribution of ventilation-perfusion ratio is more uniform in prone than supine posture in the normal human lung. J Appl Physiol (1985). 2013;115:313–24.
23. Sud S, Friedrich JO, Taccone P, et al. Prone ventilation reduces mortality in patients with acute respiratory failure and severe hypoxemia: systematic review and meta-analysis. Intensive Care Med. 2010;36:585–99.
24. Guerin C, Reignier J, Richard JC, et al. Prone positioning in severe acute respiratory distress syndrome. N Engl J Med. 2013;368:2159–68.
25. Fan E, Del Sorbo L, Goligher EC, et al. An Official American Thoracic Society/European Society of Intensive Care Medicine/Society of Critical Care Medicine Clinical Practice Guideline: Mechanical ventilation in adult patients with acute respiratory distress syndrome. Am J Respir Crit Care Med. 2017;195:1253–63.
26. Cressoni M, Chiumello D, Algieri I, et al. Opening pressures and atelectrauma in acute respiratory distress syndrome. Intensive Care Med. 2017;43:603–11.
27. Ferguson ND, Cook DJ, Guyatt GH, et al. High-frequency oscillation in early acute respiratory distress syndrome. N Engl J Med. 2013;368:795–805.
28. Meade MO, Young D, Hanna S, et al. Severity of hypoxemia and effect of high-frequency oscillatory ventilation in acute respiratory distress syndrome. Am J Respir Crit Care Med. 2017;196:727–33.
29. Combes A, Hajage D, Capellier G, et al. Extracorporeal membrane oxygenation for severe acute respiratory distress syndrome. N Engl J Med. 2018;378:1965–75.
30. Vaquer S, de Haro C, Peruga P, Oliva JC, Artigas A. Systematic review and meta-analysis of complications and mortality of veno-venous extracorporeal membrane oxygenation for refractory acute respiratory distress syndrome. Ann Intensive Care. 2017;7:51.
31. Albert SP, Dirocco J, Allen GB, et al. The role of time and pressure on alveolar recruitment. J Appl Physiol (1985). 2009;106:757–65.
32. Hasan D, Satalin J, van der Zee P, et al. Excessive extracellular ATP desensitizes P2Y2 and P2X4 ATP receptors provoking surfactant impairment ending in ventilation-induced lung injury. Int J Mol Sci. 2018;19:1185.
33. Kollisch-Singule M, Emr B, Smith B, et al. Airway pressure release ventilation reduces conducting airway micro-strain in lung injury. J Am Coll Surg. 2014;219:968–76.
34. Zhou Y, Jin X, Lv Y, et al. Early application of airway pressure release ventilation may reduce the duration of mechanical ventilation in acute respiratory distress syndrome. Intensive Care Med. 2017;43:1648–59.

ARDS in Obese Patients: Specificities and Management

6

A. De Jong, D. Verzilli, and S. Jaber

6.1 Introduction

Obesity is a global healthcare problem that has risen to epidemic proportions worldwide [1, 2]. It is now common to admit obese medical or surgical patients to the intensive care unit (ICU) [3]. It is estimated that at least 20% of patients admitted to the ICU are obese [4, 5]. One of the main challenges of the critical care management of obese patients is successful respiratory system management. The negative effects of thoracic wall weight and abdominal fat mass on pulmonary compliance, leading to decreased functional residual capacity and arterial oxygenation, are exacerbated by a supine position and further worsened after general anesthesia and mechanical ventilation. Obese patients are at risk of developing lung de-recruitment and then atelectasis. The incidence of acute respiratory distress syndrome (ARDS) is increased in obese patients [6, 7].

However, while obesity contributes to many diseases and is often associated with higher all-cause mortality in the general (non-selected) population [1], obese patients with ARDS have a similar or lower mortality risk when compared with non-obese patients with ARDS [7–9]. Obese patients therefore represent a specific population of ICU patients, and could differ from non-obese patients. The main aim of this chapter is to summarize the most recent data on the

A. De Jong · S. Jaber (✉)
PhyMedExp, University of Montpellier, INSERM U1046, CNRS UMR 9214, Montpellier, France

Anesthesia and Critical Care Department B, Saint Eloi Teaching Hospital, Centre Hospitalier Universitaire Montpellier, Montpellier, France
e-mail: s-jaber@chu-montpellier.fr

D. Verzilli
PhyMedExp, University of Montpellier, INSERM U1046, CNRS UMR 9214, Montpellier, France

J.-L. Vincent (ed.), *Annual Update in Intensive Care and Emergency Medicine 2019*, Annual Update in Intensive Care and Emergency Medicine,
https://doi.org/10.1007/978-3-030-06067-1_6

epidemiology, outcomes, pathophysiology, ventilatory support and adjuvant therapies of the obese patient with ARDS.

6.2 Epidemiology and Pathophysiology

6.2.1 Obesity and Risk of ARDS

Obese patients are particularly at risk of ARDS. In 1795 patients admitted from 1997 to 2009 to two centers, Gong et al. [6] reported that obesity was associated with ARDS compared with normal weight (odds ratio [OR] 1.66 [95% confidence interval (CI) 1.21–2.28] for obese; OR 1.78 [95% CI 1.12–2.92] for severely obese). Higher body mass index (BMI) and obesity were associated with longer lengths of stay but not ARDS mortality after adjusting for baseline clinical factors. Similar to these results, in a secondary analysis from a prospective, multicenter, international cohort in 2004 of 4968 adult patients in 349 ICUs, Anzueto et al. [7] observed a higher incidence of ARDS and acute renal failure in obese patients. After adjustment, obesity was significantly associated with the development of ARDS with ORs of 1.69 (95% CI 1.07–2.69) for obese and 2.38 (95% CI 1.15–4.89) for severely obese compared with normal weight; however, there were no associations with increased duration of mechanical ventilation, length of stay or mortality. These results were confirmed in a recent meta-analysis [10], which showed that obesity was associated with a significantly increased risk of ARDS (pooled OR 1.89 [95% CI 1.45–2.47], $I^2 = 50\%$, $p < 0.00001$, $n = 30{,}583$).

The respiratory physiology of the obese patient might explain the increased incidence of ARDS criteria in obese patients. Anatomic and physiological alterations are observed in obese patients, affecting the face, neck, pharynx, chest wall and lungs. Excess abdominal fat may increase abdominal pressure. The displacement of the diaphragm upward, added to the increased chest wall weight, may raise baseline pleural pressure [11]. While total lung capacity and spirometric values usually remain normal, there is a decrease in functional residual capacity. Reduced functional residual capacity can trigger the closure of peripheral dependent airways during tidal ventilation, and decreased lung compliance due to tidal ventilation below the lower inflection point of the inspiratory pressure–volume curve. These changes result in atelectasis and ventilation–perfusion mismatch and hypoxemia, these effects being increased in the supine position. These modifications pave the way for infections and associated ARDS. The increased prevalence of gastroesophageal reflux disease and difficult intubation [12] can also increase aspiration incidence during intubation, and the underlying insult of ARDS [13].

It is worth noting that despite the increased incidence of ARDS in obese patients, only two of the four prospective scores predicting lung injury, the Lung Injury Prediction Score (LIPS) [14] and the Emergency Department Lung Injury Prediction Score (EDLIPS) [15], include obesity as a prognostic factor. Obesity status is not included in the surgical lung injury prediction score (SLIP-2 score) [16] or the early acute lung injury score (EALI score) [17].

6.2.2 Prognosis of Obese Patients with ARDS

Although the prognosis of obese ARDS patients remains debated, it seems that obese patients with ARDS have a similar or better prognosis than non-obese patients. Table 6.1 shows the main observational studies that have reported epidemiology and outcome in obese patients with ARDS. Ni et al. [23] showed in a meta-analysis performed in ARDS patients that compared with normal weight, being underweight was associated with higher mortality (OR 1.59, 95% CI 1.22–2.08, $p = 0.0006$), while obesity (OR 0.68, 95% CI 0.57–0.80, $p < 0.00001$) and morbid obesity (OR 0.72, 95% CI 0.56–0.93, $p = 0.01$) were more likely to result in lower mortality. These results were similar to those of another meta-analysis performed by Zhi et al. [10]: obesity was significantly associated with reduced risk of ARDS mortality. However, longer prognosis is more uncertain. In a recent analysis of 144 candidate predictors in a large, multicenter, prospective cohort of ARDS survivors, obesity at admission was associated with worse 6-month quality of life (EQ-5D) [24].

There are several potential explanations for these findings, although data delineating mechanisms are lacking. Obese patients may have been misclassified as ARDS in case of interpretation of atelectasis as bilateral infiltrates. Although Gong and colleagues [6] found that increased frequency of PaO_2/FiO_2 <200 was the criterion responsible for the higher ARDS incidence in obese patients, rather than radiographic findings, atelectasis is also associated with a low PaO_2/FiO_2 ratio [25]. Despite a similar pulmonary injury, obese patients might be more prone to hypoxemia because of a greater incidence of atelectasis, which could result in a lower PaO_2/FiO_2 ratio compared with normal weight patients, and therefore a misdiagnosis of ARDS. Reduced functional residual capacity could participate in atelectrauma in case of non-appropriate ventilatory settings (positive end-expiratory pressure [PEEP] too low), worsening hypoxemia. Furthermore, recent evidence suggests that obesity induces a low-grade inflammation, generating a process that may subsequently protect the lung against further insults, through a mechanism of pre-conditioning [4]. However, two important confounding factors limit the extrapolation of these observational studies and could explain their discrepancy. The type of obesity (grade, repartition of fat [android vs. gynoid], sarcopenic/non-sarcopenic obesity) is not indicated and muscular strength and function and the metabolic status of the patients (insulin sensitivity) were not evaluated. Diaphragmatic force may also be stronger in obese patients, as recently suggested by an experimental study performed in obese Zucker rats [26]. In obese rats, the diaphragmatic force was increased at baseline and after mechanical ventilation, compared to non-obese rats, which might be a protective factor in case of ARDS onset, facilitating liberation from mechanical ventilation. Another key element when considering the relationship between obesity and ARDS is that clinicians might consider obese patients to be at high risk of worse outcome; this belief could result in earlier admission to the ICU. Increased monitoring, associated with an increased use of prophylactic measures, could then explain the better prognosis observed in obese patients [4]. The medical or surgical status of the patients could also be a confounding factor. Our team evaluated the impact of medical admission as opposed to surgical admission on the short and long term outcome of obese ICU patients, in a prospective, observational cohort study of 791 obese patients

Table 6.1 Main observational studies reporting epidemiology and outcomes in obese patients with acute respiratory distress syndrome (ARDS)

	O'Brien et al. (2004) [18]	O'Brien et al. (2006) [9]	Morris et al. (2007) [19]	Gong et al. (2010) [6]	Stapleton et al. (2010) [20]	Anzueto et al. (2011) [7]	Soto et al. (2012) [21]	De Jong et al. (2018) [22]
Type of study	Prospective multicenter	Retrospective multicenter	Prospective multicenter	Prospective multicenter	Retrospective multicenter	Prospective multicenter	Retrospective multicenter	Retrospective single center
Country	USA	USA	USA	USA	USA	International	USA	France
Purpose	To examine the association between excess BMI and outcome in mechanically ventilated ARDS patients	To describe the influence of admission BMI on outcome of critical illness in mechanically ventilated ARDS patients	To clarify the relationship between BMI and ICU outcomes, particularly in patients with ARDS	To determine if BMI and obesity are associated with development of ARDS and mortality in ARDS	To assess if cytokine response might be attenuated in patients who are obese and critically ill or if obesity might modify the relationship between plasma cytokines and clinical outcomes in ARDS	To describe the influence of BMI on clinical outcomes in a large cohort of mechanically ventilated patients	To evaluate whether BMI was associated with AKI in the ARDS patients	To evaluate the relationship between 90-day mortality and driving pressure in ARDS patients according to obesity status
Main endpoints	Mortality at 28 days	Hospital mortality	Mortality, hospital LOS, ICU LOS	Development of ARDS and all-cause 60-day mortality	Plasma cytokine levels	Incidence of ARDS, ICU and hospital mortality	Mortality at 60 days after ARDS	Mortality at day 90
Included patients	902 mechanically ventilated patients with ARDS	1488 mechanically ventilated adults with ARDS included in the Project IMPACT database	825 mechanically ventilated patients with ARDS	1795 patients	1409 mechanically ventilated patients with ARDS	4968 adult patients who received mechanical ventilation for more than 12 h	751 patients with ARDS	362 mechanically ventilated ARDS patients

Period of inclusion	1996–1999	1995–2001	1999–2000	1999–2007	1996–2002	2004	1999–2010	2009–2017
Main result	After risk adjustment, excess BMI was not associated with death	BMI was independently associated with hospital mortality ($p < 0.0001$) when modeled as a continuous variable. The adjusted odds were highest for the lowest BMIs and then declined to a minimum between 35 and 40 kg/m^2	No ICU mortality difference. Severely obese patients had longer hospital LOS than normal weight patients	BMI was associated with ARDS on multivariable analysis. Among patients with ARDS, increasing BMI was associated with increased LOS ($p = 0.007$) but not with mortality	Obese patients with ALI had lower levels of several pro-inflammatory cytokines. Unadjusted 90-day mortality was highest in patients who were underweight (45.9%) and lowest in patients who were obese (27.6%) ($p < 0.05$). After adjustment, BMI was not associated with mortality	After adjustment, the BMI was significantly associated with the development of ARDS. No differences in outcomes (duration of mechanical ventilation, LOS or ICU/hospital mortality	The prevalence of AKI increased significantly with increasing weight. On multivariable analysis, AKI was associated with increased ARDS mortality whereas BMI was associated with decreased mortality	Contrary to non-obese ARDS patients, driving pressure was not associated with mortality in obese ARDS patients. Mortality rate did not differ between obese and non-obese patients, before or after multivariable analysis

ICU intensive care unit, *BMI* body mass index, *AKI* acute kidney injury, *LOS* length of stay, *ALI* acute lung injury

admitted over 14 years, using a propensity-score-matched analysis [27]. Twenty percent of the patients included had ARDS. The main results were that ICU mortality in the medical group was higher than that in the surgical group and remained significantly higher 365 days post-ICU admission. After adjustment for category of admission, ICU mortality did not differ in obese and non-obese patients [22). The current notion that all obese patients have similar ICU outcomes should be reconsidered.

6.3 Ventilator Support

A summary of the recommendations for ventilatory management of the obese patient with ARDS is given in Box 6.1.

6.3.1 Positioning

A reverse Trendelenburg position, in which the supine patient's head is placed higher than the feet at an angle of 45°, might help to liberate the obese patient

Box 6.1 Recommendations for ventilatory management of the obese patient with acute respiratory distress syndrome (ARDS)

1. Ventilatory settings
- No difference between pressure and volume modes
- Low tidal volume (6 mL/kg based on ideal body weight)
- High positive end-expiratory pressure (PEEP)
- Recruitment maneuvers
- Assess transpulmonary pressures using esophageal pressure rather than driving pressure

2. Neuromuscular blockers
- In case of severe ARDS
- Be careful of accidental awareness during general anesthesia (more frequent in obese patients) using appropriate sedation-analgesia with monitoring of depth of sedation
- May contribute to reduce mortality in severe ARDS

3. Prone position
- In case of severe ARDS
- Feasible without increased complications compared to non-obese patients when performed by a trained team
- Particular caution for abdominal positioning to avoid increased intra-abdominal pressure and organ compression; use reverse Trendelenburg position if possible
- Allows improvement in PaO_2/FiO_2 ratio
- May help to reduce mortality in ARDS

4. Extracorporeal membrane oxygenation (ECMO)
- Feasible with appropriate cannulas
- May help to reduce mortality in severe ARDS

5. Extracorporeal carbon dioxide removal ($ECCO_2R$)
- Feasible in obese patients
- May help to reduce tidal volume in mild to moderate ARDS

from the ventilator [28]. The reverse Trendelenburg position could act by reducing transdiaphragmatic pressure and atelectasis, resulting in improved gas exchange.

6.3.2 Ventilator Settings

Protective ventilation should be applied, using low tidal volume, moderate to high PEEP, and recruitment maneuvers [29]. As the lungs do not grow with weight gain [3], tidal volume should be set according to ideal body weight, based on height and sex, and not actual body weight [3, 12]. In the 2010s, these recommendations of low tidal volume according to ideal body weight were poorly applied [30]. In 580 mechanically ventilated adult patients admitted to three ICUs between February 1, 2006 and January 31, 2008, O'Brien et al. [30] reported that morbidly obese patients were often ventilated with significantly higher tidal volumes based on the predicted body weight compared with patients of normal body weight. Similarly, in the study by Anzueto et al. [7], a retrospective analysis of prospective data collected in 2004, severely obese patients were more likely to receive low tidal volumes based on actual body weight but high volumes based on predicted body weight. The ventilatory management of obese patients has probably changed since the periods of inclusion of these two studies. In the French center of Montpellier, we performed an analysis of ventilator settings in obese and non-obese ARDS patients from 2009 to 2017 [22]. Four hundred patients with ARDS were included, 295 non-obese patients and 105 obese patients. In contrast to the two previous studies [7, 30], we observed that ventilator settings were appropriate in obese and non-obese patients: tidal volume based on ideal body weight was not significantly different between obese and non-obese patients [22].

To take into account the increased abdominal pressure and chest wall mass and to limit atelectasis occurrence, higher PEEP is needed in obese patients compared to non-obese patients [31]. In a recent study, Pirrone et al. [32] showed that PEEP values commonly used by clinicians (11.6 ± 2.9 cmH_2O) was inadequate for optimal mechanical ventilation for morbidly obese ICU patients. A recruitment maneuver followed by end-expiratory pressure titration significantly improved lung volumes, respiratory system elastance and oxygenation. These authors assessed the effects of two approaches for titrating PEEP (a decremental PEEP trial and an end-expiratory transpulmonary pressure approach), and reported no significant differences on end-expiratory lung volume, respiratory mechanics or gas exchange. The two methods of evaluating PEEP identified the same optimal PEEP levels (20.7 ± 4.0 vs. 21.3 ± 3.8 cmH_2O; $p = 0.40$). Similar results were reported in obese patients in the operating room under general anesthesia in the study by Nestler et al. [33]. The authors [33] performed individualized PEEP titration using electrical impedance tomography and noted that a mean PEEP value of 18 cmH_2O was required to optimize end-expiratory lung volume. However, patients receiving optimized PEEP had greater need for intravenous fluids and vasopressors [33].

6.3.3 Driving, Transpulmonary and Transthoracic Pressures

Some studies have suggested that higher driving pressure (driving pressure = plateau pressure − PEEP) was associated with higher mortality in ARDS [34, 35]. However, the relationship between driving pressure and mortality has been poorly studied in obese patients with ARDS. The respiratory system (Fig. 6.1) includes the lung and the chest wall, and the airway pressure is related to both transpulmonary pressure (lung assessment, =alveolar pressure − pleural pressure) and transthoracic pressure (chest and abdomen assessment, =pleural pressure − atmospheric pressure), which differ in obese compared to the non-obese patients [12]. The relative part of pressure due to transthoracic pressure is higher in the obese patient than in the non-obese patient (elevated pleural pressure, which can be estimate by esophageal pressure) [36]. The key factor generating ventilator-induced lung injury (VILI) is regional lung overdistension with high transpulmonary pressure (Fig. 6.1). These lesions are usually apprehended by the evaluation of the plateau pressure, which

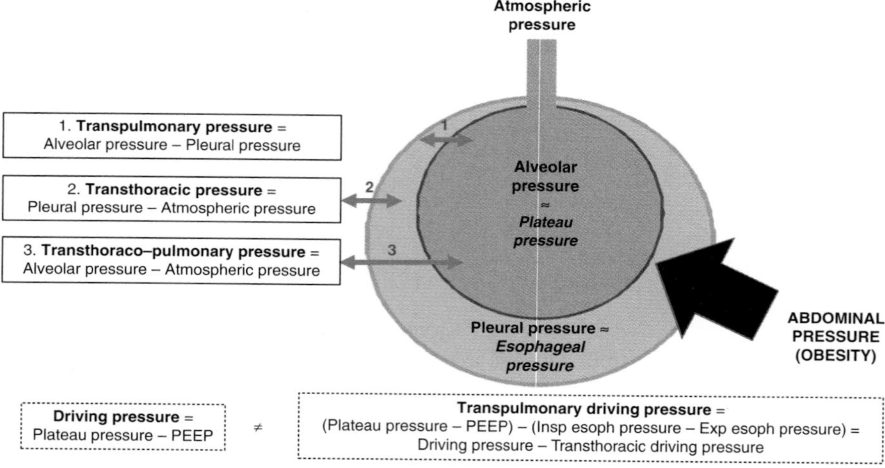

Fig. 6.1 Pressures of the respiratory system. The respiratory system includes the lung and the chest wall, and the airway pressure is related to both transpulmonary pressure (lung assessment, =alveolar pressure − pleural pressure) and transthoracic pressure (chest and abdomen assessment, =pleural pressure − atmospheric pressure), which differ in the obese patient compared to the non-obese patient. The relative portion of pressure due to transthoracic pressure is higher in the obese patient than in the non-obese patient (elevated pleural pressure, which can be estimated by esophageal pressure). The plateau pressure represents the pressure used to distend the chest wall plus lungs. In obese patients, elevated plateau pressure may be related to an elevated transthoracic pressure, rather than an increase in transpulmonary pressure with accompanying lung overdistension. Usual driving pressure, i.e., transthoraco-pulmonary driving pressure (plateau pressure − positive end-expiratory pressure [PEEP]), may not be appropriate to assess the severity of obese patients with acute respiratory distress syndrome (ARDS). To differentiate the chest wall pressure from the lung pressure, assessing transpulmonary pressure (plateau pressure − PEEP − (inspiratory esophageal pressure − expiratory esophageal pressure)) using esophageal pressure may be appropriate in obese ARDS patients. *insp* inspiratory, *exp* expiratory, *esoph* esophageal

represents the pressure used to distend the chest wall plus lungs. As seen earlier, obese patients have a very stiff chest wall, with elevated baseline pleural pressure, and much of the pressure that is applied by the ventilator will be used to distend the chest wall rather than the lung. An elevated plateau pressure may be related to an elevated transthoracic pressure, rather than an increase in transpulmonary pressure, with accompanying lung overdistension. We hypothesized that in obese patients with ARDS, with limited ventilated lung area and stiff chest wall, driving pressure would not be representative of the real pressure applied to the lungs and would not be associated with mortality [22]. We observed that the driving pressure at day 0 in non-obese patients was significantly lower in survivors at day 90 (11.9 ± 4.2 cmH_2O) than in non-survivors (15.2 ± 5.2 cmH_2O, $p < 0.001$). However, in obese patients, driving pressure at day 0 was not significantly different in survivors at day 90 (13.7 ± 4.5 cmH_2O) than in non-survivors (13.2 ± 5.1 cmH_2O, $p = 0.41$). These results were confirmed in multivariable analysis, showing that driving pressure was not an independent factor for mortality in obese patients [22]. The results of this recent study suggest that driving pressure could not be appropriate to assess the severity or prognosis of obese patients with ARDS [22].

To differentiate the chest wall pressure from the lung pressure, assessing transpulmonary pressure using transesophageal pressure may be appropriate in these patients. A recent study examined the relationships between the respiratory system and transpulmonary driving pressure (the difference between airway plateau minus PEEP and inspiratory esophageal pressure minus expiratory esophageal pressure), pulmonary mechanics and 28-day mortality [37]. The results suggest that using PEEP titration to target positive transpulmonary pressure via esophageal manometry causes both improved elastance and driving pressures. Treatment strategies leading to decreased respiratory system and transpulmonary driving pressure at 24 h were associated with improved 28 day mortality. This strategy could be applied in obese patients, using esophageal pressure monitoring. Eichler et al. [38] showed that during laparoscopic bariatric surgery, patients require high peroperative levels of PEEP to maintain a positive transpulmonary pressure throughout the respiratory cycle. In the critical care setting, Fumagalli et al. [39] aimed to determine the relationship between transpulmonary pressure, lung mechanics, and lung morphology in obese patients with acute respiratory failure. They reported that, in obesity, low-to-negative values of transpulmonary pressure predict lung collapse and intratidal recruitment/derecruitment. These results further support, for some authors, the use of transpulmonary pressure, using esophageal pressure monitoring, to monitor obese patients in ARDS.

6.3.4 Neuromuscular Blockers

Neuromuscular blockers can be used in obese patients. When neuromuscular blockers are used, special care must be taken to prevent awareness during general anesthesia [40], because of rapid redistribution of sedatives in fat. Bispectral index (BIS) monitoring may help prevent accidental awareness during general anesthesia, although its efficacy for this purpose remains debated.

6.3.5 Adjuvant Therapies

6.3.5.1 Prone Position

Prone positioning enables recruitment of more tissue in the dorsal region than can be derecruited in ventral regions, and lung inflation is more homogeneously distributed along the dorsoventral axis of the lung with a decrease in ventilation perfusion inequalities. In a non-obese population, Guérin et al. [41] showed that in patients with severe ARDS, early application of prolonged prone positioning sessions significantly decreased 28-day and 90-day mortality. As pointed out earlier, obese patients are particularly prone to atelectasis with a decreased functional residual capacity and may be more likely to respond to prone positioning. In a specific population of obese patients, the safety and efficiency of prone position in obese patients, defined using a BMI >35 kg/m^2, were analyzed [8]. The primary endpoint was to evaluate the rate of complications of prone positioning and the secondary endpoint was to assess the effect on gas exchange, the nosocomial infection rate and mortality. For the 66 patients evaluated, at least one complication occurred in 20 patients, at similar rates in obese and non-obese patients (10/33 vs. 10/33, $p = 1.00$). The PaO_2/FiO_2 ratio was significantly increased with prone compared to supine positioning in the two groups ($p < 0.0001$). In obese patients, the PaO_2/FiO_2 ratio was significantly higher with prone positioning than in non-obese patients ($p = 0.03$), whereas there was no statistically significant difference for the supine position. This study was a single center study performed by a trained team. Particular care was needed to avoid increased abdominal pressure and associated complications, such as renal failure and hypoxic hepatitis [42], which might be triggered by prone positioning. To avoid these side-effects, the reverse Trendelenburg position and optimal abdominal fat positioning can be used. The technique is described in Fig. 6.2.

6.3.5.2 Extracorporeal Membrane Oxygenation

The use of venovenous extracorporeal membrane oxygenation (VV-ECMO) has reemerged as an option for ARDS refractory to conventional support [43]. In addition to cannulation difficulty, obtaining sufficient circuit flow can be challenging in morbid obese patients [44]. There remains significant hesitancy in many centers to offer ECMO support to the obese population. However, class III obesity was not associated with poorer outcomes in obese ECMO patients in a recent study [45]. Among the 55 patients with ARDS placed on ECMO during the study period, 12 were morbidly obese (BMI >40 kg/m^2). Pre-ECMO mechanical ventilatory support and indices of disease severity were similar between the two groups, as were cannulation strategy and duration of ECMO support. Nine (75%) morbidly obese patients and 27 (63%) non-morbidly obese patients were successfully weaned from ECMO support, and patient survival to time of discharge was 67% and 58%, respectively. In the subset of super obese patients (BMI >50 kg/m^2, n = 6), recovery and midterm survival was 100%. Transport of morbidly obese patients receiving ECMO is also safe [46]. In the recent EOLIA study [47] performed in patients with very severe ARDS, including obese patients (only patients with BMI >45 kg/m^2 were excluded), 60-day mortality was not significantly lower

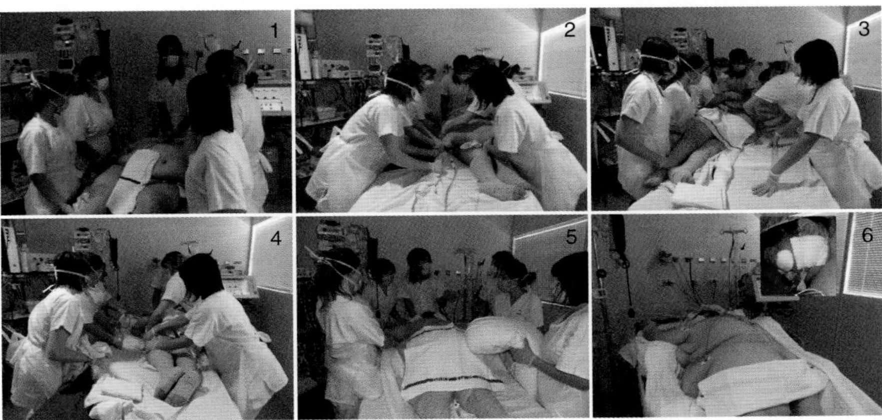

Fig. 6.2 Prone positioning of obese patients. Step 1: The patient is lying down, under deep sedation and analgesia. One operator is at the head of the patient to secure the airway access, three operators are on the right, two on the left, and one is mobile. Step 2: The monitor is checked. The patient is then turned on the left side first. Step 3: The patient is then moved to the other side of the bed. Step 4: The patient is turned. Step 5: Upper chest and pelvic supports are placed to avoid abdominal compression. Step 6: Finally, compression points are checked regularly, and the head is turned every 2 h. Bed is positioned in a reverse Trendelenburg position

with ECMO than with a strategy of conventional mechanical ventilation that included ECMO as rescue therapy. However, 28% of the patients in the control group crossed over to ECMO for refractory hypoxemia. Based on these data, also reported by others [48], ECMO support in ARDS patients should not be withheld from the obese patient population.

6.3.5.3 Extracorporeal Carbon Dioxide Removal

Use of extracorporeal carbon dioxide removal ($ECCO_2R$) in non-obese and obese patients with ARDS is under evaluation [43, 49]. A recent pilot [50] study performed in 20 patients with mild to moderate ARDS and a mean BMI of 30 ± 7 kg/m^2 showed that a low-flow $ECCO_2R$ device enabled very low tidal volume ventilation with moderate increase in $PaCO_2$ in patients with mild-to-moderate ARDS. $ECCO_2R$ is promising in this setting in the obese population, to further avoid volutrauma using very low tidal volumes associated with high PEEP with the aim of avoiding closed alveoli and atelectasis.

6.4 Research Agenda

Because obesity status is often an exclusion criterion in the major randomized controlled studies in ARDS, specific outcome studies are needed in obese patients with ARDS. Results from the main randomized controlled studies assessing effects of mechanical ventilation settings (optimal ventilatory mode, tidal volume, PEEP value, recruitment maneuver type and modalities) cannot be generalized to obese patients. Future randomized controlled trials are necessary to evaluate the effect of different strategies of ARDS management on outcomes in this population. Similar evaluations should be conducted in obese patients without ARDS at admission to the ICU with the aim of preventing development of ARDS. The most recent physiologic studies suggest that an individualized approach should be evaluated in obese patients with ARDS.

6.5 Conclusion

Obese patients have an increased risk of ARDS. Atelectasis formation, increased baseline oxygen consumption and iatrogenic ventilator management could explain the higher incidence of ARDS in obese patients. Lung volumes are not increased in obese patients compared to non-obese patients, and settings of protective ventilation should be applied, based on the ideal body weight and not on the real body weight. Transthoracic pressure is higher in obese patients than in non-obese patients, so driving pressure may be not appropriate to assess the severity of ARDS and to guide ventilatory management in obese patients. Monitoring of eesophageal pressure seems particularly interesting in morbidly obese patients, in order to assess the real transpulmonary pressure and set optimal PEEP levels. To counteract the onset of atelectasis in the dependent region of the lungs, prone positioning may be advised in obese patients with ARDS, by a trained team. Individualized treatment remains the best option for optimal outcomes, taking into account the pathophysiology of the obese patient.

References

1. Afshin A, Forouzanfar MH, Reitsma MB, et al. Health effects of overweight and obesity in 195 countries over 25 years. N Engl J Med. 2017;377:13–27.
2. Hales CM, Fryar CD, Carroll MD, et al. Differences in obesity prevalence by demographic characteristics and urbanization level among adults in the United States, 2013–2016. JAMA. 2018;319:2419–29.
3. Pepin JL, Timsit JF, Tamisier R, et al. Prevention and care of respiratory failure in obese patients. Lancet Respir Med. 2016;4:407–18.
4. Ball L, Serpa Neto A, Pelosi P. Obesity and survival in critically ill patients with acute respiratory distress syndrome: a paradox within the paradox. Crit Care. 2017;21:114.
5. De Jong A, Molinari N, Pouzeratte Y, et al. Difficult intubation in obese patients: incidence, risk factors, and complications in the operating theatre and in intensive care units. Br J Anaesth. 2015;114:297–306.
6. Gong MN, Bajwa EK, Thompson BT, Christiani DC. Body mass index is associated with the development of acute respiratory distress syndrome. Thorax. 2010;65:44–50.
7. Anzueto A, Frutos-Vivar F, Esteban A, et al. Influence of body mass index on outcome of the mechanically ventilated patients. Thorax. 2011;66:66–73.
8. De Jong A, Molinari N, Sebbane M, et al. Feasibility and effectiveness of prone position in morbidly obese patients with ARDS: A case-control clinical study. Chest. 2013;143:1554–61.

9. O'Brien JM Jr, Phillips GS, Ali NA, et al. Body mass index is independently associated with hospital mortality in mechanically ventilated adults with acute lung injury. Crit Care Med. 2006;34:738–44.
10. Zhi G, Xin W, Ying W, et al. "Obesity paradox" in acute respiratory distress syndrome: asystematic review and meta-analysis. PLoS One. 2016;11:e0163677.
11. Shashaty MG, Stapleton RD. Physiological and management implications of obesity in critical illness. Ann Am Thorac Soc. 2014;11:1286–97.
12. De Jong A, Chanques G, Jaber S. Mechanical ventilation in obese ICU patients: from intubation to extubation. Crit Care. 2017;21:63.
13. Hibbert KRM, Malhotra A. Obesity and ARDS. Chest. 2012;142:785–90.
14. Gajic O, Dabbagh O, Park PK, et al. Early identification of patients at risk of acute lung injury: evaluation of lung injury prediction score in a multicenter cohort study. Am J Respir Crit Care Med. 2011;183:462–70.
15. Elie-Turenne MC, Hou PC, Mitani A, et al. Lung injury prediction score for the emergency department: first step towards prevention in patients at risk. Int J Emerg Med. 2012;5:33.
16. Kor DJ, Lingineni RK, Gajic O, et al. Predicting risk of postoperative lung injury in high-risk surgical patients: a multicenter cohort study. Anesthesiology. 2014;120(5):1168–81.
17. Levitt JE, Calfee CS, Goldstein BA, et al. Early acute lung injury: criteria for identifying lung injury prior to the need for positive pressure ventilation. Crit Care Med. 2013;41:1929–37.
18. O'Brien JM Jr, Welsh CH, Fish RH, et al. Excess body weight is not independently associated with outcome in mechanically ventilated patients with acute lung injury. Ann Intern Med. 2004;140:338–45.
19. Morris AE, Stapleton RD, Rubenfeld GD, et al. The association between body mass index and clinical outcomes in acute lung injury. Chest. 2007;131:342–8.
20. Stapleton RD, Dixon AE, Parsons PE, et al. The association between BMI and plasma cytokine levels in patients with acute lung injury. Chest. 2010;138:568–77.
21. Soto GJ, Frank AJ, Christiani DC, Gong MN. Body mass index and acute kidney injury in the acute respiratory distress syndrome. Crit Care Med. 2012;40:2601–8.
22. De Jong A, Cossic J, Verzilli D, et al. Impact of the driving pressure on mortality in obese and non-obese ARDS patients: a retrospective study of 362 cases. Intensive Care Med. 2018;44:1106–14.
23. Ni YN, Luo J, Yu H, et al. Can body mass index predict clinical outcomes for patients with acute lung injury/acute respiratory distress syndrome? A meta-analysis. Crit Care. 2017;21:36.
24. Brown SM, Wilson E, Presson AP, et al. Predictors of 6-month health utility outcomes in survivors of acute respiratory distress syndrome. Thorax. 2017;72:311–7.
25. Pelosi P, Croci M, Ravagnan I, et al. The effects of body mass on lung volumes, respiratory mechanics, and gas exchange during general anesthesia. Anesth Analg. 1998;87:654–60.
26. De Jong A, Carreira S, Na N, et al. Diaphragmatic function is enhanced in fatty and diabetic fatty rats. PLoS One. 2017;12:e0174043.
27. De Jong A, Verzilli D, Sebbane M, et al. Medical versus surgical ICU obese patient outcome: a propensity-matched analysis to resolve clinical trial controversies. Crit Care Med. 2018;46:e294–301.
28. Burns SM, Egloff MB, Ryan B, et al. Effect of body position on spontaneous respiratory rate and tidal volume in patients with obesity, abdominal distension and ascites. Am J Crit Care. 1994;3:102–6.
29. Jaber S, Bellani G, Blanch L, et al. The intensive care medicine research agenda for airways, invasive and noninvasive mechanical ventilation. Intensive Care Med. 2017;43:1352–65.
30. O'Brien JM Jr, Philips GS, Ali NA, et al. The association between body mass index, processes of care, and outcomes from mechanical ventilation: a prospective cohort study. Crit Care Med. 2012;40:1456–63.
31. Bime C, Fiero M, Lu Z, et al. High positive end-expiratory pressure is associated with improved survival in obese patients with acute respiratory distress syndrome. Am J Med. 2017;130:207–13.

32. Pirrone M, Fisher D, Chipman D, et al. Recruitment maneuvers and positive end-expiratory pressure titration in morbidly obese ICU patients. Crit Care Med. 2016;44:300–7.
33. Nestler C, Simon P, Petroff D, et al. Individualized positive end-expiratory pressure in obese patients during general anaesthesia: a randomized controlled clinical trial using electrical impedance tomography. Br J Anaesth. 2017;119:1194–205.
34. Amato MB, Meade MO, Slutsky AS, et al. Driving pressure and survival in the acute respiratory distress syndrome. N Engl J Med. 2015;372:747–55.
35. Guerin C, Papazian L, Reignier J, et al. Effect of driving pressure on mortality in ARDS patients during lung protective mechanical ventilation in two randomized controlled trials. Crit Care. 2016;20:384.
36. Behazin N, Jones SB, Cohen RI, Loring SH. Respiratory restriction and elevated pleural and esophageal pressures in morbid obesity. J Appl Physiol (1985). 2010;108:212–8.
37. Baedorf Kassis E, Loring SH, Talmor D. Mortality and pulmonary mechanics in relation to respiratory system and transpulmonary driving pressures in ARDS. Intensive Care Med. 2016;42:1206–13.
38. Eichler L, Truskowska K, Dupree A, Busch P, Goetz AE, Zöllner C. Intraoperative ventilation of morbidly obese patients guided by transpulmonary pressure. Obes Surg. 2018;28:122–9.
39. Fumagalli J, Berra L, Zhang C, et al. Transpulmonary pressure describes lung morphology during decremental positive end-expiratory pressure trials in obesity. Crit Care Med. 2017;45:1374–81.
40. Pandit JJ, Andrade J, Bogod DG, et al. 5th National Audit Project (NAP5) on accidental awareness during general anaesthesia: summary of main findings and risk factors. Br J Anaesth. 2014;113:549–59.
41. Guérin C, Reignier J, Richard JC, et al. Prone positioning in severe acute respiratory distress syndrome. N Engl J Med. 2013;368:2159–68.
42. Weig T, Janitza S, Zoller M, et al. Influence of abdominal obesity on multiorgan dysfunction and mortality in acute respiratory distress syndrome patients treated with prone positioning. J Crit Care. 2014;29:557–61.
43. Combes A, Brodie D, Chen YS, et al. The ICM research agenda on extracorporeal life support. Intensive Care Med. 2017;43:1306–18.
44. Schmid C, Philipp A, Hilker M, et al. Venovenous extracorporeal membrane oxygenation for acute lung failure in adults. J Heart Lung Transplant. 2012;31:9–15.
45. Kon ZN, Dahi S, Evans CF, et al. Class III obesity is not a contraindication to venovenous extracorporeal membrane oxygenation support. Ann Thorac Surg. 2015;100:1855–60.
46. Salna M, Chicotka S, Biscotti M 3rd, et al. Morbid obesity is not a contraindication to transport on extracorporeal support. Eur J Cardiothorac Surg. 2018;53:793–8.
47. Combes A, Hajage D, Capellier G, et al. Extracorporeal membrane oxygenation for severe acute respiratory distress syndrome. N Engl J Med. 2018;378:1965–75.
48. Swol J, Buchwald D, Dudda M, et al. Veno-venous extracorporeal membrane oxygenation in obese surgical patients with hypercapnic lung failure. Acta Anaesthesiol Scand. 2014;58:534–8.
49. Morelli A, Del Sorbo L, Pesenti A, et al. Extracorporeal carbon dioxide removal (ECCO2R) in patients with acute respiratory failure. Intensive Care Med. 2017;43:519–30.
50. Schmidt M, Jaber S, Zogheib E, et al. Feasibility and safety of low-flow extracorporeal CO2 removal managed with a renal replacement platform to enhance lung-protective ventilation of patients with mild-to-moderate ARDS. Crit Care. 2018;22:122.

Part III

Extracorporeal Respiratory Support

7 ECMO After EOLIA: The Evolving Role of Extracorporeal Support in ARDS

M. Salna, D. Abrams, and D. Brodie

7.1 Introduction

Over the past decade, the rapidly expanding use of extracorporeal membrane oxygenation (ECMO) for the acute respiratory distress syndrome (ARDS) has outpaced the evidence. Before 2018, there had only been one large, randomized clinical trial involving relatively modern extracorporeal technology that evaluated the impact of ECMO on acute respiratory failure, predominately ARDS. Advances in ECMO technology, coupled with improvements in the management of ARDS, made it apparent that in order to clarify the role of ECMO for patients with severe forms of ARDS, further high-quality evidence would be needed [1]. The ECMO to rescue Lung Injury in severe ARDS (EOLIA) trial compared the impact of early venovenous ECMO (VV-ECMO) in patients with severe forms of ARDS against optimal conventional standard-of-care management [2]. Despite failing to meet the primary outcome of improved survival with ECMO at 60 days, the results of EOLIA are more nuanced than the trial conclusion might suggest. A comprehensive analysis of EOLIA provides valuable insights into the evolving role of ECMO and its future use in ARDS. This chapter will summarize the rationale for the trial, provide an in-depth interpretation of the results, and explore their implications on the role of ECMO in the management of ARDS.

M. Salna
Division of Cardiothoracic Surgery, Department of Surgery, Columbia University Medical Center/NewYork-Presbyterian Hospital, New York, NY, USA

D. Abrams · D. Brodie (✉)
Division of Pulmonary, Allergy, and Critical Care Medicine, Columbia University Medical Center/NewYork-Presbyterian Hospital, New York, NY, USA
e-mail: hdb5@cumc.columbia.edu

J.-L. Vincent (ed.), *Annual Update in Intensive Care and Emergency Medicine 2019*, Annual Update in Intensive Care and Emergency Medicine, https://doi.org/10.1007/978-3-030-06067-1_7

7.2 Background

ECMO provides oxygenation and carbon dioxide removal in respiratory failure and both gas exchange and circulatory support for patients in cardiac failure. Much like dialysis for renal failure, this form of extracorporeal organ support (ECOS) was developed as an adjunct to mechanical ventilation in refractory respiratory failure [3]. In most approaches to ECMO, a cannula is placed in a central vein from which venous blood is removed by an external pump, passes through an oxygenator that removes carbon dioxide and directly oxygenates the blood, and is then reinfused back into the patient. When the drainage and reinfusion cannulae are both located in central veins, the circuit is referred to as VV-ECMO. This is in contrast to venoarterial ECMO (VA-ECMO), whereby blood is drained from a vein and reinfused into an artery to provide hemodynamic support.

The most common indication for VV-ECMO in respiratory failure is severe ARDS [4]. ARDS is characterized by an acute, diffuse inflammatory lung injury causing increased alveolar permeability and impaired gas exchange, resulting in hypoxemia, decreased respiratory system compliance and increased physiologic deadspace [5]. Clinically, it is defined by the presence of bilateral infiltrates on chest imaging within seven days of an inciting event, impaired oxygenation, and cannot entirely be explained by cardiogenic pulmonary edema. The grading of severity depends on the extent of hypoxemia, with severe ARDS characterized by the ratio of the partial pressure of arterial oxygen to the fraction of inspired oxygen (PaO_2/FiO_2) ≤ 100 mmHg in the presence of at least 5 cmH_2O of positive end-expiratory pressure (PEEP) [6].

Globally, ARDS accounts for over 10% of all ICU admissions and 24% of patients receiving mechanical ventilation [7]. This translates into approximately three million patients developing ARDS annually, with hospital mortality ranging from 35% to 46% for the categories of mild to severe ARDS. Importantly, survivors may have significant quality of life impairment long after recovery [8].

Although invasive mechanical ventilation remains the standard of care in the most severe forms of ARDS, patients in whom gas exchange is refractory to conventional ventilation, or who have especially low respiratory system compliance with excessively high airway pressures despite optimal ventilator management, may benefit from the addition of ECMO.

The incorporation of ECMO into the management of respiratory failure traces its roots to the 1970s, with the first reported use by Hill et al. in 1972 [9]. However, a subsequent randomized, controlled trial failed to demonstrate a survival benefit with ECMO [10]. Another negative trial, often included as part of the early experience with ECMO, was actually performed with a related technique - extracorporeal carbon dioxide removal ($ECCO_2R$) - and it, too, demonstrated no survival benefit over conventional management [11].

Until 2018, the only randomized, controlled trial that incorporated relatively modern ECMO technology in adults with respiratory failure was the Conventional ventilation or ECMO for Severe Adult Respiratory failure (CESAR) trial [12]. A summary of the randomized controlled ECMO trials can be found in Table 7.1. Although there was a reduction in death or severe disability at 6 months in the CESAR ECMO referral

Table 7.1 Randomized controlled trials of extracorporeal membrane oxygenation (ECMO)

Authors [Ref]	Year	No. of patients	Inclusion criteria	ECMO group survival (%)	Non-ECMO group survival (%)
Zapol et al. [10]	1979	90	PaO_2/FiO_2 <50 mmHg for >2 h PaO_2/FiO_2 <83 mmHg for >12 h	9.5	8.3
Peek et al. (CESAR) [12]	2009	180	Murray Score ≥3.0[a] Hypercapnia with pH <7.2	63[c,d]	47
Combes et al. (EOLIA) [2]	2018	249	PaO_2/FiO_2 <50 mmHg for >3 h PaO_2/FiO_2 <80 mmHg for >6 h pH <7.25 with $PaCO_2$ ≥60 mmHg for >6 h[b]	65[e]	54

[a]Mean PaO_2/FiO_2 of 75 mmHg
[b]As a result of ventilator adjustments to maintain plateau pressure (Pplat) ≤32 cmH_2O
[c]Statistically significant difference in survival between groups
[d]22 of 90 (24%) patients within the ECMO referral group did not receive ECMO
[e]35 of 125 (28%) control group patients crossed over to ECMO, 20 (57%) of whom died within 60 days

group (37% vs. 53%, relative risk [RR] 0.69, 95% CI 0.05–0.97, p = 0.03), there were important aspects to the trial that limit the interpretation of the results. With only 76% of patients in the ECMO referral arm actually receiving ECMO, and a lack of mandated lung-protective ventilation in the control arm (only 70% of control subjects received lung-protective ventilation at any time during the trial), this was not truly a randomized trial of ECMO versus standard-of-care mechanical ventilation. One conclusion that can be drawn from CESAR, however, is that patients with severe acute respiratory failure, including ARDS, may benefit from referral to expert centers that adhere to standard-of-care lung-protective ventilatory strategies, and are also capable of providing ECMO as part of a defined management algorithm.

At around the same time the CESAR trial was published, there happened to be a high rate of severe ARDS associated with influenza A(H1N1), presenting a unique opportunity to study the adjunctive benefits of ECMO in severe respiratory failure seemingly refractory to conventional ventilator management. A multicenter observational study in Australia and New Zealand reported a 75% rate of survival to discharge among 68 patients treated with ECMO for influenza A(H1N1)-associated severe ARDS [13, 14]. Subsequent matched-pairs analyses of distinct European influenza A(H1N1)-associated ARDS cohorts generated conflicting data about the benefit of ECMO [15, 16].

A meta-analysis of eight studies involving 266 influenza A(H1N1)-associated ARDS patients who received ECMO identified the benefit of a short duration between the start of mechanical ventilation and the initiation of ECMO (median 2 days), and highlighted the potential importance of referral to specialized ECMO centers [17].

7.3 Resurgence of ECMO and the Need for More Data

With the publication of the CESAR trial and the H1N1 studies, rates of adult ECMO usage for respiratory failure surged, as evidenced by a 433% increase in the United States from 2006 to 2011 [18], and a threefold increase from 2007 to 2012 in Germany [19]. Despite growing enthusiasm for ECMO, overall in-hospital mortality in these studies reached nearly 60%, considerably higher than reports from specialized ECMO centers worldwide. These data suggested that the rate of increased use of ECMO may not have been entirely justified based on the available evidence at the time [20] or that ECMO was not being uniformly applied. An inconclusive body of evidence supporting the use of ECMO in patients with ARDS largely relegated ECMO to a last-resort, salvage therapy in ARDS management [21].

7.4 Lung-Protective Ventilation

A major limitation in interpreting prior ECMO trials was a lack of strict adherence to modern standards of lung-protective ventilation in all patients, which represents the current standard of care for invasive mechanical ventilation in ARDS [22, 23]. However, the hypercapnia and respiratory acidosis that may arise from low-volume, low-pressure ventilation strategies have been cited as reasons for nonadherence with lung-protective ventilation [24].

Recent literature has suggested that tidal volumes less than the standard-of-care 4–8 mL/kg predicted body weight (PBW), may offer even greater lung protection, particularly given the correlation between lower tidal volumes and airway pressures and reductions in inflammatory cytokines associated with ventilator-induced lung injury (VILI) [25–27]. Typically, achieving very low tidal volumes or very low airway pressures would be limited by unacceptable levels of hypercapnia and respiratory acidosis. However, ECMO (or $ECCO_2R$) mitigates this problem by directly removing carbon dioxide from the blood. A comparison between very low tidal volume ventilation (3 mL/kg PBW) with $ECCO_2R$ and low tidal volume ventilation (6 mL/kg PBW) without $ECCO_2R$ in overall less severe ARDS patients revealed a significant reduction in ventilator-free days in the $ECCO_2R$ patients [28]. This so-called "ultra-lung-protective" ventilation strategy could also be achieved with the aid of ECMO in the most severe forms of ARDS. In fact, it has become common practice at ECMO centers to lower tidal volumes and airway pressures beyond traditional lung-protective ventilation goals when using ECMO for the management of severe ARDS [29].

Adjunctive strategies, including prone positioning (for which there is very strong data) and neuromuscular blocking agents (NMBAs), when used in conjunction with lung-protective ventilation, have been found to have survival benefits in randomized, controlled trials [30, 31]. High-frequency oscillatory ventilation (HFOV), thought to limit volutrauma while recruiting atelectatic lung regions, failed to demonstrate a benefit in two large randomized, controlled trials in moderate to severe ARDS and is no longer routinely recommended [32, 33].

The data supporting the use of recruitment maneuvers and inhaled vasodilators remains controversial [34–36]. Modern ARDS management strategies defined the standard of care against which ECMO would ideally be compared in the EOLIA trial in order to best assess the true efficacy of ECMO over optimal conventional management. Although enrollment in EOLIA preceded the establishment of some of this standard of care, especially prone positioning, the trial anticipated the use of what is now considered optimal management of patients with severe forms of ARDS.

7.5 ECMO to rescue Lung Injury in severe ARDS (EOLIA) Trial

The primary objective of the EOLIA trial was to compare the effect of early initiation of ECMO to optimal conventional management on 60-day mortality in patients with the most severe forms of ARDS within seven days of starting invasive mechanical ventilation. Several important considerations went into the design of EOLIA, informed by limitations from previous studies. Recruitment was limited to centers with extensive experience with ARDS management and the ability to either initiate ECMO soon after enrollment or promptly transport patients to ECMO-capable centers. In order to optimize safe and timely transfer, a mobile ECMO team would be deployed to the non-ECMO center where patients would be initiated on ECMO and transported back to an ECMO center [37]. Additionally, it was mandated that centers strictly adhere to pre-specified invasive mechanical ventilation strategies, which included standard of care lung-protective ventilation and adjunctive therapies (especially prone positioning and NMBAs) in the control arm and an ultra-lung-protective ventilation strategy in the ECMO arm.

Patients included in the study met one of the following three criteria: (1) PaO_2/FiO_2 ratio <50 mmHg for >3 h despite optimization of mechanical ventilation and the potential use of adjunctive therapies (inhaled nitric oxide or prostacyclin, recruitment maneuvers, HFOV, or almitrine infusion); (2) PaO_2/FiO_2 <80 mmHg for >6 h (otherwise, as above); or (3) pH <7.25 with a $PaCO_2$ ≥60 mmHg for >6 h (with respiratory rate increased to 35 breaths per minute) resulting from mechanical ventilation settings adjusted to keep plateau airway pressure (Pplat) ≤32 cmH_2O. Physicians were strongly encouraged to use NMBAs and prone positioning prior to randomization in all patients. A full list of exclusion criteria can be found in the EOLIA supplementary appendix [2].

Patients randomized to the ECMO arm underwent percutaneous venovenous cannulation. To limit VILI, mechanical ventilation was set to: volume-assist control, FiO_2 0.3–0.6, PEEP ≥10 cmH_2O, tidal volume adjusted for Pplat ≤24 cmH_2O, with a respiratory rate of 10–30 breaths per minute, or a version of airway pressure release ventilation (APRV) mode with a high pressure level ≤24 cmH_2O and a low pressure level ≥10 cmH_2O.

Patients in the control arm were managed according to the settings outlined by the "pulmonary recruitment" group of the Express trial with volume-assist control, tidal volumes of 6 mL/kg PBW and PEEP set so as not to exceed a Pplat of 28–30

cmH_2O. Crossover to ECMO was permitted in patients with refractory hypoxemia defined as a saturation of arterial oxygen (SaO_2) <80% for >6 h despite the use of prone positioning, NMBAs and other adjunctive therapies as feasible, and only in the absence of irreversible multiple organ failure and when the treating clinician felt that ECMO could change the outcome of the patient.

Controversially, at the recommendation of the Data Safety Monitoring Board (DSMB), enrollment was stopped in April 2017 after continuation was determined to be futile in achieving the primary endpoint based on pre-specified criteria. Of the 249 patients who had been randomized, 124 had been assigned to the ECMO group and 125 to the control group. Among the control patients, 35 (28%) crossed over to ECMO for refractory hypoxemia.

At 60 days, 44 patients (35%) in the ECMO group and 57 (46%) in the control group had died (RR 0.76, 95% CI: 0.55–1.04, $p = 0.09$). The Kaplan-Meier survival estimates for the primary outcome are presented in Fig. 7.1.

Of the three inclusion criteria described above, one potentially important signal occurred among patients meeting Criteria #3—those with an arterial pH <7.25 with a $PaCO_2 \geq 60$ mmHg for >6 h. In this group, mortality was 24% (6/25 patients) for ECMO-supported patients compared with 55% for control (11/20) patients. Although clearly underpowered to detect a statistically significant difference, this observation suggests that patients with severely reduced respiratory system compliance may receive the greatest benefit from ECMO through a ventilation strategy that is beyond standard of care low-volume, low-pressure ventilation; a hypothesis that warrants further investigation.

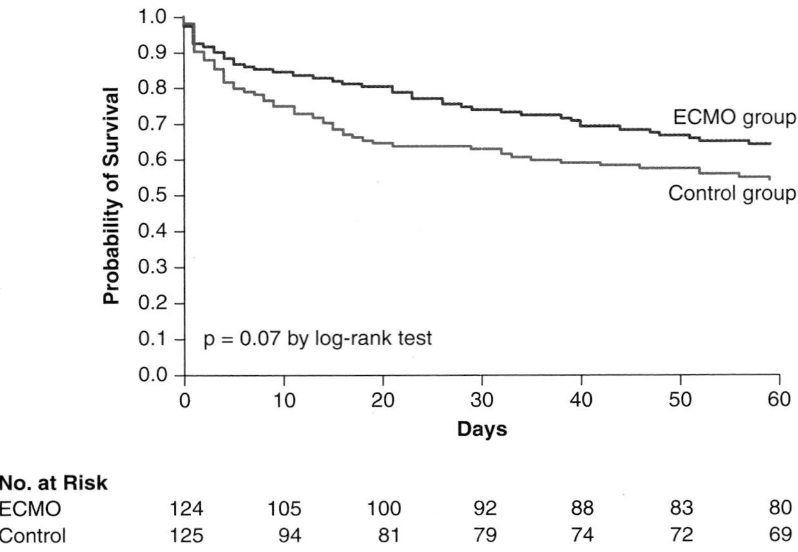

Fig. 7.1 Kaplan-meier survival estimates in the intention-to-treat population during the first 60 days of EOLIA. From [2] with permission. Copyright © (2018) Massachusetts Medical Society

The predicted mortalities in the conventional treatment and ECMO groups were 60% and 40%, respectively. With observed mortalities of 46% and 35%, the study was underpowered to achieve significance based on prespecified calculations. The high prevalence of proning (90%) in the control arm, even prior to the adoption of prone positioning as the ideal standard of care [30], likely contributed to these lower than predicted mortality rates, further diminishing the ability to detect a statistically significant difference between the groups. One limiting factor in conducting a larger study than in the past was the anticipated low rate of enrollment in EOLIA (less than 1 patient/unit/year). It has been estimated that 624 patients would have been required to have enough power to achieve statistical significance based on the actual mortality rates in EOLIA [38]. Even if 100 units had participated, such a study would take approximately 9 years to complete, which may be considered an impractical amount of time, especially given rapidly evolving changes in technology and practice.

Another controversial feature of EOLIA was the high rate of crossover from the control group to the ECMO group (28%), much higher than the anticipated 5% rate of crossover. These patients were noted, after the fact, to have markers of more severe ARDS at baseline, with higher plateau and driving pressures, lower respiratory system compliance, and more extensive infiltrates on chest radiography. Before crossing over, 25% of these patients had cardiac arrests, 20% had severe right heart failure, and 17% received ECMO while undergoing cardiopulmonary resuscitation (CPR). Sixty-day mortality was 57% for the crossover patients, compared with 41% for control patients who did not cross over and 35% for the ECMO group.

Allowing patients to cross over from control to intervention dilutes the estimated treatment effect, if any, when analyzing the data as intention-to-treat. However, at the time EOLIA was designed, there was insufficient clinical equipoise at most ECMO centers to conduct a trial of ECMO versus conventional management without the option for crossover, the very centers where EOLIA would need to be conducted. This then begs the question, how would the effect estimate have changed if these crossover patients had not received ECMO? Of the 35 patients who crossed over from conventional therapy to salvage ECMO, 15 (43%) survived. It is impossible to know what would have happened to those patients had they not received ECMO. At the very least, among those who received ECMO during cardiac arrest, the likelihood of survival would assuredly have been very low. In order to account for this uncertainty, *post hoc* sensitivity analysis of treatment failure at 60 days was conducted for different hypothetical survival rates in the crossover group, ranging from 0 to 33%. A survival rate of 33% or less in the crossover group had they not received ECMO (rather than the observed rate of 43% with crossover to ECMO) would have led to a statistically significant relative risk of death favoring the ECMO arm. Moreover, a rank-preserving structural failure time model, used to adjust for the effect of crossover, estimated a hazard ratio for death within 60 days that approached statistical significance (0.51 [95% CI: 0.24–1.02, $p = 0.055$]), further suggesting that there was a true effect of ECMO in reducing mortality, contrary to what the p value alone would traditionally indicate.

7.6 Lessons Learned from EOLIA

Overall, the EOLIA trial was a negative study, having failed to achieve a statistically significant improvement in survival with ECMO compared with conventional mechanical ventilation. This result, in combination with low enrollment rates and an unexpectedly high rate of crossover, may lead clinicians to conclude that ECMO has no advantage over optimal conventional management in very severe forms of ARDS. However, the results of the EOLIA trial are informative in how ECMO may be paired with lung-protective ventilation strategies beyond the current standard of care to improve outcomes (Box 7.1).

The implementation of ECMO permitted considerable reductions in mechanical ventilatory parameters. Patients receiving ECMO were able to have their tidal volumes, plateau airway pressures, driving pressures, and respiratory rates decreased well below those in the control groups. Specifically, after one day on ECMO, tidal volumes were reduced by more than 40%, driving pressures by 25%, plateau pressures by nearly 20%, and respiratory rates by nearly 25%. These changes inevitably translated into a marked reduction in the mechanical forces applied to the lungs, compared with the conventional arm, very likely with an associated decrease in the risk or degree of VILI.

The design and results of EOLIA point to the importance of ARDS management by experienced centers. Volume-outcome relationships in healthcare have been well established, including in the use of mechanical ventilation for respiratory failure [39]. This association seemed to hold true in the CESAR trial in which patients with severe acute respiratory failure transferred to a regional ECMO referral center had better outcomes and were more likely to receive lung-protective ventilation, regardless of whether or not they received ECMO, compared to non-transferred, control patients. Poor adherence to lung-protective ventilation, as well as an inability to perform more advanced maneuvers, such as prone positioning, at less experienced centers, suggests that transferring patients with ARDS to more experienced respiratory failure centers would optimize outcomes [3]. A proposed algorithm for ARDS management is outlined in Fig. 7.2.

Box 7.1 Findings from the EOLIA trial in favor of and against the use of extracorporeal membrane oxygenation (ECMO) in severe acute respiratory distress syndrome (ARDS)

In favor of ECMO	Against ECMO
Trend towards decreased mortality in ECMO versus control group (35% vs. 46%, relative risk 0.76; 95% CI: 0.55–1.04, p = 0.09)	Primary outcome failed to reach statistical significance
Rapid improvement in gas exchange compared with non-ECMO arm	Trial stopped early by DSMB for futility in reaching primary outcome
Potential to permit greater lung-protective ventilation (tidal volumes reduced by >40%, driving pressures by 25%, respiratory rate by >20%)	Unknown economic implications of ECMO use
Significantly more days free from renal failure, renal replacement therapy, and cardiac failure. No increased rate of stroke	Significantly more severe thrombocytopenia and bleeding events requiring transfusion

DSMB Data Safety Monitoring Board

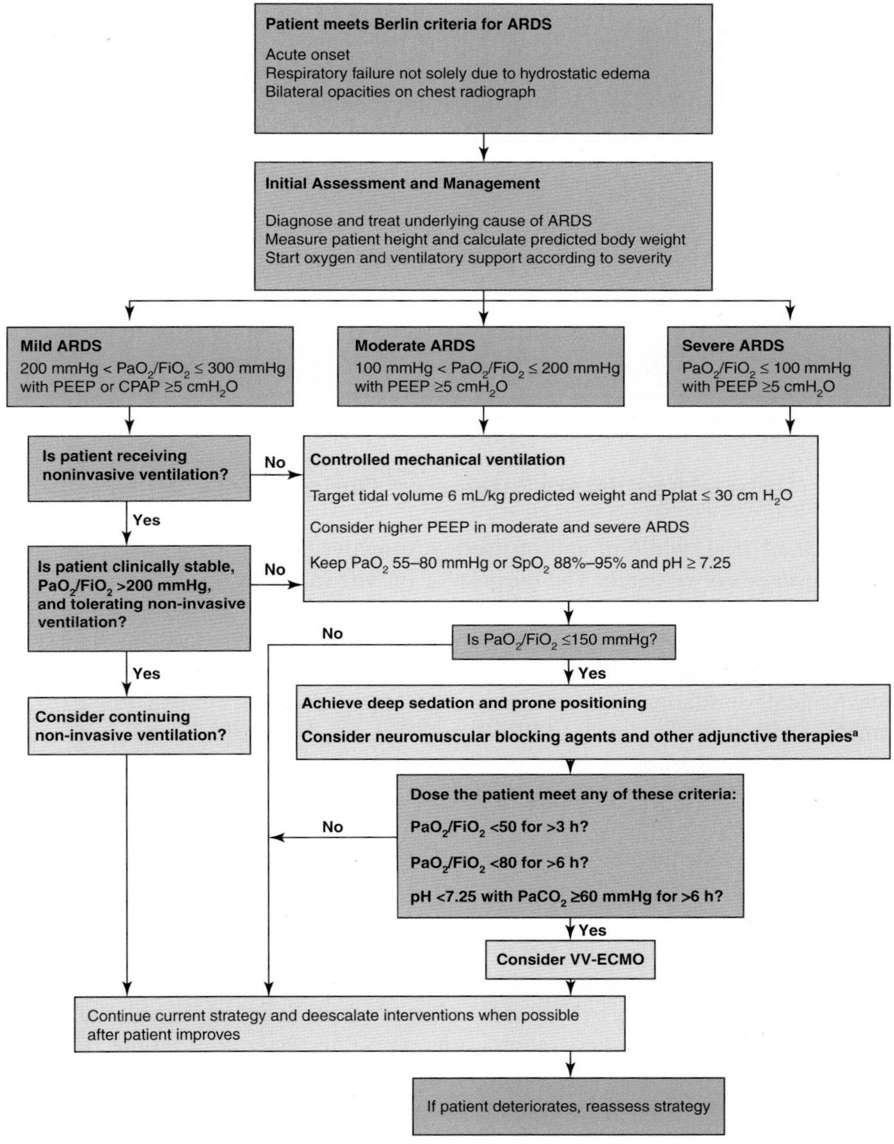

Fig. 7.2 Suggested algorithm for management of acute respiratory distress syndrome (ARDS). Adapted from [5] with permission. *CPAP* continuous positive airway pressure, FiO_2 fraction of inspired oxygen, *PEEP* positive end-expiratory pressure, *Pplat* plateau pressure measured after a 0.5 s end-inspiratory pause when there is no flow, SpO_2 oxygen saturation measured by pulse oximetry, *VV-ECMO* venovenous extracorporeal membrane oxygenation. [a]Adjunctive therapies, in addition to prone positioning and the use of neuromuscular blocking agents, as used in the EOLIA trial, including: inhaled nitric oxide or prostacyclin, recruitment maneuvers, high-frequency oscillatory ventilation, or almitrine infusion

Given the complex, resource-intensive nature of ECMO, it is not surprising that a favorable volume-outcome relationship has been suggested both by data from the influenza A(H1N1) pandemic and more recently by an international registry-based study of over 50,000 patients [15, 40]. These findings, along with the results of EOLIA, further support the regionalization of ECMO programs in many settings for patients with respiratory failure to ensure the safe use of ECMO and adherence to the highest standards of care [41]. The reassuringly low rate of complications in the EOLIA trial is likely to be, at least in part, a reflection of the level of experience with ECMO at participating sites. If a patient warrants ECMO support but ECMO is unavailable at that hospital, referral to a center with ECMO transport capabilities should be considered [42].

7.7 Future Directions and Areas of Uncertainty

7.7.1 Optimal Ventilatory Parameters During ECMO

The EOLIA trial, while in and of itself informative, opens the door to multiple future avenues of research. The purpose of ECMO in the EOLIA trial was not to replace conventional mechanical ventilation, but rather to demonstrate how the two could be used synergistically to improve outcomes, mostly through the use of a very-lung-protective ventilation strategy to minimize VILI. EOLIA used a mechanical ventilation approach in the ECMO group that limited Pplat to 24 cmH_2O, with moderate levels of PEEP and what may be considered by some to be only a modest reduction in the respiratory rate (compared to what may be achievable with $ECCO_2R$). It remains to be determined what the optimal ventilator settings are during ECMO support for severe ARDS in order to maximally reduce VILI, and whether reductions in parameters beyond those used in EOLIA could offer additional benefit. Questions remain as to whether the use of $ECCO_2R$ to achieve similar reductions in mechanical ventilation in patients with less severe forms of ARDS can likewise improve outcomes. The feasibility and effects of $ECCO_2R$-facilitated ultra-lung-protective ventilation in less severe forms of ARDS are currently being evaluated by a large prospective randomized trial (pRotective vEntilation with veno-venouS lung assisT in respiratory failure [REST]; ClinicalTrials.gov identifier: NCT02654327). Additionally, an international, multicenter pilot study (Strategy of UltraProtective lung ventilation with Extracorporeal CO_2 Removal for New-Onset moderate to seVere ARDS [SUPERNOVA]; ClinicalTrials.gov Identifier: NCT02282657T) assessing the safety and feasibility of 4 mL/kg tidal volumes with the use of $ECCO_2R$ was recently completed and has helped inform the design of an upcoming randomized control trial. There have also been consensus statements by groups of ECMO experts calling for an ECMO research agenda to address transfusion policies, anticoagulation strategies, and the role of early mobilization during ECMO support, among other areas of uncertainty [1].

7.7.2 The Economics of ECMO

In the current era of value-based healthcare, the costs of ECMO will be under scrutiny. Unadjusted cost-analysis of the 2009 influenza A(H1N1) pandemic in Australia and New Zealand found the use of ECMO to be associated with a five-fold increase in costs compared with those who did not receive ECMO [43]. Moreover, an economic evaluation of the CESAR trial in the United Kingdom found that the average cost per ECMO-referred patient was more than double the average cost of non-referred patients. However, when assessed as a lifetime prediction of cost per quality-adjusted life year, the costs were within the values regarded as affordable by many healthcare systems [12]. A later Brazilian study reported similarly appropriate cost-utility ratios [44]. While regionalization of ECMO at select centers may reduce costs, future studies across a variety of countries and healthcare systems are needed to assess the true global economic impact of ECMO to better guide policymaking in healthcare.

7.8 Conclusion

The EOLIA trial compared the use of ECMO to optimal conventional management in the most severe forms of ARDS. While considered a traditionally negative study statistically, owing in part to a high rate of crossover to ECMO, and a mortality rate in the control arm that was less than anticipated in the setting of high rates of prone positioning, it nonetheless remains highly informative [45]. The effect size and confidence intervals, along with *post hoc* analyses and secondary outcomes favoring the ECMO arm, all suggest a clinical benefit to the use of ECMO in this setting. EOLIA demonstrated relatively low complication rates with ECMO, identified a subset of patients (i.e., those with more severe reductions in respiratory system compliance) who may receive greater benefit from extracorporeal support, and highlighted the importance of ARDS (and ECMO) management at expert centers.

Research networks, such as the international ECMO Network (ECMONet; www.internationalecmonetwork.org), have been established to better define the role of ECMO in respiratory and cardiac failure by facilitating high-quality, collaborative research, along with the Extracorporeal Life Support Organization (ELSO; www.elso.org) and others. With the results of EOLIA and growing momentum for additional ECMO and $ECCO_2R$ trials, there will likely be greater acceptance of including ECMO in the management algorithm of ARDS.

References

1. Combes A, Brodie D, Chen YS, et al. The ICM research agenda on extracorporeal life support. Intensive Care Med. 2017;43:1306–18.
2. Combes A, Hajage D, Capellier G, et al. Extracorporeal membrane oxygenation for severe acute respiratory distress syndrome. N Engl J Med. 2018;378:1965–75.

3. Ranieri VM, Brodie D, Vincent JL. Extracorporeal organ support: from technological tool to clinical strategy supporting severe organ failure. JAMA. 2017;318:1105–6.
4. Brodie D, Bacchetta M. Extracorporeal membrane oxygenation for ARDS in adults. N Engl J Med. 2011;365:1905–14.
5. Fan E, Brodie D, Slutsky AS. Acute respiratory distress syndrome: advances in diagnosis and treatment. JAMA. 2018;319:698–710.
6. Ranieri VM, Rubenfeld GD, Thompson BT, et al. Acute respiratory distress syndrome: the Berlin Definition. JAMA. 2012;307:2526–33.
7. Bellani G, Laffey JG, Pham T, et al. Epidemiology, patterns of care, and mortality for patients with acute respiratory distress syndrome in intensive care units in 50 countries. JAMA. 2016;315:788–800.
8. Herridge MS, Tansey CM, Matte A, et al. Functional disability 5 years after acute respiratory distress syndrome. N Engl J Med. 2011;364:1293–304.
9. Hill JD, O'Brien TG, Murray JJ, et al. Prolonged extracorporeal oxygenation for acute post-traumatic respiratory failure (shock-lung syndrome). Use of the Bramson membrane lung. N Engl J Med. 1972;286:629–34.
10. Zapol WM, Snider MT, Hill JD, et al. Extracorporeal membrane oxygenation in severe acute respiratory failure. A randomized prospective study. JAMA. 1979;242:2193–6.
11. Morris AH, Wallace CJ, Menlove RL, et al. Randomized clinical trial of pressure-controlled inverse ratio ventilation and extracorporeal CO_2 removal for adult respiratory distress syndrome. Am J Respir Crit Care Med. 1994;149:295–305.
12. Peek GJ, Mugford M, Tiruvoipati R, et al. Efficacy and economic assessment of conventional ventilatory support versus extracorporeal membrane oxygenation for severe adult respiratory failure (CESAR): a multicentre randomised controlled trial. Lancet. 2009;374:1351–63.
13. Davies A, Jones D, Bailey M, et al. Extracorporeal membrane oxygenation for 2009 influenza A(H1N1) acute respiratory distress syndrome. JAMA. 2009;302:1888–95.
14. Freebairn R, McHugh G, Hickling K. Extracorporeal membrane oxygenation for ARDS due to 2009 influenza A(H1N1). JAMA. 2010;303:941–2; author Reply 2
15. Noah MA, Peek GJ, Finney SJ, et al. Referral to an extracorporeal membrane oxygenation center and mortality among patients with severe 2009 influenza A(H1N1). JAMA. 2011;306:1659–68.
16. Pham T, Combes A, Roze H, et al. Extracorporeal membrane oxygenation for pandemic influenza A(H1N1)-induced acute respiratory distress syndrome: a cohort study and propensity-matched analysis. Am J Respir Crit Care Med. 2013;187:276–85.
17. Zangrillo A, Biondi-Zoccai G, Landoni G, et al. Extracorporeal membrane oxygenation (ECMO) in patients with H1N1 influenza infection: a systematic review and meta-analysis including 8 studies and 266 patients receiving ECMO. Crit Care. 2013;17:R30.
18. Sauer CM, Yuh DD, Bonde P. Extracorporeal membrane oxygenation use has increased by 433% in adults in the United States from 2006 to 2011. ASAIO J. 2015;61:31–6.
19. Karagiannidis C, Brodie D, Strassmann S, et al. Extracorporeal membrane oxygenation: evolving epidemiology and mortality. Intensive Care Med. 2016;42:889–96.
20. Tramm R, Ilic D, Davies AR, Pellegrino VA, Romero L, Hodgson C. Extracorporeal membrane oxygenation for critically ill adults. Cochrane Database Syst Rev. 2015;1:CD010381.
21. Abrams D, Brodie D. Extracorporeal circulatory approaches to treat acute respiratory distress syndrome. Clin Chest Med. 2014;35:765–79.
22. Brower RG, Matthay MA, Morris A, Schoenfeld D, Thompson BT, Wheeler A. Ventilation with lower tidal volumes as compared with traditional tidal volumes for acute lung injury and the acute respiratory distress syndrome. N Engl J Med. 2000;342:1301–8.
23. Mercat A, Richard JC, Vielle B, et al. Positive end-expiratory pressure setting in adults with acute lung injury and acute respiratory distress syndrome: a randomized controlled trial. JAMA. 2008;299:646–55.
24. Rubenfeld GD, Cooper C, Carter G, Thompson BT, Hudson LD. Barriers to providing lung-protective ventilation to patients with acute lung injury. Crit Care Med. 2004;32:1289–93.

25. Hager DN, Krishnan JA, Hayden DL, Brower RG. Tidal volume reduction in patients with acute lung injury when plateau pressures are not high. Am J Respir Crit Care Med. 2005;172:1241–5.
26. Terragni PP, Del Sorbo L, Mascia L, et al. Tidal volume lower than 6 ml/kg enhances lung protection: role of extracorporeal carbon dioxide removal. Anesthesiology. 2009;111:826–35.
27. Needham DM, Colantuoni E, Mendez-Tellez PA, et al. Lung protective mechanical ventilation and two year survival in patients with acute lung injury: prospective cohort study. BMJ. 2012;344:e2124.
28. Bein T, Weber-Carstens S, Goldmann A, et al. Lower tidal volume strategy (approximately 3 mL/kg) combined with extracorporeal CO_2 removal versus 'conventional' protective ventilation (6 mL/kg) in severe ARDS: the prospective randomized Xtravent-study. Intensive Care Med. 2013;39:847–56.
29. Marhong JD, Munshi L, Detsky M, Telesnicki T, Fan E. Mechanical ventilation during extracorporeal life support (ECLS): a systematic review. Intensive Care Med. 2015;41:994–1003.
30. Guerin C, Reignier J, Richard JC, et al. Prone positioning in severe acute respiratory distress syndrome. N Engl J Med. 2013;368:2159–68.
31. Papazian L, Forel JM, Gacouin A, et al. Neuromuscular blockers in early acute respiratory distress syndrome. N Engl J Med. 2010;363:1107–16.
32. Young D, Lamb SE, Shah S, et al. High-frequency oscillation for acute respiratory distress syndrome. N Engl J Med. 2013;368:806–13.
33. Ferguson ND, Cook DJ, Guyatt GH, et al. High-frequency oscillation in early acute respiratory distress syndrome. N Engl J Med. 2013;368:795–805.
34. Hodgson CL, Tuxen DV, Davies AR, et al. A randomised controlled trial of an open lung strategy with staircase recruitment, titrated PEEP and targeted low airway pressures in patients with acute respiratory distress syndrome. Crit Care. 2011;15:R133.
35. Cavalcanti AB, Suzumura EA, Laranjeira LN, et al. Effect of lung recruitment and titrated positive end-expiratory pressure (PEEP) vs. low PEEP on mortality in patients with acute respiratory distress syndrome: a randomized clinical trial. JAMA. 2017;318:1335–45.
36. Artigas A, Camprubi-Rimblas M, Tantinya N, Bringue J, Guillamat-Prats R, Matthay MA. Inhalation therapies in acute respiratory distress syndrome. Ann Transl Med. 2017;5:293.
37. Combes A, Brechot N, Luyt CE, Schmidt M. Indications for extracorporeal support: why do we need the results of the EOLIA trial? Med Klin Intensivmed Notfmed. 2018;113:21–5.
38. Gattinoni L, Vasques F, Quintel M. Use of ECMO in ARDS: does the EOLIA trial really help? Crit Care. 2018;22:171.
39. Kahn JM, Goss CH, Heagerty PJ, Kramer AA, O'Brien CR, Rubenfeld GD. Hospital volume and the outcomes of mechanical ventilation. N Engl J Med. 2006;355:41–50.
40. Barbaro RP, Odetola FO, Kidwell KM, et al. Association of hospital-level volume of extracorporeal membrane oxygenation cases and mortality. Analysis of the extracorporeal life support organization registry. Am J Respir Crit Care Med. 2015;191:894–901.
41. Combes A, Brodie D, Bartlett R, et al. Position paper for the organization of extracorporeal membrane oxygenation programs for acute respiratory failure in adult patients. Am J Respir Crit Care Med. 2014;190:488–96.
42. Salna M, Chicotka S, Biscotti M 3rd, et al. Management of surge in extracorporeal membrane oxygenation transport. Ann Thorac Surg. 2018;105:528–34.
43. Higgins AM, Pettila V, Harris AH, et al. The critical care costs of the influenza A/H1N1 2009 pandemic in Australia and New Zealand. Anaesth Intensive Care. 2011;39:384–91.
44. Park M, Mendes PV, Zampieri FG, et al. The economic effect of extracorporeal membrane oxygenation to support adults with severe respiratory failure in Brazil: a hypothetical analysis. Rev Bras Ter Intensiva. 2014;26:253–62.
45. Harrington D, Drazen JM. Learning from a trial stopped by a data and safety monitoring board. N Engl J Med. 2018;378:2031–2.

Physiological and Technical Considerations of Extracorporeal CO_2 Removal

8

C. Karagiannidis, F. Hesselmann, and E. Fan

8.1 Introduction

Extracorporeal systems are increasingly used in severe hypoxemic and/or hypercapnic respiratory failure [1]. Although recent data have shown an advantage of high-flow veno-venous extracorporeal membrane oxygenation (VV-ECMO) in severe acute respiratory distress syndrome (ARDS) [2, 3], there is a paucity of evidence regarding the utility of extracorporeal CO_2 removal ($ECCO_2R$, often similarly used: low-flow ECMO) in patients with respiratory failure. Despite this fact, the number of available systems is dramatically increasing. In this chapter, we therefore provide an overview of the currently used technologies with advantages and disadvantages in the light of physiology.

8.2 Physiology of Carbon Dioxide (CO_2)

Most of the CO_2 of our body is stored as bicarbonate (HCO_3^-) in slow reacting compartments such as bones and therefore not directly accessible for CO_2 removal. Only 1–5% of the total CO_2 content is dissolved in the blood and thus can be removed with an extracorporeal system. The only way to increase the soluble CO_2 content in

C. Karagiannidis (✉)
Department of Pneumology and Critical Care Medicine, Cologne-Merheim Hospital, ARDS and ECMO Centre, Witten/Herdecke University Hospital, Cologne, Germany
e-mail: Christian.Karagiannidis@uni-wh.de

F. Hesselmann
Department of Cardiovascular Engineering, Institute of Applied Medical Engineering, Helmholtz Institute Aachen, RWTH Aachen University, Aachen, Germany

E. Fan
Interdepartmental Division of Critical Care Medicine, University of Toronto and the Extracorporeal Life Support Program, Toronto General Hospital, Toronto, Canada

J.-L. Vincent (ed.), *Annual Update in Intensive Care and Emergency Medicine 2019*, Annual Update in Intensive Care and Emergency Medicine,
https://doi.org/10.1007/978-3-030-06067-1_8

plasma is to further dissolve it from HCO_3^-. This has been achieved experimentally through electrodialysis, an interesting technology with the ability to increase the efficiency of CO_2 removal with low blood flow rates [4]. However, the diffusion capacity for CO_2 is far higher than for oxygen, facilitating the opportunity for effective CO_2 removal even with lower blood flow rates than required for oxygenation. Moreover, in regard the different compartments of CO_2 storage, long-term CO_2 removal may at least theoretically reduce the amount of stored of CO_2 in the body, which is approximately 120 L and therefore about 10 times more than oxygen.

Among all the physiological effects of CO_2, the effect on the pulmonary vasculature is of major importance. CO_2 is one of the strongest vasoconstrictors of the pulmonary arterial vessels. Removing CO_2 extracorporeally may therefore lead to lowering of the mean pulmonary arterial pressure by vasodilatation of the pulmonary vessels [5], but might have the disadvantage that reversing the vasoconstrictive effect may lead to unselective vasodilatation in all areas of the lung, leading to increased shunt fraction in some patients with atelectasis.

8.3 Control of Respiratory Drive

A further effect of CO_2 is its function as the strongest stimulus of the central respiratory drive [6], which is sometimes hard to control in daily clinical practice in patients with severe lung failure. Therefore, $ECCO_2R$ may serve as a powerful tool to control this drive. This might be important in patients with ARDS [7] particularly by reducing high transpulmonary pressure and therefore 'spontaneous breathing induced, and ventilator-associated' lung failure (i.e., patient self-inflicted lung injury) [8]. Furthermore, $ECCO_2R$ may facilitate spontaneous breathing even in patients with severe respiratory failure being bridged to lung transplantation [9]. However, clinical experience supports the notion that regulation of the respiratory drive is independent of CO_2 in some critically ill patients (e.g., patients with stiff or fibrotic lungs and strong respiratory drive stimulated by the Hering-Breuer reflex) [10, 11].

8.4 $ECCO_2R$ Systems and Cannulas

Increasing numbers of different $ECCO_2R$ systems are becoming available on the market, nearly all of them for veno-venous access. Historically, these systems evolved on the one hand from very low-flow renal-replacement therapy, operating at blood flow rates between 200 and 400 mL/min and driven by roller pumps [12], and on the other hand from high-flow ECMO systems with variable blood flow rates, driven by centrifugal pumps. The membrane lungs (often similarly used: oxygenator) available are usually not specifically designed for $ECCO_2R$ systems. Therefore, a large variety of membrane lungs with surface areas from 0.32 m^2 to more than 1 m^2 are available on the market and in use. Most systems outside the operating room are coated with heparin and, as an alternative, with phosphorylcholine/phosphatidylcholine or albumin. Furthermore, many membrane lungs designed for ECMO offer the opportunity to heat the patient. Although this is often not necessary in low-flow systems, some patients (e.g., with low body mass index [BMI]), such as some patients with chronic obstructive pulmonary disease (COPD), tend to have a decrease in body temperature even with low blood flow rates.

For vascular access, different cannulas are in use. Very low-flow systems often utilize dual-lumen dialysis catheters. Although the price is very low, the recirculation rate is high with these catheters [13], limiting the efficiency of CO_2 removal. For higher blood flow rates, specifically designed double lumen cannulas can be used, usually in the range from 14.5 to 20 Fr. It is important to note that adapters for these smaller cannulas are often 1/4 inch (0.6 cm) whereas larger cannulas (>20 Fr) usually use 3/8 inch (1 cm) adapters, as is used for high flow ECMO. As an alternative to expensive and specifically designed double lumen cannulas, two small single lumen cannulas can be used offering the advantage of lower implantation risk and cost, and nearly no recirculation, whereas the main disadvantage is that two vessels have to be cannulated. Finally, smaller diameter tubing is often more flexible than typical 3/8 inch tubing, leading sometimes to unexpected kinking in daily clinical practice.

8.5 Pump Technology

As mentioned earlier, $ECCO_2R$ systems with blood flow rates between 200 and 400 mL/min are typically driven by roller pumps—with the exception of the specifically designed Hemolung RAS system (ALung Technologies, Pittsburgh, PA, USA)—and those with blood flow rates above 500 mL/min are usually driven by centrifugal pumps, also called rotary blood pumps. A direct comparison of the hemolysis, coagulation, and inflammatory response potential, and thus a universal preference between roller pumps and centrifugal pumps appears difficult due to the various systems and versatile fields of application. However, centrifugal pumps play a major role in extracorporeal lung assist systems, especially due to their ability to increase the blood flow far above 400 mL/min if necessary.

From an engineering perspective, several critical aspects related to the functionality of centrifugal pumps at different operating conditions are important. As with the large, industrially used turbomachines, rotary blood pumps are developed for a specific design point. The respective components of the pump are dimensioned for this design point to allow for optimal flow guidance, as loss-free and efficient as possible. In contrast to the large turbomachinery in industry, blood pumps operate in a wide range of flow rates and pressures (e.g., 0.5–10 L/min, 0–800 mmHg) instead of a specific operating or design point. This broad application range can be achieved, in very simplified terms, by shifting the design point to high pump flows and by oversizing the hydraulic pump components. Although this reduces the flow-induced friction losses with large pump flows, it can show increased blood damage at small pump flows [14].

The hemolysis index (HI), defined as the ratio of the increase in plasma free hemoglobin (ΔHb) to the total hemoglobin concentration, is dependent on the operating point of rotary blood pumps (Fig. 8.1a). The HI appears to increase in a nonlinear fashion for decreasing flows. It can be expressed as a functional relationship of the main factors exposure time, t (estimated as the ratio of priming volume and pump flow), and the effective stress, τ [15]:

$$HI(\%) = \frac{\Delta Hb}{Hb} \times 100 = C\tau^{\alpha} t^{\beta},$$

Whereas the shear stress increases with increasing pump speed and pump flow (Fig. 8.1b), the exposure time is positively associated with pump flow (Fig. 8.1c) and is correlated with the HI at low pump flows [16].

A high priming volume, as is required for the desired application in a large operating range of blood pumps, can therefore negatively affect the exposure time and hence the HI. Another reason why the HI is dependent on the operating point of rotary blood pumps is the high degree of blood recirculation in the gaps at low flows (the ratio of main pump flow to gap flow and or pump-internal return flow), which is also displayed as low hydraulic efficiency. The Rotaflow pump (Getinge AB, Gothenburg, Sweden) illustrates why rotary blood pumps do not operate equally well at every operating point from a hemocompatibility point of view. The gap flows increase for high speeds and corresponding high pressures and towards low flow rates, whereby the ratio between pump flow and the sum of the two gap flows can easily be 1–10 (Fig. 8.2a, b). This means that the majority of blood recirculates through the gaps multiple times before leaving the pump, significantly reducing the hydraulic efficiency of the pump to <10% (Fig. 8.2c). This multiple exposure flow can lead to increased hemolysis in the blood.

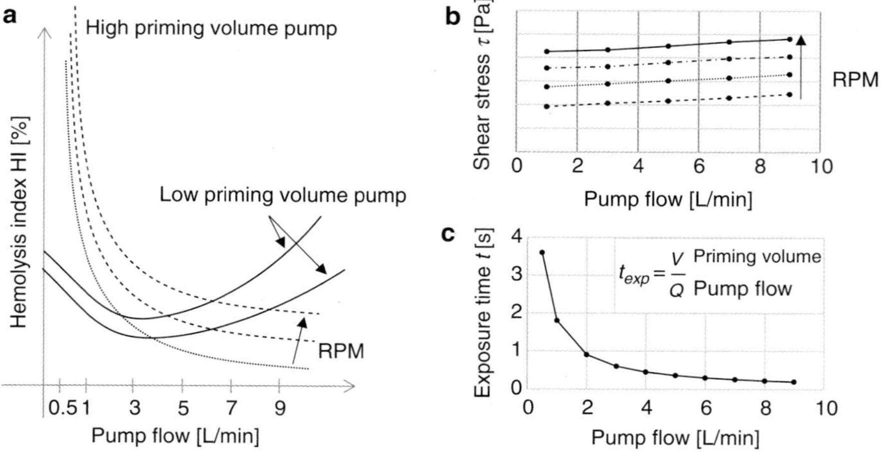

Fig. 8.1 Operating points of rotary blood pumps with corresponding hemolysis index (HI) (panel **a**), shear stress (panel **b**) and exposure time (t_{exp}) (panel **c**) *RPM* revolutions per minute

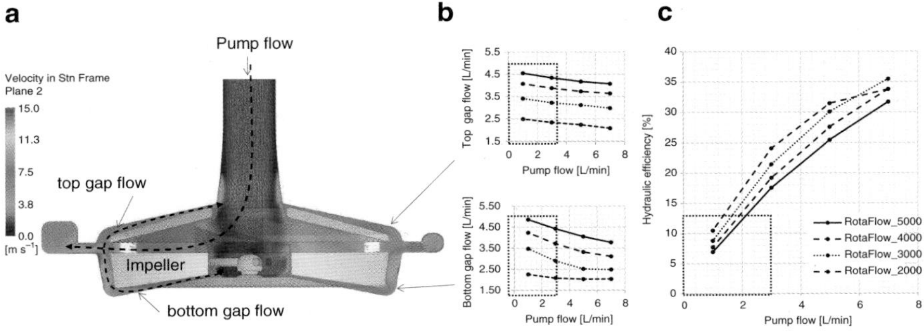

Fig. 8.2 Gap flow (panels **a** and **b**) and hydraulic efficiency (panel **c**) of rotary blood pumps

In conclusion, the authors recommend that industry consider the design of new low-flow pumps featuring smaller filling volumes (Fig. 8.1a) to decrease the amount of flow recirculation and the exposure time and ultimately reduce the risk of hemolysis at low flow rates.

8.6 Membrane Lung Technology

Nearly all $ECCO_2R$ systems use established membrane lungs, typically designed for different applications than $ECCO_2R$. However, this may lead to increased clotting as observed in some clinical reports [17]. Therefore, specifically designed membrane lungs for $ECCO_2R$ may be of particular importance. From an engineering point of view, adequate gas exchange and high hemocompatibility are the main goals of the design process of a membrane lung. Depending on the application, a low pressure drop and low priming volume would also be favorable.

Gas exchange is mainly determined by the membrane surface area in artificial lungs [18]. The exchange area is commonly estimated based on empirical values or simulated oxygen transfer predictions [19] and then validated experimentally. However, a large membrane surface area has increased thrombotic potential due to its artificial character. Progressive or acute clot formation in the membrane lung is the reason for an acute or elective system exchange in up to a third of cases [20]. The thrombotic potential of membrane lungs correlates with low flow states [21, 22]. Therefore, sufficient washout and homogeneous flow distribution is the key to reduce the risk of thrombus formation and clots.

As a preliminary indicator, the theoretical washout, N_{wo}, depends on the priming volume and determines the washout capabilities in the intended flow range of different membrane lungs:

$$N_{wo} = \frac{\dot{V}}{V_{pr}}$$

In this equation, $\dot{V}$ is the flow rate and V_{pr} is the priming volume of the membrane lung. The theoretical washout describes the amount of volume exchange at a given flow rate. An overview of different commercially available devices and their volume exchange rate at maximum and, most importantly, minimum flow rate is given in Table 8.1. Of note, the minimum theoretical washout is typically around 2/min. However, for current devices, many of which were designed for ECMO applications, operating at such low flows is associated with an elevated risk of thrombus formation inside the devices with all the associated problems: elevated pressure drop, decreased gas transfer efficiency, or ultimately mechanical failure and the need for a system exchange. For example, operating a Hilite 7000 LT (see Table 8.1) at a flow of 0.5 L/min would yield a theoretical, potentially insufficient, washout <2/min.

There are two principle configurations of membrane lungs that determine the flow path (see Table 8.2). The fiber matrices are either wound around an inner cylinder or stacked and glued into a rectangular housing. Examples of a wound membrane lung are the Hilite product line (Xenios AG, Heilbronn, Germany) and CAPIOX Oxygenator (Terumo, Tokyo, Japan). One of the advantages is the

Table 8.1 Priming volume and theoretical washout (data for commercially available devices were obtained from manufacturers' manuals)

Device	Priming volume (mL)	Flow range (L/min)	Theoretical washout (/min)
Novalung iLA	175	0.5–4.5	2.86–25.71
Quadrox-i Pediatric	99	0.2–2.8	2.02–28.28
Quadrox-i Small Adult	175	0.5–5	2.86–28.57
Quadrox-i Adult	215	0.5–7	2.33–32.56
Capiox RX05	43	0.1–1.5	2.36–34.88
Hilite 800 LT	55	0.1–0.8	1.82–14.55
Hilite 2400 LT	95	0.35–2.4	3.68–25.26
Hilite 7000 LT	320	1–7	3.13–21.88

Table 8.2 Advantages and disadvantages of most common configurations of membrane lungs for CO_2 retention applications

	Stacked	Wound
Advantages	– Low pressure drop through higher permeability in flow direction – Unidirectional flow – Increased convectional gas transfer through cross-layered fiber arrangement	– Countercurrent flow possible
Disadvantages	– Inhomogeneous wash out of the corners and higher risk of thrombus formation – Allows only crosscurrent flow	– Prone to clogging through washed in debris due to its smaller cross-sectional area – Mostly long fibers and long flow path
Examples	– iLA (Novalung, Germany) – Quadrox series (Maquet, Germany)	– Hilite product line (Medos Medizintechnik AG, Germany) – CAPIOX oxygenator (Terumo, Japan)

possibility of countercurrent gas flow, which allows a constant driving force for the diffusion of the gas. On the other hand, the fiber length is usually longer. The stacked design has a wide cross-sectional area and a rather short flow path through the fiber bundle. The bigger cross-sectional area makes this design comparably more resistant to clogging through washed in debris and it offers lower pressure drop. However, it is obviously more challenging to distribute a tubular flow profile at the inlet connector equally over the full cross-sectional area of the fiber bundle. Consequently, the corners experience lower blood flow velocities and thus are usually prone to clotting. The Quadrox product line (Getinge AB, Gothenburg, Sweden) and iLA (Xenios AG, Heilbronn, Germany) are prominent examples of stacked membrane lung design.

For CO_2 retention applications, further design parameters require attention. The driving force for the gas exchange according to Fick's law of diffusion is the partial pressure difference between blood and sweep gas. Although the pressure gradient for oxygen is approximately 650 mmHg [23], the gradient for CO_2 is usually only 45–90 mmHg. Along the fiber, the CO_2 content will adjust to the blood content and the diffusive driving force declines. To obtain an efficient membrane lung with the lowest necessary amount of membrane surface, a design incorporating short fibers and allowing high sweep gas ratios keeps the gradient over the full length of the fiber at the highest possible level.

In addition, various attempts to increase CO_2 elimination on membrane lungs have been made. Eash et al. recognized that the major resistance to gas transfer in membrane lungs lay in the blood-sided laminar boundary layer on the membrane surface and was proportional to the thickness of this layer [24]. Active and passive approaches have been investigated to disrupt the boundary layer and overcome the diffusive resistance. The most prominent example for active mixing is the Hemolung RAS device (ALung Technologies Inc., Pittsburgh, PA, USA). Svitek et al. documented an increase in CO_2 removal by 133% by rotation of the fiber bundle with 1500 RPM [25]. A passive approach was evaluated by developing a membrane lung with circular blood flow paths that promote gas transfer through secondary flow [26].

In conclusion, the authors recommend that membrane lungs should be specifically designed for $ECCO_2R$ with target blood flow rates <500 mL/min and 500–1500 mL/min with optimized blood flow paths aiming for faster washout and lowest possible clotting rate.

8.7 Blood Flow Rates and Treatment Goals

Considering all the possible modifications of the circuit, the blood flow rate is the main determinant and easiest way to increase the CO_2 removal rate. Human and animal data suggest that a blood flow rate of 250 mL/min removes 40–60 mL CO_2/min [27–32], accounting for 20–25% of total CO_2 production in patients at rest, whereas an increase in the blood flow rate up to 1000 mL/min removes approximately 150 mL CO_2/min. In most patients, this blood flow rate is enough to remove approximately 50–60% of total CO_2, which may be associated with an important clinical impact. Furthermore, the CO_2 removal capacity is independent of the oxygen content of the sweep gas flow, with even 21% oxygen (ambient air) sweep gas having no impact on CO_2 removal capacity compared to 100% oxygen (own unpublished data). Therefore, under defined circumstances, ambient air can be used for $ECCO_2R$ systems, only loosing 10–30 mL oxygen transfer/min compared to use of 100% oxygen as sweep gas. By contrast, in high-flow ECMO, CO_2 removal capacity is linearly correlated with the sweep gas flow rate; sweep gas flow rates >5–6 L/min have only a minor impact on CO_2 removal in low flow systems, and this is more pronounced in systems with large membrane lung surfaces [13, 18].

In general, in choosing the 'right' system for the 'right' patient, one has to consider that the discrepancy between a low blood flow rate and large surface area may lead to more clotting, since the passing time through the membrane lung is slow. To avoid the vicious circle of clotting, associated loss of coagulation factors (particularly fibrinogen) and secondary bleeding, anticoagulation with a target activated partial thromboplastin time (aPTT) of 1.8–2 times the reference is often necessary. Nevertheless, optimizing the membrane lung surface area and new developments focusing on specific designs for low blood flow rates with faster transit times through the membrane lung represent promising opportunities to avoid the potential adverse effects of anticoagulation. Importantly, use of lower blood flow rates and systems is not necessarily less invasive or less risky!

8.8 Which CO_2 Removal Capacity Is Appropriate?

In our opinion, there is no right or wrong blood flow rate. The amount of CO_2 removal is dependent on the treatment goals for the patient. A blood flow rate of 1000 mL/min removes half of the CO_2 and may correct even severe respiratory acidosis [13], whereas very low blood flow rates have a less pronounced effect. Thus, low flow rates may be more appropriate in patients with less severe respiratory acidosis or to reduce the invasiveness of mechanical ventilation in ARDS. However, there are currently no high-quality data for an evidence-based recommendation in COPD or in ARDS. The authors therefore recommend attempting to include all patients with potential indications for $ECCO_2R$ into large observational registries or clinical trials when possible.

8.9 Conclusion

Despite the lack of rigorous data, the use of extracorporeal support devices for respiratory failure is increasing at an exponential rate around the world. $ECCO_2R$ represents a promising technology that may be useful in patients with hypercapnic respiratory failure, or to reduce the intensity of mechanical ventilation delivered to patients with ARDS. Current systems available on the market are typically hybrid constructs, made up of components that were not necessarily designed or optimized for the delivery of low flow rates. The development of purpose-driven $ECCO_2R$ devices—with custom pumps, membrane lungs, cannula, and tubing—may improve the risk/benefit profile for these devices. Clinical trials are urgently needed to confirm the potential efficacy of $ECCO_2R$ in patients with respiratory failure.

Acknowledgements We are grateful to Sascha Groß-Hardt, Institute of Applied Medical Engineering, Helmholtz Institute Aachen, RWTH Aachen University, Germany for his contribution to the current work. The current work was supported by the German Federal Ministry of Education and Research (13GW0219B; Verbundprojekt tragbare Langzeitunterstützung der Lunge zur Behandlung der schweren COPD [p-ECCO2R]).

References

1. Karagiannidis C, Brodie D, Strassmann S, et al. Extracorporeal membrane oxygenation: evolving epidemiology and mortality. Intensive Care Med. 2016;42:889–96.
2. Combes A, Hajage D, Capellier G, et al. Extracorporeal membrane oxygenation for severe acute respiratory distress syndrome. N Engl J Med. 2018;378:1965–75.
3. Peek GJ, Mugford M, Tiruvoipati R, et al. Efficacy and economic assessment of conventional ventilatory support versus extracorporeal membrane oxygenation for severe adult respiratory failure (CESAR): a multicentre randomised controlled trial. Lancet. 2009;374:1351–63.
4. Zanella A, Castagna L, Salerno D, et al. Respiratory electrodialysis. A novel, highly efficient extracorporeal CO_2 removal technique. Am J Respir Crit Care Med. 2015;192:719–26.
5. Karagiannidis C, Strassmann S, Philipp A, Muller T, Windisch W. Veno-venous extracorporeal CO_2 removal improves pulmonary hypertension in acute exacerbation of severe COPD. Intensive Care Med. 2015;41:1509–10.
6. Schaefer KE. Respiratory pattern and respiratory response to CO_2. J Appl Physiol. 1958;13:1–14.
7. Karagiannidis C, Lubnow M, Philipp A, et al. Autoregulation of ventilation with neurally adjusted ventilatory assist on extracorporeal lung support. Intensive Care Med. 2010;36:2038–44.
8. Brochard L, Slutsky A, Pesenti A. Mechanical ventilation to minimize progression of lung injury in acute respiratory failure. Am J Respir Crit Care Med. 2017;195:438–42.
9. Biscotti M, Gannon WD, Agerstrand C, et al. Awake extracorporeal membrane oxygenation as bridge to lung transplantation: a 9-year experience. Ann Thorac Surg. 2017;104:412–9.
10. Crotti S, Bottino N, Ruggeri GM, et al. Spontaneous breathing during extracorporeal membrane oxygenation in acute respiratory failure. Anesthesiology. 2017;126:678–87.
11. Crotti S, Bottino N, Spinelli E. Spontaneous breathing during veno-venous extracorporeal membrane oxygenation. J Thorac Dis. 2018;10:S661–9.
12. Jeffries RG, Lund L, Frankowski B, Federspiel WJ. An extracorporeal carbon dioxide removal (ECCO2R) device operating at hemodialysis blood flow rates. Intensive Care Med Exp. 2017;5:41.
13. Karagiannidis C, Kampe KA, Sipmann FS, et al. Veno-venous extracorporeal CO_2 removal for the treatment of severe respiratory acidosis: pathophysiological and technical considerations. Crit Care. 2014;18:R124.
14. Liu GM, Jin DH, Jiang XH, et al. Numerical and in vitro experimental investigation of the hemolytic performance at the off-design point of an axial ventricular assist pump. ASAIO J. 2016;62:657–65.
15. Giersiepen M, Wurzinger LJ, Opitz R, Reul H. Estimation of shear stress-related blood damage in heart valve prostheses—in vitro comparison of 25 aortic valves. Int J Artif Organs. 1990;13:300–6.

16. Fraser KH, Zhang T, Taskin ME, Griffith BP, Wu ZJ. A quantitative comparison of mechanical blood damage parameters in rotary ventricular assist devices: shear stress, exposure time and hemolysis index. J Biomech Eng. 2012;134:081002.
17. Del Sorbo L, Pisani L, Filippini C, et al. Extracorporeal CO_2 removal in hypercapnic patients at risk of noninvasive ventilation failure: a matched cohort study with historical control. Crit Care Med. 2015;43:120–7.
18. Karagiannidis C, Strassmann S, Brodie D, et al. Impact of membrane lung surface area and blood flow on extracorporeal CO_2 removal during severe respiratory acidosis. Intensive Care Med Exp. 2017;5:34.
19. Zhang J, Chen X, Ding J, et al. Computational study of the blood flow in three types of 3D hollow fiber membrane bundles. J Biomech Eng. 2013;135:121009.
20. Lubnow M, Philipp A, Foltan M, et al. Technical complications during veno-venous extracorporeal membrane oxygenation and their relevance predicting a system-exchange—retrospective analysis of 265 cases. PLoS One. 2014;9:e112316.
21. Gartner MJ, Wilhelm CR, Gage KL, Fabrizio MC, Wagner WR. Modeling flow effects on thrombotic deposition in a membrane oxygenator. Artif Organs. 2000;24:29–36.
22. Funakubo A, Taga I, McGillicuddy JW, Fukui Y, Hirschl RB, Bartlett RH. Flow vectorial analysis in an artificial implantable lung. ASAIO J. 2003;49:383–7.
23. Kaesler A, Rosen M, Schmitz-Rode T, Steinseifer U, Arens J. Computational modeling of oxygen transfer in artificial lungs. Artif Organs. 2018;42:786–99.
24. Eash HJ, Jones HM, Hattler BG, Federspiel WJ. Evaluation of plasma resistant hollow fiber membranes for artificial lungs. ASAIO J. 2004;50:491–7.
25. Svitek RG, Frankowski BJ, Federspiel WJ. Evaluation of a pumping assist lung that uses a rotating fiber bundle. ASAIO J. 2005;51:773–80.
26. Fernando UP, Thompson AJ, Potkay J, et al. A membrane lung design based on circular blood flow paths. ASAIO J. 2017;63:637–43.
27. Schmidt M, Jaber S, Zogheib E, Godet T, Capellier G, Combes A. Feasibility and safety of low-flow extracorporeal CO_2 removal managed with a renal replacement platform to enhance lung-protective ventilation of patients with mild-to-moderate ARDS. Crit Care. 2018;22:122.
28. de Villiers Hugo J, Sharma AS, Ahmed U, Weerwind PW. Quantification of carbon dioxide removal at low sweep gas and blood flows. J Extra Corpor Technol. 2017;49:257–61.
29. Peperstraete H, Eloot S, Depuydt P, De Somer F, Roosens C, Hoste E. Low flow extracorporeal CO_2 removal in ARDS patients: a prospective short-term crossover pilot study. BMC Anesthesiol. 2017;17:155.
30. Batchinsky AI, Jordan BS, Regn D, et al. Respiratory dialysis: reduction in dependence on mechanical ventilation by venovenous extracorporeal CO_2 removal. Crit Care Med. 2011;39:1382–7.
31. Allardet-Servent J, Castanier M, Signouret T, Soundaravelou R, Lepidi A, Seghboyan JM. Safety and efficacy of combined extracorporeal CO_2 removal and renal replacement therapy in patients with acute respiratory distress syndrome and acute kidney injury: The Pulmonary and Renal Support in Acute Respiratory Distress Syndrome Study. Crit Care Med. 2015;43:2570–81.
32. Burki NK, Mani RK, Herth FJF, et al. A novel extracorporeal CO(2) removal system: results of a pilot study of hypercapnic respiratory failure in patients with COPD. Chest. 2013;143:678–86.

Part IV

Cardiac Arrest

9 Cardiac Arrest in the Intensive Care Unit

J. Tirkkonen, I. Efendijev, and M. B. Skrifvars

9.1 Introduction

Most in-hospital cardiac arrests (IHCAs) occur on normal general wards due to non-cardiac etiology, and the prognosis is poor with only one fifth of IHCA patients surviving to hospital discharge [1–3]. Studies from the last two decades have repeatedly highlighted the presence of abnormal vital signs preceding a clear majority of IHCAs [4, 5]. This explains the poor survival even when immediate advanced cardiac life support is provided; if the cardiac arrest occurs after hours of continuous hemodynamic and respiratory instability, efforts to recover spontaneous circulation do not solve the core problem [6]. Therefore, in-hospital advanced cardiac life support programs have shifted towards the prevention of cardiac arrest in general wards through use of rapid response systems [7]. A multitude of before-after trials have shown that IHCAs (and indeed also in-hospital deaths) may be avoided through early detection of deteriorating vital signs and timely transfers to intensive care [8].

A less investigated subgroup of IHCAs are those occurring inside the intensive care unit (ICU). Intensive care is considered cost-effective compared with other healthcare interventions, but the daily costs are nevertheless high [9]. In Finland, for example, the average one-year healthcare cost is $40,000 for a patient with

J. Tirkkonen
Department of Intensive Care Medicine and Department of Emergency, Anesthesia and Pain Medicine, Tampere University Hospital, Tampere, Finland

I. Efendijev
Division of Intensive Care Medicine, Department of Anaesthesiology, Intensive Care and Pain Medicine, University of Helsinki and HUS Helsinki University Hospital, Helsinki, Finland

M. B. Skrifvars (✉)
Department of Emergency Care and Services, University of Helsinki and HUS Helsinki University Hospital, Helsinki, Finland
e-mail: markus.skrifvars@hus.fi

J.-L. Vincent (ed.), *Annual Update in Intensive Care and Emergency Medicine 2019*, Annual Update in Intensive Care and Emergency Medicine,
https://doi.org/10.1007/978-3-030-06067-1_9

ICU-treated traumatic brain injury (TBI), whereas the average one-year healthcare cost for a patient that survives an ICU-CA with poor neurological outcome is $519,000 [10, 11].Therefore, we should acknowledge the ethical and financial burden of ICU-CAs and, as with IHCAs, shift the treatment strategy from reactive (resuscitation) to proactive (prevention). Indeed, some ICU-CAs may be iatrogenic in nature and therefore potentially avoidable. In this chapter, we provide an overview of what is currently known on the incidence, etiology and outcome of cardiac arrests occurring on the ICU. In addition, we will touch upon strategies aimed at preventing ICU-CAs.

9.2 Definition of ICU Cardiac Arrest

IHCA refers to the cessation of cardiac activity in a hospitalized patient who had a pulse at the time of admission [12]. Therefore, we suggest that ICU-CA should be defined as 'the cessation of cardiac activity in a patient admitted to the ICU who had a pulse at the time of ICU admission'. However, marked variability in ICU-CA definitions exist, which makes comparisons between different studies more complicated. Anthi et al. defined ICU-CA as "the sudden cessation of effective cardiac action resulting in brain hypoperfusion and requiring initiation of cardiopulmonary resuscitation (CPR) with compressions" [13], whereas in a study by Chang et al. it was required that "pulseless events were documented by either a duty physician or an experienced ICU nurse via carotid palpation" [14]. In a Finnish retrospective multicenter registry study, the ICU-CA cohort included also patients requiring just defibrillation, as the Therapeutic Intervention Scoring System-76 (TISS-76) documentation "requirement for CPR and/or countershock within 48 h" was used to define the ICU-CA cases [15]. Further, some studies from the 1990s also included respiratory arrests in the ICU-CA cohort [16, 17]. The more recent ICU-CA studies do not always use clear definitions either; although an Australian study clearly stated that ICU-CAs were defined according to the Utstein Statement [18], a Korean study did not define their ICU-CA cases at all [19]. It is evident that this variation in definition will make comparison between studies very difficult.

9.3 Incidence

The incidence of IHCA is between 1 and 5 events per 1000 hospital admissions [1–3, 20, 21]. These incidence counts often include, by definition, all the cardiac arrests occurring inside hospital doors, although arguably ICU-CAs form their own entity and differ substantially from general ward cardiac arrests [3, 20, 21]. The ICU-CA incidence varies greatly in the literature as presented in Table 9.1 [13–15, 18, 19, 22–28]. The data come from two decades and four continents. Galhorta et al. [25] and Chan et al. [26] report incidence rates <5 cases per 1000 ICU admissions; in contrast Efendijev et al. [15] report six-fold and Wallace et al. [23] 19-fold

Table 9.1 Incidence of intensive care unit cardiac arrests (ICU-CA)

Study	Country	ICU-CA incidence per 1000 ICU admissions
Smith et al. (1995) [22]	USA	11
Anthi et al. (1998) [13]	Greece	7.3
Wallace et al. (2002) [23]	USA	78
Enohumah et al. (2006) [24]	Germany	10
Galhorta et al. (2007) [25]	USA	4.0
Chan et al. (2008) [26]	USA	4.4
Gershengorn et al. (2012) [27]	USA	18
Skrifvars et al. (2012) [28]	Australia	5.6
Lee et al. (2013) [19]	Korea	13
Rozen et al. (2014) [18]	Australia	6.3
Efendijev et al. (2014) [15]	Finland	29

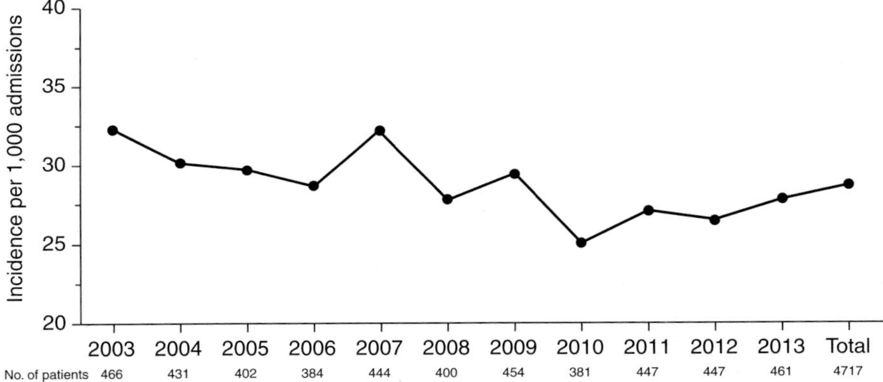

Fig. 9.1 Incidence of intensive care unit cardiac arrests in Finland between 2003 and 2013 [15]

incidence rates. How can these differences be explained? Notably the study settings are quite different, as the studies by Galhorta et al. [25] and Chan et al. [26] were prospective singe center studies mainly evaluating the effectiveness of rapid response systems whereas the study by Efendijev et al. was a retrospective 10-year registry study including data from 21 different ICUs [15]. The study by Wallace et al. was conducted in a cancer center in the 1990s, and after reporting the extremely high incidence, the authors themselves indeed debate on the ethical and financial aspects of providing CPR among ICU patients with a malignant disease [23]. Worth mentioning is the fact that only three study cohorts consist of ICU-CA patients who had their arrest within the past decade (since August 2008), including a total of only 189 cases [18, 19, 28]. Global temporal trends in ICU-CA incidence cannot be observed as the study settings vary substantially, but Efendijev et al. [15] reported that in Finland the ICU-CA incidence decreased between 2003 and 2013 (Fig. 9.1). The existing literature in any case suggests that approximately one in every hundred ICU patients had a cardiac arrest during his/her admission. In larger ICUs this translates to a weekly event.

9.4 Etiology and Primary Rhythm

Obviously, the presumed etiology of ICU-CA depends on the ICU setting. Cardiac reasons for a circulatory collapse are common in post-cardiac surgery ICUs, but rare in neurological/neurosurgical ICUs [29, 30]. In mixed ICU settings, the etiology of ICU-CA has been most commonly associated with septic shock (or respiratory failure/hypotension depending on the used definitions) and other non-cardiac reasons; in every sixth arrest at least three simultaneous conditions were associated with the ICU-CA in a large multicenter study by Tian et al. [31].

Non-shockable primary rhythms (pulseless electrical activity or asystole) are not considered to be common malignant manifestations of sudden cardiac ischemia, although autopsy findings of general ward IHCA patients have revealed perhaps higher than expected ischemic findings also among patients with non-shockable rhythms [3]. Primary rhythms in ICU-CA patients are often non-shockable as well, and the documented percentage is generally between 59 and 82 [18, 19, 24, 31].

9.5 Outcome

Survival to hospital discharge is not the most relevant of patient outcomes (as 1-year survival with good neurological outcome is, for example), but it is the most frequently reported. Although Myrianthefs et al. [32] reported that from the 111 patients resuscitated in their general ICU none even survived to hospital discharge, in general ICU-CA patient prognosis is not so hopeless. Other studies have reported survival to hospital discharge rates between 2 and 79% [13–16, 18, 22–24, 27–30, 33–35]. Anthi et al. [13] and Guney et al. [30] reported the highest survival to hospital discharge percentages of >60 and 79, and also good long-term outcomes, but both these studies were conducted among post-cardiac surgery ICU patients who are known to have better ICU-CA prognosis compared with other ICU patient groups [15]. The survival percentages from general ICUs are lower, although the two most recent studies reported identical survival to hospital discharge ratios of 44% [15, 18]. In general, the earlier studies report lower survival rates to hospital discharge compared with the more recent ICU-CA studies [13–16, 18, 22–24, 27–31, 33–35]. Indeed, in the Finnish multicenter registry study, Efendijev et al. reported that ICU-CA in-hospital mortality decreased during the 10-year study period in Finland [15].

Seven studies have reported the one-year survival after an ICU-CA, with a prognosis of 1.8–39% when the results from the one previously mentioned study with post-cardiac surgery patients are excluded [11, 13, 14, 16, 33–35]. Figure 9.2 shows the one-year survival rates with study cohort sizes and study years. Although no strong deductions should be drawn from these data, it appears that the one-year survival of ICU-CA patients has improved over time. Kutsogiannis et al. have conducted the longest follow-up of ICU-CA patients; they reported that 16% of the ICU-CA patients were alive 5 years after the event [35]. However, almost all data on long-term survival is over 10 years old. The outcome data that we are most

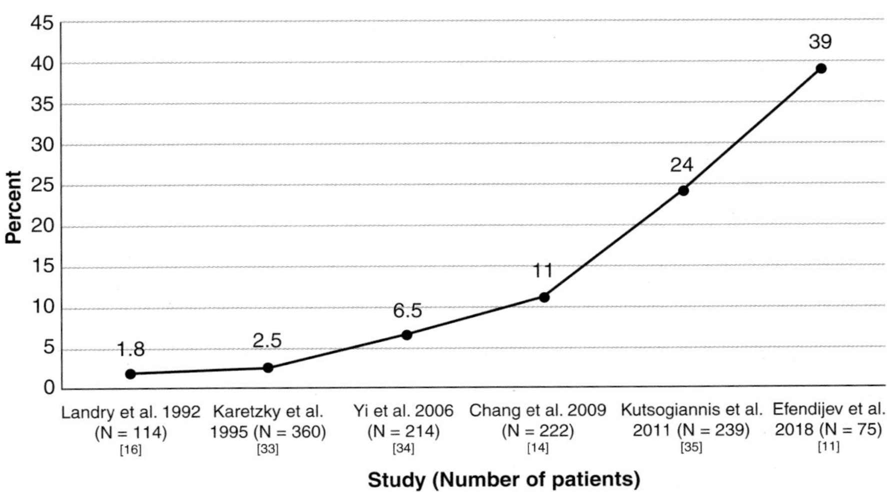

Fig. 9.2 Six studies have reported the one-year survival rate after an intensive care unit cardiac arrest

interested in is similarly rare; only Lee et al. [19] and Efendijev et al. [11] have published long-term neurological outcome data since 2006. Lee et al. [19] reported that 10% of ICU-CA patients had a cerebral performance category score (CPC) of 1–2 90 days after the event, and Efendijev et al. [11] reported that 36% of the ICU-CA patients had a CPC of 1–2 at one-year control.

9.6 Factors Associated with Outcome and Outcome Prediction

As in OHCAs and in-hospital general ward cardiac arrests, 'traditional' factors (initial shockable rhythm, short resuscitation time, lower morbidity) predict better outcome among ICU-CA patients also [3, 19, 36]. Non-operative, non-cardiovascular ICU-CA patients have the highest mortality rates, while postoperative cardiovascular ICU-CA patients have the lowest in-hospital and one-year mortality rates [13, 15]. The probability of survival to hospital discharge decreases as the number and severity of vital dysfunctions before an IHCA increases [5]. ICU-CAs do not differ in this aspect either; several studies have documented that, as expected, preceding hemodynamic and/or respiratory instability decreases the chances of survival after an ICU-CA. Tian et al. [31] reported that patients on vasopressors had half the probability of survival compared to non-vasopressor patients, and 96% of the patients on vasopressors either died or were discharged to rehabilitation or extended care facilities. Rabinstein et al. [29] reported that in their cohort no patient survived ICU-CA after a preceding deteriorating clinical course.

Early prediction of definitive outcome in cardiac arrest patients is often inconclusive. To date three specific cardiac arrest prediction scores exist. These are the

OHCA score, the Cardiac Arrest Hospital Prognosis (CAHP) score and the recently published Target Temperature Management (TTM) risk score [37–39]. All three scores are designed to predict outcomes in OHCA patients based on the data available at admission. Despite initially promising results, the predictive performance of the OHCA score was not reproducible in later studies and the score showed only moderate predictive accuracy in ICU-CA patients [28, 40]. The CAHP and TTM risk scores have not been tested in the ICU-CA population. As numerous peri-arrest factors can influence mortality and neurological outcome, the clinical utility of outcome prediction scores based solely on admission data is questionable. None of the above mentioned specific cardiac arrest prediction scores has been validated for clinical use in out-of-hospital, in-hospital or in-ICU settings [39].

Several studies have evaluated the predictive performance of the more common ICU severity-of-illness scores, the Acute Physiology and Chronic Health Evaluation (APACHE) and the Simplified Acute Physiology Score (SAPS), in cardiac arrest populations. Due to the modest discriminative abilities, neither APACHE nor SAPS scores are recommended as clinical prediction tools for mortality and neurological outcome in OHCA and IHCA patients [41–44]. The Sequential Organ Failure Assessment (SOFA) score and Multiple Organ Dysfunction Score (MODS) are both repetitive scores with day-by-day assessment of patient condition, and thus could be more suitable for outcome prediction. To the best of our knowledge, however, no study has evaluated SAPS, SOFA or MODS scores as predictors of outcome in ICU-CA patients. The study by Skrifvars et al. is so far the only study that has evaluated the APACHE III score in a cohort including ICU-CA patients, and the APACHE III had moderate predictive performance for poor outcome at hospital discharge [28].

9.7 Cost of ICU Cardiac Arrest

In addition to the increased suffering of the patient and the relatives, ICU-CA consumes financial resources whether the patient survives with a favorable neurological outcome or not. However, few data have been published on this subject. Wallace et al. analyzed 406 ICU-CAs in a cancer center between 1993 and 2000 [23]. They found that only seven patients (2%) survived to hospital discharge, whereas 104 patients survived the first 24 h but died later during their hospitalization. In today's currency (2018 US dollars), the mean ICU costs (from the date of CPR to the date of death) for these patients that died a mean 4.3 days after the event were $64,000 [23]. Efendijev et al. evaluated the total one-year healthcare-associated costs of 75 ICU-CA patients in a single center study between 2005 and 2013 [11]. The mean cost per ICU-CA patient was $112,000 (2018 US dollars). Mean cost per hospital survivor was $171,000. Importantly, however, the mean cost for a one-year survivor with a good neurological outcome was $129,000, whereas the mean cost for a one-year survivor with substantial neurological disability was $519,000 [11].

9.8 Prevention of ICU Cardiac Arrests

It is clear that many ICU-CA events are unavoidable. A severely ill patient who continues to deteriorate despite receiving maximum life-support will not benefit from resuscitation measures in case of further deterioration into cardiac arrest. Indeed, Myrianthefs et al. described their ICU's policy of refraining from CPR among ICU patients who are already on maximum vasopressor and inotropic support with underlying acute or chronic untreatable disease [32]. This policy appears reasonable, ethically sound and also comparable to that of the ideology of rapid response systems. One key element in the rapid response system is the appropriate implementation of treatment limitations in order to avoid futile resuscitation attempts [7, 8]. Currently there are no exact data on the percentage of ICU-CA cases where CPR should not have been conducted, although Wallace et al. state in their ICU-CA study that, "The application of CPR to cancer patients receiving life support is costly and typically does not lead to long-term survival" [23].

Certain ICU-CA events, however, could and should be actively prevented. A small prospective single center case-control study with 36 ICU-CA patients documented in detail the hemodynamic and respiratory variables preceding the arrests [18]. In that study, ICU-CA patients had higher median maximum and minimum respiratory rates, lower median mean arterial pressures, lower mean systolic blood pressures and lower mean bicarbonate levels in the 12 h prior to the arrests as compared with the controls (worth noting: no statistical difference in vasopressor usage) [18]. Furthermore, in 25% of ICU-CA patients, their respiratory rate was higher than 34 breaths/min, heart rate higher than 130 beats/min, median arterial pressure less than 56 mmHg or systolic blood pressure less than 80 mmHg in the 12 h prior to the arrest. While these results from a small cohort should be interpreted with caution, in 2018 these are the only data we have describing in detail the pre-arrest physiological variables of ICU CA patients. We should also acknowledge that some ICU-CAs are probably iatrogenic, associated with, for example, certain interventions, which underlines the possibility of preventable events. In the same study by Rozen et al. [18], 50% of the arrests were preceded by events such as airway manipulation, administration of sedation in non-intubated patients, immediate complications of a procedure or delirium/bleeding. Compared with the control population, there was a non-statistical trend towards a higher incidence of these preceding events among the patients who subsequently had a cardiac arrest [18].

What can be done? First and foremost, more data are urgently needed on the factors preceding cardiac arrests on the ICU. Second, proactive and highly specific warning systems independent of human factors could help redirect treatment strategies and stop the deterioration over time. It is possible, that the first trends in patient deterioration are also missed in the ICU setting, when some vital signs are prioritized at the expense of the others. Rapid response systems, for example, are based on the early detection of patient deterioration by the ward staff [7, 8]. Several activation criteria, based on patients' vital signs, have been implemented to enable the ward staff to react in time, but the more effective ones are not fixed on single parameters [45]. The early warning scores, such as the National Early

Warning Score (NEWS) in the United Kingdom, take into account all the vital signs and create a more comprehensible picture of the patient's prevailing physical state: oxygenation, ventilation and tissue perfusion [45, 46]. While rapid response team activation criteria would be of limited value in the ICU setting, other automated systems that can evaluate patient condition as a physiologic entity in relation to the clinical context (with the subsequent calculation of the early warning score-like risk profile) could have potential benefits compared to today's automatic monitor alarms. Indeed, Subbe et al. found that an electronic automated advisory vital signs monitoring and notification system reduced IHCAs and in-hospital deaths in a general ward setting [47]. Further, the severity of illness in patients admitted to the ICU was reduced as was their ICU mortality. Third, as mentioned earlier, some of the ICU-CAs might have an iatrogenic etiology. Development of less invasive, less complex and safer procedures and techniques and active implication of procedural check-lists and simulation training in high-risk procedures seem justified [48].

9.9 Future Research

We should look beyond the descriptive ICU-CA data. The whole concept of rapid response systems is based on the idea that some IHCAs on general wards may be prevented and some should be regarded as unavoidable deaths. This is likely the case in the ICU-CA sub-population also, although in ICUs, unobserved/unrecognized patient deterioration appears less likely. We need substantially more data on the events preceding ICU-CAs in order to evaluate the incidence of those that are potentially preventable. A national multicenter study by a French study group will hopefully shed some light on these questions (ClinicalTrials.gov identifier: NCT03021564).

9.10 Conclusion

We have no up-to-date data on the incidence and outcome of cardiac arrests occurring in the ICU. Indeed, almost all existing ICU-CA studies were conducted before 2010. Approximately one in every hundred ICU patients has a cardiac arrest in the ICU. Short-term survival seems better than survival from IHCAs in general, but there are few data on long-term survival. Based on a few descriptive studies, we know some of the risk factors associated with ICU-CA (and factors associated with poorer survival after ICU-CA), but more data are urgently needed on possible predisposing factors that are either iatrogenic or otherwise treatable. Twenty years ago, we began to implement rapid response systems in order to prevent IHCAs and improve the outcome of patients transferred to the ICU from general wards through timely ICU transfer. We suggest that it is time to discuss whether we could avoid some of the ICU-CAs as well, either through prevention or allowing death if maximal intensive care cannot change the course of the illness.

References

1. Sandroni C, Nolan J, Cavallaro F, Antonelli M. In-hospital cardiac arrest: incidence, prognosis and possible measures to improve survival. Intensive Care Med. 2007;33:237–45.
2. Nolan J, Soar J, Smith GB, et al. Incidence and outcome of in-hospital cardiac arrest in the United Kingdom National Cardiac Arrest Audit. Resuscitation. 2014;85:987–92.
3. Tirkkonen J, Hellevuo H, Olkkola KT, Hoppu S. Aetiology of cardiac arrest on general wards. Resuscitation. 2016;107:19–24.
4. Nurmi J, Harjola VP, Nolan J, Castrén M. Observations and warning signs prior to cardiac arrest: should a medical emergency team intervene earlier. Acta Anaesthesiol Scand. 2005;49:702–6.
5. Andersen LW, Kim WY, Chase M, et al. The prevalence and significance of abnormal vital signs prior to in-hospital cardiac arrest. Resuscitation. 2016;98:112–7.
6. Skrifvars MB, Nurmi J, Ikola K, Saarinen K, Castrén M. Reduced survival following resuscitation in patients with documented clinically abnormal observations prior to in-hospital cardiac arrest. Resuscitation. 2006;70:215–22.
7. Jones D, DeVita M, Bellomo R. Rapid-response teams. N Engl J Med. 2011;365:139–46.
8. Maharaj R, Raffaelle I, Wendon J. Rapid response systems: a systematic review and meta-analysis. Crit Care. 2015;19:254.
9. Ridley S, Morris S. Cost effectiveness of adult intensive care in the UK. Anaesthesia. 2007;62:547–54.
10. Raj R, Bendel S, Reinikainen M, et al. Temporal trends in healthcare costs and outcome following ICU admission after traumatic brain injury. Crit Care Med. 2018;46: 302–9.
11. Efendijev I, Folger D, Raj R, et al. Outcomes and healthcare-associated costs one year after intensive care-treated cardiac arrest. Resuscitation. 2018;131:128–34.
12. Jacobs I, Nadcari V, Bahr J, et al. Cardiac arrest and cardiopulmonary resuscitation outcome reports: update and simplification of the Utstein templates for resuscitation registries. A statement for healthcare professionals from a task force of the international liaison committee on resuscitation (American Heart Association, European Resuscitation Council, Australian Resuscitation Council, New Zealand Resuscitation Council, Heart and Stroke Foundation of Canada, InterAmerican Heart Foundation, Resuscitation Council of Southern Africa). Resuscitation. 2004;63:233–49.
13. Anthi A, Tzelepis GE, Alivizatos P, Michalis A, Palatianos GM, Geroulanos S. Unexpected cardiac arrest after cardiac surgery: incidence, predisposing causes, and outcome of open chest cardiopulmonary resuscitation. Chest. 1998;113:15–9.
14. Chang SH, Huang CH, Shih CL, et al. Who survives cardiac arrest in the intensive care units? J Crit Care. 2009;24:408–14.
15. Efendijev I, Rag R, Reinikainen M, Hoppu S, Skrivars MB. Temporal trends in cardiac arrest incidence and outcome in Finnish intensive care units from 2003 to 2013. Intensive Care Med. 2014;40:1853–61.
16. Landry FJ, Parker JM, Phillips YY. Outcome of cardiopulmonary resuscitation in the intensive care setting. Arch Intern Med. 1992;152:2305–8.
17. Peterson MW, Geist LJ, Schwartz DA, Konicek S, Moseley PL. Outcome after cardiopulmonary resuscitation in a medical intensive care unit. Chest. 1991;100:168–74.
18. Rozen TH, Mullane S, Kaufman M, et al. Antecedents to cardiac arrests in a teaching hospital intensive care unit. Resuscitation. 2014;85:411–7.
19. Lee HK, Lee H, No JM, et al. Factors influencing outcome in patients with cardiac arrest in the ICU. Acta Anaesthesiol Scand. 2013;57:784–92.
20. Bergum D, Nordseth T, Mjølstad OC, Skogvoll E, Haugen BO. Causes of in-hospital cardiac arrest—incidences and rate of recognition. Resuscitation. 2015;87:63–8.
21. Wallmuller C, Meron G, Kurkciyan I, Schober A, Stratil P, Sterz F. Causes of in-hospital cardiac arrest and influence on outcome. Resuscitation. 2012;83:1206–11.

22. Smith DL, Kim K, Cairns BA, Fakhry SM, Meyer AA. Prospective analysis of out-come after cardiopulmonary resuscitation in critically ill surgical patients. J Am Coll Surg. 1995;180:394–401.
23. Wallace S, Ewer MS, Price KJ, Feeley TW. Outcome and cost implications of cardiopulmonary resuscitation in the medical intensive care unit of a comprehensive cancer center. Support Care Cancer. 2002;10:425–9.
24. Enohumah KO, Moerer O, Kirmse C, Bahr J, Neumann P, Quintel M. Outcome of cardiopulmonary resuscitation in the intensive care units of a university hospital. Resuscitation. 2006;71:161–70.
25. Galhorta S, DeVita MA, Simmons RL, et al. Mature rapid response system and potentially avoidable cardiopulmonary arrests in hospital. Qual Saf Health Care. 2007;16:260–5.
26. Chan P, Khalid A, Longmore LS, et al. Hospital-wide code rates and mortality before and after implementation of a rapid response team. JAMA. 2008;300(21):2506–13.
27. Gershengorn HB, Li G, Kramer A, Wunsch H. Survival and functional outcomes after cardiopulmonary resuscitation in the intensive care unit. J Crit Care. 2012;27:9–17.
28. Skrifvars MB, Varghese B, Parr MJ. Survival and outcome prediction using the Apache III and the out-of-hospital cardiac arrest (OHCA) score in patients treated in the intensive care unit (ICU) following out-of-hospital, in-hospital or ICU cardiac arrest. Resuscitation. 2012;83:728–33.
29. Rabinstein AA, McClelland RL, Wijdicks EF, Manno EM, Atkinson JL. Cardiopulmonary resuscitation in critically ill neurologic-neurosurgical patients. Mayo Clin Proc. 2004; 79:1391–5.
30. Guney MR, Ketenci B, Yapici F, et al. Results of treatment methods in cardiac arrest following coronary artery bypass grafting. J Card Surg. 2009;24:227–33.
31. Tian J, Kaufman DA, Zarich S, et al. American Heart Association National Registry for Cardiopulmonary Resuscitation I. Outcomes of critically ill patients who received cardiopulmonary resuscitation. Am J Respir Crit Care Med. 2010;182:501–6.
32. Myrianthefs P, Kalafati M, Lemonidou C, et al. Efficacy of CPR in a general, adult ICU. Resuscitation. 2003;57:43–8.
33. Karetzky M, Zubair M, Parikh J. Cardiopulmonary resuscitation in intensive care unit and non-intensive care unit patients. Immediate and long-term survival. Arch Intern Med. 1995;155:1277–80.
34. Yi HJ, Kim YS, Ko Y, Oh SJ, Kim KM, Oh SH. Factors associated with survival and neurological outcome after cardiopulmonary resuscitation of neurosurgical intensive care unit patients. Neurosurgery. 2006;59:836–8.
35. Kutsogiannis DJ, Bagshaw SM, Laing B, Brindley PG. Predictors of survival after cardiac or respiratory arrest in critical care units. CMAJ. 2011;183:1589–95.
36. Andrew E, Nehme Z, Bernard S, Smith K. The influence of comorbidity on survival and long-term outcomes after out-of-hospital cardiac arrest. Resuscitation. 2017;110:42–7.
37. Adrie C, Cariou A, Mourvillier B, et al. Predicting survival with good neurological recovery at hospital admission after successful resuscitation of out-of-hospital cardiac arrest: the OHCA score. Eur Heart J. 2006;27:2840–5.
38. Maupain C, Bougouin W, Lamhaut L, et al. The CAHP (Cardiac Arrest Hospital Prognosis) score: a tool for risk stratification after out-of-hospital cardiac arrest. Eur Heart J. 2006;37:3222–8.
39. Martinell L, Nielsen N, Herlitz J, et al. Early predictors of poor outcome after out-of-hospital cardiac arrest. Crit Care. 2017;21:96.
40. Oksanen T, Tiainen M, Skrifvars MB, et al. Predictive power of serum NSE and OHCA score regarding 6-month neurologic outcome after out-of-hospital ventricular fibrillation and therapeutic hypothermia. Resuscitation. 2009;80:165–70.
41. Niskanen M, Kari A, Nikki P, et al. Acute physiology and chronic health evaluation (APACHE II) and Glasgow coma scores as predictors of outcome from intensive care after cardiac arrest. Crit Care Med. 1991;19:1465–73.

42. Donnino MW, Salciccioli JD, Dejam A, et al. APACHE II scoring to predict outcome in post-cardiac arrest. Resuscitation. 2013;84:651–6.
43. Salciccioli JD, Cristia C, Chase M, et al. Performance of SAPS II and SAPS III scores in post-cardiac arrest. Minerva Anestesiol. 2012;78:1341–7.
44. Bisbal M, Jouve E, Papazian L, et al. Effectiveness of SAPS III to predict hospital mortality for post-cardiac arrest patients. Resuscitation. 2014;85:939–44.
45. Smith GB, Prytherch DR, Meredith P, Schmidt PE, Featherstone PI. The ability of the National Early Warning Score (NEWS) to discriminate patients at risk of early cardiac arrest, unanticipated intensive care unit admission, and death. Resuscitation. 2013;84:465–70.
46. Tirkkonen J, Olkkola KT, Huhtala H, Tenhunen J, Hoppu S. Medical emergency team activation: performance of conventional dichotomised criteria versus national early warning score. Acta Anaesthesiol Scand. 2014;58:411–9.
47. Subbe CP, Duller B, Bellomo R. Effect of an automated notification system for deteriorating ward patients on clinical outcomes. Crit Care. 2017;21:52.
48. Treadwell JR, Lucas S, Tsou AY. Surgical checklists: a systematic review of impacts and implementation. BMJ Qual Saf. 2014;23:299–318.

Targeted Temperature Management After Cardiac Arrest: Where Are We Now?

10

A. Ray, S. Paulich, and J. P. Nolan

10.1 Introduction

Targeted temperature management (TTM) is now recognized as a cornerstone of management to minimize neurological injury following return of spontaneous circulation (ROSC) after out-of-hospital cardiac arrest (OHCA).

Although induced mild hypothermia has been used as a strategy to protect against cerebral hypoxic-ischemic injury secondary to cardiac arrest since the 1950s, this was largely reserved for open-heart surgery until the publication of two prospective randomized controlled trials (RCTs) in 2002 [1, 2]. These trials compared mild hypothermia to standard treatment following ROSC in comatose survivors of OHCA (the European study included a few in-hospital cardiac arrest [IHCA] patients) with an initial rhythm of ventricular fibrillation (VF). Both trials showed increased survival with favorable neurological outcomes in patients who were treated with mild hypothermia (32–34 °C) for 12–24 h compared with control patients not treated with mild hypothermia.

On the basis of the evidence provided by these two RCTs, as well as supporting animal data, the Advanced Life Support (ALS) Task Force of the International Liaison Committee on Resuscitation (ILCOR) made the following recommendations in October 2002 [3]:

- Unconscious adult patients with spontaneous circulation after OHCA should be cooled to 32–34 °C for 12–24 h when the initial rhythm is VF
- Such cooling may also be beneficial for other rhythms or in IHCA

A. Ray · S. Paulich
Department of Anaesthesia and Intensive Care Medicine, Royal United Hospital, Bath, UK

J. P. Nolan (✉)
Department of Anaesthesia and Intensive Care Medicine, Royal United Hospital, Bath, UK

Bristol Medical School, University of Bristol, Bristol, UK
e-mail: jerry.nolan@nhs.net

J.-L. Vincent (ed.), *Annual Update in Intensive Care and Emergency Medicine 2019*, Annual Update in Intensive Care and Emergency Medicine,
https://doi.org/10.1007/978-3-030-06067-1_10

This initial statement was followed by a broader advisory statement in 2003 [3]. This statement outlined the discussions and opinions of the ALS Task Force and explored the limitations of the data from the RCTs, advising that further evidence was required to:

- Establish the role of TTM following IHCA.
- Determine the optimum duration of TTM, the optimum target temperature and optimum rates of cooling/rewarming.
- Determine the role for TTM in pediatric cardiac arrest.

10.2 The Targeted Temperature Management Trial and Its Impact on Clinical Practice

The TTM trial, which was published in 2013, enrolled 950 unconscious adult patients admitted to 36 intensive care units (ICUs) in Europe and Australia after OHCA [4]. Patients were randomized to be treated with TTM at a target temperature of either 33 °C or 36 °C (a temperature of 36 °C rather than 'normothermia' was selected to ensure that no patients developed fever, which was widely accepted at the time to be harmful in the presence of brain injury). There was no difference in all-cause mortality through to the end of the trial (the primary outcome) between the groups (50% mortality in 33 °C group, 48% mortality in 36 °C group, hazard ratio with a temperature of 33 °C = 1.06, 95% confidence interval [CI] 0.89–1.28; p = 0.51). Neurological outcome was the same in both groups (52% of both groups were dead or had poor neurological function according to cerebral performance category (CPC) at 180 days; risk ratio 1.01, 95% CI 0.89–1.14, p = 0.87). The investigators concluded that a target temperature of 33 °C did not confer a benefit compared with 36 °C and the lead investigator has subsequently recommended 36 °C as the preferred target temperature for neurological protection following cardiac arrest [5].

Following the TTM trial, the ALS Task Force of ILCOR undertook a systematic review to address the question of whether mild hypothermia or TTM should be used, when this should be instituted and for how long it should be implemented [6]. The Task Force recommended:

- That adults with OHCA with an initial shockable rhythm be treated with TTM at a constant temperature between 32 and 36 °C for at least 24 h.
- Similar suggestions were made for OHCA with a non-shockable rhythm and for IHCA.
- That prehospital cooling with rapid infusion of large volumes of cold intravenous fluid should not be used.

10.3 Clinical Practice Before the TTM Study

Although international resuscitation guidelines recommended the use of TTM 15 years ago [3], there is some evidence that implementation was initially relatively poor [7–9]. However, just before publication of the 2013 TTM trial there is evidence that many ICUs had adopted TTM for the treatment of post-cardiac arrest patients, especially those with VF OHCA. A survey of ICUs in France undertaken between October 2010 and May 2011 documented that 99% of 119 ICUs used TTM after VF OHCA; however, the poor response rate of just 37% indicates likely bias among the respondents [10]. Respondents reported use of targeted temperatures of 33 °C (58% [49–67%]), 34 °C (23% [16–30%]) and 32 °C (8% [3–13%]).

A telephone survey of practice in UK ICUs undertaken between October 2013 and March 2014 collected responses from 208 of the 235 units and is thus more reliably reflective of national practice before any impact of the TTM trial [11]. This telephone survey attempted to document practice in every UK ICU by asking the duty ICU consultant a set of standardized questions about the management of comatose survivors of both IHCA and OHCA. At the time of the survey, 189 units (90.9%) had a temperature control policy, 5.8% relied on individual consultant decisions for target temperature and 3.4% had no policy in place. One unit reportedly targeted a temperature of <32 °C, with 76.9% of units targeting a temperature of 33–34 °C, 7.7% units targeting 35 °C and 11.5% of units targeting 36–37 °C. The duration of TTM was most commonly 24 h (76.9%).

Although these data suggest that 77% of units were targeting a temperature of ≤34 °C, further studies have demonstrated that the actual temperatures recorded show less compliance with TTM than this survey would suggest. An analysis of the United Kingdom Intensive Care National Audit and Research Centre (UK ICNARC) database documented the proportion of patients achieving a temperature of ≤34 °C in the first 24 h of ICU admission. The proportion of patients with a temperature ≤34 °C increased each year with the highest proportion occurring in 2013; however, only 47% of all OHCA and IHCA patients achieved a lowest recorded temperature of ≤34 °C. Although it is possible that there were a disproportionate number of small units adhering to a strict TTM regime, it seems more likely that there was only moderate overall implementation of the international guidelines recommending TTM. These findings are replicated in an analysis of the Australian and New Zealand Intensive Care Society (ANZICS) database, which documented a lowest temperature of ≤34 °C among 57.1% of patients admitted after OHCA before publication of the TTM trial in December 2013 [12].

As further work is done to identify the optimum temperature for TTM following cardiac arrest, it is important to ensure that international guidelines are implemented in clinical practice. In many respects, this may have a more important role in improving overall outcomes than further studies aiming to identify optimum temperature.

10.4 Changes in Practice Since the TTM Study

Whilst a target temperature of 33 °C was widely adopted following the two RCTs in 2002, the TTM trial posed significant questions about the optimal target temperature and has led to a split of opinion within the international community.

There have been several criticisms of the TTM trial including the possibility of selection bias, delays in initiation of cooling of up to 4 h, an average time of 8 h to achieve target temperature following initiation of TTM, and poor temperature control with wide error bars [5, 13].

International guidelines now recommend a constant target temperature between 32 and 36 °C (as opposed to no temperature management) but have moved away from specifying TTM at 32–34 °C [6, 14]. This has given individual ICUs the scope to adopt the TTM strategy of their choice and has led to several publications assessing the impact of a potential change in target temperature. A declarative survey using the webmail database of the French Intensive Care Society achieved responses from 518 individuals, including 264 ICUs in 11 countries [15]. Among respondents, 37% stated that they had changed their target temperature for TTM, with 23% moving to 35–36 °C and 14% targeting 36 °C. A telephone survey of 268 European ICUs spanning 14 countries documented that 68% of ICUs were continuing to provide TTM at 32–34 °C but 33% had revised their target temperature to 36 °C [16].

Whilst both of these studies are suggestive of a partial change in behavior, the 2010 European Resuscitation Council (ERC) guidelines [17] were still in effect at the time they were conducted and there is a strong possibility that more units will have changed their target temperature since this study was published. It is not clear whether some units may have abandoned TTM altogether in order to aim for normothermia. The 2016 French survey suggests that a small proportion (6%) of responders did not specifically undertake TTM [15]. The question of mild induced hypothermia vs. fever control only is being addressed by the TTM-2 trial (see later; ClinicalTrials.gov identifier: NCT02908308) [4, 18].

Findings from a survey of large teaching and university hospitals in 14 European countries [16] appear to mirror the conclusions drawn from other papers including the review of data from the UK ICNARC and the ANZICS databases [12, 19]. The UK ICNARC study analyzed patient characteristics and outcomes for all patients admitted to the ICU after cardiac arrest and clearly demonstrated increasing compliance with TTM for both OHCA and IHCA between 2004 and 2013 (use of TTM was identified from the available data as a lowest temperature of ≤34 °C within the first 24 h of ICU admission) [19]. The proportion of patients receiving TTM after OHCA increased from 13.1% in 2004 to 60.2% in 2013 and from 8.6% to 35.3% after IHCA. However, the proportion with lowest temperature ≤34 °C in the first 24 h decreased significantly in 2014 from 60.2 to 38.9% after OHCA and from 35.3 to 22.8% after IHCA. This appears to suggest that a significant number of UK ICUs have changed their target temperature for TTM or have abandoned TTM altogether following publication of the TTM trial (Fig. 10.1).

These findings are consistent with those reported from Australia and New Zealand [12]. Characteristics and outcome for patients admitted to an adult ICU for active treatment following OHCA were compared in two 3-year periods: before and after the TTM trial (4450 patients from January 2011 to December 2013 compared with 5184 patients from January 2014 to December 2016). The primary outcome was the lowest recorded temperature in the first 24 h of ICU admission. They demonstrated that the mean (±SD) pre-TTM trial temperature was 33.8 °C (±1.71 °C) compared with 34.7 °C (±1.39 °C) after the TTM trial. Data from an extended

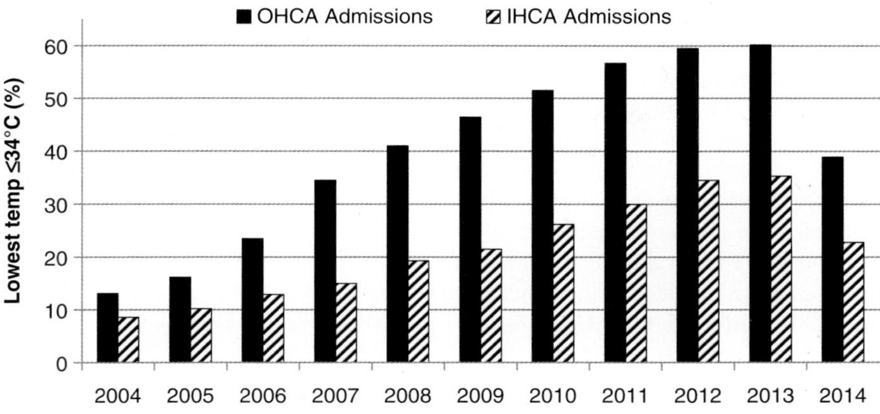

Fig. 10.1 Proportion of post-cardiac arrest patients with lowest documented temperature ≤34 °C in the first 24 h (2004–2014). *OHCA* out-of-hospital cardiac arrest, *IHCA* in-hospital cardiac arrest. p value for trend <0.001 for both OHCA and IHCA admissions. From [19]

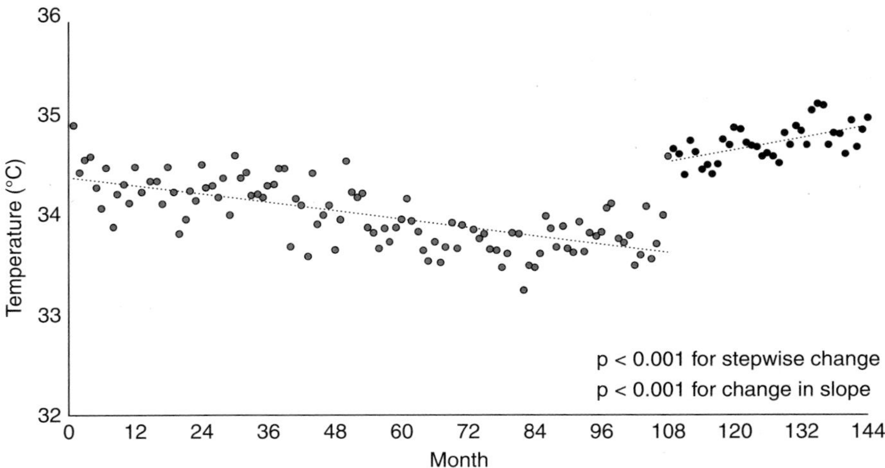

Fig. 10.2 Lowest body temperature in the first 24 h in the ICU by month. Gray dots: January 2005 to December 2013; black dots: January 2014 to December 2016. From [12] with permission

period demonstrated a trend of decreasing lowest temperature in the first 24 h from 2005 to 2013 (in keeping with the results of the UK ICNARC study) (Fig. 10.2).

Given that the above studies all demonstrate indirect evidence of some ICUs revising their target temperature in response to the TTM trial, it is important to understand the impact of these changes on outcome among these post-cardiac arrest patients.

The impact of a change in target temperature was assessed for 76 patients admitted to an ICU in Melbourne, Australia after VF OHCA [20]. Despite the relatively small cohort, these investigators showed that increasing the target temperature from 33 to 36 °C was associated with reduced compliance with the target temperature (87% vs. 50%, $p < 0.001$) and increased incidence of fever (0% vs. 19%, $p = 0.03$). The mortality rate was numerically higher (29% vs. 42%, $p = 0.31$) and neurological outcome numerically poorer (CPC 1–2 71% vs. 56%, $p = 0.22$) but neither of these differences were statistically significant.

More recently, the secondary outcomes derived from the analysis of the ANZICS database have given more detailed information about clinical outcomes after publication of the TTM trial [12]. The increase in the lowest recorded temperature in the first 24 h was associated with an increased risk of fever in the post-TTM group (16.5 vs. 12.8%, OR 1.35, 99% CI 1.16–1.57; $p < 0.001$), which is consistent with the findings of the Melbourne group [20]. In the ANZICS study, pre-TTM mortality was 52.4% compared with post-TTM mortality of 53.4% (OR 1.04, 99% CI 0.94–1.16, $p = 0.31$). Although these mortality rates are not significantly different, a segmented regression analysis of the extended data (2005–2016) demonstrated a 1.3 percentage point annual reduction in mortality after OHCA from 2005 to 2013 (99% CI −1.8 to −0.9), followed by a 0.6 percentage point annual increase in mortality from 2014 to 2016 (99% CI −1.4 to 2.6) (Fig. 10.3) [12]. Furthermore, when adjusted for Australia and New Zealand Risk of Death (ANZROD) model variables, the post-TTM trial period was associated with a statistically significant increase in mortality (adjusted OR 1.27, 99% CI 1.13–1.43; $p < 0.001$). However, when all temperature-associated variables of ANZROD are removed, this association does not reach statistical significance (adjusted OR 1.06, 99% CI 0.95–1.19, $p = 0.18$). Nonetheless, the ANZICS data show a worrying reversal of the trend for improving survival following OHCA.

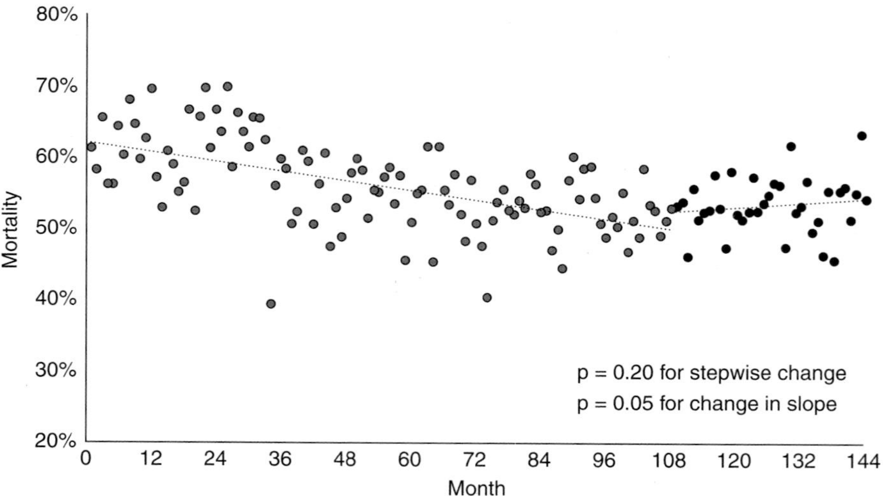

Fig. 10.3 In-hospital mortality by month. Gray dots: January 2005 to December 2013; black dots: January 2014 to December 2016. From [12] with permission

10.5 Pre-hospital TTM

Although international guidelines strongly support the use of TTM following OHCA, when to initiate cooling remains uncertain. Animal data suggest that cooling is more effective the earlier it is started [21] and laboratory and preliminary clinical studies have suggested that therapeutic hypothermia may be most effective when started during cardiopulmonary resuscitation (CPR) rather than delayed until after ROSC [22, 23]. However, recent RCTs do not support this [24, 25].

In the Rapid Infusion of Cold Normal Saline (RINSE) trial, 1202 patients in three Australian cities were randomized to either initiation of cooling before ROSC or standard care with initiation of cooling in hospital after ROSC [25]. All patients received initial resuscitation treatment, including defibrillation for shockable rhythms, intravenous cannulation, administration of an initial dose of epinephrine and ventilation with 100% oxygen. If cardiac arrest persisted, patients were randomized to receive 30 mL/kg of cold (3 °C) saline or standard treatment—i.e., no pre-hospital cold saline. There was no significant difference in the primary outcome of survival to hospital discharge (10.2% vs. 11.4%; $p = 0.51$). Of concern, if the initial presentation was a shockable rhythm, there were significantly fewer patients achieving ROSC in the cold saline group, (41% vs. 50%; $p = 0.031$). There was also an increase in the number of patients developing pulmonary edema in the group receiving cold saline intra-arrest (10% vs. 4.5%; $p < 0.001$).

The RINSE trial was designed to detect an absolute increase in survival of 7% with a power of 80% and required 2512 patients. Unfortunately, the trial was stopped early after reaching only 48% of the recruitment target. This was because of changes in TTM strategy by the receiving hospitals—from a target of 33 to 36 °C following the publication of the TTM trial [4]. Given the results at the time the trial was stopped, it seems highly unlikely that the infusion of cold saline intra-arrest would have resulted in a statistically significant increase in the primary outcome even if all 2512 patients had been recruited. There is some evidence that infusion of fluid *per se* during cardiac arrest may be harmful because of the high right heart pressures generated [26]. The RINSE trial data do not exclude the possibility that other techniques for intra-arrest cooling may be beneficial.

A recent meta-analysis of pre-hospital TTM vs. no pre-hospital TTM included 10 RCTs with a total of 4220 patients from 2002 to 2017 (including the RINSE trial) [27]. The majority of the RCTs used cold fluids; however, surface cooling and transnasal evaporative cooling were also used. There were no significant differences between the two groups for the primary outcome of neurological recovery (risk ratio [RR] 1.04; 95% CI 0.93–1.15) or the secondary outcome of survival to hospital discharge (RR 1.01; 95% CI 0.92–1.11). However, there was an increased risk of re-arrest in the therapeutic hypothermia group (RR 1.19; 95% CI 1.00–1.41).

Currently, there are few data to support the use of pre-hospital cooling. Some evidence indicates that pre-hospital cooling may reduce the chance of successful defibrillation or even increase the likelihood of re-arrest. Most patients present relatively hypothermic (<36.0 °C), so one option might be to institute TTM with a target of 36 °C and let these patients reach this temperature passively.

10.6 TTM After In-hospital Cardiac Arrest

There are several major differences between IHCA and OHCA. First, 80% of IHCA patients have an initial monitored rhythm of pulseless electrical activity (PEA) or asystole, for which there are no RCTs for TTM (although there is an ongoing trial among patients with non-shockable rhythm OHCA—NSE-HYPERION study, ClinicalTrials.gov identifier: NCT02722473) [28]. Second, after IHCA there is typically a much shorter interval to commencing CPR and other key interventions such as defibrillation and epinephrine; this might minimize the potential for TTM to reduce hypoxemic-ischemic brain injury. There are currently no RCTs examining the effectiveness of TTM after IHCA.

A retrospective propensity matched analysis of the US Get-With-The-Guidelines-Resuscitation (GWTG-R) registry compared outcomes among patients treated with TTM vs. those not treated with TTM during 2002 and 2014 (n = 26,183) [29]. After adjustment, TTM was associated with reduced survival to hospital discharge (27.4% vs. 29.2%; RR 0.88 (95% CI 0.80–0.97); risk difference (RD) −3.6% (95% CI −6.3% to −0.9%); p = 0.01) and lower rates of favorable neurological survival (17.0% vs. 20.5%; RR 0.79 (95% CI 0.69–0.90); RD −4.4% (95% CI −6.8% to −2.0%); p < 0.001). Although the authors used robust statistical methods to try to eliminate bias, that only 6% of the 26,183 patients underwent TTM implies a considerable selection bias, i.e., it is likely that only those patients at highest risk of cerebral injury were treated with TTM whereas those patients with uncomplicated short arrest times may have been selected as not requiring TTM. Although propensity matching would address some of these issues, it is very possible that there were residual confounders that were not accounted for. It will probably require an RCT to answer with high certainty whether TTM is beneficial for comatose patients after IHCA [13].

10.7 Duration of TTM

The current ILCOR recommendations are that when TTM is used, a constant temperature in the range 32–36 °C is maintained for at least 24 h [6]. However, the optimal duration is still under debate. Most centers cool patients for 24 h [16]; in contrast, neonates with anoxic asphyxia are normally cooled for 72 h [30].

In a recent RCT, TTM at 33 °C for 24 h was compared with 33 °C for 48 h among 355 patients in 10 European ICUs during 2013 and 2016 [31]. The primary outcome—favorable neurologic outcome at 6 months—was available for 351 patients: 69% (95% CI 62–75%) in the 48-h group vs. 64% (95% CI 56–71%) in the 24-h group (absolute difference 4.9%; 95% CI −5% to 14.8%; RR 1.08; 95% CI 0.93–1.25; p = 0.33). Patients who received TTM for 48 h had a higher incidence of adverse events (97% vs. 91%, p = 0.04) and a longer ICU length of stay.

This study was powered to be able to detect an absolute difference between groups of 15%. Many would deem this to be an optimistic treatment effect—very few interventions in modern intensive care show such a large effect. Detection of an absolute difference of 5% between groups would have required enrolment of 3000 patients. Outcomes were better than expected in both groups: a good neurological outcome had been predicted in 50% of the patients in the 24-h TTM group instead of the 64% that was ultimately documented. This may be explained by the exclusion of unwitnessed non-shockable rhythms, higher rates of bystander CPR, greater use of pre-hospital automated external defibrillators (AEDs), and a higher proportion of patients receiving immediate coronary angiographic intervention in comparison with previous studies. A helpful summary in an accompanying editorial concluded that this trial excluded the possibility that TTM for 48 h results in outcomes that are 15% better or 5% worse than TTM for 24 h [32].

10.8 TTM After Cardiac Arrest in Children

Two RCTs of TTM have been completed in children. These Therapeutic Hypothermia after Pediatric Cardiac Arrest (THAPCA) trials have been completed in the out-of-hospital setting (THAPCA-OH) and in the in-hospital setting (THAPCA-IH) [33]. The THAPCA trials recruited from almost 40 hospitals in the United States, Canada and the United Kingdom. Children between the ages of 2 days and 18 years old were randomized to either 48 h of TTM at 33 °C (32–34 °C) or normothermia at 36.8 °C (36–37.5 °C). After 48 h, patients underwent a further 3 days of TTM to maintain normothermia, i.e., fever prevention. In both studies, the primary outcome was survival at 12 months after cardiac arrest with a Vineland Adaptive Behavior Scales second edition (VABS-II) score of 70 or higher (on a scale from 20 to 160); those with a VABS-II score <70 before cardiac arrest were excluded.

The OHCA trial had 85% power to detect an absolute treatment effect of 20%. Among the 260 patients with data that could be evaluated, there was no significant difference in the primary outcome between the hypothermia group and the normothermia group (20% vs. 12%; relative likelihood, 1.54; 95% CI 0.86–2.76; $p = 0.14$). Although this 8% difference in the primary outcome was not statistically significant, many would argue that this trial was underpowered and that such a difference would be considered clinically significant.

The IHCA trial was powered to 90% to detect an absolute difference of 15%—requiring 558 patients. However, the trial was stopped early, after recruitment of 329 patients, on the grounds of futility. At this point, there was no difference in good neurological outcomes at 12 months (36% in the hypothermic group and 39% in the normothermic group), nor in survival at 12 months (49% in the hypothermic group and 46% in the normothermic group).

These trials differ significantly from the early trials, which showed benefit for TTM in adults [1, 2]. These early trials compared hypothermia against no fever prevention—the patients in the control arms developed fever. The effect of hypothermia compared with fever prevention may be much smaller and therefore not shown in the THAPCA trials. Larger trials are required to see if therapeutic hypothermia is superior or equivalent to therapeutic normothermia in children but these would be extremely challenging to deliver.

10.9 Ongoing Studies

There are several domains within the topic of TTM for which the evidence is unclear. One of the most important of these knowledge gaps remains the optimal target temperature and whether this should involve some degree of hypothermia or strict normothermia. Two large RCTs are currently underway which will hopefully shed more light on this issue. The targeted hypothermia vs. targeted normothermia after OHCA (TTM-2) trial began recruiting in 2018 and is due to be completed at the end of 2021. It is a multinational RCT aiming to recruit 1900 OHCA patients and is the follow up to the TTM trial that did not demonstrate any difference in survival between target temperatures of 33 and 36 °C. Patients are randomized to either TTM of 33 °C for up to 28 h, with rewarming over 12 h or standard care to avoid a temperature greater than or equal to 37.8 °C using conservative measures (fever control). If a single temperature of 37.8 °C or greater is measured, active temperature control is initiated to maintain a target temperature of 37.5 °C until 40 h after randomization. The primary outcome is 180-day survival.

The HYPERION (therapeutic hypothermia after non-shockable cardiac arrest) trial is a French multicenter RCT that is currently recruiting [28]. It is comparing therapeutic hypothermia (33 °C) with therapeutic normothermia (37 °C) for 24 h, followed by a further 24 h of therapeutic normothermia in both groups. The trial includes IHCA and OHCA patients with non-shockable rhythms. The primary outcome is good neurological outcome at 90 days and the study is powered to detect an absolute difference of 9% between groups.

10.10 Conclusion

We are now 16 years on from the landmark RCTs showing improved neurological outcome with mild induced hypothermia after OHCA [1, 2]. Whilst overall survival from OHCA has improved significantly since then, many of the same questions remain from those posed by the 2003 advisory statement published by the ALS task force [3].

Although the TTM trial provides evidence that there is no difference in mortality or neurological outcome between target temperatures of 33 and 36 °C, the recent analysis of the ANZICS database suggests that use of higher target temperatures results in increased fever and a trend towards increasing mortality [12]. This may be a cause for concern given the evidence that following the TTM trial many units have changed their practice to aim for a target temperature of 36 °C [16]. Whilst the outcomes of the TTM-2 trial are awaited, it seems prudent to at least avoid fever and ensure tight control of target temperature.

References

1. Hypothermia After Cardiac Arrest Study Group. Mild therapeutic hypothermia to improve the neurologic outcome after cardiac arrest. N Engl J Med. 2002;346:549–56.
2. Bernard SA, Gray TW, Buist MD, et al. Treatment of comatose survivors of out-of-hospital cardiac arrest with induced hypothermia. N Engl J Med. 2002;346:557–63.
3. Nolan JP, Morley PT, Vanden Hoek TL, Hickey RW. Therapeutic hypothermia after cardiac arrest. An advisory statement by the Advancement Life support Task Force of the International Liaison committee on Resuscitation. Resuscitation. 2003;57:231–5.
4. Nielsen N, Wetterslev J, Cronberg T, et al. Targeted temperature management at 33 degrees C versus 36 degrees C after cardiac arrest. N Engl J Med. 2013;369:2197–206.
5. Nielsen N. The target temperature for post cardiac arrest patients should be 36 degrees C. Crit Care Med. 2017;45:1552–4.
6. Donnino MW, Andersen LW, Berg KM, et al. Temperature management after cardiac arrest: An Advisory Statement by the Advanced Life Support Task Force of the International Liaison Committee on Resuscitation and the American Heart Association Emergency Cardiovascular Care Committee and the Council on Cardiopulmonary, Critical Care, Perioperative and resuscitation. Resuscitation. 2016;98:97–104.
7. Laver SR, Padkin A, Atalla A, Nolan JP. Therapeutic hypothermia after cardiac arrest: a survey of practice in intensive care units in the United Kingdom. Anaesthesia. 2006;61:873–7.
8. Merchant RM, Soar J, Skrifvars MB, et al. Therapeutic hypothermia utilization among physicians after resuscitation from cardiac arrest. Crit Care Med. 2006;34:1935–40.
9. Bigham BL, Dainty KN, Scales DC, Morrison LJ, Brooks SC. Predictors of adopting therapeutic hypothermia for post-cardiac arrest patients among Canadian emergency and critical care physicians. Resuscitation. 2010;81:20–4.
10. Orban JC, Cattet F, Lefrant JY, et al. The practice of therapeutic hypothermia after cardiac arrest in France: a national survey. PLoS One. 2012;7:e45284.
11. Ford AH, Clark T, Reynolds EC, et al. Management of cardiac arrest survivors in UK intensive care units: a survey of practice. J Intensive Care Soc. 2016;17:117–21.
12. Salter R, Bailey M, Bellomo R, et al. Changes in temperature management of cardiac arrest patients following publication of the Target Temperature Management Trial. Crit Care Med. 2018;46:1722–30.
13. Polderman KH, Varon J. Confusion around therapeutic temperature management hypothermia after in-hospital cardiac arrest? Circulation. 2018;137:219–21.
14. Nolan JP, Cariou A. Post-resuscitation care: ERC-ESICM guidelines 2015. Intensive Care Med. 2015;41:2204–6.
15. Deye N, Vincent F, Michel P, et al. Changes in cardiac arrest patients' temperature management after the 2013 "TTM" trial: results from an international survey. Ann Intensive Care. 2016;6:4.
16. Storm C, Nee J, Sunde K, et al. A survey on general and temperature management of post cardiac arrest patients in large teaching and university hospitals in 14 European countries-the SPAME trial results. Resuscitation. 2017;116:84–90.
17. Deakin CD, Nolan JP, Soar J, et al. European Resuscitation Council Guidelines for Resuscitation 2010 Section 4. Adult advanced life support. Resuscitation. 2010;81:1305–52.
18. Aneman A, Cariou A, Nolan JP. Understanding temperature goals after cardiac arrest. Intensive Care Med. 2018;44:940–3.
19. Nolan JP, Ferrando P, Soar J, et al. Increasing survival after admission to UK critical care units following cardiopulmonary resuscitation. Crit Care. 2016;20:219.
20. Bray JE, Stub D, Bloom JE, et al. Changing target temperature from 33 degrees C to 36 degrees C in the ICU management of out-of-hospital cardiac arrest: a before and after study. Resuscitation. 2017;113:39–43.
21. Colbourne F, Corbett D. Delayed postischemic hypothermia: a six month survival study using behavioral and histological assessments of neuroprotection. J Neurosci. 1995;15:7250–60.

22. Sterz F, Safar P, Tisherman S, Radovsky A, Kuboyama K, Oku K. Mild hypothermic cardiopulmonary resuscitation improves outcome after prolonged cardiac arrest in dogs. Crit Care Med. 1991;19:379–89.
23. Castren M, Nordberg P, Svensson L, et al. Intra-arrest transnasal evaporative cooling: a randomized, prehospital, multicenter study (PRINCE: Pre-ROSC IntraNasal Cooling Effectiveness). Circulation. 2010;122:729–36.
24. Debaty G, Maignan M, Savary D, et al. Impact of intra-arrest therapeutic hypothermia in outcomes of prehospital cardiac arrest: a randomized controlled trial. Intensive Care Med. 2014;40:1832–42.
25. Bernard SA, Smith K, Finn J, et al. Induction of therapeutic hypothermia during out-of-hospital cardiac arrest using a rapid infusion of cold saline: The RINSE Trial (Rapid Infusion of Cold Normal Saline). Circulation. 2016;134:797–805.
26. Ditchey RV, Lindenfeld J. Potential adverse effects of volume loading on perfusion of vital organs during closed-chest resuscitation. Circulation. 1984;69:181–9.
27. Lindsay PJ, Buell D, Scales DC. The efficacy and safety of pre-hospital cooling after out-of-hospital cardiac arrest: a systematic review and meta-analysis. Crit Care. 2018;22:66.
28. Lascarrou JB, Meziani F, Le Gouge A, et al. Therapeutic hypothermia after nonshockable cardiac arrest: the HYPERION multicenter, randomized, controlled, assessor-blinded, superiority trial. Scand J Trauma Resusc Emerg Med. 2015;23:26.
29. Chan PS, Berg RA, Tang Y, Curtis LH, Spertus JA, American Heart Association's Get with the Guidelines-Resuscitation Investigators. Association between therapeutic hypothermia and survival after in-hospital cardiac arrest. JAMA. 2016;316:1375–82.
30. Shankaran S, Laptook AR, Ehrenkranz RA, et al. Whole-body hypothermia for neonates with hypoxic-ischemic encephalopathy. N Engl J Med. 2005;353:1574–84.
31. Kirkegaard H, Soreide E, de Haas I, et al. Targeted temperature management for 48 vs 24 hours and neurologic outcome after out-of-hospital cardiac arrest: a randomized clinical trial. JAMA. 2017;318:341–50.
32. Callaway CW. Targeted temperature management after cardiac arrest: finding the right dose for critical care interventions. JAMA. 2017;318:334–6.
33. Moler FW, Silverstein FS, Holubkov R, et al. Therapeutic hypothermia after out-of-hospital cardiac arrest in children. N Engl J Med. 2015;372:1898–908.

Part V

Cardiac Function

Left Diastolic Function in Critically Ill Mechanically Ventilated Patients

11

P. Formenti, M. Brioni, and D. Chiumello

11.1 Introduction

Left ventricular (LV) diastolic dysfunction is a clinical entity that remains poorly understood and identified in the intensive care unit (ICU) setting. In general, it is a syndrome defined by the presence of symptoms of congestive heart failure without sign of reduced LV systolic dysfunction [1]. Distinguishing diastolic heart failure from systolic heart failure is important because of differences in treatment and prognosis, even if the two entities often coexist, and some authors have proposed the hypothesis that diastolic LV dysfunction is essentially a precursor of systolic failure [2]. Diastolic dysfunction has multiple causes and is associated with multiple disorders, including impaired relaxation (common in ischemia and during systemic inflammatory states), impaired peak LV filling (with inadequate transmitral pressure gradient due to raised LV pressure or inability to generate negative LV pressure), stiffness of the left ventricle (fibrosis and hypertrophy), and constriction (pericardial or compression from dilated right ventricle). Diastolic LV dysfunction is common in the ICU but often unrecognized. Identification and determination of its severity may be

P. Formenti
Unità Operativa Complessa di Anestesia e Rianimazione, Centro di Ricerca coordinata di insufficienza respiratoria, Ospedale San Paolo-Azienda Socio Sanitaria Territoriale Santi Paolo e Carlo, Milan, Italy

M. Brioni
Dipartimento di Scienze della Salute, Università degli Studi di Milano, Milan, Italy

D. Chiumello (✉)
Unità Operativa Complessa di Anestesia e Rianimazione, Centro di Ricerca coordinata di insufficienza respiratoria, Ospedale San Paolo-Azienda Socio Sanitaria Territoriale Santi Paolo e Carlo, Milan, Italy

Dipartimento di Scienze della Salute, Università degli Studi di Milano, Milan, Italy
e-mail: davide.chiumello@unimi.it

J.-L. Vincent (ed.), *Annual Update in Intensive Care and Emergency Medicine 2019*, Annual Update in Intensive Care and Emergency Medicine,
https://doi.org/10.1007/978-3-030-06067-1_11

useful to optimize circulatory support in critically ill patients. From this point of view, echocardiography is one of the most powerful diagnostic and monitoring tools available to the modern intensivist, providing the means to diagnose cardiac systolic or diastolic dysfunction, its underlying cause, and to suggest therapeutic interventions [3].

The principal aim of this chapter is to summarize the current evidence regarding the assessment of LV diastolic dysfunction in the ICU and its impact among critically ill mechanically ventilated patients. A comprehensive bibliographic search strategy was developed assessing the following databases: PubMed, CINAHL, Cochrane Library, Scopus, Web of Science, from inception to the cut-off date of July 2018. The following key-words were used, alone or combined with appropriate boolean operators, to search the different databases: 'left diastolic dysfunction', 'intensive care unit', 'mechanical ventilation', 'critical care', 'critically ill patients', 'critical illness'.

11.2 Definitions and Pathophysiology

Diastolic heart failure is defined as a condition caused by increased resistance to the filling of one or both ventricles; this leads to symptoms of congestion from the inappropriate upward shift of the diastolic pressure-volume relation [4]. Although this definition describes the principal pathophysiologic mechanism of diastolic heart failure, it is not clinically applicable. In a more practical definition, diastolic heart failure is a condition that includes classic congestive heart failure findings with normal systolic function at rest, but with alteration in diastolic function [5]. Conventionally, diastole can be divided into four phases: iso-volumetric relaxation, from closure of the aortic valve to mitral valve opening; early rapid ventricular filling, immediately after mitral valve opening; diastasis, a period of low flow during mid-diastole; and late rapid filling, during atrial contraction [6]. During the period in which the heart returns to its relaxed state, the cardiac muscle is perfused. With diastolic dysfunction, the heart is able to supply the body's metabolic requests at rest, but with a higher filling pressure [7]. The transmission of this higher end-diastolic pressure to the pulmonary circulation may cause pulmonary congestion, which leads to dyspnea. In severe cases, the ventricle becomes so stiff that the atrial muscle fails and end-diastolic volume cannot be normalized with elevated filling pressure, with a subsequent reduction in cardiac output [1] (Fig. 11.1). Thus, during diastolic dysfunction the combination of active relaxation and passive myocardial compliance that normally maintain an adequate cardiac output are altered and left atrial pressure should be increased to maintain a satisfactory cardiac output.

Different parameters have been used over the past two decades to describe diastolic dysfunction, so it is difficult to define its real incidence in critically ill patients. It seems to occur in about 30% of cases [8], and the majority of studies tend to relate it with concomitant syndromes, such as sepsis, or clinical conditions, such as respiratory weaning failure.

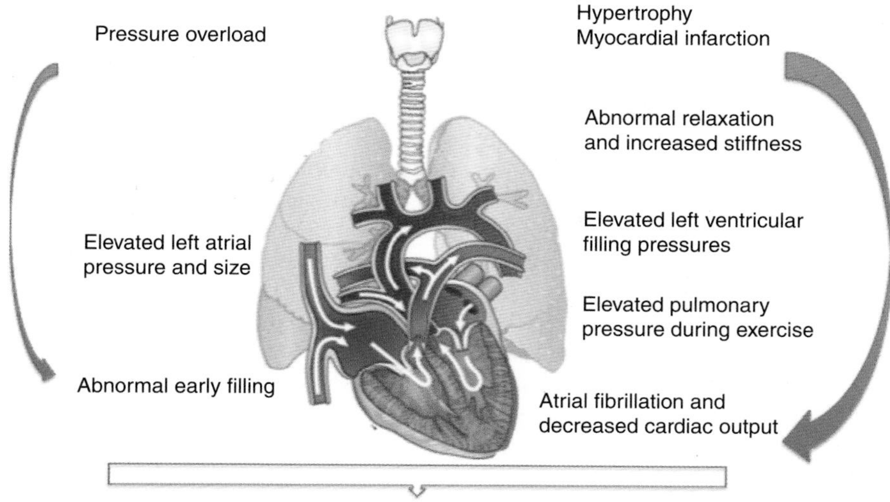

Fig. 11.1 Pathophysiology of diastolic (dys)function. The figure depicts the main pathophysiological patterns that contribute to diastolic dysfunction

11.3 Echocardiographic Diagnosis

Heart failure can present as dyspnea, orthopnea, jugular venous distention, tachycardia, third or fourth heart sounds, hepatomegaly, and edema. Cardiomegaly and pulmonary venous congestion are commonly found on chest radiography. However, these findings frequently also occur in non-cardiac conditions, such as pulmonary disease, anemia, hypothyroidism, and obesity. Furthermore, it is difficult to distinguish diastolic from systolic heart failure based on physical findings alone. Moreover, in critically ill patients, signs and symptoms of heart failure are non-specific, and differ because the severity of pathologies (such as sepsis, hypoxia and acidosis), changes in intravascular status (from intravenous fluid therapy, capillary leak syndrome, renal replacement therapies) and the large variety of treatments (such as sedatives, vasopressors, inotropes and positive pressure ventilation) result in constant fluctuations in the loading conditions of the heart, affecting most of the qualitative and quantitative methods for the measurement of LV filling pressures. Therefore, the study of cardiac function, invasively or non-invasively, is crucial for appropriate treatment of patients. Determination of atrial and ventricular pressures and volumes with cardiac catheterization remains the gold standard method to study diastolic function. However, this invasive method is not applicable as a routine screening tool [9]. Echocardiography is an alternative non-invasive method to assess cardiac function, which in recent years has become familiar also to intensivists, and its use in the study of diastolic dysfunction is well established in the literature.

11.3.1 Basic Concept

Two-dimensional (2D) echocardiography with Doppler imaging provides information on chamber size, wall thickness and motion, systolic function, valvular function and pericardial status; moreover, it can be used to evaluate the characteristics of diastolic transmitral and pulmonary venous flow patterns [10]. Among the different parameters that may be measured with 2D-echocardiography, the most important are the volume of the left atrium, which, if elevated (>34 mL/m^2) may support the presence of elevated LV filling pressures, and the LV ejection fraction and LV wall motion abnormalities, which evaluate systolic function [11] (Fig. 11.2).

Another important modality that should be used is Doppler imaging, in particular the pulsed wave Doppler (cm/s), which measures the velocity of blood flow in a specific region. Pulsed wave Doppler can be applied—only with sinus rhythm—to study transmitral blood flow patterns (Fig. 11.3). With this modality, in the time/velocity diagram, we can identify two waves: the first (E wave) corresponds to the early diastolic passive filling of the left ventricle, while the second (A wave) corresponds to the atrial contraction. The ratio between the two values can be used for the diagnosis of diastolic dysfunction, as isolated parameters are inaccurate because they depend also on volume status. Normally, the E/A ratio is 1.5 [12].

Recently, an adjunctive modality of Doppler imaging able to detect low velocities has been introduced, so called tissue Doppler imaging (TDI). This modality can be used in the apical 4 chamber view to study the movements of the mitral annular plane during the cardiac cycle, at both septal and lateral insertion sites of the mitral leaflets [13]. Normally, TDI enables the systolic (S), the early diastolic (e′) and the

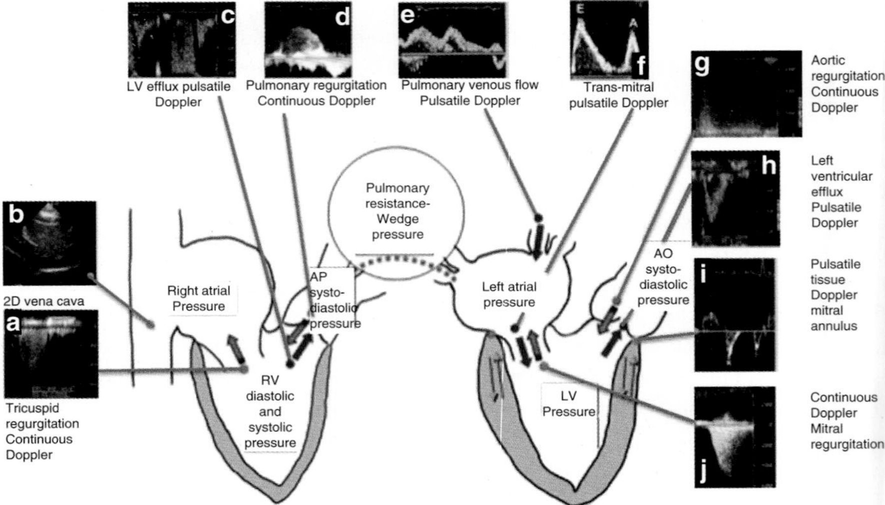

Fig. 11.2 Echocardiographic evaluation of diastolic function. The figure summarizes the different variables that can be measured by echocardiography in the evaluation of diastolic function. *LV* left ventricular, *RV* right ventricular

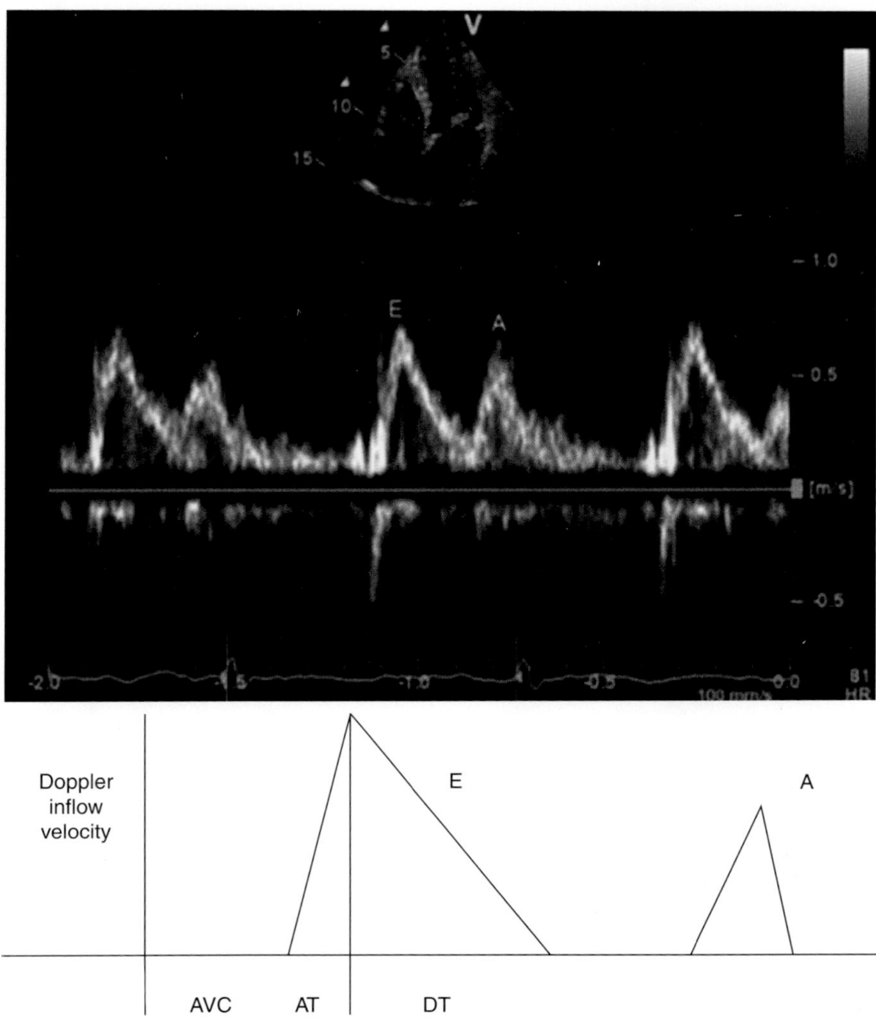

Fig. 11.3 Transmitral pulsed wave Doppler. The figure shows a schematic representation of left ventricular diastolic filling velocity with transmitral Doppler ultrasound. *AVC* acceleration velocity time, *AT* acceleration time, *DT* deceleration time, *E* diastolic filling maximal velocity, *A* telediastolic maximal filling velocity

late diastolic peak velocities (a′) to be assessed (Fig. 11.4). The e′ wave peak velocity has been validated as a relatively preload- and afterload-independent measure of LV relaxation, especially when it is measured at the lateral annulus [14]. However, it is not completely load independent and is affected by many ICU therapies. Normal minimum relaxation values are 8 cm/s at the septal mitral annulus and 10 cm/s at the lateral mitral annulus, or 9 cm/s for average e′ velocity [15]. Values below these thresholds suggest diastolic dysfunction in outpatients; however, the normal minimum values in critically ill patients is yet to be determined [16].

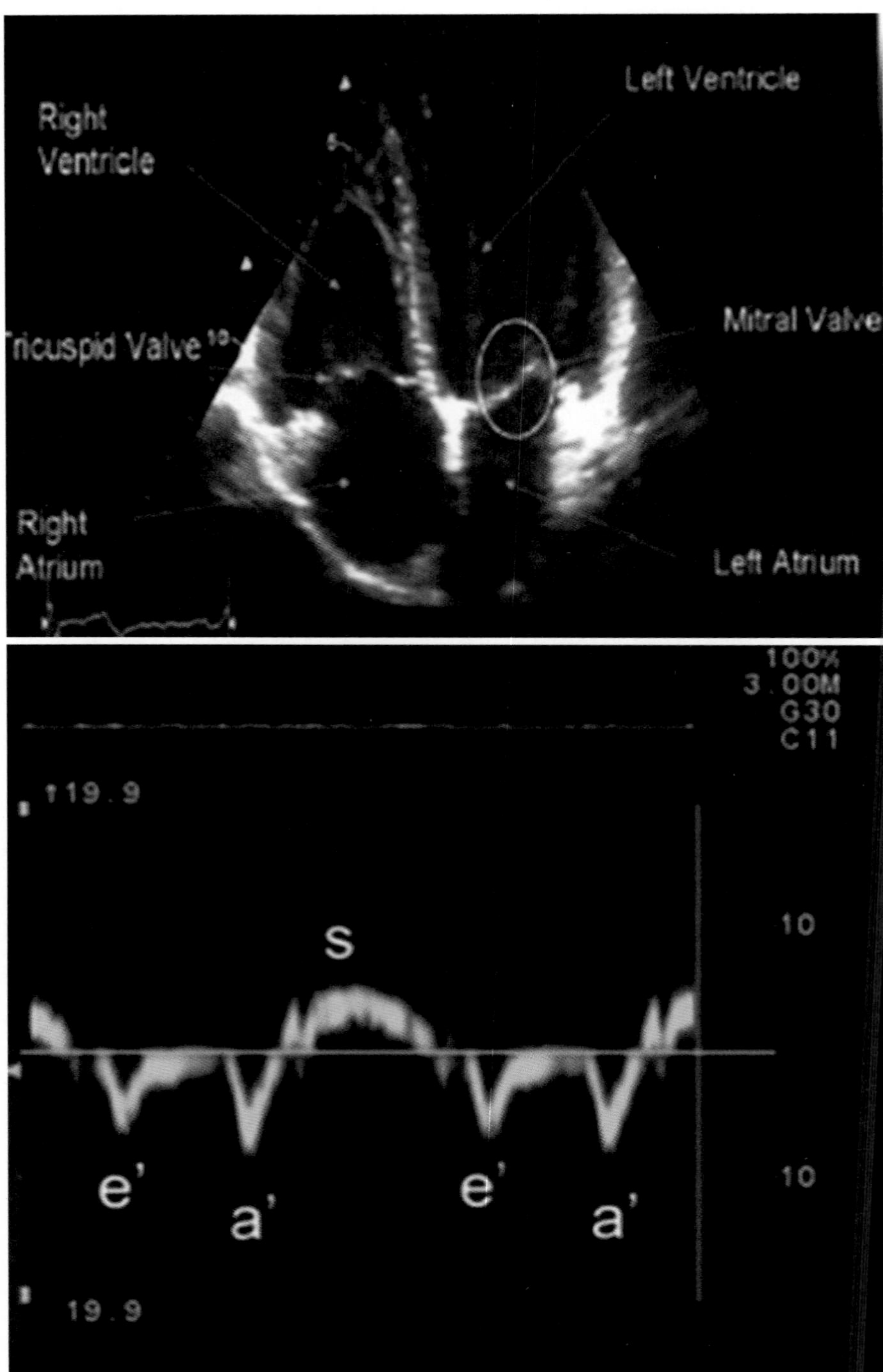

Fig. 11.4 Echocardiographic assessment of left ventricular diastolic function with tissue Doppler imaging (TDI). Upper panel: apical four-chamber view, circle shows position where tissue Doppler must be placed to measure the velocity of change in myocardial length. Lower panel: tissue Doppler measurement at the lateral insertion site of the mitral leaflets shows the diastolic e′ and a′ waves and systolic s′ wave

Finally, as impaired LV diastolic function is transmitted to the right chambers through an increase in pulmonary venous and arterial pressure, the tricuspid regurgitation should be investigated [17]. In particular, a tricuspid regurgitation peak velocity greater than 2.8 m/s is associated with diastolic dysfunction and elevated left atrial pressure.

11.3.2 Left Diastolic Dysfunction

The reported incidence of left diastolic dysfunction ranges between 1.4 and 59.4%, depending on the definition criteria adopted [13]. The new American Society of Echocardiography/European Association of Cardiovascular Imaging (ASE/EACVI) guidelines [14] recommend to take into account several specific measures when determining whether LV diastolic function is normal or abnormal in the absence of myocardial disease. Among these, the most important are the mitral annular e′ velocity (septal e′ < 8 cm/s, lateral e′ < 10 cm/s), E/e′ ratio (average >14, septal >15, lateral >13), the left atrial volume index (>34 mL/m^2), and the peak velocity of tricuspid regurgitation (>2.8 m/s). Nevertheless, some echographic parameters are difficult or impossible to measure in the presence of arrhythmias (such as tachycardia or atrial fibrillation), which are common in the critically ill, and left atrial volume and tricuspid regurgitation are influenced by positive pressure ventilation. For these reasons, Lanspa et al. [18] proposed a simplified definition of left diastolic dysfunction, which is easier to use in the ICU setting where cardiac ultrasound is often performed by intensivists. The simplified definition is based on septal e′, which is considered to be an index of myocardial relaxation, and the ratio of early diastolic velocity of mitral inflow to mitral annular velocity (E/e′), which has a strong association with left atrial pressure (Fig. 11.5). Previous studies have shown that e′ is significantly lower, and E/e′ significantly higher, in non-survivors of septic shock [19, 20].

11.4 Left Diastolic Dysfunction in the ICU

Most of the available literature has investigated left diastolic dysfunction in septic patients, and although in the majority of these studies the patients were receiving mechanical ventilation, little information is available about the role of mechanical ventilation or the acute phase of lung injury (Table 11.1).

A few pioneering papers investigated diastolic dysfunction using ancestral echocardiography. Among these, Parker et al. [35] reported combined hemodynamic and radionuclide cine-angiographic findings in 20 patients with septic shock. Survivors demonstrated initially high mean LV volumes that recovered to normal values within one week, while non-survivors had normal mean LV volumes that were unaltered with time. Similar observations were reported in a subsequent study in which

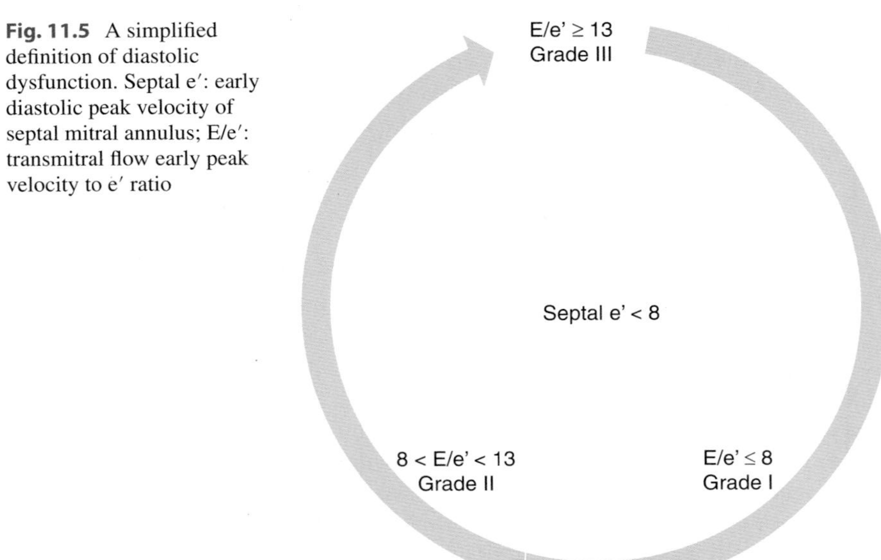

Fig. 11.5 A simplified definition of diastolic dysfunction. Septal e′: early diastolic peak velocity of septal mitral annulus; E/e′: transmitral flow early peak velocity to e′ ratio

the main purpose was to investigate right heart function [36]. The authors suggested how the combination of peripheral vascular resistance and direct depression of the myocardium may act together in depressing ejection fraction, with an increase in mortality due to the inability of ventricular dilation (increased preload). A few years later, Jafri et al. [21] reported that Doppler parameters of LV filling were abnormal in a cohort of septic patients. In this cohort, patients demonstrated an increased peak atrial velocity, a decreased E/A ratio, an increased atrial filling fraction, and a prolongation of atrial filling period as a function of the diastolic filling period, presumably because of delayed relaxation and decreased LV end-diastolic compliance. No information about mechanical ventilation settings or evolution of diastolic dysfunction is available. Munt et al. [22] used pulsed wave Doppler to measure peak filling rate normalized to mitral stroke volume in 24 septic patients and again showed an abnormality of LV relaxation in non-survivors. Furthermore, no account was made for the potential impact of mechanical ventilation on diastolic filling.

The advent of TDI has simplified echocardiographic estimation of ventricular relaxation and ventricular filling pressures and the increasing number of studies in the field has shown that diastolic dysfunction is common in critically ill patients. The significance of diastolic dysfunction was recently highlighted by studies that demonstrated that TDI parameters might be of prognostic use in the ICU population. More recent observations may help to clarify the scenario in these regard. An alteration in the E/e′ ratio has been described in patients with septic shock and, although one study found that the E/e′ ratio was an independent predictor of mortality [20], another investigation failed to find this association [23]. In a single center prospective cohort study, 53 patients were investigated by TDI each day after admission to the ICU with septic shock with the aim of assessing the prevalence of

Table 11.1 Principle studies related to echocardiographic investigation of left ventricular (LV) diastolic dysfunction and mechanical ventilation (MV) in intensive care unit (ICU) patients

	First author [ref]	Setting, no. of patients	Methods	Main remarks
Diastolic dysfunction and sepsis	Jafri et al. [21]	23 MV vs. 30 control	Transmitral pulsed Doppler	Increased peak atrial velocity, decreased E/A ratio, increased atrial filling fraction and prolongation of atrial filling period as a function of the diastolic filling period in septic vs. control
	Munt et al. [22]	24 MV	PWD	Non-survivors had a more abnormal pattern of LV relaxation (E/VTI, 4.7; deceleration time, 235) E/A showed a non-significant trend in the same direction
	Landesberg et al. [20]	262 not all MV	PWD (peak mitral inflow E and A velocity waves); apical four-chamber view; TDI (s′, e′ and a′ septal and lateral; the e′/a′ ratio and LV filling index E/e′ ratio) vs. troponin T/pro-BNP	Diastolic dysfunction only (e′-wave <8 cm/s), or combined systolic–diastolic dysfunction higher mortality and significantly higher serum levels of high-sensitivity troponin-T and N-terminal pro-BNP
	Landesberg et al. [19]	106 MV	Global strain, strain-rate imaging and 3D left and RV volume vs. standard echocardiography vs. troponin-T	LV diastolic dysfunction and RV dilatation are the echocardiographic variables correlating best with troponin elevation
	Pulido et al. [23]	106 MV; multicenter	M-mode,2-dimensional, Doppler echocardiographic study (parasternal long-short-axis views; apical 4-chamber, 2-chamber, long-axis views)	Diastolic dysfunction diagnosed in 36%; no statistically significant difference in 30-day mortality diastolic dysfunction vs. no diastolic dysfunction
	Rolando et al. [24]	53 (45 MV)	M-mode, 2-dimension and Doppler echocardiography (parasternal long- short-axis, apical 4/2-chamber long-axis and subcostal views); TDI (e′/a′ ratio and ventricular filling index E/e′ ratio)	Mortality rate 66%. Multivariate regression analysis: the E/e′ ratio = independent predictor of mortality (E/e′ ratio ROC 0.71)
	Gonzales et al. [25]	223 (204 MV)—5 years retrospective	LV ejection fraction; maximal velocity of mitral Doppler E and A, E/A ratio; tissue Doppler imaging E′ wave maximal velocity on the lateral mitral, and lateral E/E′ ratio	LV diastolic dysfunction diagnosed in 31%; lateral E′ maximal velocity = independently associated with ICU mortality
	Sanfilippo et al. [26]	Meta-analysis	TDI used for definition of diastolic dysfunction	LV diastolic dysfunction in 29.6%: a trend towards higher mortality comparing isolated diastolic dysfunction or combined systolic-diastolic dysfunction vs. normal heart function
	Mahjoub et al. [27]	83 MV	SV, mitral flow early wave velocity (E), E′ and the E/E′ ratio before and after volume expansion	Increase E/e′ after volume expansion in patients with sepsis-induced diastolic dysfunction and non-responders to fluid challenge, which translates an increase in left ventricular filling pressures

Table 11.1 (continued)

	First author [ref]	Setting, no. of patients	Methods	Main remarks
Diastolic dysfunction and MV	Roche-campo et al. [28]	67 MV	PWD early (E) and late (A) diastolic wave velocities at the mitral valve, and TDI early (e′) and late (a′) diastolic wave velocities	Diastolic dysfunction diagnosed in 39%; increased LV filling pressures (↑E/e′ ratio and diastolic relaxation in failed weaning trials e′ decreased in 93.3% of patients who failed weaning trials
	Lamia et al. [29]	39 MV	E/e′ measured before and during SBT vs. Swan-Ganz	E/E′ > 8.5 at the end of the SBT predicted weaning-induced PAOP elevation with a sensitivity of 94% and a specificity of 73%
	Ommen et al. [30]	100 MV	Doppler mitral inflow, pulmonary venous inflow, and TDI vs. Swan-Ganz	E/e′ < 8 accurately predicted normal M-LVDP, and E/e′ >15 identified increased M-LVDP
	Caille et al. [31]	117 MV	Maximal velocities of mitral E and A waves, maximal velocity of e′ wave and LV stroke volume	Patients who failed weaning exhibited at baseline a significantly lower LVEF and higher E/E′
	Papanikolaou et al. [32]	50 MV	Mitral inflow analysis; TDI (mitral/tricuspid annular velocities and color M-mode Doppler velocity of propagation (V p))	pre-SBT values of lateral E/e′ greater than 7.8 and E/V p greater than 1.51 predicted weaning failure. Lateral E/e′ = independently associated with weaning failure before SBT
	Moschietto et al. [33]	68 MV	Mitral Doppler inflow E velocity to annular tissue Doppler Ea wave velocity (E/E′) ratio measurement	E/E′ ratio was higher in weaning failed group. The cut-off value to predict weaning failure gave an E/e′ ratio during the SBT of 14.5 (sensitivity of 75%, specificity of 95.8%)
	Konomi et al. [34]	42 MV	PWD and TDI during 2 h SBT vs. BNP values	The grade of diastolic dysfunction correlated with BNP levels. Presence of diastolic dysfunction independently associated with weaning failure

PWD pulsed wave Doppler, *TDI* tissue Doppler imaging, *SBT* spontaneous breathing trial, *BNP* B-type natriuretic protein, *RV* right ventricular, *PAOP* pulmonary artery occlusion pressure, *LVEF* left ventricular ejection fraction, *M:LVDP* mean left ventricular diastolic pressure

29. Lamia B, Maizel J, Ochagavia A, et al. Echocardiographic diagnosis of pulmonary artery occlusion pressure elevation during weaning from mechanical ventilation. Crit Care Med. 2009;37:1696–701.
30. Ommen SR, Nishimura RA, Appleton CP, et al. Clinical utility of Doppler echocardiography and tissue Doppler imaging in the estimation of left ventricular filling pressures: a comparative simultaneous Doppler-catheterization study. Circulation. 2000;102:1788–94.
31. Caille V, Amiel JB, Charron C, Belliard G, Vieillard-Baron A, Vignon P. Echocardiography: a help in the weaning process. Crit Care. 2010;14:R120.
32. Papanikolaou J, Makris D, Saranteas T, et al. New insights into weaning from mechanical ventilation: left ventricular diastolic dysfunction is a key player. Intensive Care Med. 2011;37:1976–85.
33. Moschietto S, Doyen D, Grech L, Dellamonica J, Hyvernat H, Bernardin G. Transthoracic Echocardiography with Doppler Tissue Imaging predicts weaning failure from mechanical ventilation: evolution of the left ventricle relaxation rate during a spontaneous breathing trial is the key factor in weaning outcome. Crit Care. 2012;16:R81.
34. Konomi I, Tasoulis A, Kaltsi I, et al. Left ventricular diastolic dysfunction--an independent risk factor for weaning failure from mechanical ventilation. Anaesth Intensive Care. 2016;44:466–73.
35. Parker MM, Shelhamer JH, Bacharach SL, et al. Profound but reversible myocardial depression in patients with septic shock. Ann Intern Med. 1984;100:483–90.
36. Parker MM, Suffredini AF, Natanson C, Ognibene FP, Shelhamer JH, Parrillo JE. Responses of left ventricular function in survivors and nonsurvivors of septic shock. J Crit Care. 1989;4:19–25.
37. Villar J, Blanco J, Zhang H, Slutsky AS. Ventilator-induced lung injury and sepsis: two sides of the same coin. Minerva Anestesiol. 2011;77:647–53.
38. Brown SM, Pittman J, Miller Iii RR, et al. Right and left heart failure in severe H1N1 influenza A infection. Eur Respir J. 2011;37:112–8.
39. Mekontso-Dessap A, de Prost N, Girou E, et al. B-type natriuretic peptide and weaning from mechanical ventilation. Intensive Care Med. 2006;32:1529–36.
40. de Meirelles Almeida CA, Nedel WL, Morais VD, Boniatti MM, de Almeida-Filho OC. Diastolic dysfunction as a predictor of weaning failure: a systematic review and meta-analysis. J Crit Care. 2016;34:135–41.

The Effects of Disease and Treatments on Ventriculo-Arterial Coupling: Implications for Long-term Care

12

F. Guarracino, P. Bertini, and M. R. Pinsky

12.1 Introduction: Physiology of the Relationship Between the Left Ventricle and the Arterial Vasculature

Left ventricular (LV) function can be described by its pressure-volume trajectory during one cardiac cycle, with volume on the x-axis (Fig. 12.1). This LV pressure-volume representation is extremely informative of most of the determinants of LV function, describing the four phases of the cardiac cycle: diastolic filling, isovolumic contraction, ejection and isovolumic relaxation. Each pressure-volume loop defines the systolic and diastolic limits of LV pressure and volume independent of preload or afterload. LV pressure-volume points cannot exist outside the limits of diastolic compliance and the end-systolic elastance, defined as the LV end-systolic pressure-volume relationship (ESPVR), which is mostly linear over the physiologic range with a negative slope and a positive zero pressure volume intercept. The ESPVR defines the maximal LV systolic stiffness and is thus also called end-systolic elastance (Ees). At the other extreme, the end-diastolic pressure-volume relationship (EDPVR), reflecting global LV diastolic compliance is slightly curvilinear becoming steeper (stiffer) as LV volumes become large. Important to this discussion, the LV ESPVR reflects global LV systolic function, with increasing and decreasing Ees reflecting increasing and decreasing LV contractility, respectively; whereas EDPVR represents LV diastolic properties.

The position and shape of the LV pressure-volume loop depends on the preload, afterload and structural qualities of the myocardium. Preload, which reflects end-diastolic wall stretch can be approximated by LV end-diastolic pressure and

F. Guarracino (✉) · P. Bertini
Department of Anesthesia and Critical Care Medicine, Azienda Ospedaliero Universitaria Pisana, Pisa, Italy
e-mail: f.guarracino@ao-pisa.toscana.it

M. R. Pinsky
Department of Critical Care Medicine, University of Pittsburgh, Pittsburgh, PA, USA

J.-L. Vincent (ed.), *Annual Update in Intensive Care and Emergency Medicine 2019*, Annual Update in Intensive Care and Emergency Medicine,
https://doi.org/10.1007/978-3-030-06067-1_12

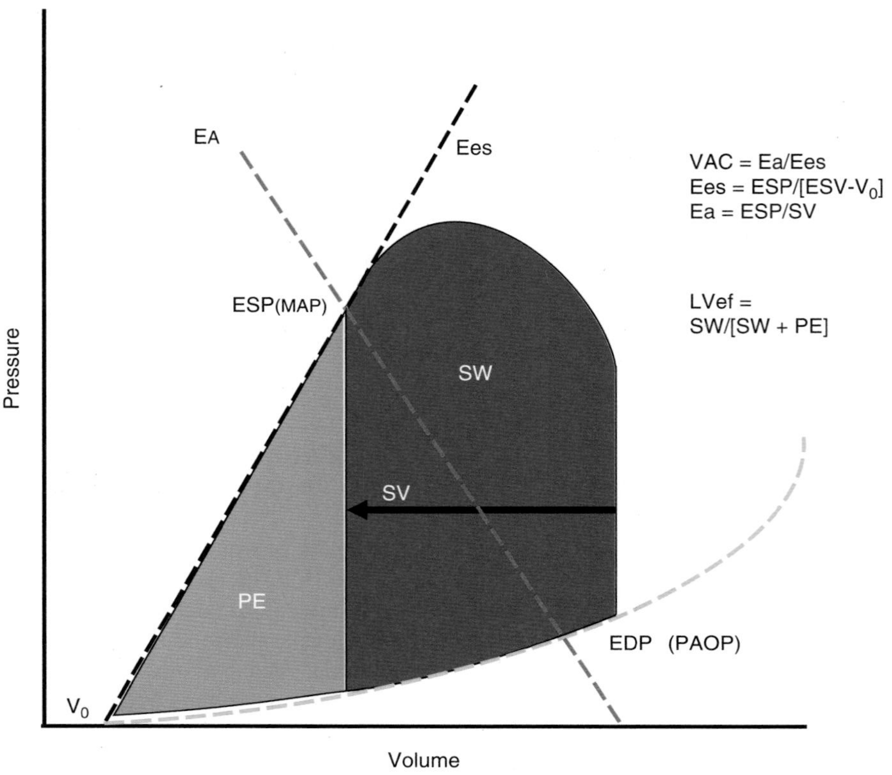

Fig. 12.1 Pressure-volume loop of a cardiac cycle. *VAC* ventriculo-arterial coupling, *Ea* arterial elastance, *Ees* ventricular elastance, *ESP* end-systolic pressure, *ESV* end-systolic volume, V_0 volume X-axis intercept, *SV* stroke volume, *LVef* left ventricular efficiency, *SW* stroke work, *PE* potential energy, *MAP* mean arterial pressure, *EDP* end-diastolic pressure, *PAOP* pulmonary artery occlusion pressure

volume. Afterload, which reflects maximal LV wall stress during active contraction is influenced more by arterial characteristics opposing LV ejection.

One of the primary determinants of LV afterload is the associated rise in arterial pressure as the left ventricle ejects during systole. On the LV pressure-volume loop diagram, this arterial elastance (Ea) can be represented by a line intersecting with LV end-diastolic volume on the volume axis and the end-systolic pressure-volume point on the pressure-volume loop. But to measure Ea one must know end-systolic pressure. End-systolic pressure is not peak systolic pressure but the LV pressure at the end of the ejection phase. How it is estimated is the subject of debate because may hydrodynamic processes contribute to the increasing arterial pressure during ejection and end-systole cannot be identified as the end of antegrade flow from the aortic valve in many disease states. For example, very early termination of flow occurs with aortic regurgitation and very delayed cessation of flow is seen during intra-aortic balloon counter-pulsation [1, 2]. Most non-invasive methods estimate end-systolic pressure as 90% of the peak systolic pressure [3, 4]. Based on this construct, Ea can therefore be calculated as the ratio of end-systolic pressure to stroke volume (SV) [3].

Importantly, the ratio between Ea and Ees, called ventriculo-arterial coupling, has been used as a measure of the mechanical ejection efficiency of the cardiovascular system and has been widely investigated in both chronic and acute conditions and their responses to pharmacologic interventions [5, 6]. Other properties and measurements, such as SV and ejection fraction (EF), can be derived from ventriculo-arterial coupling analysis.

Diastolic properties of the ventricle are much more difficult to quantify, mostly because of the non-linearity of the EDPVR. Stiffness in particular is defined by the dP/dV relationship, the change in pressure for a given change in volume. Generally, diastolic stiffness increases as end-diastolic pressure increases in a non-linear fashion. For this reason, it is difficult to estimate in clinical practice. LV capacitance has been introduced to evaluate diastolic properties, referenced to an end-diastolic pressure of 30 mmHg (V30).

Furthermore, the LV pressure-volume plane offers the ability to investigate the determinants of myocardial oxygen consumption (MVO_2). MVO_2 is linearly related to the area consumed by the LV single cycle pressure-volume loop, reflecting LV stroke work, plus the Ees-defined potential energy triangle before end-systolic volume. The sum of LV stroke work plus elastance-defined potential energy, is the LV pressure-volume area, and varies directly with MVO_2. The larger the pressure-volume area, the greater the MVO_2. The elastance-defined potential energy reflects 'wasted' cardiac work in that no LV SV occurs though energy is required. Many pharmacologic strategies have aimed to minimize this potential work while maximizing stroke work. An example of this is the use of afterload reduction in heart failure patients, which will preferentially decrease the elastance-defined potential work and may actually increase stroke work by increasing SV as ejection pressure decreases. Disease states as well may impair LV energetics by altering both Ees and Ea.

12.2 Measuring Ventriculo-Arterial Coupling

Ventriculo-arterial coupling, defined as the Ees/Ea ratio, is a dimensionless quantity often used to interpret and quantify the LV ejection efficiency. Several studies have introduced measurement using invasive and non-invasive techniques in humans and animal models of disease [7].

The original method proposed to measure Ees and Ea, and one that remains very accurate, is to measure a series of LV pressure-volume loops over several heart beats as either LV end-diastolic volume or end-systolic pressure are varied. This can be accomplished by using an end-inspiratory hold maneuver, inflating a balloon in the inferior vena cava or giving inhaled amyl nitrate to transiently reduce preload or limb muscle contraction or inflation of an aortic balloon to transiently increase afterload. These multi-beat methods allow calculation of ESPVR, EDPVR, Ees and

Ea. Ees is defined as the upper left pressure-volume domains and Ea the series of end-diastolic volume to end-systolic pressure lines. Of note, with rapid decreases in preload, Ea remains constant so the Ea values for each sequential Ea will be in parallel with those before and after it. The advantages of such multi-beat methods are accuracy and reproducibility, making them the reference method to assess other approaches. Their main disadvantage is the need to simultaneously measure both LV pressure and volume, necessitating a left heart catheterization procedure, usually requiring specialized clinical cardiac catherization equipment. Thus, this approach is not suitable for routine bedside assessments. Potentially, 3D-echocardiography can be used to assess LV volumes and experimental estimates of LV pressure have been proposed but are not clinically available [8, 9].

Single-beat methods have been developed for direct application in the clinical environment of the operating room, intensive care unit (ICU) or echocardiography laboratory. Single-beat methods do not rely on varying afterload or preload via occluding vena cava, or applying vasoactive medication [10]. Such methods presume that by measuring maximal elastance (Emax) at the end of systole, one is also measuring Ees. There are several single beat techniques to estimate Ees. Conceptually, they can be divided into volume, pressure or combined volume-pressure methods.

Volume methods assume that V_0, the zero pressure volume intercept on the x-axis of the ESPVR curve, occurs at the origin (zero pressure and zero volume) [11, 12]. This assumption usually underestimates true Ees because if V_0 is greater than 0 mL, the slope of the Ees will be less. Accordingly, this method reports inaccurate estimates of Ees, which can become very inaccurate if V_0 is much greater than zero. However, it is very useful if LV volume measurements are precise, as demonstrated in the estimate of Ees using 3D-echocardiography or magnetic resonance imaging (MRI) in the right heart [13]. In this case Ees is calculated as:

$$Ees = \frac{end\text{-}systolic\ pressure}{end\text{-}systolic\ volume}$$

Although an approximation, these simplified estimations of Ees [14] have been demonstrated to correlate well with directly measured Ees, using the multi-beat method.

Pressure methods are essentially based on the determination of Pmax (or P_{ISO}), which is considered the maximal pressure exerted by the ventricle during isovolumic contractions (ventricle squeeze if its outflow is prevented). Once obtained, Ees (or Emax) can be calculated as:

$$Ees\left(Emax\right) = \frac{Pmax}{SV}$$

This theoretical pressure can be calculated from a nonlinear extrapolation of the early and late portions of the ventricular pressure curve (Fig. 12.1) as derived from

Sunagawa et al. [15]. Takeuchi et al., in 1991, demonstrated that Emax calculated using Pmax correlates well with Ees derived from the multibeat analysis [16].

Senzaki et al. in 1996 [17] and subsequently Chen et al. in 2001 [4] proposed a combined pressure and volume method to non-invasively calculate Ees by fitting time varying elastance curves with regression analysis data extrapolated from a subset of patients with different cardiovascular conditions. In practice, Chen's algorithm needs to be fitted with data derived from echocardiographic and hemodynamic monitoring: systolic and diastolic blood pressure, ejection fraction, stroke volume, pre-ejection time and total ejection time, commonly measured at the bedside, and this is the most used so far in clinical practice [5, 18–21].

12.3 Measuring Right Ventricular Ventriculo-Arterial Coupling

The most accurate methods to assess RV ventriculo-arterial coupling are based on cardiac MRI, which is able to measure RV end-diastolic and end-systolic volumes, while assessing end-systolic pulmonary arterial pressure using a pulmonary artery catheter (PAC) [22]. These approaches have found great utility in the assessment of patients with pulmonary hypertension and their response to therapy and time.

These methods, although very accurate to assess stable patients with chronic disease, are not very useful in a critical care scenario. At the bedside, volumes can be obtained by placing conductance catheters in the right ventricle and by inserting a PAC in order to measure RV pressure at end-systole [23]. As for the left ventricle, estimation of Pmax of the RV during a theoretical RV isovolumic contraction by extrapolation of the RV pressure profile is also possible [24].

12.4 Ventriculo-Arterial Coupling in Critical Care

Many critical care scenarios can alter Ees, Ea or both, greatly influencing ventriculo-arterial coupling and thus overall cardiovascular performance. LV Ees reduction is usually seen in acute left myocardial infarction or myocarditis and may develop in sustained sepsis. Severe sepsis can cause a generalized vasoplegia thus decreasing Ea. Since septic shock is also associated with systemic hypotension, if Ea decreases enough or cardiac output is too low owing to decreased venous return or both, vasopressors are often needed to increase arterial pressure enough to sustain an adequate organ perfusion pressure. Vasopressors will increase Ea as arterial pressure increases. Thus, ventriculo-arterial coupling is often put into imbalance during many acute diseases and their treatment.

Similar ventriculo-arterial coupling imbalance can occur on the right side of the circulation. RV failure due to hypotension or ischemia will decrease RV Ees, and pulmonary embolism, aggressive ventilation and acute respiratory distress syndrome (ARDS) can all increase RV afterload increasing pulmonary arterial Ea [25]. Thus, these disease states are also often associated with ventriculo-arterial coupling imbalance.

Finally, biventricular impairment is often seen in many severe diseases making treatment options difficult and prognosis poor. Thus, assessing ventriculo-arterial coupling for both sides of the heart is an important exercise in the assessment and management of critically ill patients with cardiorespiratory insufficiency.

12.5 Disease and Treatment Influence on Ventriculo-Arterial Coupling

Therapeutic interventions in the critically ill, by altering arterial tone and contractility, have effects on ventriculo-arterial coupling. Analyzing hemodynamic states using a pathophysiological approach is useful in order to better understand the disease phenotype either created *de novo* by the disease or in combination with therapies. For example, inotropic agents are often used to support patients with acute heart failure. Based on the above discussion, one would expect inotropes to be most effective if baseline Ees is low, as compared to Ea. Dobutamine, for example, will increase Ees and decrease Ea, and if given in a setting of a low Ees relative to Ea may restore normal ventriculo-arterial coupling. In sepsis, we previously showed that although Ea is decreased, Ees is decreased more, presumably due to septic cardiomyopathy, and, because of the associated tachycardia or use of norepinephrine infusions, Ea is increased. These combined effects may lead to LV failure if ventriculo-arterial coupling imbalance is sustained for greater than 8 h. Interestingly, fluid resuscitation may restore ventriculo-arterial coupling by selectively decreasing Ea, and if present would be associated with an increase in both cardiac output and arterial pressure. Thus, patients who recouple their ventriculo-arterial coupling ratio in response to norepinephrine should increase their cardiac output whereas those who do not, will not increase cardiac output even though both may realize a similar increase in arterial pressure.

Functional hemodynamic monitoring [26], relying on dynamic indexes of preload, is useful in defining volume responders. Presumably those patients will also have a balanced ventriculo-arterial coupling, although this assumption has not been rigorously tested.

Severe sepsis and septic shock represent one of the most complex cardiovascular states to be encountered in critical care medicine. Both LV contractility (Ees) and arterial tone (Ea) are differentially altered. And, if acute lung disease is also present, as is commonly the case with patients who initiate their septic state with pneumonia, right sided ventriculo-arterial coupling imbalance can also occur. Furthermore, with the associated vasoplegia and vascular endothelial leak, decreases in absolute and effective circulating blood volume often also occur. The increased sympathetic tone also induces tachycardia, which artificially sustains a higher Ea than would otherwise be the case if heart rate were lower. Consequently, reductions in mean arterial pressure (MAP) and SV are often seen associated with an increased cardiac output.

Applying a pathophysiological approach, we would observe a huge reduction in SV and end-systolic pressure (MAP) and, surprisingly, a significant increase in Ea. This may require further explanation: Ea is often mistaken or misinterpreted as total peripheral resistance, but to be specific,

$$\text{total peripheral resistance} = \frac{MAP}{heart\ rate} \cdot \text{SV}$$

If MAP is assumed to reflect end-systolic pressure, we find

$$\text{total peripheral resistance} \propto \frac{end\text{-}systolic\ pressure}{SV} \cdot \text{heart rate}$$

However, $\frac{end\text{-}systolic\ pressure}{SV} = \text{Ea}$.

Therefore, Ea ≅ total peripheral resistance · heart rate.

Accordingly, Ea depends on both total peripheral resistance and heart rate. In fact, in situations where the arterial tone is decreased but heart rate is increased, Ea can be maintained constant or even increase.

Moreover, according to the equation

$$\text{Ea} = \frac{end\text{-}systolic\ pressure}{SV}$$

Ea is always increased if SV change is greater that the change in end-systolic pressure. This interaction between SV and end-systolic pressure is probably the reason why septic shock patients may benefit from heart rate reduction aiming to restore ventriculo-arterial coupling; the use of beta-blockers has been successful, because it simultaneously reduces Ea [27]. Theoretically, inodilators, such as levosimendan, could show beneficial effects on both Ees and Ea preventing uncoupling and hemodynamic derangement [28].

Treatment-associated ventriculo-arterial coupling imbalances may impact longer term outcomes. Those septic shock patients receiving prolonged high doses of vasopressor to sustain a higher arterial pressure and thus higher Ea have increased mortality in randomized prospective clinical trials of lower pressor doses. Ventriculo-arterial coupling imbalance has also recently been demonstrated to have prognostic value in elderly patients with sepsis or septic shock [29] and in patients following acute myocardial infarction [30].

Altered RV ventriculo-arterial coupling can be useful to determine the prognosis of a patient who has normal LV function, but increased pulmonary vascular resistance.

The long-term effects of ventriculo-arterial coupling imbalance due to critical illness are unclear. However, in cardiac patients chronic LV or RV ventriculo-arterial coupling mismatch portends a grave prognosis and is more predictive of early mortality than most other physiological or clinical markers [25, 31].

12.6 Conclusion

Cardiovascular physiology is often altered by systemic diseases like septic shock. If persistent, these changes portend a poor prognosis even if the patients survive the acute event and are discharged from the hospital. Intensivists should be cognizant of the determinants of ventriculo-arterial coupling and how to measure it and how treatments impact patient outcome.

Although hemodynamic monitoring is widely used in the critically ill [32], so far there is lack of evidence of its impact on patient outcomes. However, literature in the field of hemodynamic monitoring shows the benefits of more tailored approaches rather than customary protocols in order to properly diagnose and address the pathophysiology underlining ongoing hemodynamic alterations [33]. The study of ventriculo-arterial coupling may be the key to demonstrate how a more patient-centered approach could positively impact long-term outcomes.

References

1. Kelly RP, Ting CT, Yang TM, et al. Effective arterial elastance as index of arterial vascular load in humans. Circulation. 1992;86:513–21.
2. Marchionni N, Fumagalli S, Baldereschi G, Di Bari M, Fantini F. Effective arterial elastance and the hemodynamic effects of intraaortic balloon counterpulsation in patients with coronary heart disease. Am Heart J. 1998;135:855–61.
3. Chemla D, Antony I, Lecarpentier Y, Nitenberg A. Contribution of systemic vascular resistance and total arterial compliance to effective arterial elastance in humans. Am J Physiol Heart Circ Physiol. 2003;285:H614–20.
4. Chen CH, Fetics B, Nevo E, et al. Noninvasive single-beat determination of left ventricular end-systolic elastance in humans. J Am Coll Cardiol. 2001;38:2028–34.
5. Guarracino F, Ferro B, Baldassarri R, et al. Non invasive evaluation of cardiomechanics in patients undergoing MitrClip procedure. Cardiovasc Ultrasound. 2013;11:13.
6. Ky B, French B, May Khan A, et al. Ventricular-arterial coupling, remodeling, and prognosis in chronic heart failure. J Am Coll Cardiol. 2013;62:1165–72.
7. Chirinos JA. Ventricular-arterial coupling: Invasive and non-invasive assessment. Artery Res. 2013;7:2–14.
8. Herberg U, Gatzweiler E, Breuer T, Breuer J. Ventricular pressure-volume loops obtained by 3D real-time echocardiography and mini pressure wire-a feasibility study. Clin Res Cardiol. 2013;102:427–38.
9. Herberg U, Linden K, Dewald O, et al. 3D real-time echocardiography combined with mini pressure wire generate reliable pressure-volume loops in small hearts. PLoS One. 2016;11:e0165397.
10. Nakamoto T, Cheng CP, Santamore WP, Iizuka M. Estimation of left ventricular elastance without altering preload or afterload in the conscious dog. Cardiovasc Res. 1993;27:868–73.
11. Little WC. The left ventricular dP/dtmax-end-diastolic volume relation in closed-chest dogs. Circ Res. 1985;56:808–15.
12. Tanoue Y, Sese A, Ueno Y, Joh K, Hijii T. Bidirectional Glenn procedure improves the mechanical efficiency of a total cavopulmonary connection in high-risk fontan candidates. Circulation. 2001;103:2176–80.
13. Bellofiore A, Chesler NC. Methods for measuring right ventricular function and hemodynamic coupling with the pulmonary vasculature. Ann Biomed Eng. 2013;41:1384–98.

14. Bombardini T, Costantino MF, Sicari R, et al. End-systolic elastance and ventricular-arterial coupling reserve predict cardiac events in patients with negative stress echocardiography. Biomed Res Int. 2013;2013:235194.
15. Sunagawa K, Yamada A, Senda Y, et al. Estimation of the hydromotive source pressure from ejecting beats of the left ventricle. IEEE Trans Biomed Eng. 1980;27:299–305.
16. Takeuchi M, Igarashi Y, Tomimoto S, et al. Single-beat estimation of the slope of the end-systolic pressure-volume relation in the human left ventricle. Circulation. 1991;83:202–12.
17. Senzaki H, Chen CH, Kass DA. Single-beat estimation of end-systolic pressure-volume relation in humans. A new method with the potential for noninvasive application. Circulation. 1996;94:2497–506.
18. Bertini P, Baldassarri R, Simone V, et al. Perioperative non-invasive estimation of left ventricular elastance (Ees) is no longer a challenge; it is a reality. Br J Anaesth. 2014;112:578.
19. Di Bello V, Giannini C, De Carlo M, et al. Acute improvement in arterial-ventricular coupling after transcatheter aortic valve implantation (CoreValve) in patients with symptomatic aortic stenosis. Int J Cardiovasc Imaging. 2012;28:79–87.
20. Fournier SB, Donley DA, Bonner DE, et al. Improved arterial-ventricular coupling in metabolic syndrome after exercise training: a pilot study. Med Sci Sports Exerc. 2015;47:2–11.
21. Guarracino F, Ferro B, Morelli A, et al. Ventriculoarterial decoupling in human septic shock. Crit Care. 2014;18:R80.
22. Kuehne T, Yilmaz S, Steendijk P, et al. Magnetic resonance imaging analysis of right ventricular pressure-volume loops: in vivo validation and clinical application in patients with pulmonary hypertension. Circulation. 2004;110:2010–6.
23. Solda PL, Pantaleo P, Perlini S, et al. Continuous monitoring of right ventricular volume changes using a conductance catheter in the rabbit. J Appl Physiol. 1992;73:1770–5.
24. Brimioulle S, Wauthy P, Ewalenko P, et al. Single-beat estimation of right ventricular end-systolic pressure-volume relationship. Am J Physiol Heart Circ Physiol. 2003;284:H1625–30.
25. Simon MA, Pinsky MR. Right ventricular dysfunction and failure in chronic pressure overload. Cardiol Res Pract. 2011;2011:568095.
26. Pinsky MR, Payen D. Functional hemodynamic monitoring. Crit Care. 2005;9:566–72.
27. Morelli A, Singer M, Ranieri VM, et al. Heart rate reduction with esmolol is associated with improved arterial elastance in patients with septic shock: a prospective observational study. Intensive Care Med. 2016;42:1528–34.
28. Zangrillo A, Putzu A, Monaco F, et al. Levosimendan reduces mortality in patients with severe sepsis and septic shock: A meta-analysis of randomized trials. J Crit Care. 2015;30:908–13.
29. Yan J, Zhou X, Hu B, et al. Prognostic value of left ventricular-arterial coupling in elderly patients with septic shock. J Crit Care. 2017;42:289–93.
30. Milewska A, Minczykowski A, Krauze T, et al. Prognosis after acute coronary syndrome in relation with ventricular-arterial coupling and left ventricular strain. Int J Cardiol. 2016;220:343–8.
31. Vanderpool RR, Pinsky MR, Naeije R, et al. RV-pulmonary arterial coupling predicts outcome in patients referred for pulmonary hypertension. Heart. 2015;101:37–43.
32. Downs EA, Isbell JM. Impact of hemodynamic monitoring on clinical outcomes. Best Pract Res Clin Anaesthesiol. 2014;28:463–76.
33. Guarracino F, Bertini P, Pinsky MR. Novel applications of bedside monitoring to plumb patient hemodynamic state and response to therapy. Minerva Anestesiol. 2018;84:858–64.

Part VI

Shock

Mechanical Circulatory Support Devices for Cardiogenic Shock: State of the Art

13

L. A. Hajjar and J.-L. Teboul

13.1 Introduction

Cardiogenic shock is the clinical expression of circulatory failure, as a consequence of left, right or biventricular dysfunction. Cardiogenic shock is also defined as a state of critical end-organ hypoperfusion due to primary cardiac dysfunction [1–3]. Cardiogenic shock is not simply a decrease in cardiac contractile function, but also a multiorgan dysfunction syndrome involving the entire circulatory system, often complicated by a systemic inflammatory response syndrome with severe cellular and metabolic abnormalities [4]. The clinical presentation of cardiogenic shock varies from hemodynamic abnormalities of pre-shock to mild shock, progressing to more profound shock and finally refractory shock, which is associated with high mortality rates. Additional insults can occur, such as arrhythmias, vasodilation, ischemia and infection, acutely changing the trajectory of the disease [5]. The contemporary management of cardiogenic shock involves early diagnosis and directed therapy to optimize oxygen delivery and tissue perfusion.

The diagnosis of cardiogenic shock is based on the presence of: (1) persistent hypotension defined as systolic blood pressure <90 mmHg or mean arterial

L. A. Hajjar (✉)
Department of Cardiopneumology, Instituto do Coracao, Universidade de São Paulo, Sao Paulo, Brazil

Cardiologic Intensive Care Unit, Hospital SirioLibanes, Sao Paulo, Brazil
e-mail: ludhmila@usp.br

J.-L. Teboul
Faculté de Médecine Paris-Sud, Universite Paris-Sud, Le Kremlim-Bicêtre, France

Service de reánimation médicale, Hôpitaux Universitaires Paris-Sud, Hôpital de Bicêtre, Le Kremlin-Bicêtre, France

Inserm UMR_S999, Le Plessis-Robinson, France

J.-L. Vincent (ed.), *Annual Update in Intensive Care and Emergency Medicine 2019*, Annual Update in Intensive Care and Emergency Medicine, https://doi.org/10.1007/978-3-030-06067-1_13

pressure (MAP) 30 mmHg below baseline or requirement of vasopressors to achieve a systolic blood pressure ≥90 mmHg; and (2) signs of impaired organ perfusion (e.g., central nervous system abnormalities including confusion or lack of alertness, or even loss of consciousness; oliguria; cold, clammy skin and extremities, tachypnea, increased arterial lactate >2 mmol/L) despite normovolemia or hypervolemia [1].

Some clinical trials include hemodynamic parameters as diagnostic criteria, including low cardiac index (CI) (<1.8 L/min/m^2 without support or <2.2 L/min/m^2 with support) and adequate or elevated filling pressures (left ventricular end-diastolic pressure >15 mmHg) [1, 6]. However, the diagnosis of cardiogenic shock is mainly based on clinical examination.

The most common cause of cardiogenic shock is acute coronary syndrome. Other causes include mechanical complications of acute coronary syndrome, myocarditis, right ventricular (RV) failure and progressive heart failure from cardiomyopathies [7]. In the CardShock study [8], among 219 patients with cardiogenic shock, 68% had ST-elevation myocardial infarction (STEMI), 9% mechanical complications of myocardial infarction and 20% non-acute coronary syndrome causes, such as worsening chronic heart failure, valvular heart disease, stress-induced cardiomyopathy and myocarditis. Patients may also present with cardiogenic shock post-cardiotomy and because of significant ventricular arrhythmias, pulmonary embolism, or cardiac tamponade.

Cardiogenic shock remains a challenging condition with mortality rates of approximately 50% [4]. The field of temporary mechanical circulatory support to manage patients with cardiogenic shock has advanced in the last decade. However, indications for temporary mechanical circulatory support and device selection are part of a complex process requiring consideration of the severity of cardiogenic shock, early and prompt hemodynamic resuscitation, specific patient risk factors, technical limitations, adequate resources and training, and assessment of futility of care. Early intervention with adequate selection of the most appropriate mechanical circulatory support device may improve outcomes [5] (Fig. 13.1).

13.2 Management of Cardiogenic Shock

The focus of the treatment of cardiogenic shock is to prevent organ failure through hemodynamic resuscitation and optimization, and simultaneously to assess and treat a potential reversible cause.

13.2.1 Hemodynamic Support

Myocardial dysfunction generates a spiral of reduced stroke volume, increasing ventricular diastolic pressure and wall stress, which reduces coronary perfusion pressure. In addition, left ventricular (LV) dysfunction and ischemia increase diastolic stiffness, which elevates left atrial pressure, leading to pulmonary

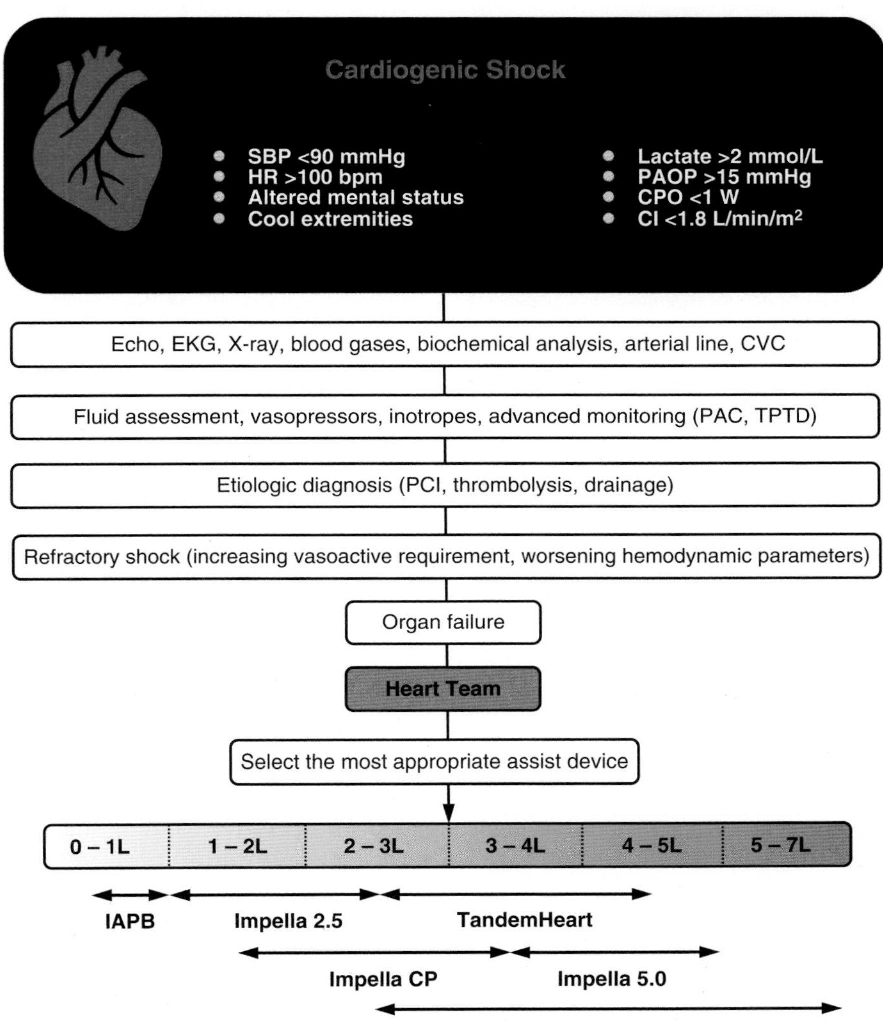

Fig. 13.1 Management of cardiogenic shock. *SBP* systolic blood pressure, *HR* heart rate, *PAOP* pulmonary artery occlusion pressure, *CPO* cardiac power output, *CI* cardiac index, *ECHO* echocardiogram, *EKG* eletrocardiogram, *CVC* central venous catheter, *PAC* pulmonary artery catheter, *TPTD* transpulmonary thermodilution, *PCI* percutaneous intervention

congestion, hypoxia, and worsening ischemia. Initial compensatory mechanisms result in activation of the sympathetic nervous system and the renin–angiotensin–aldosterone system. In about 40–50% of cases, there is a concomitant activation of cytokines, increased inducible nitric oxide synthase (iNOS), increasing levels of NO and subsequent vasodilation and hypotension. Activation of the inflammatory cascade is associated with myocardial depression. Cytokines such as interleukin

(IL)-1, IL-6 and tumor necrosis factor (TNF)-α and reactive oxygen species (ROS) can disturb regional autoregulation leading to impaired microcirculation. This might also contribute to reduced oxygen extraction at the tissue level [7]. Improvement in hemodynamic parameters, which reflects normalization of the macrocirculation, does not always result in restoration of the microcirculation [9]. This has been shown by studies in conditions of a loss of hemodynamic coherence where resuscitation resulted in normalization of systemic hemodynamic variables but did not lead to an improvement in microcirculatory perfusion and oxygenation [10, 11].

We can divide the hemodynamic management of patients with cardiogenic shock into three steps.

13.2.1.1 Step 1: Initial Assessment (Salvage Phase)

Recognition of cardiogenic shock should trigger a rapid assessment of the etiology and hemodynamic profile based on history, physical examination, laboratory investigations, electrocardiogram (EKG), and echocardiography. The initial assessment and management are performed wherever the patient is—emergency room, hemodynamic lab, surgical room or intensive care unit (ICU). Even in cases of prehospital diagnosis, adequate management should be started in this salvage phase.

Arterial line: arterial blood pressure must be monitored using a continuously transduced arterial line. The initial target MAP should be at least 65 mmHg, taking into account individual variability. Radial or femoral access is preferred in this setting. An arterial line also allows blood gas analysis and arterial lactate monitoring. The arterial catheter provides calculation of pulse pressure variation (PPV), which is a predictor of fluid responsiveness in mechanically ventilated patients when applicable. Minimally invasive cardiac output might be useful in the initial management of patients, using devices based on arterial waveform analysis. However, a number of studies have shown inconsistent performance of these devices in the setting of acute/very low cardiac output states and cardiogenic shock [12].

Central venous catheter: the central venous catheter (CVC) allows fluids, inotropes and vasopressors to be administered in a timely fashion. From the CVC, important hemodynamic variables, such as the central venous pressure (CVP), the central venous oxygen saturation ($ScvO_2$) and the central venous carbon dioxide pressure ($PcvCO_2$) can be obtained. The CVC must be inserted preferentially in the internal jugular vein, using ultrasound guidance.

Echocardiography: in the context of cardiogenic shock, transthoracic echocardiography is essential for diagnosis and to follow therapy. In the ICU, repeated echocardiography is recommended for evaluation of left and right ventricular function, valve dysfunction, and exclusion/diagnosis of mechanical complications. Echocardiography is also emerging as a hemodynamic monitoring tool in the ICU for estimation of cardiac output, cardiac filling pressures, to predict volume responsiveness, and determine response to critical care interventions [13]. The main advantages of echocardiography are its non-invasiveness and its ability to assess both cardiac structure and function. From measurement of the velocity–time integral (VTI) of the flow in the LV outflow tract, measurement of RV size, search for pericardial effusion and search for respiratory variations in vena cava diameter, intensivists can quickly confirm and/or define the type of shock. Moreover, changes in cardiac output induced by therapeutic tests of fluid responsiveness or by fluid administration can be reliably estimated by the changes in VTI, as the area of the LV outflow tract remains unchanged over a short time period [12].

Vasopressors: norepinephrine is considered the vasopressor of choice in cardiogenic shock. Subgroup analysis of patients with cardiogenic shock suggested lower mortality with norepinephrine compared to dopamine [14]. It is speculated that the increased heart rate associated with dopamine use may contribute to increased ischemic events. In a recent study of patients with septic shock, norepinephrine administration during early resuscitation increased cardiac systolic function despite the presumed increase in LV afterload secondary to the increased arterial pressure [15]. In patients with vasodilatory shock refractory to norepinephrine (doses >0.2 μg/kg/min), vasopressin should be initiated. This drug is associated with reduced rates of atrial fibrillation and lower requirement of renal replacement therapy (RRT) in vasodilatory shock [16]. Epinephrine should not be used in cardiogenic shock due to its effect in increasing lactate levels, in increasing oxygen consumption and arrythmias and also due to the association with higher mortality rates [17, 18].

In a recent randomized clinical trial, norepinephrine was superior to epinephrine in achieving hemodynamic goals, and epinephrine increased lactate levels in patients with cardiogenic shock after acute myocardial infarction [19]. A meta-analysis of individual data from 2584 patients showed that epinephrine use for hemodynamic management of patients with cardiogenic shock was associated with a threefold increased risk of death [20].

Inotropes: The addition of an inotropic agent may help to improve stroke volume after hemodynamic stabilization with a vasopressor in cardiogenic shock. Dobutamine is the initial therapy and (starting dose 2.5 μg/kg/min) may act rapidly to restore stroke volume [1]. Levosimendan and milrinone, due to their vasodilator properties, should not be used in the management of cardiogenic shock.

Fluids and red blood cells: due to the vasodilation that can occur in cardiogenic shock, many patients may develop hypovolemia. In these cases, dynamic assessment of fluid status should be performed, through echocardiography parameters and cardiac output monitors. A fluid challenge identifies and simultaneously treats volume depletion, whilst avoiding deleterious consequences of fluid overload through its small volume and targeted administration [21].

Red blood cell transfusion is recommended on an individual basis, according to hemodynamic parameters after the administration of inotropes and vasopressors and fluid status assessment. Usually, hemoglobin levels >8 g/dL are needed to optimize oxygen delivery in patients with shock. However, the value is dependent on hemodynamic circumstances, patient age, comorbidities and compensatory response to anemia and shock [22, 23].

13.2.1.2 Step 2: Optimization and Stabilization

The second phase of the hemodynamic management of cardiogenic shock aims to optimize the hemodynamic goals and stabilize the patient to prevent complications. In this setting, accurate hemodynamic monitoring is recommended, and re-evaluation of therapies and patient response should be performed. The objectives of care are to optimize fluid status, and to adjust doses of inotropes and vasopressors to improve oxygen delivery and tissue perfusion.

Hemodynamic monitoring: after collecting information from clinical examination, CVP, arterial blood pressure, heart rate, gas analysis, echocardiography and minimally invasive cardiac output assessment, in most cases it is possible to make valid therapeutic decisions and select the most appropriate hemodynamic therapy. If the response of the patient is positive and shock is resolving, there is no need to add any further monitoring device. If the response is inadequate, it is recommended that more information be obtained using an advanced hemodynamic monitoring technique. It is also recommended that advanced hemodynamic monitoring should be used earlier when acute respiratory distress syndrome (ARDS) is associated with shock because in this situation fluid management is even more challenging. The two hemodynamic monitoring technologies considered as advanced are the pulmonary artery catheter (PAC) and transpulmonary thermodilution systems [12, 24]. PAC use has fallen out of favor over the last two decades because of the difficulty measuring and interpreting the hemodynamic variables as well as failure to demonstrate any benefit of its use in critically ill patients in randomized clinical trials [25]. Nevertheless, it has been recently suggested that the PAC may still have a key role in the hemodynamic monitoring of critically ill patients [26, 27]. Currently, the PAC is recommended in patients with refractory shock, in shock patients with RV dysfunction and/or with ARDS, and when selecting the ideal mechanical circulatory support device. Its advantage is that it can be used to measure the pulmonary artery pressure, and to provide an estimation of pulmonary vascular resistance and other potentially useful hemodynamic variables, such as right atrial pressure, left and right ventricular work, pulmonary artery occlusion pressure (PAOP), mixed venous oxygen saturation (SvO_2), oxygen delivery, oxygen consumption and extraction [12].

The use of transpulmonary thermodilution is recommended in patients with severe shock, especially in the case of ARDS [12, 24]. This technique measures cardiac output in an intermittent way, but transpulmonary thermodilution devices can also provide a real-time measurement of cardiac output through pressure waveform analysis after initial calibration. Pressure waveform analysis also continuously provides PPV and/or stroke volume variation (SVV), two dynamic markers of preload responsiveness. The cardiac output measurement is accurate and precise, even in patients with high blood flow RRT. The mathematical analysis of the thermodilution curve provides other hemodynamic variables, such as the global end-diastolic volume (GEDV), a marker of cardiac preload, the cardiac function index and the global ejection fraction, markers of cardiac systolic function. The extravascular lung water (EVLW) is a quantitative measure of pulmonary edema and the pulmonary vascular permeability index (PVPI), a marker of the lung capillary leak. Thus, such devices are particularly appropriate for guiding fluid management in patients with concomitant acute circulatory and respiratory failure as they help clinicians assess the benefit/risk ratio of fluid administration. The benefit can be evaluated by the preload responsiveness indices that these devices provide (PPV, SVV, pulse wave analysis-derived cardiac output response to passive leg raising or end-expiratory occlusion test). The recommendation to use advanced hemodynamic monitoring should apply only to the subgroup of patients with shock who do not respond to the initial treatment and/or who have associated ARDS [12, 24].

13.2.1.3 Step 3: Titrating Therapies

In this phase, patients should be carefully evaluated regarding the response to therapy. Clinical examination, macrohemodynamic and microhemodynamic variables, perfusion tissue markers and, if possible, microcirculation should be assessed in an integrative approach, trying to discern the circulatory status of patient. In the case of hemodynamic stability, vasoactive drug weaning may be started and de-escalating therapies might be a goal. However, 10–15% of patients develop refractory shock needing increased doses of vasopressors and inotropes, presenting signs of tissue hypoxia, and in many cases already developing organ failure. In this setting, mechanical circulatory support should be considered.

13.2.2 Specific Management According to the Etiology of the Cardiogenic Shock

In the case of cardiogenic shock due to acute coronary syndrome, myocardial revascularization is the only evidence-based therapy with proven survival benefit. Fibrinolysis should be reserved for patients with STEMI when timely percutaneous coronary intervention (PCI) is not feasible [2]. The SHOCK trial is one of the milestone randomized trials in cardiogenic shock [28]. Although it failed to show a reduction in 30-day mortality by early revascularization-based management either with PCI or coronary artery bypass grafting (CABG) [28], there was a significant mortality reduction at 6 months and at long-term follow-up [29]. More than 80% of patients with cardiogenic shock have multivessel or left main coronary artery disease [1]. These patients have higher mortality than patients with single-vessel disease. In recent years, immediate multivessel PCI of all high-grade lesions has been recommended in addition to the culprit lesion [2]. However, the randomized, multicenter Culprit Lesion Only PCI vs. Multivessel PCI in Cardiogenic Shock (CULPRIT-SHOCK) trial showed a significant clinical benefit of a culprit-lesion-only strategy with a reduction in the primary endpoint of 30-day mortality or severe renal failure requiring RRT (45.9% culprit-lesion-only PCI vs. 55.4% immediate multivessel PCI group; relative risk 0.83; 95% confidence interval 0.71–0.96; $p = 0.01$) which was mainly due to an absolute 8.2% reduction in 30-day mortality (43.3% vs. 51.5%; relative risk 0.84; 95%

confidence interval 0.72–0.98, p = 0.03) [30]. Two recent meta-analyses confirmed an increased mortality at short-term follow-up with multivessel PCI and similar outcome at longer follow-up [31]. Data from one-year outcomes from the CULPRIT-SHOCK trial showed that mortality did not differ significantly between the two groups at 1 year; however, the rates of rehospitalization for heart failure and repeat revascularization were higher in the culprit-lesion-only PCI group than in the multivessel PCI group at this time point [32].

Evidence comparing PCI vs. CABG showed that the type of revascularization did not influence the outcome of patients with cardiogenic shock [1]. In current clinical practice, immediate CABG is performed in less than 4% of patients [1]. Antithrombotic therapy, including antiplatelets and anticoagulation, is essential during and after PCI in patients with acute coronary syndrome. Prasugrel/ticagrelor or clopidogrel is indicated in addition to aspirin in all patients undergoing PCI. Because of the delayed and impaired onset of oral antiplatelets action in unstable patients, glycoprotein IIb/IIIa inhibitors or cangrelor may be more liberally used in cardiogenic shock [1].

Unfractionated heparin or low molecular weight heparin should also be administered with antiplatelets. There are no specific randomized trials in patients with cardiogenic shock, so the same recommendation applies as for other types of acute coronary syndrome [2]. The etiologic diagnosis is essential to improve outcomes. Echocardiography should be performed in the initial assessment of patients with cardiogenic shock to promptly diagnose and treat mechanical complications of acute myocardial infarction, cardiac tamponade, acute valve insufficiency or pulmonary embolism. Independent of the phase of therapy, organ support and maintenance must be given according to shock severity.

13.2.3 Mechanical Circulatory Support

Escalating doses of vasopressors and inotropes are associated with increased mortality. Mechanical circulatory support is an essential part of the management of cardiogenic shock and is commonly utilized as a bridge-to-decision, whether it is recovery, palliation, heart transplant or a durable mechanical circulatory support device. A comparison of technical features of the available percutaneous assist devices is shown in Table 13.1.

13.2.3.1 Intra-aortic Balloon Pump

The intra-aortic balloon (IABP) pump, a counterpulsation pump placed percutaneously in the descending aorta, is the most used assist device worldwide. It requires a native beat and a stable rhythm as the balloon is synchronized with the heart. For more than four decades, IABP has been used to improve hemodynamic parameters in patients with cardiogenic shock. An IABP reduces afterload, increases cardiac output, optimizes coronary flow and decreases oxygen consumption [33]. The insertion of an IABP is relatively easy, it has a low cost and associated vascular complications are rare. However, the increase in cardiac output is relatively small, about

Table 13.1 Technical properties of percutaneous circulatory assist devices

	IAPB	IMPELLA 2.5	IMPELLA CP	IMPELLA 5.0	TandemHeart	VA-ECMO
Mechanism	Aorta	LV → aorta	LV → aorta	LV → aorta	LA → aorta	RA → aorta
Flow (L/min)	0.3–0.5	1.0–2.5	3.7–4.0	Max. 5.0	2.5–5.0	3.0–7.0
Cannula size (Fr)	7–8	13–14	13–14	21	15–17 arterial 21 venous	14–16 arterial 18–21 venous
Femoral artery size (mm)	>4.0	5.0–5.5	5.0–5.5	8.0	8.0	8.0
Cardiac synchrony or stable rhythm	Yes	No	No	No	No	No
Maximum implant days	TBD	7–10 days	7–10 days	2–3 weeks	2–3 weeks	3–4 weeks
Cardiac power	↑	↑↑	↑↑	↑↑	↑↑	↑↑↑
Afterload	↓	↓	↓	↓	↑	↑↑↑
MAP	↑	↑↑	↑↑	↑↑	↑↑	↑↑
LVEDP	↓	↓↓	↓↓	↓↓	↓↓	↔
PAOP	↓	↓↓	↓↓	↓↓	↓↓	↔
LV preload	–	↓↓	↓↓	↓↓	↓↓	↓
Coronary perfusion	↑	↑	↑	↑	–	–

IABP intraaortic balloon pump, *VA-ECMO* veno-arterial extracorporeal membrane oxygenation, *LV* left ventricle, *LA* left atrium, *RA* right atrium, *MAP* mean arterial pressure, *LVEDP* left ventricular end-diastolic pressure, *PAOP* pulmonary artery occlusion pressure

500–800 mL/min/m^2. The IABP-SHOCK II trial randomized 600 patients with cardiogenic shock after acute myocardial infarction and early revascularization to IABP or conventional treatment and found no difference in 30-day mortality between the treatment groups [34]. These results led to a downgrading of the IABP recommendation in the ESC guidelines with a current class IIIB recommendation for routine use of IABPs in cardiogenic shock. The 2017 ESC STEMI guidelines now recommend IABP use only in patients with mechanical complications (class IIa, level C) [35].

Recent meta-analyses of IABP therapy in post-acute myocardial infarction patients with cardiogenic shock (incorporating the results of the IABP-SHOCK II trial) have further called into question the utility of IABP therapy in these patients. Analyzing data from 17 studies, Romeo et al. reported no overall differences in short- or long-term mortality in patients receiving IABP therapy. Interestingly, when stratified by initial treatment, IABP therapy significantly reduced mortality (RR 0.77, 95% CI 0.68–0.87) in patients receiving thrombolytic therapy but significant increased mortality (RR 1.18, 95% CI 1.04–1.34) in patients receiving primary PCI [36].

In spite of the evidence against the routine use of IABP, it is often used as initial mechanical support (bridge therapy) until other more sophisticated devices become available. Another field of interest is the use of IABP in patients receiving extracorporeal membrane oxygenation (ECMO) due to the afterload reduction. There are data showing benefits of IABP in patients with ECMO, with a decrease in PAOP, less pulmonary edema and increased survival [37].

13.2.3.2 TandemHeart

The TandemHeart (TandemLife, Pittsburgh, PA, USA) is a percutaneous centrifugal pump that provides mechanical circulatory support of up to 4 L/min via a continuous flow centrifugal pump. Oxygenated blood is withdrawn from the left atrium via a 21 Fr inflow cannula placed via trans-septal puncture and then re-injected into the lower abdominal aorta or iliac arteries via a 15–17 Fr outflow cannula [38]. The TandemHeart is inserted through the femoral vein and is advanced across the inter-atrial septum into the left atrium. The need for transseptal puncture is a potential limitation to its widespread use. In 2005, Thiele et al. reported their experience with TandemHeart therapy in patients with cardiogenic shock post-acute myocardial infarction [39]. Patients were randomized to hemodynamic support with either an IABP or the TandemHeart. The primary endpoint was hemodynamic improvement. While greater improvements in cardiac power and in cardiac index were seen in patients receiving the TandemHeart, 30-day mortality was similar (43% vs. 45%, $p = 0.86$) in the two groups. In 2011, Kar et al. reported outcomes following TandemHeart insertion in 80 patients with cardiogenic shock post-acute myocardial infarction [40]. Almost half of these patients had undergone cardiopulmonary resuscitation (CPR) immediately before or at the time of implantation. TandemHeart insertion was associated with significant improvements in hemodynamic indices. The 30-day and 6-month mortality rates were 40.2% and 45.3%, respectively. One patient died following wire-mediated perforation of the left atrium. Other complications included the need for blood transfusion (71%), sepsis/systemic inflammatory response syndrome [SIRS] (29.9%), bleeding around the cannula (29.1%), gastrointestinal bleeding (19.7%), coagulopathy (11%), stroke (6.8%), and device-related limb ischemia (3.4%).

13.2.3.3 Impella

The Impella (AbioMed, Danvers, MA, USA) is a continuous, non-pulsatile, axial flow Archimedes-screw pump that provides active support by expelling aspirated blood from the left ventricle into the ascending aorta. Unlike an IABP, the Impella does not require EKG or arterial waveform triggering, facilitating stability even in the setting of tachyarrhythmias or electromechanical dissociation. Reported complications include device migration, device malfunction due to thrombosis, hemolysis, bleeding requiring transfusion, arrhythmias, limb ischemia, tamponade, aortic or mitral valve injury, and stroke [1, 38].

Three versions of Impella for LV support are available: the Impella LP 2.5 that can deliver 2.5 l/min of cardiac output, the Impella CP that can deliver 3.7 L/min of cardiac output, and the Impella LP 5.0 that can deliver 5.0 l/min of cardiac output. While the Impella LP 2.5 and Impella CP can be inserted percutaneously via a 12–14 Fr sheath, insertion of the Impella LP 5.0 requires surgical cutdown of the femoral or axillary artery prior to insertion of a 22 Fr sheath [38].

The ISAR-SHOCK trial was a 2-center, randomized controlled pilot study that randomized 26 patients with cardiogenic shock post-acute myocardial infarction to Impella LP 2.5 or IABP therapy [41]. Although the cardiac index after 30 min of support was significantly increased in patients with the Impella LP 2.5 compared to those with an IABP (0.49 ± 0.46 vs. 0.11 ± 0.31 L/min/m^2 respectively; $p = 0.02$), at 4 h, no significant differences were seen in the cardiac index, modified cardiac power index (CPI), or serum lactate. After 24 h, no significant differences were seen in urine output, vasopressor requirement, or mechanical ventilation duration. Hemolysis and transfusion were significantly higher in patients with the Impella LP 2.5. Overall 30-day mortality was 46% in both groups.

Ouweneel et al., in 2017, reported the results from the IMPRESS trial, which randomized 48 patients with cardiogenic shock post-acute myocardial infarction to hemodynamic support with the Impella CP or an IABP [42]. Device placement occurred either prior to PCI, during PCI, or immediately after PCI. Notably, 92% of the study population had a history of recent cardiac arrest requiring resuscitation. At 30 days, mortality was similar (50% vs. 46% for patients receiving support with the Impella CP or IABP, respectively; $p = 0.92$). More bleeding events occurred in patients receiving support with the Impella CP. In a recent meta-analysis including 148 patients, Tandemheart or Impella use was not associated with increased survival in patients with cardiogenic shock [43].

13.2.3.4 Right Ventricular Support

Acute RV failure may occur in multiple settings, including acute myocardial infarction, myocarditis, acute decompensated heart failure, acute pulmonary embolism, pulmonary hypertension, post-cardiotomy, post-transplantation, and following LVAD implantation. Devices currently available for RV support are CentriMag (St Jude Medical, Waltham, MA), a centrifugal pump with a magnetically levitated propeller, Impella RP, an axial catheter-based pump, and the PROTEK Duo (Cardiac Assist Inc., Pittsburgh, PA) catheter with an extracorporeal centrifugal pump [38].

The RECOVER RIGHT study evaluated the safety and efficacy of the Impella RP (4.0 L/min of cardiac support) in 30 patients with RV failure refractory to medical therapy [44]. The cohort was divided into patients with RV failure following LVAD implantation and patients with RV failure following acute myocardial infarction or cardiotomy. The primary endpoint of survival to 30 days or hospital discharge was achieved in 73.3% of the overall study population, with 83.3% of patients with RV failure following LVAD implantation and 58.3% of patients with RV failure following cardiogenic shock post-acute myocardial infarction or cardiotomy alive at 30 days or discharge. All discharged patients were alive at 180 days. These results are particularly compelling when considering that prior studies of RVAD devices in patients with cardiogenic shock reported survival rates of 42–57% at discharge. In 2015, the Impella RP received approval from the FDA for adult and pediatric patients with a body surface area (BSA) $\geq$1.5 m^2 with a diagnosis of acute RV failure following LVAD implantation, acute myocardial infarction, heart transplantation or cardiotomy [38].

The CentriMag (Levitronix LLC, Waltham, MA, USA) is a short- to intermediate support device composed of a centrifugal pump, an electric motor, and a console. It can generate up to 9.9 L/min continuous flow at 5000 rpm. The cannulae are inserted through a midline sternotomy, with the inflow cannula in the left ventricle or right superior pulmonary vein and the outflow cannula in the aorta. It is a therapeutic choice for bridging patients with acute cardiogenic shock to longer term mechanical support or transplantation or when inotropic and IABP support fail [45].

13.2.3.5 VA-ECMO

VA-ECMO is a form of heart-lung bypass machine that offers extended support to patients whose heart and/or lungs are unable to sustain life in the acute setting. VA-ECMO provides cardiopulmonary support for patients in refractory cardiogenic shock as a bridge to myocardial recovery, bridge to decision, bridge to durable mechanical circulatory support, bridge to heart transplant or bridge to decision for palliative therapy. Important advances in pump and oxygenator technology, percutaneous cannulation techniques and critical care management have enabled ECMO to be considered as a viable lifesaving modality [46].

Over 87,000 patients have been enrolled in the Extracorporeal Life Support Organization (ELSO) registry, including 12,566 adults with VA-ECMO, with the number of VA-ECMO centers increasing considerably in the last decade [46]. In a VA-ECMO circuit, deoxygenated blood is pulled from the venous circulation by a pump via a large cannula. Patients may be cannulated centrally (open chest) or peripherally. Blood passes through the pump into an oxygenator where gas exchange occurs (carbon dioxide removal and oxygenation). Oxygenated blood returns via another cannula to the arterial circulation using a centrifugal pump. Modern centrifugal pumps cause less blood damage, reduced heat generation, cause less thrombogenicity and are smaller than old roller pumps. Polymethyl pentene-coated nonporous hollow fiber membrane oxygenators require lower priming volumes and have better gas exchange capability, improved blood compatibility, and show greater stability and preservation of coagulation factors and platelets.

Modern percutaneous approaches have resulted in wider utilization of ECMO, including in-hospital based programs that place patients in cardiac arrest on ECMO support (extracorporeal cardiopulmonary resuscitation [eCPR]), delivery programs with 'in the field' ECMO cannulation, and periprocedural ECMO in cardiac catheterization laboratories, in the surgical room and in the ICU [47]. Distal perfusion catheters that direct a proportion of the returned oxygenated blood flow from the ECMO circuit to the cannulated leg decrease the risks of critical limb ischemia in femoral cannulation.

Survival among patients on VA-ECMO support remains modest, with hospital mortality rates of 50–60% and 6-month survival as low as 30% [38]. This may be a consequence of inadequate selection of potential candidates and insufficient training of the involved professionals.

The appropriate selection of patients for ECMO is challenging, because it should consider the adequate support, patient characteristics and the time of the procedure regarding potential reversibility of the shock state. There are few clinical studies evaluating VA-ECMO in adults. Of 12 studies, 7 are retrospective, 2 are meta-analyses and 3 are prospective studies [46]. Patients with potentially reversible causes of shock, such as fulminant myocarditis or primary graft failure, have better survival than patients with cardiogenic shock after surgery or acute myocardial infarction [48, 49]. Patients for whom ECMO is deployed during or immediately after cardiac arrest have an especially poor prognosis. Pre-ECMO risk factors independently associated with poor outcomes include older age, female sex, and higher body mass index, as well as markers of illness severity including renal, hepatic, or central nervous system dysfunction, longer duration of mechanical ventilation, elevated lactate levels, and reduced prothrombin activity [48].

The management of patients receiving ECMO is based on predefined protocols, which include adequate set and flow control, management of gas exchange, reduction of LV preload, monitoring volume status and anticoagulation and evaluation for weaning [50]. Echocardiography is recommended on a daily basis to evaluate patients receiving VA-ECMO.

13.3 Role of a Cardiogenic Shock Team

Cardiogenic shock is a disease with high mortality and its management is complex, so it is essential to make an early diagnosis and to mobilize adequate resources. The availability of a shock team facilitates timely interventions and avoids futility. The shock team comprises a multidisciplinary group involving an interventional cardiologist, cardiologist, cardiothoracic surgeon, a critical care physician and specialized nurses. The shock team must be ready not only to select and insert the appropriate device in the acute setting, but must also consider long-term strategies, such as permanent devices and transplantation. The shock team must also be prepared to recommend against a mechanical circulatory support device in special settings, such as the occurrence of multiple organ failure, or in the presence of advanced comorbidities.

13.4 Conclusion: The Future

Cardiogenic shock should be considered a high-mortality disease that develops as a continuum from the initial insult to the occurrence of organ failure and death. Many advances have contributed to improve diagnosis and therapy of cardiogenic shock. However, these have not led to improved outcomes. In the future, to obtain better results, we should learn how to deliver existing effective therapies within a timely and multifaceted strategy.

Early utilization of mechanical circulatory support instead of escalating doses of inotropes and vasopressors might avoid the downward spiral seen in patients with cardiogenic shock and resulting in high mortality rates. Appropriate device selection is still a complex decision process and we expect to obtain more objective data in the near future to help in the decision process, taking into account simultaneously the severity of cardiogenic shock, goals of care, patient-specific risks and technical limitations along with assessment for futility of care.

References

1. Mebazaa A, Combes A, Van Diepen S, et al. Management of cardiogenic shock complicating myocardial infarction. Intensive Care Med. 2018;44:760–73.
2. Ibanez B, James S, Agewall S, et al. 2017 ESC guidelines for the management of acute myocardial infarction in patients presenting with ST-segment elevation: the Task Force for the management of acute myocardial infarction in patients presenting with ST-segment elevation of the European Society of Cardiology (ESC). Eur Heart J. 2018;39:119–77.
3. van Diepen S, Katz JN, Albert NM, et al. Contemporary management of cardiogenic shock: a scientific statement from the American Heart Association. Circulation. 2017;136:e232–68.
4. Mandawat A, Rao SV. Percutaneous mechanical circulatory support devices in cardiogenic shock. Circ Cardiovasc Interv. 2017;10:e004337.
5. Bellumkonda L, Gul B, Masri SC. Evolving concepts in diagnosis and management of cardiogenic shock. Am J Cardiol. 2018;122:1104–10.
6. Hochman JS, Buller CE, Sleeper LA, et al. Cardiogenic shock complicating acute myocardial infarction—etiologies, management and outcome: a report from the SHOCK Trial Registry. SHould we emergently revascularize Occluded Coronaries for cardiogenic shocK? J Am Coll Cardiol. 2000;36(3 Suppl A):1063–70.
7. Reynolds HR, Hochman JS. Cardiogenic shock: current concepts and improving outcomes. Circulation. 2008;117:686–97.
8. Harjola VP, Lassus J, Sionis A, et al. Clinical picture and risk prediction of short-term mortality in cardiogenic shock. Eur J Heart Fail. 2015;17:501–9.
9. Ince C. Hemodynamic coherence and the rationale for monitoring the microcirculation. Crit Care. 2015;19:S8.
10. Edul VS, Enrico C, Laviolle B, et al. Quantitative assessment of the microcirculation in healthy volunteers and in patients with septic shock. Crit Care Med. 2012;40:1443–8.
11. Trzeciak S, McCoy JV, Phillip Dellinger R, et al. Early increases in microcirculatory perfusion during protocol-directed resuscitation are associated with reduced multi-organ failure at 24 h in patients with sepsis. Intensive Care Med. 2008;34:2210–7.
12. Jozwiak M, Monnet X, Teboul JL. Less or more hemodynamic monitoring in critically ill patients. Curr Opin Crit Care. 2018;24:309–15.
13. Price S, Platz E, Cullen L, et al. Expert consensus document: echocardiography and lung ultrasonography for the assessment and management of acute heart failure. Nat Rev Cardiol. 2017;14:427–40.
14. De Backer D, Biston P, Devriendt J, et al. Comparison of dopamine and norepinephrine in the treatment of shock. N Engl J Med. 2010;362:779–89.
15. Hamzaoui O, Jozwiak M, Geffriaud T, et al. Norepinephrine exerts an inotropic effect during the early phase of human septic shock. Br J Anesth. 2018;120:517–24.
16. McIntyre WF, Um KJ, Alhazzani W, et al. Association of vasopressin plus catecholamine vasopressors vs catecholamines alone with atrial fibrillation in patients with distributive shock: a systematic review and meta-analysis. JAMA. 2018;319:1889–900.
17. Levy B, Perez P, Perny J, et al. Comparison of norepinephrine-dobutamine to epinephrine for hemodynamics, lactate metabolism, and organ function variables in cardiogenic shock. A prospective, randomized pilot study. Crit Care Med. 2011;39:450–455 48.
18. Tarvasmaki T, Lassus J, Varpula M, et al. Current real-life use of vasopressors and inotropes in cardiogenic shock—adrenaline use is associated with excess organ injury and mortality. Crit Care. 2016;20:208.
19. Levy BC, Clere-Jehl R, Legras A, et al. Epinephrine versus norepinephrine in cardiogenic shock after acute myocardial infarction. J Am Coll Cardiol. 2018;72:173–82.

20. Léopold V, Gayat E, Pirracchio R, et al. Epinephrine and short-term survival in cardiogenic shock: an individual data meta-analysis of 2583 patients. Intensive Care Med. 2018;44: 847–56.
21. Toscani L, Aya HD, Antonakaki D, et al. What is the impact of the fluid challenge technique on diagnosis of fluid responsiveness? A systematic review and meta-analysis. Crit Care. 2017;21:207.
22. Nakamura RE, Vincent JL, Fukushima JT, et al. A liberal strategy of red blood cell transfusion reduces cardiogenic shock in elderly patients undergoing cardiac surgery. J Thorac Cardiovasc Surg. 2015;150:1314–20.
23. Hajjar LA, Fukushima JT, Almeida JP, et al. Strategies to reduce blood transfusion: a Latin-American perspective. Curr Opin Anaesthesiol. 2015;28:81–8.
24. Cecconi M, De Backer D, Antonelli M, et al. Consensus on circulatory shock and hemodynamic monitoring.Task force of the European Society of Intensive Care Medicine. Intensive Care Med. 2014;40:1795–815.
25. Marik PE. Obituary: pulmonary artery catheter 1970 to 2013. Ann Intensive Care. 2013;3:38.
26. De Backer D, Hajjar LA, Pinsky MR. Is there still a place for the Swan–Ganz catheter? We are not sure. Intensive Care Med. 2018;44:960–2.
27. De Backer D, Bakker J, Cecconi M, et al. Alternatives to the Swan-Ganz catheter. Intensive Care Med. 2018;44:730–41.
28. Hochman JS, Sleeper LA, Webb JG, et al. Early revascularization in acute myocardial infarction complicated by cardiogenic shock. SHOCK investigators. Should we emergently revascularize occluded coronaries for cardiogenic shock. N Engl J Med. 1999;341:625–34.
29. Hochman JS, Sleeper LA, Webb JG, et al. Early revascularization and long-term survival in cardiogenic shock complicating acute myocardial infarction. JAMA. 2006;295:2511–5.
30. Thiele H, Akin I, Sandri M, et al. PCI strategies in patients with acute myocardial infarction and cardiogenic shock. N Engl J Med. 2017;377:2419–32.
31. de Waha S, Jobs A, Pöss J, et al. Multivessel versus culprit lesion only percutaneous coronary intervention in cardiogenic shock complicating acute myocardial infarction: a systematic review and meta-analysis. Eur Heart J. 2018;7:28–37.
32. Thiele H, Akin I, Sandri M, et al. One-year outcomes after PCI strategies in cardiogenic shock. N Engl J Med. 2018;379:1699–710.
33. Kapelios CJ, Terrovitis JV, Nanas JN. Current and future applications of the intra-aortic balloon pump. Curr Opin Cardiol. 2014;29:258–65.
34. Thiele H, Zeymer U, Neumann FJ. Intraaortic balloon support for myocardial infarction with cardiogenic shock. N Engl J Med. 2012;367:1287–96.
35. Ibanez B, James S, Agewall S, et al. 2017 ESC Guidelines for the management of acute myocardial infarction in patients presenting with ST-segment elevation. Eur Heart J. 2017;9:119–77.
36. Romeo F, Acconcia MC, Sergi D, et al. The outcome of intra-aortic balloon pump support in acute myocardial infarction complicated by cardiogenic shock according to the type of revascularization: a comprehensive meta-analysis. Am Heart J. 2013;165:679–92.
37. Aso S, Matsui H, Fushimi K, et al. The effect of intraaortic balloon pumping under venoarterial extracorporeal membrane oxygenation on mortality of cardiogenic patients: an analysis using a nationwide inpatient database. Crit Care Med. 2016;44:1974–9.
38. Mandawat A, Rao SV. Percutaneous mechanical circulatory support devices in cardiogenic shock. Circ Cardiovasc Interv. 2017;10:e004337.
39. Thiele H, Sick P, Boudriot E, et al. Randomized comparison of intra-aortic balloon support with a percutaneous left ventricular assist device in patients with revascularized acute myocardial infarction complicated by cardiogenic shock. Eur Heart J. 2005;26:1276–83.
40. Kar B, Gregoric ID, Basra SS, et al. The percutaneous ventricular assist device in severe refractory cardiogenic shock. J Am Coll Cardiol. 2011;57:688–96.
41. Seyfarth M, Sibbing D, Bauer I, et al. A randomized clinical trial to evaluate the safety and efficacy of a percutaneous left ventricular assist device versus intra-aortic balloon pumping for treatment of cardiogenic shock caused by myocardial infarction. J Am Coll Cardiol. 2008;52:1584–8.

42. Ouweneel DM, Eriksen E, Sjauw KD, et al. Percutaneous mechanical circulatory support versus intra-aortic balloon pump in cardiogenic shock after acute myocardial infarction. J Am Coll Cardiol. 2017;69:278–87.
43. Thiele H, Jobs A, Ouweneel DM, et al. Percutaneous short-term active mechanical support devices in cardiogenic shock: a systematic review and collaborative meta-analysis of randomized trials. Eur Heart J. 2017;38:3523–31.
44. Anderson MB, Goldstein J, Milano C, et al. Benefits of a novel percutaneous ventricular assist device for right heart failure: the prospective RECOVER RIGHT study of the Impella RP device. J Heart Lung Transplant. 2015;34:1549–60.
45. Hsu PL, Parker J, Egger C. Mechanical circulatory support for right heart failure: current technology and future outlook. Artif Organs. 2012;36:332–47.
46. Kleeber ME, Haddad EV, Choi CW, et al. Venoarterial extracorporeal membrane oxygenation in cardiogenic shock. JACC Heart Fail. 2018;6:503–16.
47. Maxhera B, Albert A, Ansari E, et al. Survival predictors in ventricular assist device patients with prior extracorporeal life support: selecting appropriate candidates. Artif Organs. 2014;38:727–32.
48. Ouweneel DM, Schotborogh JV, Limpens J, et al. Extracorporeal life support during cardiac arrest and cardiogenic shock: a systematic review and metaanalysis. Intensive Care Med. 2016;42:1922–34.
49. Marasco SF, Lukas G, McDonald M, et al. Review of ECMO (extra corporeal membrane oxygenation) support in critically ill adult patients. Heart Lung Circ. 2008;17(Suppl 4):S41–7.
50. Extracorporeal Life Support Organization (ELSO). Guidelines for adult cardiac failure. https://www.elso.org/Portals/0/IGD/Archive/FileManager/e76ef78eabcusersshyerdocumentselsoguidelinesforadultcardiacfailure1.3.pdf. Accessed 31 Oct 2018.

Sodium Thiosulfate: A New Player for Circulatory Shock and Ischemia/Reperfusion Injury?

14

M. Bauer, P. Radermacher, and M. Wepler

14.1 Introduction

Sodium thiosulfate ($Na_2S_2O_3$) is a cation-chelating agent and has various application areas in the chemical industry, e.g., in processes of water purification and in the mining industry. In medicine, sodium thiosulfate is a recognized drug since its identification as an antidote for minimum lethal doses of sodium cyanide back in 1933 [1]. Sodium thiosulfate acts as a sulfur donor for sulfurtransferase to convert cyanide to thiocyanide, which is less toxic and can be eliminated via the urine. Therefore, sodium thiosulfate still serves as a treatment for cyanide poisoning worldwide. Besides its use as a treatment for cyanide poising, sodium thiosulfate is also used as an antioxidant, has chelating properties, and induces release of hydrogen sulfide (H_2S) and nitric oxide (NO) *in vivo,* causing vasodilation (Fig. 14.1) [2]. Due to these chemical properties, sodium thiosulfate is an accepted drug for the treatment of chronic renal failure-induced calciphylaxis [3] and cisplatin poising [4], and has recently been recognized to lower the incidence of cisplatin-induced hearing loss among children with hepatoblastoma [5]. Furthermore, the anti-oxidant and the H_2S-releasing properties of sodium thiosulfate have prompted a study in patients with acute coronary syndrome (ClinicalTrials.gov Identifiers NCT03017963 and NCT02899364).

M. Bauer
Department of Anesthesiology and Intensive Care Medicine, University Hospital Jena, Jena, Germany

P. Radermacher
Institute for Anesthesiologic Pathophysiology and Process Development, University Hospital Ulm, Ulm, Germany

M. Wepler (✉)
Department of Anesthesiology, University Hospital Ulm, Ulm, Germany
e-mail: martin.wepler@uni-ulm.de

J.-L. Vincent (ed.), *Annual Update in Intensive Care and Emergency Medicine 2019*, Annual Update in Intensive Care and Emergency Medicine,
https://doi.org/10.1007/978-3-030-06067-1_14

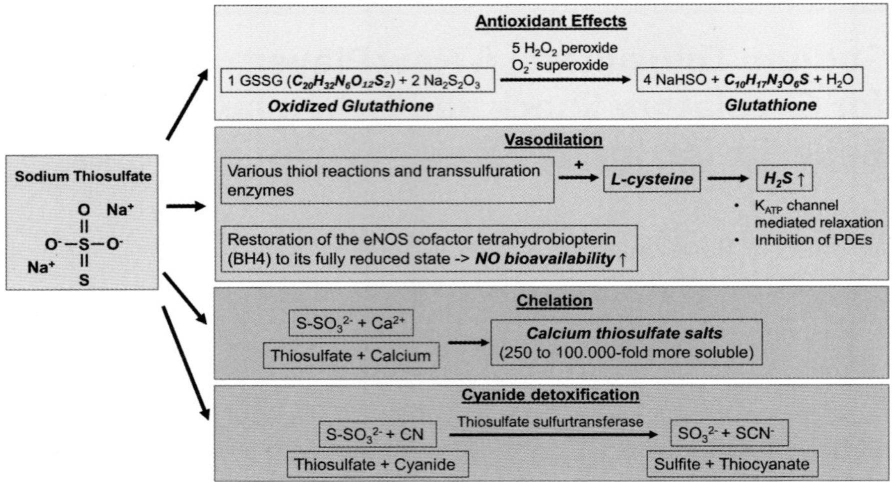

Fig. 14.1 Effects of sodium thiosulfate ($Na_2S_2O_3$, left) in clinical use (right). *GSSG* glutathione disulfide, *H_2S* hydrogen sulfide, *eNOS* endothelial nitric oxide synthase, *NO* nitric oxide, *PDE* phosphodiesterase

H_2S, as one of the three endogenous gaseous mediators, can be produced endogenously by the enzymes cystathionine γ-lyase (CSE), cystathionine β-synthase (CBS) and 3-mercaptopyruvate sulfurtransferase (3-MST) [6] and is metabolized *in vivo* by oxidation to persulfate, thiosulfate, sulfite and sulfate. Thiosulfate ($S_2O_3^{2-}$) is a derivative of the more unstable thiosulfuric acid ($H_2S_2O_3$) and as a sodium salt ($Na_2S_2O_3$) that is significantly more stable and highly water soluble. H_2S can be regenerated from thiosulfate by the enzymes 3-MST or rhodanase (Rde) in the presence of other reducing disulfides such as thioredoxin (Trx) or dihydrolipoic acid (DHLA) [7]. Therefore, sodium thiosulfate acts as a potent H_2S-releasing compound [8], especially under hypoxic conditions [7]. The very short half-life of less than a minute limits the clinical use of H_2S itself and has led to the development and use of H_2S-releasing compounds like GYY4137, hydrogen sulfite (NaHS), or sodium sulfide (Na_2S) with better pharmacokinetic properties. However, these compounds also have certain limitations for clinical use, e.g., toxic adverse effects or a very narrow therapeutic margin [9]. In contrast, the relatively low toxicity, high therapeutic margin and excellent solubility [10] make sodium thiosulfate a favorable H_2S-releasing compound.

14.2 Sodium Thiosulfate Dose-Dependently Affects Mitochondrial Respiration *In Vitro*

At the molecular level, H_2S exerts different effects on mitochondrial respiration, mainly determined by its dose, but also dependent on enzymatic reactions. On the one hand, at high concentrations, H_2S reversibly and competitively binds to mitochondrial complex IV (cytochrome C oxidase), thereby inhibiting the binding of oxygen, resulting in a shutdown of mitochondrial electron transport and cellular ATP generation [6]. At moderate concentrations, it is proposed that H_2S binds to the reduced cytochrome C oxidase active site and acts as a competitive inhibitor of the enzyme. As H_2S competes with cytochrome C oxidase's substrate, O_2, it can be subsequently replaced by O_2. At lower concentrations, H_2S does not compete with the substrate O_2, but can still reduce the active side of cytochrome C oxidase and thus inhibit the enzyme [6]. Therefore, the inhibiting effect of H_2S on mitochondrial complex IV becomes even more relevant under hypoxia. On the other hand, H_2S can serve as a physiological mitochondrial substrate. Its functional effect is comparable to Krebs cycle-derived electron donors, such as nicotinamide adenine dinucleotide (in the reduced form abbreviated as NADH) or flavin adenine dinucleotide (hydroquinone form $FADH_2$) [6]. The enzymes involved in this process are sulfide quinone reductase (SQR), dioxygenase, and sulfurtransferase (rhodanase), which can be summed as the sulfide oxidation unit [6]. Electrons donated from H_2S most likely enter the mitochondrial respiratory chain through the sulfide oxidation unit, a reaction that (1) reduces coenzyme Q and transfers electrons between complex I, II, and III; and (2) releases an oxidized form of sulfur, thiosulfate ($H_2S_2O_3$), with (1) and (2) being reactions that both consume oxygen [6]. Of note, some of these reactions can take place in one direction or the other. When thiosulfate is present or administered, e.g., through sodium thiosulfate, H_2S can be produced from thiosulfate by the enzyme rhodanase. In detail, formation of H_2S from thiosulfate is favored by the oxidation states of the sulfur molecules in thiosulfate, possible most likely due to the presence of sulfur molecules in different oxidation states [11]. Hypoxia increases the reducing conditions of the mitochondrial matrix and, under reducing conditions, H_2S can be generated from thiosulfate in the mitochondria [7]. Therefore, mitochondria are intimately involved in the oxygen-sensing process.

To examine the effects of sodium thiosulfate on mitochondrial respiration, we prepared primary cultures of cortical neurons from fetal rat brains (embryonic day 18; E18). The brains were collected in Hanks' balanced salts solution (HBSS). Tissue of the fronto-temporal cortex was carefully dissected out. Cell suspensions were prepared by treating the tissue with 0.25% trypsin for 20 min at 37 °C, followed by homogenization. After preparation, the cortical neurons were seeded on poly-L-lysine-coated (0.1 mg/mL) culture flasks. The cells were grown in neurobasal medium, complemented with B27 supplement, L-glutamine, and penicillin/streptomycin. Cell culture experiments were performed between day 22–24. Sodium thiosulfate was applied to the cell culture media of primary cortical rat neurons in various doses (4, 20, and 100 mM). Cells were harvested after 4 hours for the assessment of mitochondrial oxygen consumption (JO_2) in terms of ETS capacity (maximum respiratory activity of the electron transfer system in the uncoupled state). The incubation of neuronal cells with sodium thiosulfate *in vitro* showed that the increase in mitochondrial respiration at the uncoupled state was highest at doses of 4 and 20 mM *in vitro* (Fig. 14.2). Expecting a volume of distribution in humans of 15 L and a molecular weight of 158 g/mol of sodium thiosulfate, 4 mM would equal a dose of 0.125 g/kg sodium thiosulfate in adult humans. Indeed, 4 mM of sodium

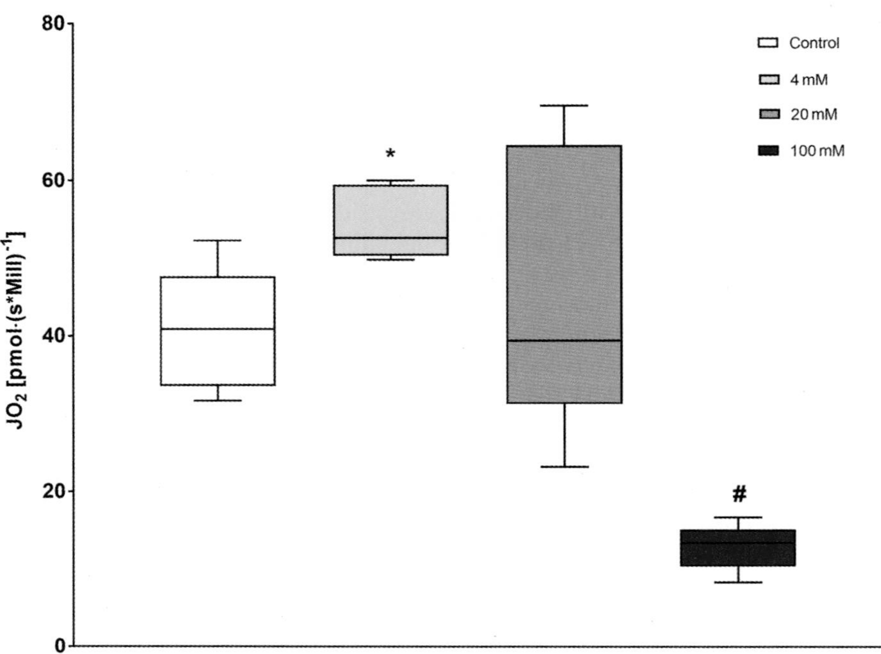

Fig. 14.2 Effects of different concentrations of sodium thiosulfate on mitochondrial respiration (JO_2) in cultured cortical neurons from fetal rat brains. N = 6 measurements in each group. *$p < 0.01$ and #$p < 0.0001$ vs. control (Mann-Whitney-Test between the two groups), respectively. Data are expressed as median and interquartile range

thiosulfate *in vitro* is a rather high dose based on the existing *in vitro* studies (Table 14.1), whereas an *in vivo* dose of roughly 0.125 g/kg sodium thiosulfate is well within the effective and non-toxic range (Table 14.1). Although we cannot finally prove it, it is most likely that sodium thiosulfate at a dose of 4 or 20 mM *in vitro* increases mitochondrial respiration compared to a control group by donating electrons to the respiratory chain at complex I, II, or III, but decreases mitochondrial respiration at higher doses of 100 mM by inhibiting complex IV [6] in a dose-dependent manner (Fig. 14.2).

14.3 Sodium Thiosulfate Exerts Beneficial Effects in Chronic Renal Dysfunction

As mentioned above, sulfate and thiosulfate are metabolites of H_2S. Recently, in a sub-study of the Prevention of Renal and Vascular End-stage Disease (PREVEND) study (n = 6839), it was shown that urinary sulfate, but not thiosulfate, excretion was inversely associated with risk of all-cause mortality [25]. The strong association between sulfate excretion and mortality in the study population emphasizes the importance of sulfate, or its precursor H_2S, on patient outcome. End-stage kidney

Table 14.1 Beneficial effects of sodium thiosulfate in different animal models of acute critical illness

Species	Experimental model	Effect of sodium thiosulfate	References
Models of lung injury			
Mouse	LPS and systemic inflammation (CLP)-induced lung injury	Sodium thiosulfate (2 g/kg i.p. at LPS injection) reduced cytokine levels, lung permeability, histologic lung injury, and ROS production	[12]
Rabbit	Hyperoxia and L-arginine-induced pulmonary hypertension and lung edema in isolated perfused lungs	Reduction in pulmonary hypertension and lung edema by sodium thiosulfate (12 mM)	[13]
Rat	Cisplatin-treated metastatic lung tumor and inoculation of the transitional cell carcinoma into the lung	Sodium thiosulfate (1581 mg/kg i.v. 10 min. after cisplatin administration) induced a better anti-tumor effect than seen in the group given cisplatin alone as evaluated by the number of lung tumor nodules and survival time	[14]
Rat	Model of experimental tuberculosis	Sodium thiosulfate (100 or 150 mg/kg) induced a marked anti-inflammatory and anti-sclerogenic effect, rearrangement of fibrous connective tissue into loose shapeless tissue with increased number of cell elements, changes in the structure of collagen fibers down to granular degeneration, and typical properties of the connective tissues were observed in different periods of tuberculosis development	[15]
Models of ischemia/reperfusion injury			
Rat	Model of isolated heart subjected to ischemia/reperfusion injury	Postconditioning with sodium thiosulfate (1 mM) preserved mitochondrial structure, function, and number, reduction in metabolic demand of the re-perfused heart, reduction in free radical release	[16]
Rat	Model of adenine-induced vascular calcification in combination with heart ischemia/reperfusion injury	Increased infarct size, lactate dehydrogenase, and creatine kinase release in the coronary perfusate and altered hemodynamics as well as mitochondrial dysfunction compared to control rats (without vascular calcification) treated with sodium thiosulfate (400 mg/kg for 28 days) and subjected to ischemia/reperfusion injury; improvement in cardio-protection only when sodium thiosulfate was combined with nicorandil	[17]

(continued)

Table 14.1 (continued)

Species	Experimental model	Effect of sodium thiosulfate	References
Rat	Isolated mitochondria from adenine-induced vascular calcified kidneys, sodium thiosulfate was administered for 28 days before isolation, isolated mitochondria were subjected to oxidative stress by nitrogen gas purging (hypoxia/ischemia/reperfusion injury) to assess mitochondrial recovery	Reduced oxidative stress and augmented mitochondrial enzyme activities in sodium thiosulfate-treated (400 mg/kg) animals	[18]
Rat	Glucose oxidase/catalase-induced apoptosis in cardiomyocytes in vitro, in vivo using both isolated rat heart and intact left anterior descending artery (LAD) occlusion model of ischemia/reperfusion injury	Sodium thiosulfate of 1 mM reduced apoptosis in cardiomyocytes *in vitro*. Isolated rat hearts treated with sodium thiosulfate prior to ischemic/reperfusion injury showed improved hemodynamics and a reduced infarct size. Cardiac fibers from LAD-occluded rat hearts showed less derangement when treated with sodium thiosulfate	[19]
Rat	Myocardial ischemia/reperfusion injury in an isolated heart model	Sodium thiosulfate at a dose of 1 mM given at reperfusion significantly reduced infarct size and showed a reduction of apoptosis as evidenced from decreased activity of caspase-3 in the myocardium, lowered expression of casp-3 and PARP, and showed less DNA fragmentation and histological derangement of fibers compared to the injury control	[20]
Mouse	Global cerebral ischemia/reperfusion injury induced by 40 min of bilateral common carotid artery occlusion with microsurgical clips	Systemic administration of sodium thiosulfate (10 mg/kg i.p.) improved survival and neurological function, which was associated with a marked increase of thiosulfate in plasma and brain tissues and with inhibition of caspase-3 activity by persulfidation at Cys163 in caspase-3	[21]
Dog	Model of experimental tourniquet shock and experimental myocardial infarction	Sodium thiosulfate (500 mg/kg i.v.) augmented hemodynamics under acute circulatory disturbances both in tourniquet shock and myocardial infarction. Sodium thiosulfate increased cardiac discharge, minute blood flow volume, the threshold of ventricular fibrillation, improved the heart work, and decreased and normalized the general peripheral resistance	[22]

Table 14.1 (continued)

Species	Experimental model	Effect of sodium thiosulfate	References
Models of inflammation			
Mouse	LPS-induced systemic inflammation	Dose-dependent improved survival in sodium thiosulfate-treated animals (1 or 2 g/kg i.p. at LPS injection)	[23]
Mouse	Model of acute liver failure induced by D-Galactosamine (GalN, 300 mg/kg) and LPS (1 μg/kg) i.p.	Administration of sodium thiosulfate (2 g/kg i.p. at 30 min before and 3 h after GalN/LPS challenge) attenuated GalN/LPS-induced liver injury via activation of Akt and Nrf2-dependent signaling and inhibition of GalN/LPS-induced JNK phosphorylation in wild-type mice	[24]

LPS lipopolysaccharide, *CLP* cecal-ligation and puncture, *ROS* reactive oxygen species, *i.p.* intraperitoneal, *i.v.* intravenous, *LAD* left anterior descending artery, *PARP* poly [ADP-ribose] polymerase

disease (ESKD), for which renal replacement therapy (RRT) is needed, is a major factor impacting patient outcome. Most patients reach ESKD not because of an acute event, but because of a chronic, gradual decline in kidney function over decades. In most western countries, the primary causes of ESKD are diabetes, hypertension and renal vascular disorders. Renal vascular disorders may be triggered by oxalate and the subsequent formation of calcium oxalate crystals, which can result from excessive nutritional intake (e.g., chocolate or nuts) or pathological overproduction of oxalate (e.g., due to primary hyperoxaluria, enteric hyperoxaluria, or excessive vitamin C ingestion). A renal vascular disorder itself is most likely caused by oxidative stress and antioxidant depletion, which cause a corresponding injury to the renal epithelium. Oxidants, which appear to be mainly mitochondria-derived, could impair the intracellular antioxidant defense system including the activity of superoxide dismutase (SOD). In a rat model of ethylene glycol-induced hyperoxaluria and renal injury, treatment with sodium thiosulfate (0.4 g/kg) preserved renal function by maintaining creatinine clearance. This effect was accompanied by maintained tissue SOD activity in the sodium thiosulfate group. Because sodium thiosulfate is mainly eliminated by the kidney [26] and partially exchanged and metabolized by proximal tubular cells [27], the preserved renal function in the sodium thiosulfate group was potentially mediated via the maintained tissue SOD activity. In general, free radical oxidants are short lived and their very rapid dismutation to H_2O_2 represents one of the major oxidant stresses. The exposure of a porcine proximal tubular kidney cell line in the study by Bijarnia et al. led to a pronounced increase in H_2O_2 [28]. In their study, sodium thiosulfate dose-dependently reduced H_2O_2 levels, which they assume took place according to the chemical reaction: $4H_2O_2 + S_2O_3^{2-} \rightarrow 2SO4^{2-} + 2H^+ + 3H_2O$ [28]. H_2O_2 has previously been shown to promote osteogenic differentiation of vascular smooth muscle cells and thereby to trigger vascular calcification [29]. Sodium thiosulfate can prevent this type of vascular calcification in uremic rats [30], and, recently, endogenous urinary thiosulfate excretion was demonstrated to be associated with a favorable cardiovascular risk profile and a survival benefit of renal transplant recipients [31], which is in line with the association between sulfate excretion and mortality in the subgroup of the PREVEND study [25]. In another study in rats with angiotensin II (Ang II)-induced hypertensive renal disease, treatment with sodium thiosulfate (1 g/kg per day for three weeks) reduced hypertension, proteinuria, oxidative stress and improved renal function (Fig. 14.3 [32]). This study also investigated the effects of NaHS as an H_2S donor. Interestingly, in an *ex vivo* isolated perfused kidney setup, NaHS, but not sodium thiosulfate, reduced intrarenal pressure. Therefore, also in this model, the beneficial effects of sodium thiosulfate are more likely to be related to the antioxidant effects of sodium thiosulfate.

14.4 Sodium Thiosulfate Exerts Beneficial Effects in Acute Models of Ischemia/Reperfusion Injury

In contrast to the above-mentioned chronic organ dysfunctions, acute-on-chronic injuries are of primary concern in the intensive care unit (ICU). For example, hypoxemia and tissue ischemia during hemorrhagic shock trigger systemic hyper-inflammation, which leads to multiorgan failure (MOF) [33]. The restoration of blood

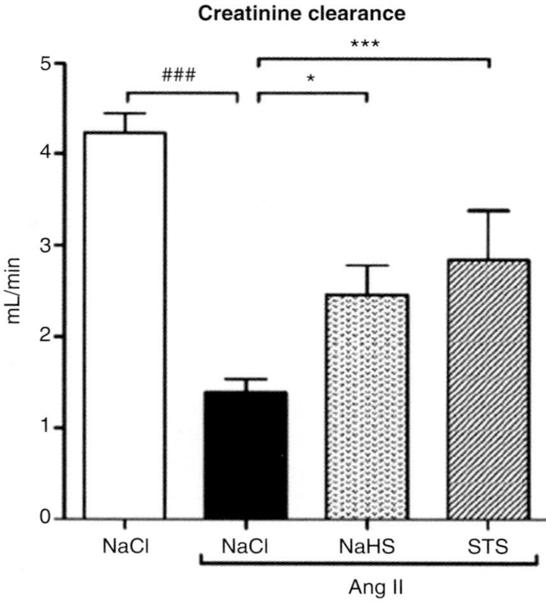

Fig. 14.3 Reduction of renal function loss in sodium hydrosulfate (NaHS) and sodium thiosulfate (STS)-treated rats. Three weeks of angiotensin II (Ang II) infusion decreased renal function as evidenced by a 67% decrease in creatinine clearance. Treatment with NaHS and STS reduced renal function loss by preserving the creatinine clearance. (###$p < 0.001$ vs. control, *$p < 0.05$, ***$p < 0.001$ vs. Ang II + NaCl). From [32] with permission

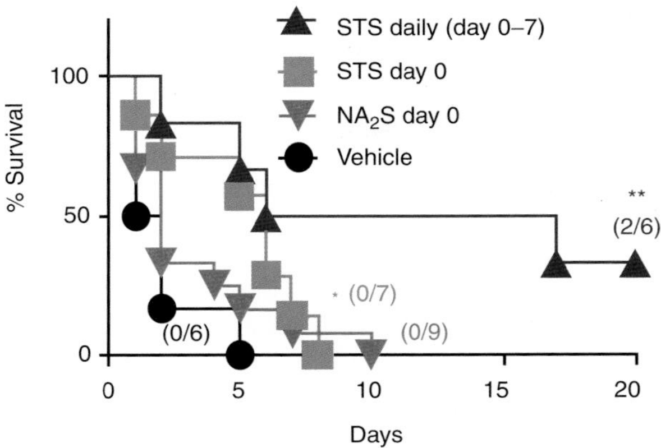

Fig. 14.4 Effects of thiosulfate in brain ischemia/reperfusion injury. Percent survival for 20 days after reperfusion of mice subjected to 40 min of bilateral common carotid artery occlusion (BCAO). Mice were given saline or sodium thiosulfate (STS) at 10 mg/kg intra-peritoneally 1 min after reperfusion or 1 min plus every 24 h after reperfusion for 7 days. n = 6 or 7, $^{**}p < 0.01$. From [21]

flow during resuscitation after hemorrhagic shock represents an ischemia/reperfusion injury, which may further aggravate organ dysfunction by development of acidosis, coagulopathy and systemic inflammation [34], and induces further tissue damage by oxidative stress [35]. H_2S itself has been studied in various models of ischemia/reperfusion injury including myocardial infarction, cerebral ischemia, and transplant-associated renal ischemia (Table 14.1). The beneficial effects are broad and often show end-organ protection, which could lead to a survival benefit (Fig. 14.4) [21]. However, one mechanism of H_2S-related organ protection in animal models of ischemia/reperfusion injury is the reduction in acidosis by lowering lactate levels [34], most likely due to the activation of mitochondrial adenosine triphosphate (ATP)-sensitive potassium channels and, hence, a shift to aerobic glycolysis [36]. Another beneficial effect of H_2S is vasodilation (Fig. 14.1), but this clearly depends on the cause of disease. On the one hand, in a mouse model of intestinal ischemia, H_2S was shown to lower mucosal injury scores due to vasodilatory effects, which improved mesenteric perfusion [37]. On the other hand, in a mouse model of hemorrhagic shock, the vasodilatory effects of H_2S dose-dependently worsened animal outcome [38]. The vasodilatory effects of H_2S are mediated through an interaction with the endothelial NO synthase and its production of the vasodilator, NO [2]. Under physiological conditions, H_2S can dissociate to hydrosulfide (HS^-). The latter reacts with RS-NO (S-nitrosylated cysteine) and releases NO to produce RS-SH (S-sulfhydrated cysteine) via the proposed following reaction: $HS^- + RSNO \rightarrow NO + RS\text{-}SH$ [39]. This reaction would also explain the finding of Altaany et al. that S-sulfhydration can reverse S-nitrosylation but not the other way around. NO cannot interact with the cysteine residue once a stable RS-SH is formed [39].

In addition to organ protective effects due to an increase in aerobic glycolysis and vasodilation, H_2S also acts as a potent antioxidant. H_2S can directly scavenge reactive oxygen species (ROS), increase intracellular glutathione levels, and reduce the amount of ROS produced through modulation of mitochondrial ROS production [40]. Glutathione in its reduced form (GSH) is a very potent intracellular antioxidant, and the ratio of reduced to oxidized glutathione (GSSG) corresponds to the capacity of a cell to attenuate oxidative stress. Thioredoxin also acts as regulator of cellular oxidation/reduction (redox) status and has antioxidant properties, which was shown in mice that were protected against a renal ischemia/reperfusion injury when they over expressed the human thioredoxin gene [41]. In a study by Jha et al., H_2S preserved GSH levels and thioredoxin-1 expression in mice subjected to hepatic ischemia/reperfusion injury [42]. The injury to hepatocytes depends to a great extent on the restoration of oxygen supply upon reperfusion [43]. Therefore, mitochondria as cell organelles, whose function highly depends on oxygen availability, determine cellular fate and death. H_2S can exert potential mito-protective actions at low concentrations, but shows significant toxicity at higher concentrations, e.g., inhibition of the respiratory chain (Fig. 14.2). Also, the very short half-life of H_2S and the disadvantages of common H_2S-releasing compounds, including toxic adverse effects or a very narrow therapeutic margin [9], limit their clinical use. In contrast, the relatively low toxicity, high therapeutic margin and excellent solubility [10] make sodium thiosulfate a favorable H_2S-releasing compound. Therefore, we tested whether administration of sodium thiosulfate can serve as a strategy to achieve the mitochondrial protection observed with donors of H_2S, but with a substantially improved safety profile. CSE knockout mice ($CSE^{-/-}$) and wild-type controls ($CSE^{+/+}$) were studied using a standardized hepatic ischemia/reperfusion injury model. Ischemia was induced in the left lateral lobe of the liver by clamping the branch of the hepatic artery and portal vein using a microaneurysm clamp. This procedure resulted in a segmental (30%) ischemia. After 1 h, the clamp was removed to initiate reperfusion. The reperfusion time points were set to 1 h or 24 h. In this model, we investigated the effect of sodium thiosulfate on hepatic ischemia/reperfusion injury *in vivo* using intravital microscopy to analyze the early ischemia/reperfusion injury in $CSE^{-/-}$ and $CSE^{+/+}$ mice. Sodium thiosulfate (0.0456 g/kg) injected into the tail vein 10 min before the onset of reperfusion led to a significant recovery of mitochondrial granularity in the $CSE^{+/+}$ group at the beginning of reperfusion (60 min). This effect was also detected at the end of reperfusion (120 min) for both genotypes ($CSE^{-/-}$ and $CSE^{+/+}$ mice). In a further experiment, mice underwent 6 h or 24 h reperfusion in order to analyze the degree of necrosis and hepatocyte injury. Sodium thiosulfate caused a significant reduction of plasma alanine aminotransferase (ALT) levels in $CSE^{+/+}$ mice after 6 h and in $CSE^{-/-}$ mice after 24 h. After treatment with sodium thiosulfate, $CSE^{-/-}$ mice exhibited a significant reduction in necrotic areas (47%). This effect was not significant in $CSE^{+/+}$ mice. However, a reduction (from 28% to 17%) was detected, underlining the potential therapeutic value of sodium thiosulfate for the treatment of hepatic ischemia/reperfusion injury (unpublished data).

14.5 Sodium Thiosulfate Improves Lung Function in a Porcine Model of Hemorrhagic Shock

Whereas *in vitro* and small animal studies, with the possibility of examining the effects of a certain gene (e.g., by studying knockout mice) are generally used to study specific mechanisms more in detail, larger animal models are more able to mimic clinical scenarios, in part due to human-sized animals and the possibility to more reliably use invasive measurements of organ function and resuscitation methods. We therefore established a porcine model of hemorrhagic shock [9] to study the effects of post-shock treatment with sodium thiosulfate. As stated above, systemic hyperinflammation due to hypoxemia and tissue ischemia during hemorrhagic shock increases the risk of MOF [33]. The ischemia/reperfusion injury during restoration of blood flow may further aggravate tissue damage by oxidative stress [35]. Acute respiratory failure leads to hypox(em)ia, which can further enhance systemic inflammation [44]. Increasing H_2S availability has been shown to be protective in various shock models, in particular after acute lung injury (ALI) and/or ischemic/reperfusion injury [45, 46], in part due to better maintenance or even improved mitochondrial function. However, as stated above, older as well as newly developed H_2S-releasing compounds still have potential drawbacks including a very narrow dosing and time window (Na_2S [9]) or hemodynamic adverse effects (AP39 [38]). To our knowledge, sodium thiosulfate has been studied in two mouse models of systemic inflammation-induced ALI [12, 23] (Table 14.1), but large animal studies are still missing. Therefore, in a randomized, controlled, blinded experimental study, we tested the effects of sodium thiosulfate in an established porcine *in vivo* model of hemorrhagic shock. Anesthetized, mechanically ventilated, and surgically instrumented hypercholesterolemic pigs with preexisting coronary artery disease underwent 3 h of hemorrhagic shock (removal of 30% of the calculated blood volume and subsequent titration of mean arterial blood pressure [MAP] $\approx 40\,\text{mmHg}$). This animal strain is of particular importance while studying H_2S-releasing compounds like sodium thiosulfate, because these animals have reduced expression of the H_2S producing enzyme, CSE, in coronary arteries and therefore can be considered as a large animal analogy to CSE-knockout mice [47]. Post-shock resuscitation (72 h) in our large animal model of hemorrhagic shock comprised re-transfusion of shed blood, crystalloids (balanced electrolyte solution) and norepinephrine support. Pigs were randomly assigned to "treatment" (0.1 g/kg/h intravenous sodium thiosulfate [Köhler Chemie, Bensheim, Germany] for 24 h after post-shock resuscitation) and "vehicle" (same amount of 0.9% intravenous sodium chloride for 24 h after post-shock resuscitation).

Animals that were treated with sodium thiosulfate during resuscitation from hemorrhagic shock had improved gas exchange expressed as the Horovitz-Index compared to the vehicle-treated animals (Fig. 14.5a). Additionally, lung mechanics expressed as positive end-expiratory pressure (PEEP) values were preserved in sodium thiosulfate-treated animals (Fig. 14.5b). Strikingly, this effect was only manifest when standard treatment had been resumed, i.e., after the sodium thiosulfate infusion had already been stopped. We also measured sulfide concentrations in whole swine blood by gas chromatography–mass spectrometry [48] before, during, and after hemorrhagic shock with resuscitation. Sodium thiosulfate (0.1 g/kg/h intravenously) led to a significant increase in blood sulfide concentrations at the end of the sodium thiosulfate treatment (Fig. 14.5c) compared to the vehicle-treated animals.

In rodents, H_2S itself is known to diminish lung injury [49], at least in part due to cytoprotective effects by reducing systemic inflammation [23, 50]. In 2014,

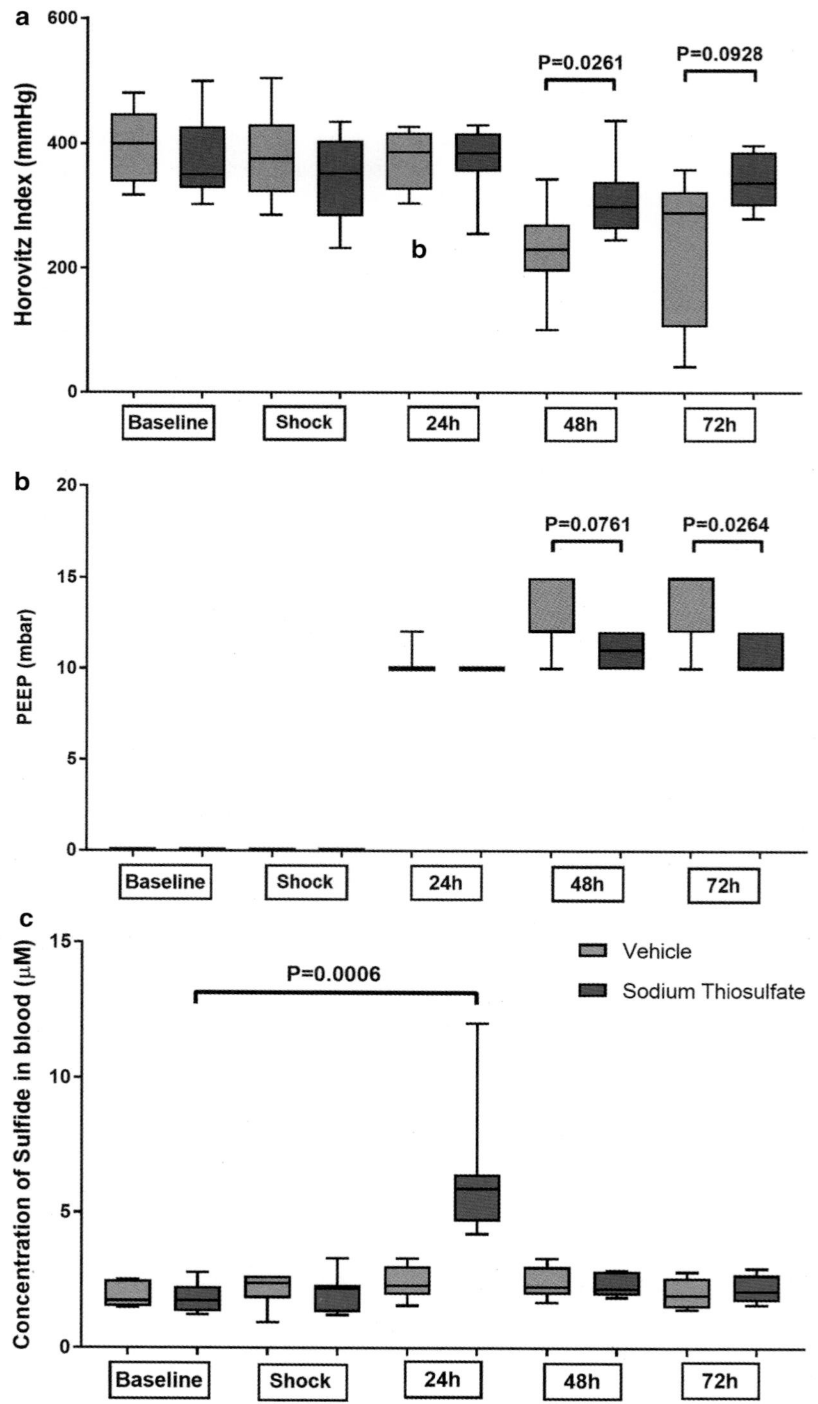
a
Horovitz Index (mmHg)
600
400
200
0
P=0.0261
P=0.0928
b
Baseline
Shock
24h
48h
72h
b
PEEP (mbar)
20
15
10
5
0
P=0.0761
P=0.0264
Baseline
Shock
24h
48h
72h
c
Concentration of Sulfide in blood (μM)
15
10
5
0
P=0.0006
Vehicle
Sodium Thiosulfate
Baseline
Shock
24h
48h
72h

Sakaguchi et al. studied the effects of sodium thiosulfate in a mouse model of lipopolysaccharide (LPS)-induced ALI [12]. In their study, mice were challenged with 2 mg/kg LPS intratracheally and treated with sodium thiosulfate (2 g/kg) at 0 and 12 h after intratracheal LPS. Sodium thiosulfate significantly decreased the influx of cells into the alveolar space as well as myeloperoxidase levels in mice challenged with LPS. By measuring bronchoalveolar lavage (BAL) fluid protein content and lung wet-dry weight ratio, Sakaguchi et al. also showed that sodium thiosulfate attenuated the pulmonary vascular leakage and lung edema in LPS-challenged mice. Furthermore, sodium thiosulfate exerted anti-inflammatory effects by reducing cytokine levels in lung tissue. The anti-inflammatory effects of sodium thiosulfate are most likely mediated through an inhibition of LPS-induced activation of nuclear factor-kappa B (NF-κB) signaling by inhibiting IκB phosphorylation [12]. This is consistent with the hypothesis that sulfide also exerts anti-inflammatory effects via inhibition of NF-κB. Sodium thiosulfate administration in the study by Sakaguchi et al. led to an increase in plasma sulfide levels in mice challenged with LPS or saline (56 ± 16 μM and 46 ± 22 μM, respectively) [12]. Sakaguchi et al. also measured levels of sulfide in human umbilical vein endothelial cells (HUVEC) and observed that sodium thiosulfate increased intracellular sulfide levels within 2 h after the start of incubation of HUVEC with LPS and sodium thiosulfate. Since LPS triggered NF-κB activation within 1 h, and sodium thiosulfate markedly inhibited NF-κB activation, their data suggest that the anti-inflammatory effects of sodium thiosulfate are primarily mediated by intracellular sulfide converted from sodium thiosulfate [12]. The proposed hypotheses that the *in vivo* effects of sodium thiosulfate are mediated by intracellular effects is further supported by the finding that thiosulfate can be converted to H_2S via 3-MST, which is expressed in the vascular endothelium.

Fig. 14.5 (**a**) Gas exchange expressed as the Horovitz-Index; (**b**) lung mechanics expressed as positive end-expiratory pressure (PEEP) values; and (**c**) concentration of sulfide in whole blood. Gas exchange expressed as the Horovitz-Index (**a**) is preserved in animals treated with sodium thiosulfate at 48 h after hemorrhagic shock ($n = 10$) when compared to vehicle-treated animals ($n = 9$). Lung mechanics expressed as PEEP values (**b**) are preserved in animals treated with sodium thiosulfate at 72 h after hemorrhagic shock ($n = 10$) when compared to vehicle-treated animals ($n = 9$). Concentration of sulfide in whole blood is increased at the end of the 24 h treatment with sodium thiosulfate ($n = 7$) compared to vehicle-treatment ($n = 6$). Time is expressed as hours (h) after reperfusion following hemorrhagic shock with start of therapy. It should be noted that baseline and shock PEEP were set to zero with a fraction of inspired oxygen concentration (FiO_2) of 21% to mimic a clinical scenario where the patient would be treated first after the injury. At start of reperfusion, FiO_2 was set to 30% and PEEP to 10 mbar, because swine are particularly susceptible to atelectasis formation due to the lack of alveolar collateral ventilation. During resuscitation, PEEP was adjusted according to the arterial partial pressure of oxygen (PaO_2/FiO_2 <300 or <200 mmHg, I/E ratio was increased to 1:1, and PEEP increased to 12 or 15 mbar, respectively) [9, 36, 47]. Data are expressed as median and interquartile range

14.6 Conclusion

The therapeutic use of the gaseous transmitter H_2S is highly limited in clinical settings due to its narrow therapeutic window and potential toxic adverse effects at high concentrations. Sodium thiosulfate ($Na_2S_2O_3$) is an approved and recognized drug that is used to treat cyanide poisoning, chronic renal failure-induced calciphylaxis, cisplatin overdosing, and has recently been recognized to lower the incidence of cisplatin-induced hearing loss among children with hepatoblastoma. The results of our present studies show that: (1) sodium thiosulfate is a potent mediator of mitochondrial respiration *in vitro*; (2) sodium thiosulfate offers potential as a drug to treat hepatic ischemia/reperfusion injury, e.g., during tumor surgery and hemorrhagic shock; and (3) sodium thiosulfate attenuates lung injury that develops after resuscitation from hemorrhagic shock, most likely involving a sulfur/H_2S-dependent mechanism.

In conclusion, sodium thiosulfate, as a non-toxic, clinically applicable donor of H_2S, should be considered as a new therapeutic approach for the treatment of critical care diseases involving an ischemia/reperfusion injury, as in the currently ongoing study in patients with acute coronary syndrome, and, due to our preliminary results, especially in critical care involving ischemia/reperfusion injury of the liver or lung.

Acknowledgements Supported by the CRC1149, the German MoD, and an unrestricted grant by Köhler Chemie.

References

1. Chen KK, Rose CL. Nitrite and thiosulfate therapy in cyanide poisoning. JAMA. 1952;2:113–9.
2. Szabo C, Papapetropoulos A. International Union of Basic and Clinical Pharmacology. CII: Pharmacological modulation of H2S levels: H2S donors and H2S biosynthesis inhibitors. Pharmacol Rev. 2017;4:497–564.
3. Nigwekar SU, Thadhani R, Brandenburg VM. Calciphylaxis. N Engl J Med. 2018;4:399–400.
4. Tsang RY, Al-Fayea T, Au HJ. Cisplatin overdose: toxicities and management. Drug Saf. 2009;12:1109–22.
5. Brock PR, Maibach R, Childs M, et al. Sodium thiosulfate for protection from cisplatin-induced hearing loss. N Engl J Med. 2018;25:2376–85.
6. Szabo C, Ransy C, Módis K, et al. Regulation of mitochondrial bioenergetic function by hydrogen sulfide. Part I. Biochemical and physiological mechanisms. Br J Pharmacol. 2014;8:2099–122.
7. Olson KR, Deleon ER, Gao Y, et al. Thiosulfate: a readily accessible source of hydrogen sulfide in oxygen sensing. Am J Physiol Regul Integr Comp Physiol. 2013;6:R592–603.
8. Snijder PM, Frenay AR, de Boer RA, et al. Exogenous administration of thiosulfate, a donor of hydrogen sulfide, attenuates angiotensin II-induced hypertensive heart disease in rats. Br J Pharmacol. 2015;6:1494–504.
9. Bracht H, Scheuerle A, Gröger M, et al. Effects of intravenous sulfide during resuscitated porcine hemorrhagic shock. Crit Care Med. 2012;7:2157–67.
10. Salmhofer H, Franzen M, Hitzl W, et al. Multi-modal treatment of calciphylaxis with sodium-thiosulfate, cinacalcet and sevelamer including long-term data. Kidney Blood Press Res. 2013;4–5:346–59.
11. Vairavamurthy A, Manowitz B, Luther GW, Jeon Y. Oxidation state of sulfur in thiosulfate and implications for anaerobic energy metabolism. Geochim Cosmochim Acta. 1993;7:1619–23.

12. Sakaguchi M, Marutani E, Shin HS, et al. Sodium thiosulfate attenuates acute lung injury in mice. Anesthesiology. 2014;6:1248–57.
13. Nozik-Grayck E, Piantadosi CA, van Adelsberg J, Alper SL, Huang YC. Protection of perfused lung from oxidant injury by inhibitors of anion exchange. Am J Phys. 1997;2. (Pt 1:L296–304.
14. Iwamoto Y, Aoki K, Kawano T, Baba T. Upper hemibody infusion of cis-diamminedichloroplatinum (II) followed by systemic antidote, sodium thiosulfate, for lung metastasis in rats. Clin Exp Metastasis. 1984;3:261–70.
15. Novoselova VP, Andrzheiuk NI. Vliianie tiosul'fata natriia na morfologicheskie proiavleniia eksperimental'nogo tuberkuleza. Arkh Patol. 1983;6:67–73.
16. Ravindran S, Kurian GA. Effect of sodium thiosulfate postconditioning on ischemia-reperfusion injury induced mitochondrial dysfunction in rat heart. J Cardiovasc Transl Res. 2018;3:246–58.
17. Ravindran S, Ramachandran K, Kurian GA. Sodium thiosulfate mediated cardioprotection against myocardial ischemia-reperfusion injury is defunct in rat heart with co-morbidity of vascular calcification. Biochimie. 2018;147:80–8.
18. Mohan D, Balasubramanian ED, Ravindran S, Kurian GA. Renal mitochondria can withstand hypoxic/ischemic injury secondary to renal failure in uremic rats pretreated with sodium thiosulfate. Indian J Pharmacol. 2017;4:317–21.
19. Ravindran S, Boovarahan SR, Shanmugam K, Vedarathinam RC, Kurian GA. Sodium thiosulfate preconditioning ameliorates ischemia/reperfusion injury in rat hearts via reduction of oxidative stress and apoptosis. Cardiovasc Drugs Ther. 2017;5–6:511–24.
20. Ravindran S, Jahir Hussain S, Boovarahan SR, Kurian GA. Sodium thiosulfate post-conditioning protects rat hearts against ischemia reperfusion injury via reduction of apoptosis and oxidative stress. Chem Biol Interact. 2017;274:24–34.
21. Marutani E, Yamada M, Ida T, et al. Thiosulfate mediates cytoprotective effects of hydrogen sulfide against neuronal ischemia. J Am Heart Assoc. 2015;11:e002125.
22. Oksman TM, Levandovskii IV, Epishin IN, Vrana M, Blazhek Z. Sodium thiosulfate in the treatment of early postischemic disorders. Biull Eksp Biol Med. 1981;9:275–8.
23. Tokuda K, Kida K, Marutani E, et al. Inhaled hydrogen sulfide prevents endotoxin-induced systemic inflammation and improves survival by altering sulfide metabolism in mice. Antioxid Redox Signal. 2012;1:11–21.
24. Shirozu K, Tokuda K, Marutani E, Lefer D, Wang R, Ichinose F. Cystathionine γ-lyase deficiency protects mice from galactosamine/lipopolysaccharide-induced acute liver failure. Antioxid Redox Signal. 2014;2:204–16.
25. van den Born JC, Frenay ARS, Koning AM, et al. Urinary excretion of sulfur metabolites and risk of cardiovascular events and all-cause mortality in the general population. Antioxid Redox Signal. 2018 Jul 25. https://doi.org/10.1089/ars.2017.7040. [Epub ahead of print].
26. Farese S, Stauffer E, Kalicki R, et al. Sodium thiosulfate pharmacokinetics in hemodialysis patients and healthy volunteers. Clin J Am Soc Nephrol. 2011;6:1447–55.
27. Ullrich KJ, Rumrich G, Kloss S. Bidirectional active transport of thiosulfate in the proximal convolution of the rat kidney. Pflugers Arch. 1980;2:127–32.
28. Bijarnia RK, Bachtler M, Chandak PG, van Goor H, Pasch A. Sodium thiosulfate ameliorates oxidative stress and preserves renal function in hyperoxaluric rats. PLoS One. 2015;4:e0124881.
29. Byon CH, Javed A, Dai Q, et al. Oxidative stress induces vascular calcification through modulation of the osteogenic transcription factor Runx2 by AKT signaling. J Biol Chem. 2008;22:15319–27.
30. Pasch A, Schaffner T, Huynh-Do U, Frey BM, Frey FJ, Farese S. Sodium thiosulfate prevents vascular calcifications in uremic rats. Kidney Int. 2008;11:1444–53.
31. van den Berg E, Pasch A, Westendorp WH, et al. Urinary sulfur metabolites associate with a favorable cardiovascular risk profile and survival benefit in renal transplant recipients. J Am Soc Nephrol. 2014;6:1303–12.
32. Snijder PM, Frenay A-RS, Koning AM, et al. Sodium thiosulfate attenuates angiotensin II-induced hypertension, proteinuria and renal damage. Nitric Oxide. 2014;42:87–98.

33. Cannon JW. Hemorrhagic shock. N Engl J Med. 2018;4:370–9.
34. Satterly SA, Salgar S, Hoffer Z, et al. Hydrogen sulfide improves resuscitation via non-hibernatory mechanisms in a porcine shock model. J Surg Res. 2015;1:197–210.
35. Eltzschig HK, Eckle T. Ischemia and reperfusion—from mechanism to translation. Nat Med. 2011;11:1391–401.
36. Simon F, Giudici R, Duy CN, et al. Hemodynamic and metabolic effects of hydrogen sulfide during porcine ischemia/reperfusion injury. Shock. 2008;4:359–64.
37. Jensen AR, Drucker NA, Khaneki S, Ferkowicz MJ, Markel TA. Hydrogen sulfide improves intestinal recovery following ischemia by endothelial nitric oxide-dependent mechanisms. Am J Physiol Gastrointest Liver Physiol. 2017;5:G450–6.
38. Wepler M, Merz T, Wachter U, et al. The mitochondria-targeted H2S-donor AP39 in a murine model of combined hemorrhagic shock and blunt chest trauma. Shock. 2018. Jun 20. https://doi.org/10.1097/SHK.0000000000001210. [Epub ahead of print].
39. Altaany Z, Ju Y, Yang G, Wang R. The coordination of S-sulfhydration, S-nitrosylation, and phosphorylation of endothelial nitric oxide synthase by hydrogen sulfide. Sci Signal. 2014;342:ra87.
40. Bos EM, Wang R, Snijder PM, et al. Cystathionine γ-lyase protects against renal ischemia/reperfusion by modulating oxidative stress. J Am Soc Nephrol. 2013;5:759–70.
41. Kasuno K, Nakamura H, Ono T, Muso E, Yodoi J. Protective roles of thioredoxin, a redox-regulating protein, in renal ischemia/reperfusion injury. Kidney Int. 2003;4:1273–82.
42. Jha S, Calvert JW, Duranski MR, Ramachandran A, Lefer DJ. Hydrogen sulfide attenuates hepatic ischemia-reperfusion injury: role of antioxidant and antiapoptotic signaling. Am J Physiol Heart Circ Physiol. 2008;2:H801–6.
43. Paxian M, Bauer I, Rensing H, et al. Recovery of hepatocellular ATP and "pericentral apoptosis" after hemorrhage and resuscitation. FASEB J. 2003;9:993–1002.
44. Eltzschig HK, Carmeliet P. Hypoxia and inflammation. N Engl J Med. 2011;7:656–65.
45. Ikeda K, Marutani E, Hirai S, Wood ME, Whiteman M, Ichinose F. Mitochondria-targeted hydrogen sulfide donor AP39 improves neurological outcomes after cardiac arrest in mice. Nitric Oxide. 2015;49:90–6.
46. Ahmad A, Szabo C. Both the H_2S biosynthesis inhibitor aminooxyacetic acid and the mitochondrially targeted H_2S donor AP39 exert protective effects in a mouse model of burn injury. Pharmacol Res. 2016;113(Pt A):348–55.
47. Merz T, Stenzel T, Nussbaum B, et al. Cardiovascular disease and resuscitated septic shock lead to the downregulation of the H_2S-producing enzyme cystathionine-gamma-lyase in the porcine coronary artery. Intensive Care Med Exp. 2017;5:17.
48. McCook O, Radermacher P, Volani C, et al. H_2S during circulatory shock: some unresolved questions. Nitric Oxide. 2014;41:48–61.
49. Francis RC, Vaporidi K, Bloch KD, Ichinose F, Zapol WM. Protective and detrimental effects of sodium sulfide and hydrogen sulfide in murine ventilator-induced lung injury. Anesthesiology. 2011;5:1012–21.
50. Whiteman M, Li L, Rose P, Tan CH, Parkinson DB, Moore PK. The effect of hydrogen sulfide donors on lipopolysaccharide-induced formation of inflammatory mediators in macrophages. Antioxid Redox Signal. 2010;10:1147–54.

15 Lactate in Critically Ill Patients: At the Crossroads Between Perfusion and Metabolism

M. Greco, A. Messina, and M. Cecconi

15.1 Introduction: Lactate in Shock

Lactic acidosis is a common finding in critically ill patients, including patients with septic shock, cardiogenic or hypovolemic shock, trauma and liver failure [1–3]. In these conditions, hyperlactatemia occurs when production of lactic acid significantly exceeds lactate consumption. Lactate levels have been associated with patient outcomes in a large number of studies, either at patient admission or presentation or during the course of recovery [3–5]. In a study including more than 10,000 patients with septic shock, peak lactate concentration was associated with a near linear increase in patient mortality [6]. Outcome prediction was confirmed not only for absolute lactate values, but change in serum lactate levels was also independently associated with mortality [4].

The pivotal importance of lactate for the clinician resides in the possibility to use it as a target to guide resuscitation in patients with shock, or as a marker for early recognition of tissue hypoperfusion and worse prognosis, prompting immediate treatment. Lactate measurement is also easy and fast to obtain using point-of-care testing (most arterial blood gas analyzers offer the possibility to measure lactate). For this reason, current sepsis guidelines recommend using lactate as a target for resuscitation in patients with septic shock [7]. However, despite the unquestioned association between lactate and prognosis in critical care patients, clinical interpretation of lactate elevation is difficult.

By classic teaching, an increase in lactate is generally perceived as an increase in production due to a shift toward anaerobic metabolism related to reduced organ perfusion. However, in critical care patients, measured lactate levels are the sum of

M. Greco · A. Messina · M. Cecconi (✉)
Department of Anesthesia and Intensive Care,
Humanitas Clinical and Research Center - IRCCS, Milan, Italy
e-mail: maurizio.cecconi@hunimed.eu

J.-L. Vincent (ed.), *Annual Update in Intensive Care and Emergency Medicine 2019*, Annual Update in Intensive Care and Emergency Medicine,
https://doi.org/10.1007/978-3-030-06067-1_15

several metabolic and catabolic processes, and lactate elevation may be due to an increase in production or a reduction in clearance. In addition, lactate can be elevated in critically ill patients without necessarily being related to tissue dysoxia [8]. Lactate clearance is a common but imprecise term to refer to lactate metabolism, because lactate is a molecule widely produced, and metabolized by several organs. Like glucose, it is at the crossroads of several metabolic pathways [9, 10].

15.2 Lactate Metabolism

The correct interpretation of lactate synthesis and excretion is crucial to avoid misunderstandings regarding lactate increase in the blood. Lactatemia (the concentration of lactate in the blood) reflects the balance between production and consumption of lactate. As a physiological consequence, for the same etiological mechanism determining an increase in lactate, one can either observe hyperlactatemia (if metabolism decreases) or normolactatemia [11].

15.2.1 Synthesis

The normal daily production of about 1500 mmol of lactate is mainly determined by the metabolism of different organs, such as muscles (25%), the skin (25%), the brain (20%), the intestine (10%) and red blood cells (20%), which are devoid of mitochondria [11]. Lactate is produced according to the following cytoplasmic reaction:

$$\text{Pyruvate} + \text{NADH} + \text{H}^+ \leftrightarrow \text{Lactate} + \text{NAD}^+$$

This biochemical reaction promotes lactate formation, causing a ten-fold lactate/pyruvate ratio. Hence, the lactate increase in the blood is due to pyruvate production exceeding its utilization by the mitochondria. Because the pyruvate is essentially produced via glycolysis, any increase in glycolysis, regardless of its origin, can cause lactatemia. Pyruvate is principally metabolized into the mitochondria by means of the aerobic oxidation pathway, using the Krebs cycle. This reaction is extremely efficient in terms of energetic performance, leading to the production of 36 molecules of ATP for one molecule of pyruvate:

$$\text{Pyruvate} + \text{CoA} + \text{NAD} \rightarrow \text{acetyl-CoA} + \text{NADH} + \text{H}^+ + \text{CO}_2$$

The synthesis of lactate in the cell is dependent on the ATP/ADP and NADH/NAD ratios, which are both related to the oxygen utilization in the mitochondria. In fact, hypoxia inhibits mitochondrial oxidative phosphorylation [12], leading to a decrease in the ATP/ADP ratio and an increase in the NADH/NAD ratio. This metabolic condition inhibits both the pyruvate carboxylase (converting pyruvate into oxaloacetate) and the pyruvate dehydrogenase (converting pyruvate into acetyl-CoA). When the physiological pathway of pyruvate use is affected by alterations in the redox potential of the cell, the excess pyruvate concentration is shifted to lactate production and to the less efficient anaerobic glycolysis.

However, not just the increase in the NADH/NAD ratio, but also a drop in cytosolic pH triggers an increase in the lactate/pyruvate ratio. In fact, from the first equation:

$$\text{Pyruvate} + \text{NADH} + \text{H}^+ \leftrightarrow \text{Lactate} + \text{NAD}^+$$

at equilibrium:

$$\text{Lactate / pyruvate} = K\left(\text{dissociation constant}\right) \times \left(\text{NADH / NAD}\right) \times \text{H}^+$$

Hence, changing the H^+ concentration affects the lactate/pyruvate ratio. The use of this NADH/NAD ratio has been proposed to distinguish hypoxia-related hyperlactatemia from hyperlactataemia resulting from an increase in glycolytic flux without hypoxic stress [13, 14].

15.2.2 Metabolism

The metabolism of the lactate produced in the mitochondria follows different biochemical pathways:

1. transformed into oxaloacetate or alanine via the pyruvate pathway;
2. consumed directly by periportal hepatocytes (60%) to produce glycogen and glucose (neoglycogenesis and neoglucogenesis via the Cori cycle). Neoglucogenesis is associated with a lower energetic efficiency (two ATP molecules produced per molecule of glucose to generate lactate, while six molecules of ATP are consumed for every molecule of glucose generated from lactate). However, this process allows the liver to use the ATP generated by fatty acid beta-oxidation to produce glucose. Moreover, this pathway has been shown to be a pivotal mechanism by which various tissues share an energetic substrate as a common source of carbons for oxidation, the so-called "lactate shuttle" theory [11];
3. the cortex of the kidney also participates in the metabolism of lactate (30%). The threshold of renal excretion is about 5–6 mmol/L, implying that, within the physiological range of blood concentration, lactate is not actually excreted in the urine.

Elevated lactate levels are the net effect of an increase in lactate production from organs and a reduction in metabolism by liver, kidney and muscle. The interaction of these aspects in critical care conditions varies widely, and is still a matter of debate.

15.3 Lactate in Septic Shock

In septic shock patients, there is a mismatch between oxygen demand and oxygen consumption, leading to tissue hypoxia. With tissue hypoxia, mitochondrial oxidation ceases to work, leading to a switch toward lactate hyperproduction and underutilization. There is overwhelming evidence on the association between lactate and mortality in this condition and, as a paradigm, this has been related to oxygen debt [15]. However, the classic view of reduced hypoxia as the sole cause of tissue hypoperfusion has been challenged in recent years [16]. When athletes are subjected to life-threatening hypoxia (e.g., on the summit of Mouth Everest), lactate levels may be normal or only slightly elevated [17]. A reduction in lactate following acute exposure to hypoxia at high altitude in climbers has been described as the "lactate paradox", first described in 1930 [18].

Two studies have demonstrated that peripheral muscle tissue is not subject to hypoxia in septic shock patients. Boekstegers et al. measured a higher oxygen level in muscle tissue from patients with sepsis than from healthy patients. Unexpectedly, tissue oxygen levels were increased -not decreased- with increasing severity of sepsis [19]. Similarly, a microdialysis study showed an increased concentration of lactate and normal oxygen tension in muscle tissue from septic shock patients [20]. Thus, a reduction in oxygen delivery and consequent switch to anaerobiosis are not the sole factors responsible for lactate production in sepsis. In this case, when glycolysis rate exceeds mitochondrial capacity due to hypoxia, tissue lactate levels increase. However, at least two other processes are implicated [21]. The first is increased lactate levels due to increased aerobic glycolysis in skeletal muscle, through β2-receptor stimulation. Increased epinephrine release in shock states could stimulate sarcolemmal Na+/K+ ATPase, enhancing lactate production in muscle. In the study by Levy et al., inhibition of Na+/K+ ATPase normalized muscular lactate levels in septic shock patients [20]. These data were confirmed by a study by Ronco et al., in which no association was demonstrated between arterial lactate concentration and oxygen delivery (DO_2) in a physiological study on patients with sepsis [22]. The shift in metabolism related to epinephrine production can play a significant role in lactate production [23].

A second process is related to decreased lactate metabolism secondary to regional hypoperfusion and hypoxia or organ dysfunction. While this latter mechanism may be a major contributor to elevated lactate levels in the first phases of shock, more often it is involved later on, after the primary phase of resuscitation. In patients with hyperlactatemia at 24 h from the initial signs of shock, there is usually 'normal' production with decreased clearance of lactate [10].

15.4 Lactate and Organ Metabolism in Sepsis

The liver is responsible for 60% of lactate clearance. Despite this, a failure in liver metabolism is deemed responsible for elevated lactate level in sepsis only in case of hepatic ischemia and advanced cirrhosis [24]. Alterations in liver flow, more than in liver function, may be responsible for the overall increase in lactate. Liver or splanchnic hypoperfusion may indeed persist despite global hyperdynamic flow status. Organ dysfunction due to sepsis or sepsis-related hypoperfusion may modify metabolism to the point of transforming the liver, the principal organ for lactate metabolism, to a lactate-producing organ during sepsis [25]. When comparing different animal models of shock, van Genderen et al. demonstrated that regional perfusion was in a certain measure independent from cardiac output and hyperdynamic flow. Perfusion deficit was normalized by an increase in cardiac output in other models, but persisted in the sepsis model [26]. To distinguish between an increase in production of lactate or a decrease in clearance, Levraut et al. assessed hepatic clearance by infusing lactate (1 mmol/kg) in septic shock patients with mild hyperlactatemia. Patients with elevated lactate demonstrated reduced clearance [10]. Persistence of lactate elevation after resuscitation in sepsis should also be considered as a possible sign of altered clearance rather than evidence of persisting tissue hypoxia, especially in the context of 'normalized' variables such as central venous ($ScvO_2$) or mixed venous (SvO_2) oxygen saturation and central venous-to-arterial CO_2 difference (PCO_2gap).

In addition to the liver, other organs are affected by sepsis in terms of lactate metabolism. The lungs release a substantial amount of lactate during septic shock. Although it has been demonstrated that lactate is released during acute lung injury and acute respiratory distress syndrome (ARDS) [27], the presence of hypoxia in a highly oxygenated organ like the lung seems unlikely. Moreover, in this study, no correlation was found between venous lactate levels and arterial-venous mixed difference [28]. This suggests that oxygen consumption and lactate release during septic shock are not the results of the same process.

Lactate increase in sepsis may also be a protective mechanism more than a maladaptive response, due to the use of lactate as a substrate for energy production in organs like the brain and heart. During shock, as in exercise, myocardial lactate levels increase. Brain cells switch to lactate metabolism in case of increased metabolic demand. Moreover, septic shock is not the only category of shock in which lactate elevation has been proposed as a marker of prognosis and as a target for therapy. In trauma patients, lactate has been used as a prognostic marker for mortality and massive bleeding, and as a target for resuscitation and timing of surgery. Lactate trend was deemed more important than the lactate peak in trauma patients. The use of lactate trend to opt for damage control surgery versus early total care has been termed lactate-controlled early total care [29].

15.5 Non Hypoperfusion-Related Causes of Hyperlactatemia: Type B Hyperlactatemia

In a patient with hyperlactatemia, hypoperfusion and shock should be considered as the most frequent causes of the raised blood lactate, while several other causes of lactate elevation should be ruled out. Malignancy, seizures, shivering and intoxication lead to increased lactate levels. Those conditions were classically referred to as Type B hyperlactatemia and are reported in Box 15.1 [6].

Box 15.1: Causes of Hyperlactatemia

Tissue dysoxia	Other causes of lactic acidosis	
Inadequate DO_2	*Adequate DO_2*	
Septic shock	Gut ischemia	Metformin acidosis
Hemorrhagic shock	Seizures	Thiamine deficiency
Obstructive shock	Hematological malignancies	Intoxication[a]
Hypovolemic shock	β-adrenergic stimulation	Hypothermia
Anemia	Large quantities of Ringer's lactate	Dysfunction of mitochondrial chains
Hypoxia	Liver failure	Traumatic brain injury
Intoxication[a]	Shivering	

[a]Intoxication may affect both oxygen delivery (DO_2) and uptake

Lactate is increased in patients with traumatic brain injury (TBI), due to an increased release of lactate and various other mediators and a shift in cerebral metabolism. In a study by Ferreruela et al., peak lactate concentration after TBI was around 6.5 mmol/L [6].

Patients with diabetes may present with hyperlactatemia due to a direct increase in pyruvate production, or to the more frequent mechanism of biguanide toxicity. Diabetes has been defined as an independent risk factor for lactic acidosis [30].

Hematologic malignancies may be associated with lactic acidosis. The pathogenesis of lactic acidosis in this setting is not well understood, but may be due to a shift toward aerobic glycolysis (the Warburg effect). Chemotherapy and tumor mass reduction generally resolve or reduce lactic acidosis in these patients [31].

Thiamine deficiency is another rare cause of lactic acidosis, which may be present in hematologic patients or patients with malnutrition or on total parental nutrition. Thiamine deficiency may lead to severe acidosis and mortality if not suspected and treated accordingly [32].

Acute liver failure, cirrhosis in critical illness and hepatic surgery have long been known to be sources of hyperlactatemia. The liver plays a crucial role in lactate metabolism, but it can transform to a lactate-producing organ in case of hypoxia or direct insult [33].

Studies have found an association between infusion of Ringer's lactate and lactate levels. However, the rise in lactate is generally clinically insignificant. A massive infusion of Ringer's lactate (60 mL/kg) was associated with an increase of 2.0 mmol/L of lactate levels in healthy patients undergoing gynecologic surgery [34].

15.6 The Prognostic Value of Lactate in ICU Patients

Since the early studies of the 1960s and 1970s [35, 36], blood lactate concentrations have been used extensively as a biochemical marker of damaged tissue perfusion in critically ill patients admitted to the intensive care unit (ICU). In 1965, Peretz et al. described a mortality rate of 100% when lactate levels exceeded 13.3 mmol/L in patients with shock [37]. Regardless of the underlying mechanism, hyperlactatemia, and especially the persistence of hyperlactatemia during the ICU stay, remains a major negative prognostic factor in critically ill patients. In fact, a lactate level of >2 mmol/L at ICU admission or during the ICU stay was associated with mortality rates of up to 40% [38, 39], whereas values >10 mmol/L are associated with high mortality rates of 80% or more [3, 37, 40].

As general indications:

1. the prognostic value is better for lactate than for pyruvate or the lactate/pyruvate ratio, suggesting that the complex mechanism associated with impaired cellular function during shock cannot only be explained by tissue hypoxia;
2. progression of blood lactate concentrations has a better prognostic value than absolute baseline concentration at admission. In fact, persistent hyperlactatemia, increasing lactate levels and/or reduced lactate clearance [41] are consistently associated with a worse outcome [42].

The relationship between increased lactatemia and mortality in ICU patients was already reported more than 20 years ago by Bernardin et al. in a small cohort of ICU patients with septic shock. These authors reported 62% mortality for those patients with both a mean arterial pressure <85 mmHg and lactate >3 mmol/L [43]. More recently, Nichol et al. assessed the relationship between ICU admission lactate, maximal lactate and time-weighted lactate levels and hospital outcome, by analyzing the data of an intensive care database of 7155 consecutive critically ill patients admitted to the ICUs of four Australian university hospitals [3]. The authors reported that a lactate level >8 mmol/L and a peak of lactate >10 mmol/L were both associated with an ICU and in-hospital mortality rate of about 80% [3].

Haas et al. [40] studied, in a retrospective analysis, 400 patients with a serum lactate concentration of >10 mmol/L documented on at least one occasion (2.8% of the total ICU cohort admitted to a tertiary Dutch ICU during an observational period of 22 months). Patients with lactate levels >10 mmol/L had an ICU mortality of 78.2% (compared to 9.8% of overall mortality) and in-hospital mortality of 78.5%. In the subgroup of 91 patients who had hyperlactatemia >10 mmol/L for more than 24 h, ICU mortality was 95.6% and in the 53 patients who had this degree of hyperlactatemia for more than 48 h, ICU mortality was 100%. Interestingly, the area under the receiver operating characteristics curve (AUC) for prediction of ICU mortality using the 12 h lactate clearance (calculated considering the blood lactate concentration 12 h after the first measurement of lactate >10 mmol/L) was 0.91 and, a threshold value of 12 h lactate clearance of 32.8% had a sensitivity of 89.6% and a specificity of 82.8% for predicting ICU mortality. By contrast, when severe hyperlactatemia had a reversible cause associated with a higher lactate clearance in the first 12 h, the ICU mortality was less than 25%.

The prognostic value of hyperlactatemia reported by Ferreruela et al. in a retrospective cohort study of patients admitted to a tertiary Spanish ICU was modest [6]. In the 1373 patients included, the AUC of lactate concentration and the optimal cut off to predict in-hospital mortality were 0.72 (0.70–0.75) and 8.6 mmol/L, respectively, with a sensitivity of 59.9% and a specificity of 78.1%. Lactatemia >20 mmol/L resulted in a mortality rate >80% [6]. Varis et al. reported comparable results in a post-hoc analysis of the FINNAKI study [44]. This study showed a 90-day mortality rate of 43.4% for the subgroup of patients admitted with a lactate level ≥2 mmol/L and 45.9% for a level ≥3 mmol/L, compared to 22.6% for those patients admitted with a lactate level <2 mmol/L. However, the sensitivity and specificity in predicting the outcome were 67% and 56% for lactatemia ≥2 mmol/L and 49% and 71% for lactatemia ≥3 mmol/L [44].

15.7 Lactate as a Target for Resuscitation

Lactate-guided resuscitation has been included in sepsis guidelines [7]. While this approach may be useful in several situations, the systematic use of lactate to guide fluid therapy over the full course of ICU admission is increasingly questioned. In a randomized controlled study on lactate-guided therapy in patients with septic shock, patients treated according to lactate measurements had lower mortality and reached lower sequential organ failure assessment (SOFA) scores than controls. However, despite receiving more fluids and vasodilators, there was no difference in lactate levels in the two groups [45].

Lactate metabolism is not linear, as it exhibits two-phase kinetics. Hernandez and colleagues demonstrated that lactate levels decrease rapidly in the first 6 h of resuscitation in patients with septic shock, and distinguished two phases of flow-responsive and flow-independent hyperlactatemia [46]. A similar pattern was shown for the capillary refill time and venous-to-arterial CO_2 difference. In this study, 50% of patients reached normal lactate levels by 24 h. Of the 40 remaining patients, 24 (60%) had normalized lactate at 48 h, and 16 (40%) by 48 h. The biphasic curve in lactate levels implies that resuscitation with fluids should not be continued until lactate normalizes. The second phase is more related to reduced lactate clearance than to lactate hyperproduction due to fluid hypoperfusion. Lactate levels should not be used as the sole target for fluid perfusion. Clinical variables, including capillary refill time and diuresis, and metabolic targets (SvO_2 and PCO_2gap) should guide resuscitation in this setting [15].

More than lactate levels, physicians should target lactate trend when managing patients with shock. The normalization trend is more important than the absolute normal value. This strategy should be used to avoid over-resuscitation and detrimental fluid overload [46]. In a prospective study in critically ill patients, a lactate reduction >10% in the first two hours after emergency room admission predicted survival in patients with septic shock [47]. The ongoing ANDROMEDA-SHOCK randomized trial will determine whether perfusion-targeted resuscitation is superior to lactate-guided resuscitation in patients enrolled in the early phase of septic shock [48]. A simple bedside measure such as capillary refill time may thus guide fluid resuscitation using a holistic view of reperfusion in place of targeting lactate levels, which are currently widely used but more challenging to interpret.

15.8 Implications for Clinicians

Shock is a form of acute circulatory failure associated with the imbalance between oxygen delivery and systemic oxygen demand [15]. The first variable is defined as the product of oxygen content and cardiac output, whereas inadequate cellular oxygen utilization derives from a tissue oxygen demand that exceeds the DO_2 or to the cellular inability to use oxygen. This latter condition is due to mitochondrial dysfunction and deregulated cell-signalling pathways associated with multiple organ damage. In the last few decades, several hemodynamic tools, more or less invasive, have been developed in order to achieve a clear picture of macroscopic cardiovascular system function at the bedside. Assessment and monitoring of microscopic cellular response to the unbalanced oxygen metabolism is still lacking.

Although serum lactate concentrations should not be considered a direct measure of tissue perfusion [11], they remain an easily achievable, cheap and well-validated surrogate of tissue hypoxia. Lactate levels should be measured and used to identify patients with adverse prognosis and need for 'intensive' care, either in the ICU or on the ward. They should prompt further measures to identify the cause of hyperlactatemia, and monitoring of both lactate level and other markers of perfusion. When no other apparent cause of hyperlactatemia is identified (see Table 15.1), clinicians should consider hypoperfusion as the likely cause.

Lactate trend more than absolute lactate levels should then be considered as a target of resuscitation, with the object of achieving a reduction in lactate in the first hours. Afterwards, whether lactate should be used as a target for further resuscitation is debated. Lactate should not be considered alone, but with other markers of hypoperfusion in critical care patients, including capillary refill time, SvO_2, PCO_2gap, and diuresis. These patients should benefit from hemodynamic monitoring or repeated echocardiography.

As general indications, the literature agrees regarding two main issues:

1. Even a small increase in lactate (i.e., >2–4 mmol/L) can indicate shock, which should be aggressively treated to obtain a reduction to normal levels in a few hours.
2. The persistence of high values of plasma lactate in already resuscitated patients (i.e., >8–10 mmol/L after 24 h of intensive therapy, with the exception of some reversible conditions (such as post-cardiac surgical patients or seizures) is predictive of very poor outcome.

We propose a general algorithm to guide resuscitation in a patient with signs of hypoperfusion and elevated lactate levels (Fig. 15.1).

ICU patients showing no trend toward reduction of hyperlactatemia after initial resuscitation should be considered at risk of developing multiorgan failure, irrespective of the cause of shock. In this subgroup, continuous hemodynamic monitoring can provide valuable information for functional hemodynamic assessment of fluid responsiveness and cardiac function. Echocardiography and hemodynamic monitoring can be used to monitor fluid responsiveness and perform a focused fluid

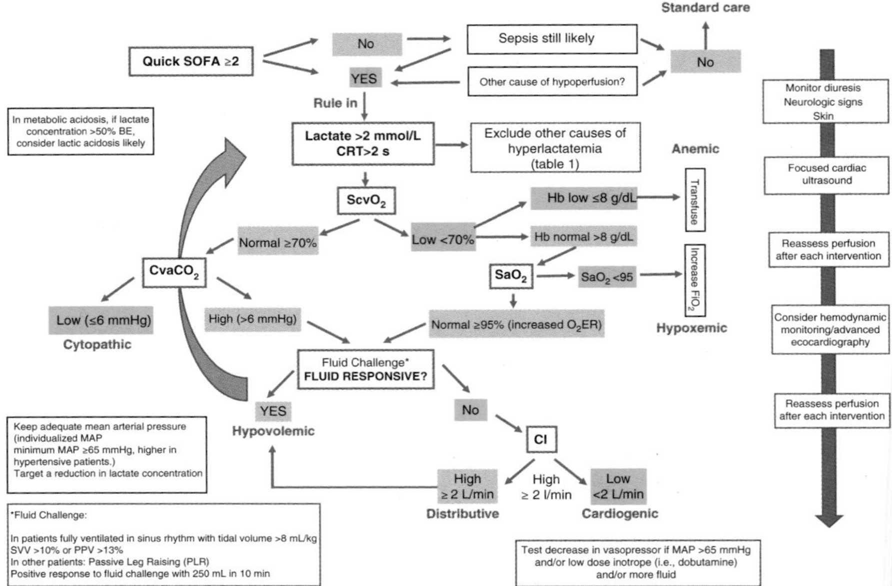

Fig. 15.1 Proposed flowchart for the management of patients with sepsis and hyperlactatemia. *MAP* mean arterial pressure, *PPV* pulse pressure variation, *CRT* capillary refill time, *SVV* stroke volume variation, $ScvO_2$ central venous oxygen saturation, *Hb* hemoglobin, *BE* base excess, *CI* cardiac index, SaO_2 arterial oxygen saturation, $CvaCO_2$ central venous-arterial carbon dioxide

therapy strategy using fluid challenges when indicated (targeting predefined criteria and respecting strict safety limits). Cardiac function should also be monitored and the need for inotropic agents evaluated.

Whether extreme levels of lactate should be considered an additional indication for ending critical care therapy is unclear. The persistence of very high plasma lactate concentrations indicates the systemic impairment of oxygen utilization, often associated with unstoppable severe systemic acidosis and cardiovascular instability. This complex decision is usually based on multifactorial criteria including clinical judgment of the underlying disease state, pre-admission frailty, daily clinical parameters and laboratory findings, information regarding presumed patient wishes and, finally, local directives and laws. Available observational data suggest use of lactate as an adjunctive criterion for considering withdrawal of intensive care support. However, the sensitivity and specificity of levels <8–10 mmol/L are too low to indicate progression to death, when used alone.

15.9 Conclusion

Lactate is a unique metabolite central to several metabolic processes in physiological and pathologic states, and its elevation is clearly related to detrimental prognosis in critically ill patients. However, interpretation of lactate levels is not univocal, and lactate concentration should be monitored and prompt further evaluation if hyperlactatemia is detected. During resuscitation, lactate should be considered not as an absolute value, but as a trend, and should never be used alone as the sole indicator of perfusion or as the unique target for patient therapy. We propose a comprehensive algorithm that can be used to guide resuscitation. In case of lactate elevation, clinicians should start comprehensive evaluation of other markers of hypoperfusion, including capillary refill time, SvO_2, and PCO_2gap, with timely initiation of hemodynamic monitoring and goal-directed therapy using both static and dynamic indices of fluid responsiveness.

References

1. Kraut JA, Madias NE. Lactic acidosis. N Engl J Med. 2014;371:2309–19.
2. Shapiro NI, Howell MD, Talmor D, et al. Serum lactate as a predictor of mortality in emergency department patients with infection. Ann Emerg Med. 2005;45:524–8.
3. Nichol AD, Egi M, Pettila V, et al. Relative hyperlactatemia and hospital mortality in critically ill patients: a retrospective multi-centre study. Crit Care. 2010;14:R25.
4. Nichol A, Bailey M, Egi M, et al. Dynamic lactate indices as predictors of outcome in critically ill patients. Crit Care. 2011;15:R242.
5. Wacharasint P, Nakada TA, Boyd JH, Russell JA, Walley KR. Normal-range blood lactate concentration in septic shock is prognostic and predictive. Shock. 2012;38:4–10.
6. Ferreruela M, Raurich JM, Ayestarán I, Llompart-Pou JA. Hyperlactatemia in ICU patients: Incidence, causes and associated mortality. J Crit Care. 2017;42:200–5.
7. Rhodes A, Evans LE, Alhazzani W, et al. Surviving Sepsis Campaign: International Guidelines for Management of Sepsis and Septic Shock: 2016. Intensive Care Med. 2017;43:304–77.
8. Hernandez G, Bruhn A, Castro R, Regueira T. The holistic view on perfusion monitoring in septic shock. Curr Opin Crit Care. 2012;18:280–6.
9. Hernandez G, Bellomo R, Bakker J. The ten pitfalls of lactate clearance in sepsis. Intensive Care Med. 2018. May 12. https://doi.org/10.1007/s00134-018-5213-x. [Epub ahead of print].
10. Levraut J, Ciebiera JP, Chave S, et al. Mild hyperlactatemia in stable septic patients is due to impaired lactate clearance rather than overproduction. Am J Respir Crit Care Med. 1998;157:1021–6.
11. Levy B. Lactate and shock state: the metabolic view. Curr Opin Crit Care. 2006;12:315–21.
12. Alberti KG. The biochemical consequences of hypoxia. J Clin Pathol Suppl (R Coll Pathol). 1977;11:14–20.
13. Levy B, Sadoune LO, Gelot AM, Bollaert PE, Nabet P, Larcan A. Evolution of lactate/pyruvate and arterial ketone body ratios in the early course of catecholamine-treated septic shock. Crit Care Med. 2000;28:114–9.
14. Leverve XM. From tissue perfusion to metabolic marker: assessing organ competition and co-operation in critically ill patients? Intensive Care Med. 1999;25:890–2.
15. Cecconi M, De Backer D, Antonelli M, et al. Consensus on circulatory shock and hemodynamic monitoring. Task force of the European Society of Intensive Care Medicine. Intensive Care Med. 2014;40:1795–815.
16. Garcia-Alvarez M, Marik P, Bellomo R. Sepsis-associated hyperlactatemia. Crit Care. 2014;18:503.
17. Grocott MP, Martin DS, Levett DZ, et al. Arterial blood gases and oxygen content in climbers on Mount Everest. N Engl J Med. 2009;360:140–9.
18. Lundby C, Saltin B, van Hall G. The 'lactate paradox', evidence for a transient change in the course of acclimatization to severe hypoxia in lowlanders. Acta Physiol Scand. 2000;170: 265–9.
19. Boekstegers P, Weidenhofer S, Kapsner T, Werdan K. Skeletal muscle partial pressure of oxygen in patients with sepsis. Crit Care Med. 1994;22:640–50.

20. Levy B, Gibot S, Franck P, Cravoisy A, Bollaert PE. Relation between muscle Na+K+ ATPase activity and raised lactate concentrations in septic shock: a prospective study. Lancet. 2005;365:871–5.
21. Hernandez G, Regueira T, Bruhn A, et al. Relationship of systemic, hepatosplanchnic, and microcirculatory perfusion parameters with 6-hour lactate clearance in hyperdynamic septic shock patients: an acute, clinical-physiological, pilot study. Ann Intensive Care. 2012;2:44.
22. Ronco JJ, Fenwick JC, Tweeddale MG, et al. Identification of the critical oxygen delivery for anaerobic metabolism in critically ill septic and nonseptic humans. JAMA. 1993;270:1724–30.
23. James JH, Luchette FA, McCarter FD, Fischer JE. Lactate is an unreliable indicator of tissue hypoxia in injury or sepsis. Lancet. 1999;354:505–8.
24. Tapia P, Soto D, Bruhn A, et al. Impairment of exogenous lactate clearance in experimental hyperdynamic septic shock is not related to total liver hypoperfusion. Crit Care. 2015;19:188.
25. Douzinas EE, Tsidemiadou PD, Pitaridis MT, et al. The regional production of cytokines and lactate in sepsis-related multiple organ failure. Am J Respir Crit Care Med. 1997;155:53–9.
26. van Genderen ME, Klijn E, Lima A, et al. Microvascular perfusion as a target for fluid resuscitation in experimental circulatory shock. Crit Care Med. 2014;42:e96–e105.
27. Kellum JA, Kramer DJ, Lee K, Mankad S, Bellomo R, Pinsky MR. Release of lactate by the lung in acute lung injury. Chest. 1997;111:1301–5.
28. Opdam H, Bellomo R. Oxygen consumption and lactate release by the lung after cardiopulmonary bypass and during septic shock. Crit Care Resusc. 2000;2:181–7.
29. Moran CG, Forward DP. The early management of patients with multiple injuries: an evidence-based, practical guide for the orthopaedic surgeon. J Bone Joint Surg Br. 2012;94:446–53.
30. Scale T, Harvey JN. Diabetes, metformin and lactic acidosis. Clin Endocrinol. 2011;74:191–6.
31. Sillos EM, Shenep JL, Burghen GA, Pui CH, Behm FG, Sandlund JT. Lactic acidosis: a metabolic complication of hematologic malignancies: case report and review of the literature. Cancer. 2001;92:2237–46.
32. Ramsi M, Mowbray C, Hartman G, Pageler N. Severe lactic acidosis and multiorgan failure due to thiamine deficiency during total parenteral nutrition. BMJ Case Rep. 2014;2014:bcr2014205264.
33. Drolz A, Horvatits T, Roedl K, et al. Acid-base status and its clinical implications in critically ill patients with cirrhosis, acute-on-chronic liver failure and without liver disease. Ann Intensive Care. 2018;8:48.
34. Orbegozo Cortes D, Rayo Bonor A, Vincent JL. Isotonic crystalloid solutions: a structured review of the literature. Br J Anaesth. 2014;112:968–81.
35. Broder G, Weil MH. Excess lactate: an index of reversibility of shock in human patients. Science. 1964;143:1457–9.
36. Weil MH, Afifi AA. Experimental and clinical studies on lactate and pyruvate as indicators of the severity of acute circulatory failure (shock). Circulation. 1970;41:989–1001.
37. Peretz DI, Scott HM, Duff J, Dossetor JB, MacLean LD, McGregor M. The significance of lacticacidemia in the shock syndrome. Ann N Y Acad Sci. 1965;119:1133–41.
38. Khosravani H, Shahpori R, Stelfox HT, Kirkpatrick AW, Laupland KB. Occurrence and adverse effect on outcome of hyperlactatemia in the critically ill. Crit Care. 2009;13:R90.
39. Juneja D, Singh O, Dang R. Admission hyperlactatemia: causes, incidence, and impact on outcome of patients admitted in a general medical intensive care unit. J Crit Care. 2011;26:316–20.
40. Haas SA, Lange T, Saugel B, et al. Severe hyperlactatemia, lactate clearance and mortality in unselected critically ill patients. Intensive Care Med. 2016;42:202–10.
41. Levraut J, Ichai C, Petit I, Ciebiera JP, Perus O, Grimaud D. Low exogenous lactate clearance as an early predictor of mortality in normolactatemic critically ill septic patients. Crit Care Med. 2003;31:705–10.
42. De Backer D. Lactic acidosis. Intensive Care Med. 2003;29:699–702.
43. Bernardin G, Pradier C, Tiger F, Deloffre P, Mattei M. Blood pressure and arterial lactate level are early indicators of short-term survival in human septic shock. Intensive Care Med. 1996;22:17–25.

44. Varis E, Pettila V, Poukkanen M, et al. Evolution of blood lactate and 90-day mortality in septic shock. a post hoc analysis of the FINNAKI study. Shock. 2017;47:574–81.
45. Jansen TC, van Bommel J, Schoonderbeek FJ, et al. Early lactate-guided therapy in intensive care unit patients: a multicenter, open-label, randomized controlled trial. Am J Respir Crit Care Med. 2010;182:752–61.
46. Hernandez G, Luengo C, Bruhn A, et al. When to stop septic shock resuscitation: clues from a dynamic perfusion monitoring. Ann Intensive Care. 2014;4:30.
47. Nguyen HB, Rivers EP, Knoblich BP, et al. Early lactate clearance is associated with improved outcome in severe sepsis and septic shock. Crit Care Med. 2004;32:1637–42.
48. Hernandez G, Cavalcanti AB, Ospina-Tascon G, et al. Early goal-directed therapy using a physiological holistic view: the ANDROMEDA-SHOCK-a randomized controlled trial. Ann Intensive Care. 2018;8:52.

Part VII

Hemodynamic and Respiratory Monitoring

16 Continuous Non-invasive Monitoring of Cardiac Output and Lung Volume Based on CO_2 Kinetics

F. Suarez-Sipmann, G. Tusman, and M. Wallin

16.1 Introduction

The gas exchange properties of the lung have long been known to theoretically support the non-invasive measurement of cardiac output and lung volume [1]. Methods based on carbon dioxide (CO_2) elimination kinetics are among the first and most extensively studied [2]. From a clinical perspective, they are also the most attractive not only because of the particular physiologic and physical-biochemical characteristics of CO_2, but also because of its universal availability. Furthermore, CO_2-based methods are perfectly adaptable to clinical simplified measurement devices and modern intensive care unit (ICU) equipment such as mechanical ventilators or anesthesia machines. In this chapter, we will review characteristic features of CO_2 kinetics and its measurement and present a novel capnodynamic method for the continuous and non-invasive measurement of end-expiratory lung volume and effective pulmonary blood flow.

F. Suarez-Sipmann (✉)
Hedenstierna Laboratory, Department of Surgical Sciences, Uppsala University, Uppsala, Sweden

Department of Intensive Care Medicine, Hospital Universitario de La Princesa, Madrid, Spain
e-mail: fsuarez.sipmann@surgsci.uu.se

G. Tusman
Department of Anesthesiology, Hospital Privado de Comunidad, Mar del Plata, Argentina

M. Wallin
Department of Physiology and Pharmacology (FYFA), C3, Eriksson I Lars Group, Karolinska Institute, Stockholm, Sweden

Maquet Critical Care AB, Solna, Sweden

J.-L. Vincent (ed.), *Annual Update in Intensive Care and Emergency Medicine 2019*, Annual Update in Intensive Care and Emergency Medicine,
https://doi.org/10.1007/978-3-030-06067-1_16

16.2 Carbon Dioxide Kinetics

CO_2 is the principal catabolite of aerobic metabolism and is produced continuously in large amounts daily. Its level in blood and body fluids depends on the equilibrium between production and elimination. There is a continuous body gradient of CO_2 from its site of production, the mitochondria, to the expired gas at the airway opening [3]. Once produced, it diffuses out of the cell and is collected by the microcirculation and transported via the bloodstream mainly as bicarbonate (HCO_3^-), to the right heart that distributes it through the lungs (i.e., pulmonary blood flow) in an amount equal to total cardiac output. When it reaches the pulmonary capillary network, the hemoglobin-bound carbonic anhydrase catalyzes the release of CO_2 that then diffuses to the ventilated alveoli that are perfused, entering the alveolar gas and finally being eliminated by alveolar ventilation to the atmosphere.

CO_2 kinetics can be evaluated in steady-states, when CO_2 output equals production, or non-steady states as, for example, during hemodynamic or ventilatory changes. Its dependence on the mentioned physiological processes, its blood solubility and transport particularities, its availability and ease of measurement, its high diffusivity and necessary total elimination by the lungs are special features that give this gas unique properties to be used as a tracer for physiologically and clinically relevant processes.

16.3 Antecedents of CO_2-Based Cardiac Output Methods

All gas exchange methods to calculate cardiac output are based on the conservation of mass represented by the classical Fick principle [4], which in its form for CO_2 can be written as:

$$Q = VCO_2 / \left(CvCO_2 - CaCO_2\right) \tag{16.1}$$

where Q is the cardiac output that when measured by expired CO_2 kinetics is referred to as effective pulmonary blood flow (CO_{EPBF}), VCO_2 the minute production of CO_2 (mL/min) and $CvCO_2$ and $CaCO_2$ the mixed venous and arterial contents of CO_2, respectively. Strictly speaking, CO_{EPBF} refers to the non-shunted portion of cardiac output that in normal physiological conditions approximates total cardiac output.

As for oxygen, the mixed venous content of CO_2 can traditionally only be measured invasively by means of a pulmonary artery catheter (PAC), which imposes obvious limitations for the clinical application of the Fick principle. In the last few decades, several methods to estimate $CvCO_2$, such as breath-holding, single breath and rebreathing maneuvers, have been described [5, 6]. However, they never succeeded as clinical methods because of their dependency on extra equipment and/or cumbersome measurement procedures.

Several later developments have opened the clinical door to CO_2-based methods of monitoring CO_{EPBF}. First, as most diatomic gases, CO_2 absorbs infrared radiation and can thus be easily recorded at the airway opening. Infrared sensor technology was soon developed and light, easy to use mainstream infrared CO_2 sensors became available at the bedside [7]. As a consequence, capnography, the graphical display of measured expired CO_2, was rapidly adopted as a monitoring standard. Capnography can be performed in either time or volume domains, resulting in time or volumetric capnography, respectively. Time capnography is by far the most widely used in clinical practice. Volumetric capnography is, however, a more attractive and complete monitoring option. It requires the simultaneous recording of expiratory CO_2 and flow and, therefore, the CO_2 sensor must be mounted and integrated on a flow sensor at the airway opening. The result is the volumetric capnogram: the plot of the amount of CO_2 expired in one tidal breath. The development of volumetric capnography [8] made non-invasive breath-by-breath VCO_2 measurement, together with end-tidal PCO_2 ($P_{ET}CO_2$) and mixed expired CO_2 available.

Second, the impossibility of measuring $CvCO_2$ was elegantly circumvented by Gedeon et al. who introduced the differential Fick method (Eqs. (16.2) and (16.3)) [9]. By inducing a change in VCO_2 and $CaCO_2$ without affecting $CvCO_2$, Gedeon et al. reasoned that the denominator of Fick's equation could theoretically be solved.

$$CO_{EPBF} = VCO_{2[b]} - VCO_{2[a]} / \left[CvCO_2 - CaCO_2\right]_{[b]} - \left[CvCO_2 - CaCO_2\right]_{[a]} \tag{16.2}$$

Such a change creates two distinct situations, denoted with the subscripts a and b in Eq. (16.2), resulting in a $\Delta CaCO_2$ and $\Delta CvCO_2$. Provided $CvCO_2$ remains constant during the measurement period, it can then be eliminated from the denominator.

Third, since CO_2 content is difficult to measure it can be substituted by its partial pressure according to Henry's law of solubility that relates the content of a gas in a fluid to its partial pressure times its solubility constant [3]. Although not a trivial calculation, Capek and Roy proposed a robust approximation based on the slope of the CO_2 dissociation curve to estimate CO_2 solubility [10]. The final simplified expression for the calculation of pulmonary blood flow then becomes:

$$CO_{EPBF} = \Delta VCO_2 / SCO_2 \bullet \Delta PCO_2 \tag{16.3}$$

where the $\Delta CvCO_2$ of the previous equation is substituted by SCO_2, the solubility constant of CO_2 times arterial PCO_2. Arterial PCO_2 can under most circumstances be considered to be close to the alveolar PCO_2 (P_ACO_2) after capillary transit equilibration. To get rid of the need to obtain an arterial blood gas sample, Gedeon et al. proposed using $P_{ET}CO_2$, which is easily obtained by expired gas analysis, to estimate arterial PCO_2. This is based on the assumption that the end-tidal gas is composed exclusively by alveolar gas, thus providing a good estimate of P_ACO_2.

The fourth important step necessary for CO_2 methods to become clinically available was to find suitable ways to introduce a perturbation capable of modifying alveolar ventilation in order to induce the necessary changes in VCO_2 and P_ACO_2 without affecting $CvCO_2$ during the measurement period. In their early work, Gedeon et al. proposed modification of the mechanical ventilation breathing pattern by introducing variable inspiratory pauses while maintaining constant tidal volume and active inspiratory and expiratory times [9]. This led to alterations equivalent to changes in minute ventilation producing rapid modifications in $P_{ET}CO_2$ and VCO_2. However, the first method that became clinically available proposed the intermittent addition of an in-series or in-parallel instrumental dead space, a variable volume rebreathing loop, inserted in the breathing circuit close to the Y piece [11]. The first, and to date only, clinically available non-invasive CO_2 cardiac output monitor, the NICO-NM3 monitor (Respironics-Philips, Wallingford, Connecticut, USA) is based on this partial rebreathing principle. An automated valve intermittently opens a parallel rebreathing circuit increasing instrumental dead-space and reducing alveolar ventilation resulting in a transient reduction in VCO_2 and increase in $P_{ET}CO_2$ that normalizes once the valve closes the rebreathing circuit [12]. It delivers intermittent CO_{EPBF} values because an entire measurement cycle, from rebreathing to stabilization, takes around 4 min.

The technological evolution of modern mechanical ventilators and anesthesia machines with tight microprocessing electronic control has opened new possibilities to introduce automated non-invasive CO_2-based cardiac output methods into the operating room and ICU. Peyton introduced the capnotracking method in which perturbations are automatically induced by ventilator changes in the respiratory rate and inspiratory-expiratory ratio that result in suitable changes in tidal volume [13]. This method has been recently refined using an oscillating pattern of respiratory rate variation resulting in a fully automated and continuous CO_{EPBF} measurement [14].

16.4 The Capnodynamic Method

Based on the principles outlined above, recently a novel capnodynamic method that delivers continuous and non-invasive CO_{EPBF} and CO_2_based end-expiratory lung volume ($EELV_{CO_2}$) has been described [15]. As for all other CO_2-based methods, expired CO_2 is measured at the airway opening using conventional infrared sensing technology whereas the integrated gas flow is measured by the flow sensor in the ventilator. Both measurements are needed to solve the capnodynamic equation, which follows the mole balance principle for CO_2 in the lung.

$$EELV_{CO_2} \bullet \left(FACO_{2^n} - FACO_{2^{n-1}}\right) = CO_{EPBF} \bullet \Delta t^n \bullet \left(CvCO_2 - CcCO_{2^n}\right) - VTCO_{2^n} \quad (16.4)$$

where $EELV_{CO_2}$ is the end-expiratory lung volume containing CO_2, $FACO_2{}^n$ the alveolar fraction of CO_2 of the nth breath, $FACO_2{}^{n-1}$ the alveolar fraction of CO_2 of the preceding breath, CO_{EPBF} the effective pulmonary blood flow (the non-shunted blood fraction of cardiac output), Δt^n the duration of the nth respiratory cycle, $CvCO_2$ and $CcCO_2$ the central venous and capillary mixed venous content of CO_2, respectively, and $VTCO_2{}^n$ the volume of CO_2 eliminated by the nth breath. The left side of the equation describes the tidal difference in the lung's CO_2 content between two consecutive breaths, whereas on the right side, the first term reflects the amount of CO_2 supplied to the lung by the blood stream and the second, $VTCO_2{}^n$, is the amount of CO_2 eliminated from the lung by the 'n[th]' current breath. As for the differential Fick principle, $CcCO_2$ is substituted by the partial pressure but with a substantial change: the capillary partial pressure of CO_2 is not estimated by $P_{ET}CO_2$ but by measured P_ACO_2. This value is obtained from the mid-portion of phase III of the volumetric capnogram as recently described by Tusman et al. [16]. The perturbation used by the capnodynamic method consists in a minimally modified breathing pattern applying a repetitive sequence of nine breaths, in which in its latest version [17], short expiratory holds are added to the last three breaths (Fig. 16.1).

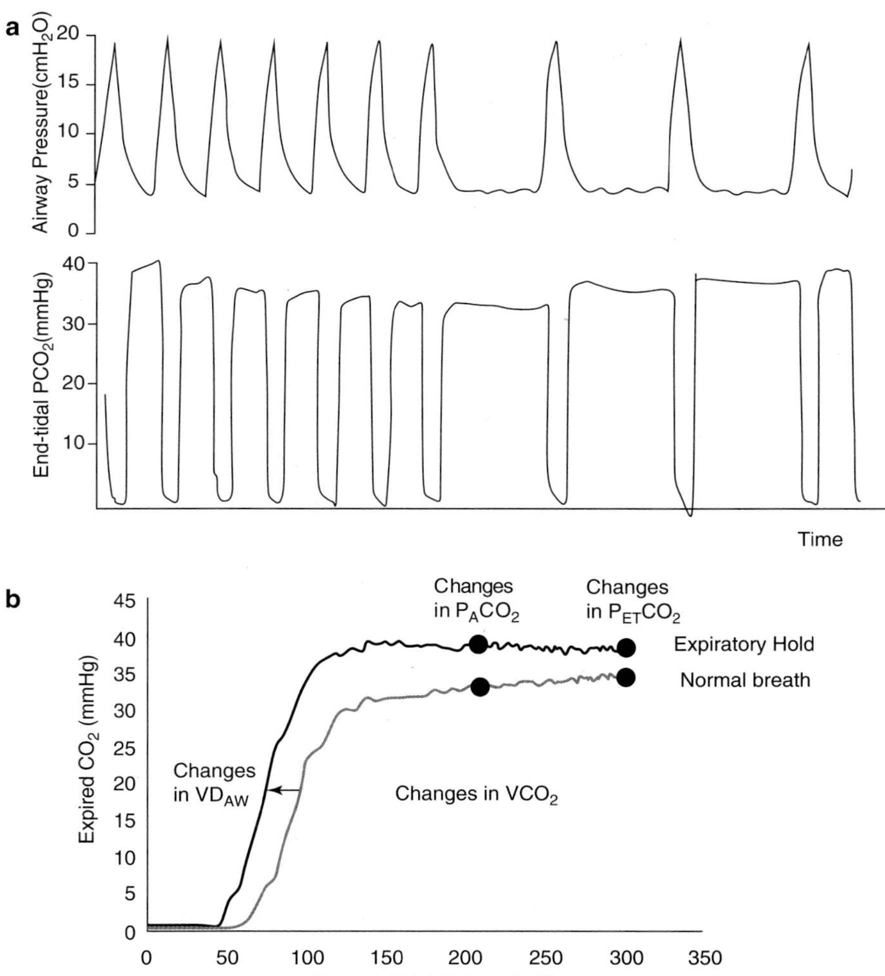

Fig. 16.1 The capnodynamic breathing pattern. Panel (**a**): The capnodynamic breathing pattern consists of a repetitive sequence of nine breaths in which an expiratory hold is added to the last three breaths. Panel (**b**): The volumetric capnogram demonstrates the changes in CO_2 elimination between a normal breath (light gray) and an expiratory hold breath (black)

That the differential Fick principle solves $CvCO_2$ as constant values can be reasonably assumed [10]. In the capnodynamic algorithm, the complete measurement cycle of nine breaths creates a set of nine equations with three unknowns where the latest breath continuously replaces the oldest one. For each new breath, the equation system is solved by numerical means, where the constant values for the three unknowns for the entire cycle which gives the best fit for the three unknowns are used.

The capnodynamic method has several theoretical advantages. It can be delivered fully automatically without any additional equipment other than a standard CO_2 sensor and a conventional mechanical ventilator or anesthesia machine. It provides non-invasive true continuous breath-by-breath estimates of cardiac output and end-expiratory lung volume at the bedside. The breathing pattern minimally interferes with the one selected by the physician. As it maintains constant tidal volume and inspiratory time it does not modify inspiratory pressures and by using expiratory instead of inspiratory holds minimizes the time on higher airway pressure, which reduces the effect on capillary blood flow and alveolar delivery of CO_2. Finally, the pattern results in improved CO_2 elimination avoiding undue increases in $PaCO_2$ as produced by the partial rebreathing method. During an expiratory hold, as described for an inspiratory hold [18], more time for CO_2 diffusion is provided, producing a small but sufficient increase in alveolar CO_2. This increase moves the stationary front between airway diffusive and convective CO_2 transport towards the airway opening resulting in transient reduced airway dead space and increased VCO_2 (Fig. 16.1).

The method, however, requires a passively breathing patient because the algorithm needs a constant breathing pattern. As for all other CO_2 based methods, CO_{EPBF} and $EELV_{CO2}$ are affected by the ventilation-perfusion status of the lung and, in conditions of increased shunt or alveolar dead space, both values divert from cardiac output and functional residual capacity (FRC) or EELV as will be discussed in the next sections.

16.5 Capnodynamic Monitoring of Effective Pulmonary Blood Flow

Cardiac output continues to be the most important monitoring parameter in hemodynamically unstable patients as the main goal of any management strategy is to preserve tissue/organ perfusion by ensuring adequate oxygen delivery [19, 20]. In recent years a myriad of new minimally invasive cardiac output monitoring options have been developed and become available to the clinician [21]. This has, however, not resulted in a more widespread adoption of cardiac output monitoring and recent reports estimate that it is used in less than 35% of patients in the perioperative setting [22]. Concerns regarding reliability, accuracy and precision of the new minimally invasive methods as well as the fact that most of these new monitoring options need extra new stand-alone devices and disposables with associated extra costs are probably partially behind the reasons for this lack of adoption.

16.5.1 CO_2-Based Methods

As explained previously, pulmonary perfusion transports all metabolically produced CO_2 to the gas exchange units. Not surprisingly, a direct relationship between pulmonary blood flow and VCO_2 has been consistently demonstrated in mathematical models [23], and in animal [24] and human studies [25]. Therefore, qualitative information regarding CO_{EPBF} can be obtained by simple visual inspection of real time changes in expired CO_2. The quantitative estimation constitutes the theoretical basis of CO_2 cardiac output methods.

From all minimally invasive cardiac output monitoring techniques, CO_2 based methods, which are in fact truly non-invasive, have been the most extensively studied and scrutinized in experimental and clinical validation studies in different populations of patients and conditions [2, 26]. In general, in all clinical studies the methods were compared to PAC thermodilution, still the reference method despite its invasiveness and its rather moderate precision and accuracy with percentage errors (i.e., normalized limits of agreement [LoA]) of up to 45% instead of the generally 30% benchmark limit of acceptability. Overall, taking these limits into account, clinical validation studies have yielded similar values of accuracy and precision for the rebreathing method with averaged bias of −0.05 and precision of 1.12 L/min and a percentage error of ±44% [26] and the capnotracking method [27] with better results for its recently improved version with a bias of −0.3 L/min, and a percentage error of ±38%, when compared to PAC thermodilution [14].

16.5.2 The Capnodynamic Method

The CO_{EPBF} obtained using the capnodynamic method has been validated experimentally and most recently in pediatric patients [28]. Experimental validations have been based on porcine models in which severe challenges, such as large changes in cardiac output, shock [15], acute lung injury [29], hypercapnia and ischemia/reperfusion [30] were tested. In addition, two different breathing patterns, using inspiratory [15] or expiratory holds [17], have been compared, in favor of the latter. All experimental validations were made with the direct measurement of cardiac output at the origin of the pulmonary artery by means of an ultrasonic flow probe, a standard experimental reference, and comparative statistical analysis was performed following current methodological recommendations [31]. Overall the method resulted in a good agreement and trending ability as determined by the 4-quadrant plot analysis and compared well to the clinical thermodilution methods. Accuracy and precision (bias and 95% LoA) and mean percentage error were 0.2 (−1.1 ± 1.2) L/min and 47% for the inspiratory hold pattern [15] and 0.05 (−1.1 ± 1.2) L/min and 36% for the expiratory hold pattern [17] with modifications under the different experimental conditions. In general, a higher bias at low cardiac output of 0.4 L/min and a lower bias −0.1 but larger LoA (−1.2 to 1.1) at high cardiac output conditions were obtained for the inspiratory hold pattern, whereas a higher bias and LoA up to −0.3 to 0.2 (−2 to 1.4) and an increase of the percentage error to 41% at higher positive end-expiratory pressure (PEEP) levels and high cardiac output conditions were obtained for the expiratory hold pattern. In the lung injury model with shunt fractions up to 36%, bias, LoA and percentage error of (uncorrected) CO_{EPBF} deteriorated from 0.2 (−1.1 to 1.5) L/min and 35% to −0.9 (−3.6 to 1.9) and 70% before and after inducing lung injury, respectively. In all studies and evaluated conditions, CO_{EPBF} demonstrated an excellent trending ability with concordance rates consistently >85% and frequently close to 100%.

Clinically, CO_{EPBF} has been compared to suprasternal two-dimensional Doppler cardiac output in children (median 8.5 months, 8.3 kg) undergoing cleft-lip-palate repair surgery [28]. The protocol included small increases in PEEP and an atropine-induced increase in cardiac output. The overall bias was −8.3 mL/kg/min with 95% LoA of −82 to 60 mL/kg/min, a mean percentage error of 49%, and a concordance rate of 64%. These accuracy and precision values were, however, not as good as expected. The authors reasoned that this was in part due to limitations of the reference method as it had a three-time worse inherent precision than CO_{EPBF}, and failed to track the reduction of cardiac output at higher PEEP levels. Their assumption was confirmed in an additional experiment in which the protocol was applied in piglets, which resulted in a minimal bias of −1 mL/kg, a percentage error of 31% and a concordance of 95% [28]. In a more recent clinical evaluation including adult patients during cardiac surgery under routine anesthetic management, CO_{EPBF} was compared to transpulmonary thermodilution resulting in a bias of 0.63, a percentage error of 34% and a concordance rate of 81% (unpublished data). Figure 16.2 illustrates an example of the performance of CO_{EPBF} and its trending ability in one of the studied patients.

As mentioned earlier, all CO_2 based methods estimate effective pulmonary blood flow, which is the non-shunted fraction of cardiac output. The correspondence with total cardiac output is therefore dependent on the ventilation-perfusion status of the lung. Accordingly, in conditions of increased shunt or alveolar dead space, total cardiac output will be underestimated by CO_{EPBF}. This problem can be handled in three ways: first, by the use of shunt correction methods. The rebreathing method implemented in the NICO monitor uses the oxygen saturation obtained by pulse-oximetry together with the inspiratory oxygen fraction value, to estimate shunt from the iso-shunt diagram [3]. The capnotracking method incorporates a minimally invasive estimation of shunt obtained from combining the shunt and the Fick equations where shunt can be solved by the measurement of oxygen uptake and pulmonary blood flow [32]. Finally, if lung function is optimized by lung recruitment and best PEEP selection, shunt can be minimized and the CO_{EPBF} then becomes closer to total cardiac output. In fact, cardiac output underestimation is of little importance when shunt values are ≤20% [29].

Second, CO_{EPBF} can be handled as an independent physiological variable that can be very relevant in patients receiving mechanical ventilation. This was already suggested by Gedeon et al., who analyzed the use of CO_{EPBF} to adjust the level of PEEP in a small group of patients with acute respiratory failure [33]. They found that CO_{EPBF} yielded PEEP levels similar to those suggested by best oxygen delivery. Third, even when CO_{EPBF} absolute values are not that close to total cardiac output, the repeatedly demonstrated capacity of maintaining a good trending ability under challenging conditions including shock and

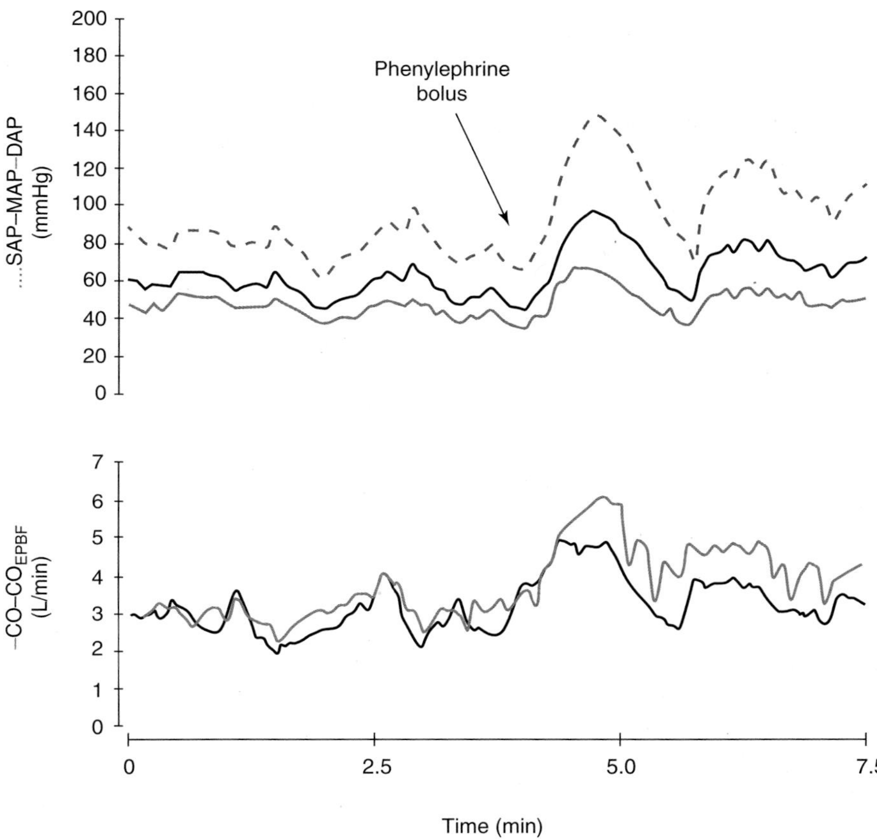

Fig. 16.2 Trending of effective pulmonary blood flow (CO_{EPBF}). Trending ability of the capnodynamic-based cardiac output method (CO_{EPBF}) compared with the reference continuous pulse contour cardiac output (PiCCO) trending in an unstable cardiac surgery patient. Arrow indicates the injection of a phenylephrine bolus to overcome a hypotensive episode. This example illustrates how continuous non-invasive CO_{EPBF} perfectly tracks changes in PiCCO in parallel to changes in invasive arterial pressure measurements. *SAP* systolic arterial pressure, *MAP* mean arterial pressure, *DAP* diastolic arterial pressure

experimental acute lung injury, is clinically useful to rapidly detect relevant cardiac output changes under routine continuous monitoring.

16.6 Capnodynamic Monitoring of End-Expiratory Lung Volume

FRC corresponds to the lung volume found at end-expiration when lung and chest-wall elastic and recoil forces equilibrate at the respiratory system's resting position. The physiological importance of FRC derives from the fact that it represents the volume of gas participating in oxygenation and CO_2 elimination and that it strongly influences the mechanical properties of the lung such as compliance and resistance [34].

From a pathophysiological perspective, FRC is of great relevance in mechanically ventilated patients because it is universally decreased due to lung collapse and increased elastic recoil. Lung collapse is one of the major contributors to reduced FRC, reaching values up to 10–15% during anesthesia [35] and 40% in severe acute respiratory distress syndrome (ARDS) [36, 37]. Collapse has an important role in the development of ventilator-induced lung injury (VILI), acting as a stress raiser by increasing lung heterogeneity, leading to amplifications of regional strain. In addition, the resultant decrease in the size of the functional lung increases the stress forces acting on the ventilated lung, which is expressed mechanically as a low compliance and higher levels of inspiratory driving pressure for a given delivered tidal volume.

Because of the use of PEEP during mechanical ventilation, FRC is generally referred to as EELV to account for this level above normal atmospheric pressure and its resultant increase in lung volume. Despite its pathophysiological relevance, measurement of FRC is rarely performed in the ICU [38]. Clinical FRC/EELV measurement has traditionally been difficult because the available methods are either logistically challenging, such as body plethysmography or cumbersome requiring additional complex-to-handle equipment, such as the inert-gas dilution and multiple breath washout techniques using gases such as helium, nitrogen, argon or sulfur-hexafluoride.

Imaging techniques, computed tomography (CT)-scan and magnetic resonance imaging (MRI) provide accurate estimates of absolute EELV but have evident practicality limitations. In current clinical practice, there are essentially two methods in use. One is electrical impedance tomography (EIT), a novel functional imaging monitoring technique that provides useful continuous relative EELV trending but does not estimate absolute values [39]. The other technique is a simplified inert-gas method based on multiple nitrogen wash in/out [40]. This fully automated method is based on the measurement of oxygen consumption and CO_2 production and does not need patient disconnection from the breathing circuit. However, it requires changes in the inspiratory fraction of oxygen and delivers intermittent measurements as it takes at least 4–5 min to obtain a value. It is also available in only one type of mechanical ventilator.

16.6.1 CO_2-Based EELV

Given the kinetics described for CO_2 and the characteristics of its simplified measurement there has been a growing interest in the development of CO_2-based methods to estimate EELV. Brewer et al. described a CO_2 wash-in method to measure FRC using the partial rebreathing principle [41]. By taking the first breath of the rebreathing period and measuring end-tidal PCO_2 and VCO_2, they proposed a method to calculate EELV. The method assumes that CO_2 elimination is at steady state during baseline before rebreathing and that the measured expired VCO_2 equals the volume of CO_2 eliminated from the blood. They added a correction factor to account for the volume of CO_2 stored in the lung tissue and the capillary blood due to its solubility as suggested by Gedeon et al. [42]. In an experimental validation, the CO_2 wash-in method resulted in an accuracy of −87 mL with LoA of ±258 mL in normal lungs and of −77 mL ±276 in injured lungs. Using the same principle as the rebreathing method implemented in the NICO-NM3 monitor, this method is totally non-invasive being able to deliver intermittent (every 3–4 min) FRC values.

16.6.2 Capnodynamic EELV

As anticipated from Eq. (16.4), $EELV_{CO_2}$ can be solved together with CO_{EPBF} using the capnodynamic method. A first experimental validation by Albu et al. [43] compared $EELV_{CO_2}$ with the helium dilution technique in healthy and lung injured rabbits. The authors observed good agreement between methods when animals were ventilated at different levels of PEEP with a mean bias of 24.8 ± 15 mL and 6.5 ± 14 mL with LoA of ±31 mL and ±29 mL in healthy and injured lungs, respectively. The difference between methods was higher at zero PEEP but became similar when PEEP was increased. This observation was not reproduced in larger animals (pigs) [44]. The authors hypothesized that as they did not add a correction factor as in the rebreathing method, such differences at low PEEP were due to the high solubility of CO_2 compared to the inert gases, so that $EELV_{CO_2}$ included the CO_2 in the capillary blood and dissolved in lung tissue [41, 42]. Accordingly, at low PEEP levels, the capillary volume is larger [45] and more CO_2 is dissolved in the lung tissue explaining the difference.

As CO_2 kinetics is highly dependent on pulmonary blood flow, hemodynamic changes can affect $EELV_{CO_2}$. Hällsjö Sander et al. tested this hypothesis in an experimental study in which animals were subjected to large decreases and increases in pulmonary blood flow [44]. $EELV_{CO_2}$, compared to the sulfur-hexafluoride wash-in/wash-out method, remained stable despite the profound changes in lung perfusion. As for CO_{EPBF}, $EELV_{CO_2}$ demonstrated an excellent trending ability with concordance rates of 100%. This finding supports the suggestion that $EELV_{CO_2}$ and CO_{EPBF} behave independently within the capnodynamic equation.

As for CO_{EPBF}, $EELV_{CO_2}$ measurement is affected by metabolism and lung perfusion (which are assumed to be stable during each measurement), as opposed to methods using insoluble inert-gases. This dependency can be regarded as a disadvantage or as an advantage depending on the intended clinical use of $EELV_{CO_2}$. From a strictly anatomical point of view, $EELV_{CO_2}$ will tend to overestimate EELV especially at low levels of PEEP. However, from a functional point of view, $EELV_{CO_2}$ represents the volume participating in gas exchange. In fact, $EELV_{CO_2}$ can be considered the functional (i.e., effective) lung volume, which may offer more relevant information in ventilated patients, such as the evaluation of a response to PEEP. For example, it may be used to monitor recruitment and de-recruitment phenomena and more importantly discriminate whether an increase in EELV in response to PEEP is due to a recruitment effect or merely an overinflation of already aerated units, something that conventional EELV methods cannot differentiate.

The unprecedented possibility to continuously and non-invasively monitor $EELV_{CO_2}$ opens interesting new options for bedside assessment of a patient's condition. We have already mentioned the importance of collapse in VILI so that $EELV_{CO_2}$ can become a useful parameter to titrate the level of PEEP and monitor VILI especially when combined with other bedside parameters. Figure 16.3 illustrates one example in which $EELV_{CO_2}$ was used in combination with respiratory

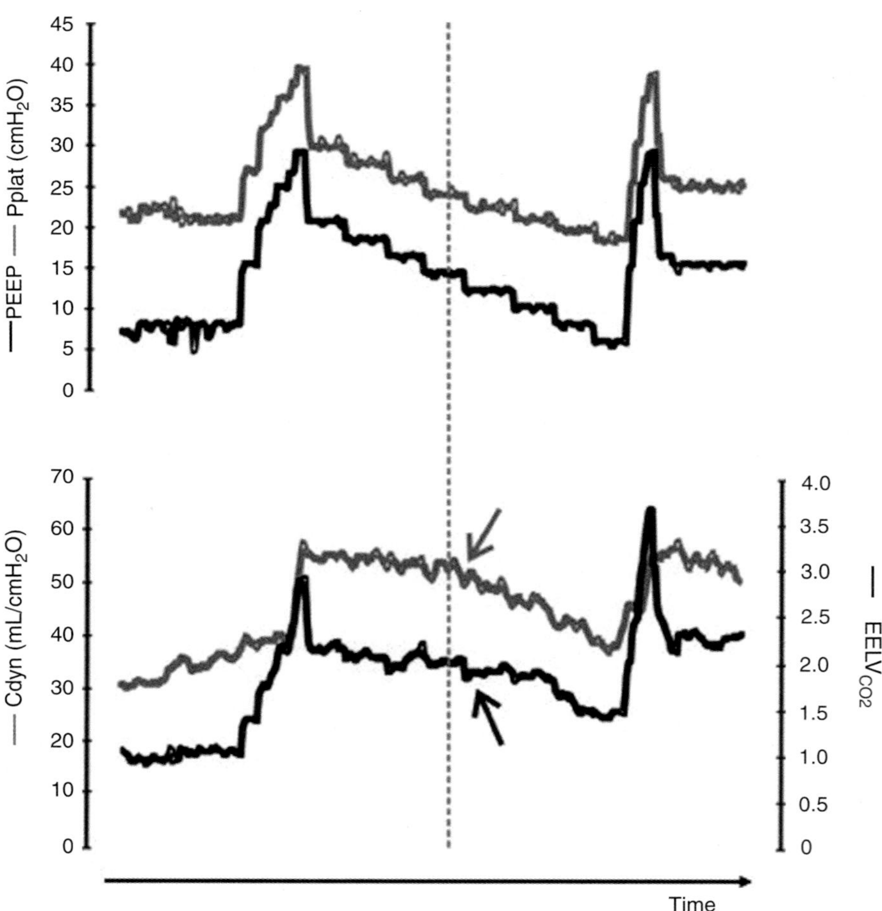

Fig. 16.3 CO_2-based end-expiratory lung volume ($EELV_{CO_2}$) trend and behavior during titration of positive end-expiratory pressure (PEEP). Real-time, breath-by-breath trend of measured $EELV_{CO_2}$ during a recruitment maneuver and decremental PEEP titration in a morbidly obese patient. The arrow marks the onset of lung collapse according to the respiratory dynamic compliance and the vertical dotted line the PEEP level at which the lung stays open. Notice how $EELV_{CO_2}$ follows the behavior of lung compliance, starting to decrease once the lung has started to collapse, highlighting its close correspondence with functional lung volume

system compliance during a PEEP titration trial after recruitment. Recently the concept of lung strain was introduced to provide a better mechanistic view of VILI [46]. Strain refers to the cyclic deformation of lung tissue during tidal inflation and is clinically calculated as the ratio between tidal volume and EELV as proposed by Gonzalez-López et al. [47]. Due to the mentioned limitations to the measurement of EELV, strain can only be measured intermittently, limitations that could be overcome by $EELV_{CO_2}$ thus providing the possibility to analyze its response to changes in ventilatory settings and gain new insight into its importance and clinical usefulness. $EELV_{CO_2}$ could also be a useful tool to analyze and monitor the effect of postural changes during surgery or ICU management including prone positioning whose physiological effects are still not completely understood.

16.7 Conclusion

In this chapter, we present a novel non-invasive and continuous capnodynamic method for monitoring effective pulmonary blood flow and EELV based on CO_2 kinetics. Experimental and initial clinical validations have confirmed that CO_{EPBF} and $EELV_{CO_2}$ are reasonable estimates of cardiac output and EELV with an acceptable accuracy and precision even in challenging clinical conditions. More importantly, both parameters consistently demonstrated an excellent trending ability when compared with reference methods. The method is minimally invasive and fully automated, being integrated into conventional ventilators and thus not requiring any additional equipment. It therefore offers the unprecedented possibility to continuously monitor these two highly relevant physiologic parameters in many patients. Clinical validation studies addressing different populations of postoperative and critically ill patients are needed to further establish the role of this promising monitoring method.

References

1. Laszlo G. Respiratory measurements of cardiac output: from elegant idea to useful test. J Appl Physiol. 2004;96:428–37.
2. Peyton PJ. Pulmonary carbon dioxide elimination for cardiac output monitoring in perioperative and critical care patients: history and current status. J Healthc Eng. 2013;4:203–22.
3. Lumb AB. Chapter 9: Carbon dioxide. In: Lumb AB, editor. Nunn's Applied Respiratory Physiology. 8th ed. London: Elsevier; 2017. p. 151–167.e2.
4. Fick A. Ueber diffusion. Annalen der Physik und Chemie. 1855;170:59–86.
5. Kim TS, Rahn H, Farhi LE. Estimation of true venous and arterial PCO_2 by gas analysis of a single breath. J Appl Physiol. 1966;21:1338–44.
6. Cade WT, Nabar SR, Keyser RE. Reproducibility of the exponential rise technique of CO_2 rebreathing for measuring $PvCO_2$ and $CvCO_2$ to non-invasively estimate cardiac output during incremental, maximal treadmill exercise. Eur J Appl Physiol. 2004;91:669–76.
7. Jaffe MB. Infrared measurement of carbon dioxide in the human breath: "breathe-through" devices from Tyndall to the present day. Anesth Analg. 2008;107:890–904.
8. Fletcher R. On-line expiratory CO_2 monitoring. Int J Clin Monit Comput. 1986;3:155–63.

9. Gedeon A, Forslund L, Hedenstierna G, et al. A new method for noninvasive bedside determination of pulmonary blood flow. Med Biol Eng Comput. 1980;18:411–8.
10. Capek JMJ, Roy RJR. Noninvasive measurement of cardiac output using partial CO_2 rebreathing. IEEE Trans Biomed Eng. 1988;35:653–61.
11. Bosman RJ, Stoutenbeek CP, Zandstra DF. Non-invasive pulmonary blood flow measurement by means of CO_2 analysis of expiratory gases. Intensive Care Med. 1991;17:98–102.
12. Haryadi DG, Orr JA, Kuck K, et al. Partial CO_2 rebreathing indirect Fick technique for non-invasive measurement of cardiac output. J Clin Monit Comput. 2000;16:361–74.
13. Peyton PJ. Continuous minimally invasive peri-operative monitoring of cardiac output by pulmonary capnotracking: comparison with thermodilution and transesophageal echocardiography. J Clin Monit Comput. 2012;26:121–32.
14. Peyton PJ. Performance of a second generation pulmonary capnotracking system for continuous monitoring of cardiac output. J Clin Monit Comput. 2018;32:1057–64.
15. Hällsjö Sander C, Hallback M, Wallin M, et al. Novel continuous capnodynamic method for cardiac output assessment during mechanical ventilation. Br J Anaesth. 2014;112:824–31.
16. Tusman G, Sipmann FS, Borges JB, et al. Validation of Bohr dead space measured by volumetric capnography. Intensive Care Med. 2011;37:870–4.
17. Sander CH, Sigmundsson T, Hallbäck M, et al. A modified breathing pattern improves the performance of a continuous capnodynamic method for estimation of effective pulmonary blood flow. J Clin Monit Comput. 2017;31:717–25.
18. Devaquet J, Jonson B, Niklason L, et al. Effects of inspiratory pause on CO_2 elimination and arterial PCO_2 in acute lung injury. J Appl Physiol. 2008;105:1944–9.
19. Vincent J-L, Rhodes A, Perel A, et al. Clinical review: update on hemodynamic monitoring--a consensus of 16. Crit Care. 2011;15:229.
20. Saugel B, Vincent JL. Cardiac output monitoring. Curr Opin Crit Care. 2018;24:165–72.
21. Mehta Y. Newer methods of cardiac output monitoring. World J Cardiol. 2014;6:1022–9.
22. Bignami E, Guarnieri M, Gemma M. Fluid management in cardiac surgery patients: pitfalls, challenges and solutions. Minerva Anestesiol. 2017;83:638–51.
23. Schwardt JD, Gobran SR, Neufeld GR, et al. Sensitivity of CO_2 washout to changes in acinar structure in a single-path model of lung airways. Ann Biomed Eng. 1991;19:679–97.
24. Tusman G, Böhm SH, Suarez Sipmann F, et al. Lung recruitment and positive end-expiratory pressure have different effects on CO_2 elimination in healthy and sick lungs. Anesth Analg. 2010;111:968–77.
25. Tusman G, Areta M, Climente C, et al. Effect of pulmonary perfusion on the slopes of single-breath test of CO_2. J Appl Physiol. 2005;99:650–5.
26. Peyton PJ, Chong SW. Minimally invasive measurement of cardiac output during surgery and critical care: a meta-analysis of accuracy and precision. Anesthesiology. 2010;113:1220–35.
27. Peyton PJ, Thompson D, Junor P. Non-invasive automated measurement of cardiac output during stable cardiac surgery using a fully integrated differential CO_2 Fick method. J Clin Monit Comput. 2008;22:285–92.
28. Karlsson J, Winberg P, Scarr B, et al. Validation of capnodynamic determination of cardiac output by measuring effective pulmonary blood flow: a study in anaesthetised children and piglets. Br J Anaesth. 2018;121:550–8.
29. Hällsjö Sander C, Hallback M, Suarez-Sipmann F, et al. A novel continuous capnodynamic method for cardiac output assessment in a porcine model of lung lavage. Acta Anaesthesiol Scand. 2015;59:1022–31.
30. Sigmundsson TS. Performance of a capnodynamic method estimating effective pulmonary blood flow during transient and sustained hypercapnia. J Clin Monit Comput. 2018;32:311–9.
31. Montenij LJ, Buhre WF, Jansen JR, et al. Methodology of method comparison studies evaluating the validity of cardiac output monitors: a stepwise approach and checklist. Br J Anaesth. 2016;116:750–8.
32. Peyton PJ, Robinson GJB, McCall PR, Thompson B. Noninvasive measurement of intrapulmonary shunting. J Cardiothorac Vasc Anesth. 2004;18:47–52.
33. Gedeon A. Non-invasive pulmonary blood flow for optimal PEEP. Clin Physiol. 1985;5:49–58.

34. Hedenstierna G. The recording of FRC--is it of importance and can it be made simple? Intensive Care Med. 1993;19:365–6.
35. Brismar B, Hedenstierna G, Lundquist H, et al. Pulmonary densities during anesthesia with muscular relaxation--a proposal of atelectasis. Anesthesiology. 1985;62:422–8.
36. Gattinoni L, Caironi P, Cressoni M, et al. Lung recruitment in patients with the acute respiratory distress syndrome. N Engl J Med. 2006;354:1775–86.
37. de Matos GF, Stanzani F, Passos RH, et al. How large is the lung recruitability in early acute respiratory distress syndrome: a prospective case series of patients monitored by computed tomography. Crit Care. 2012;16:R4.
38. Heinze H, Eicheler W. Measurements of functional residual capacity during intensive care treatment: the technical aspects and its possible clinical applications. Acta Anaesthesiol Scand. 2009;53:1121–30.
39. Frerichs I, Amato MBP, van Kaam AH, et al. Chest electrical impedance tomography examination, data analysis, terminology, clinical use and recommendations: consensus statement of the TRanslational EIT developmeNt stuDy group. Thorax. 2017;72:83–93.
40. Olegard C, Sondergaard SR, Houltz E, et al. Estimation of functional residual capacity at the bedside using standard monitoring equipment: a modified nitrogen washout/washin technique requiring a small change of the inspired oxygen fraction. Anesth Analg. 2005;101:206–12.
41. Brewer LM, Haryadi DG, Orr JA. Measurement of functional residual capacity of the lung by partial CO_2 rebreathing method during acute lung injury in animals. Respir Care. 2007;52:1480–9.
42. Gedeon A, Krill P, Osterlund B. Pulmonary blood flow (cardiac output) and the effective lung volume determined from a short breath hold using the differential Fick method. J Clin Monit Comput. 2002;17:313–21.
43. Albu G, Wallin M, Hallbäck M, et al. Comparison of static end-expiratory and effective lung volumes for gas exchange in healthy and surfactant-depleted lungs. Anesthesiology. 2013;119:101–10.
44. Hällsjö Sander C, Lönnqvist P-A, Hallbäck M, et al. Capnodynamic assessment of effective lung volume during cardiac output manipulations in a porcine model. J Clin Monit Comput. 2016;30:761–9.
45. Slutsky AR. Reduction in pulmonary blood volume during positive end-expiratory pressure. J Surg Res. 1983;35:181–7.
46. Chiumello D, Carlesso E, Cadringher P, et al. Lung stress and strain during mechanical ventilation for acute respiratory distress syndrome. Am J Respir Crit Care Med. 2008;178:346–55.
47. González-López A, García-Prieto E, Batalla-Solís E, et al. Lung strain and biological response in mechanically ventilated patients. Intensive Care Med. 2012;38:240–7.

Should We Abandon Measuring SvO_2 or $ScvO_2$ in Patients with Sepsis?

17

J.-L. Teboul, X. Monnet, and D. De Backer

17.1 Introduction

The mixed venous oxygen saturation (SvO_2) has been used to assess the adequacy of oxygen delivery (DO_2) to oxygen consumption (VO_2). Since central venous catheters (CVCs) are now more often inserted than pulmonary artery catheters (PAC) in critically ill patients, central venous oxygen saturation ($ScvO_2$) has been proposed as a substitute for SvO_2. In 2001, Rivers et al. proposed a step-by-step strategy called early goal-directed therapy (EGDT) that aimed at normalizing the $ScvO_2$ within the first 6 h of resuscitation of patients with severe sepsis or septic shock [1]. A single-center randomized controlled trial (RCT) showed that application of EGDT significantly decreased mortality in comparison with a control group, in which $ScvO_2$ was not used [1]. Following the publication by Rivers et al. [1], EGDT was endorsed by the Surviving Sepsis Campaign (SSC) in 2004 [2]. More recently, three multicenter RCTs (ProCESS [3], ARISE [4] and ProMISe [5]) compared EGDT (using $ScvO_2$) to standard care (with no use of $ScvO_2$). In none of these trials did EGDT show any benefit in terms of outcome, as confirmed by a meta-analysis [6]. Differences between the trials (design/study population/management of the control group/general management of patients with sepsis) may have contributed to the divergent results of these trials [7]. Nevertheless, the SSC experts removed $ScvO_2$ (and SvO_2) from the recommendations of the most recent version of the SSC guidelines [8]. While targeting specific predefined values in all patients may be questioned, it is probably unwise to neglect the potential interest of measuring

J.-L. Teboul (✉) · X. Monnet
Service de réanimation médicale, Univ Paris-Sud, AP-HP, Hôpitaux Universitaires Paris-Sud, Hôpital de Bicêtre, Le Kremlin-Bicêtre, France
e-mail: jean-louis.teboul@aphp.fr

D. De Backer
Department of Intensive Care, CHIREC Hospitals, Université Libre de Bruxelles, Brussels, Belgium

J.-L. Vincent (ed.), *Annual Update in Intensive Care and Emergency Medicine 2019*, Annual Update in Intensive Care and Emergency Medicine,
https://doi.org/10.1007/978-3-030-06067-1_17

$SvO_2/ScvO_2$ in patients with sepsis. In this chapter, we discuss why there is still a place for the measurement of SvO_2 or $ScvO_2$ in patients with sepsis.

17.2 Physiological Determinants and Clinical Interpretation of SvO_2

The blood flowing through the pulmonary artery is the average of all the venous returns of the body. According to the Fick equation applied to oxygen, and assuming that the mixed venous blood oxygen content is linearly correlated with SvO_2, SvO_2 is related to arterial oxygen saturation (SaO_2), VO_2, cardiac output and hemoglobin concentration (Hb) as follows:

$$SvO_2 = SaO_2 - \left[VO_2 / \left(\text{cardiac output} \times \text{Hb} \times 13.4\right)\right]$$

The SvO_2 is thus an integrative variable that reflects the balance between DO_2 and VO_2 as cardiac output, Hb and SaO_2 are the major determinants of DO_2. In healthy subjects at rest, the value of SvO_2 ranges from 70 to 75%. The SvO_2 is the result of complex interactions between its four major determinants, each of which may be altered by the disease process, compensatory mechanisms and, sometimes, therapeutic agents. For example, cardiac output should increase in face of hypoxemia or anemia and should decrease after their correction. Thus, SvO_2 can be unchanged or change less than either of its determinants.

According to the simplified Fick equation mentioned above, SvO_2 approximately equals SaO_2—(VO_2/DO_2) and thus equals SaO_2 – oxygen extraction ratio, as the oxygen extraction ratio represents the VO_2/DO_2 ratio. When SaO_2 is close to 1 (i.e., 100%), an event that occurs very often in critically ill patients, SvO_2 approximately equals 1 – the oxygen extraction ratio and thus, except in cases of very severe hypoxemia, SvO_2 can serve as a reflection of the oxygen extraction at the time it is measured.

A low SvO_2 indicates that oxygen extraction has increased to attempt to make the VO_2 match the global oxygen demand. This can occur in cases of a decrease in DO_2 (low cardiac output, anemia insufficiently compensated by elevation of cardiac output), or an increase in oxygen demand (insufficiently compensated by an elevation of cardiac output), or both. If, despite adaptive mechanisms, VO_2 does not match oxygen demand, tissue hypoxia occurs [9]. There are two important points to recognize. First, SvO_2 begins to decrease immediately when DO_2 decreases, so that a low SvO_2 does not indicate tissue hypoxia. Second, there is no unique 'critical' value of SvO_2 below which tissue hypoxia starts to develop, as SvO_2 depends on many factors [9]. As an example, a SvO_2 of 55% can be encountered in chronic heart failure patients with low cardiac output but without shock due to development of strong compensatory mechanisms aimed at increasing oxygen extraction capacities and maintaining VO_2 at the level of oxygen demand [10]. On the other hand, for similar levels of Hb and SaO_2, a SvO_2 of 55% can be associated with severe acute cardiogenic shock, where compensatory mechanisms either have no time to develop or are partly altered due to associated inflammation. In the latter case, treatment aimed at increasing cardiac output is mandatory.

Conversely, a higher than normal SvO_2 means that oxygen extraction has decreased due either to an increase in DO_2 with unchanged VO_2 or more often a decrease in VO_2 with maintained or increased DO_2. This latter situation is encountered in hyperdynamic shock states where the decrease in VO_2 does not result from a fall of DO_2 below its critical level but rather from severely altered oxygen extraction capacities [11].

17.3 Interpretation of $ScvO_2$

$ScvO_2$ has progressively replaced SvO_2 over recent years for at least two reasons: the decline in use of the PAC and, as mentioned earlier, the endorsement by the SSC [2] of the EGDT proposed by Rivers et al. [1], where $ScvO_2$ was the most important target for resuscitation. It has to be noted that in the Rivers' trial, $ScvO_2$ was continuously monitored with a fiberoptic probe placed in the superior vena cava territory [1]. Physiologically, $ScvO_2$ is expected to be a little lower than SvO_2 mostly related to the influence of the renal circulation. However, in critically ill patients, $ScvO_2$ is more frequently higher than SvO_2 [12–17], due to a higher rate of oxygen extraction by the myocardium or the splanchnic area [18] than by organs draining into the superior vena cava. Nevertheless, several studies have reported low percentage errors between the variables [12, 13], although divergent results have also been reported [15–17]. Importantly, changes in $ScvO_2$ and in SvO_2 have generally been shown to correlate well [13, 14] although not identical, suggesting that monitoring $ScvO_2$ can be a reasonable surrogate for SvO_2 especially when the latter cannot be obtained.

17.4 Usefulness of $ScvO_2$ in Sepsis: A Debatable Issue

As mentioned ealier, targeting $ScvO_2$ was integrated in the EGDT algorithm that demonstrated benefits on outcome in the pivotal study by Rivers et al. [1]. Consequently, targeting $ScvO_2$ >70% in the initial hemodynamic resuscitation of patients with severe sepsis or septic shock has for a long time been a strong recommendation of the SSC. However, since the three large multicenter RCTs (ProCESS, ARISE, ProMISe) [3–5] showed no outcome benefit with EGDT in patients with early septic shock, the recommendation to target $ScvO_2$ has been totally removed from the most recent SSC guidelines. Thus, after being idolized for more than 10 years, measuring $ScvO_2$ in sepsis has now fallen into total disgrace. As with many issues in the management of critically ill patients, the truth is probably between idolatry and disgrace and we think that measuring SvO_2 should not be totally abandoned. The arguments supporting that position are developed below.

The populations included in ProCESS [3], ARISE [4] and ProMISe [5] were far different from that included in the Rivers' study [1], in which patients were sicker as illustrated by higher severity scores at inclusion, the higher number of patients with comorbidities and the higher mortality rate in the standard care arm (57% vs. about 30% in ProCESS and ProMISe and less than 20% in ARISE). Even more importantly, the average value of $ScvO_2$ at the time of inclusion was very different in the three multicenter RCTs (above 70%) and the Rivers' study (about 48%). These striking differences can be explained by differences in the main mechanism responsible for shock and/or the treatments already received before inclusion. Data reported by Rivers et al. [1] clearly indicate that the patients (of both arms) were severely hypovolemic at the time of inclusion as suggested by the low central venous pressure (CVP) and by the markedly positive responses of mean arterial pressure and of $ScvO_2$ to the first 6 h of resuscitation, which included large amounts of fluid (on average 5000 mL in the EGDT arm versus 3500 mL in the control group). The low rate of vasopressor use (only 30% of patients) confirmed that the main component of shock was hypovolemia and not arterial tone depression.

In the three multicenter RCTs [3–5], large volumes of fluids had already been administered before inclusion (2500 mL on average) so that the hypovolemic component of shock was probably less predominant at the time of inclusion compared with the Rivers study. This explains, at least partly, why on average $ScvO_2$ was already higher than 70%. Nevertheless, by design, these three RCTs could not show any benefit of targeting $ScvO_2$ >70% since $ScvO_2$ was already above the target at the time of randomization. Thus, the question of targeting a $ScvO_2$ >70% when the $ScvO_2$ is <70% cannot be definitively answered from the results of these trials. It is thus surprising to abandon $ScvO_2$ measurements on the sole basis of such results. To find an analogy with a common issue in medicine, let us imagine an RCT comparing an antihypertensive drug with placebo in a population of patients with normal arterial blood pressure at the randomization time. Such a study would obviously not find any benefit in favor of the antihypertensive drug. Would we have concluded that antihypertensive treatment is of no interest in the treatment of patients with hypertension? By analogy, examining the potential benefits of targeting $ScvO_2$ >70% should be performed in studies of patients with low $ScvO_2$. To our knowledge, only the single-center study by Rivers et al. [1] satisfied this very basic condition, so that the utility of targeting $ScvO_2$ >70% when $ScvO_2$ is low, cannot be totally abandoned unless the evidence of negative results is provided in multicenter RCTs.

One possible argument underlying the decision to abandon the recommendation of using $ScvO_2$ in the context of septic shock, would be to consider that the large majority of patients should have already received large amounts of fluids before the first value of $ScvO_2$ is obtained. In this context, $ScvO_2$ would be already >70% in the large majority of cases, as confirmed by the three multicenter RCTs mentioned earlier [3–5]. In addition, it could be argued that since alteration of oxygen extraction is a hallmark of septic shock, $ScvO_2$ might be high, even if the patient has not been fully resuscitated. A study by Boulain et al. provides interesting findings regarding the first value of $ScvO_2$ obtained in a cohort of 363 patients with septic shock enrolled in a prospective multicenter observational study [19]. Patients had already received about 35 mL/kg fluids on average before $ScvO_2$ was obtained (8 h on average after identification of sepsis). The prevalence of low $ScvO_2$ (<70%) was not negligible (about 27%), even when clinical resuscitation endpoints were achieved and even when arterial lactate was normal [17]. In a multicenter study including 619 patients admitted to the emergency department, the percentage of patients with an initial $ScvO_2$ value <70% was 36% [20]. Therefore, at least numerically, the proportion of patients with low initial $ScvO_2$ cannot be ignored. In addition, in the study by Boulain et al., an initial $ScvO_2$ <70% was significantly and independently associated with day-28 mortality [119]. Moreover, a logistic regression analysis showed that $ScvO_2$ <70% 6 h later was still a risk factor for day-28 mortality [19]. All these findings plead against abandoning $ScvO_2$ measurements in the early phase of septic shock, at least to identify this high-risk population of patients with low $ScvO_2$. However, whether such patients could benefit from a further increase in DO_2 aimed at elevating $ScvO_2$ as suggested by the Rivers' trial [1], needs further confirmation.

Finally, measuring $ScvO_2$ could also identify patients with very high values (>80%, or even >90%), which characterize a specific population where oxygen extraction capacities are markedly impaired due to the presence of large arterio-venous shunting and/or altered microcirculation and/or reduced diffusion of oxygen from the capillaries to the cells (interstitial edema) and/or mitochondrial dysfunction. Obviously, in such a context, it is illusory to expect any correction of tissue hypoxia after increasing DO_2. Such an observation should thus discourage attempts to deliberately increase DO_2 with usual therapies (i.e., fluids, inotropes, blood transfusion), and this can reduce additional risks of over-resuscitation. Unfortunately, therapies that successfully act on functional shunting, the microcirculation or oxygen diffusion disorders and mitochondrial dysfunction are still lacking. In this regard, one clinical study in patients with septic shock showed that patients with a maximal $ScvO_2$ value >80% within the first 72 h had a higher mortality than patients with $ScvO_2$ <80% [21]. In a study by Pope et al., the mortality rate was higher than in the sub-population of patients with an initial $ScvO_2$ >90% compared to the mortality rate of those with $ScvO_2$ between 70 and 89%, even after adjustment in a multivariable analysis [20].

17.5 Clinical Use of $ScvO_2$ and SvO_2

Although targeting a given value of $ScvO_2$ predefined in therapeutic bundles is more than questionable, measurements of $ScvO_2$ can be useful for several purposes. First, it is an important warning signal. In many instances, $ScvO_2$ is one of the first, easily measured variables to be altered when perfusion to the tissues decreases.

Second, it is an important variable to help understand the hemodynamic status. It has to be combined with measurements of cardiac output, lactate and veno-arterial carbon dioxide pressure difference (PCO_2 gap) (Fig. 17.1).

- A low $ScvO_2$ (<70%) is highly informative as it suggests that DO_2 is an important contributor to the shock state, with the advantage of being potentially correctable by usual cardiovascular therapies. This, in combination with other physiological

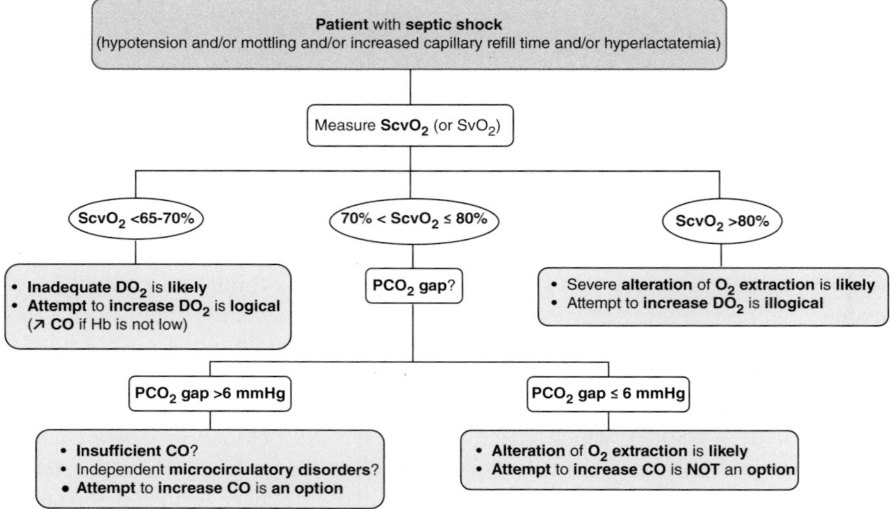

Fig. 17.1 Clinical interpretation of central venous oxygen saturation ($ScvO_2$). *Hb* hemoglobin concentration, *CO* cardiac output, *O_2* oxygen delivery, *O_2* oxygen, *PCO_2 gap* difference in carbon dioxide pressure between central venous blood and arterial blood, *SvO_2* mixed venous oxygen saturation

and hemodynamic variables, can encourage clinicians to try this therapeutic option, knowing that in patients with sepsis, there is no guarantee of significant increase in DO_2 and no guarantee of correction of microcirculatory disorders, even if DO_2 improves. In any case, we recommend making such a therapeutic decision on an individual basis.

- A high $ScvO_2$ (>80%) in the context of septic shock is also informative as it suggests marked alteration of oxygen extraction, which renders illogical any effort to increase DO_2.
- A so-called normal $ScvO_2$ (between 70 and 80%) is less informative as it neither encourages nor discourages use of therapies aimed at increasing DO_2. As an example, in a population of patients with septic shock (blood lactate = 5.5 ± 4.0 mmol/L) and mean $ScvO_2$ of 70 ± 15%, fluid infusion (500 mL of saline) was shown to increase DO_2, VO_2, and mean arterial pressure and to decrease blood lactate, all elements that suggest hemodynamic improvement [22]. In such cases of shock and 'normal' $ScvO_2$, one easy way to identify situations where increasing DO_2 can be attempted is to consider the value of the PCO_2 gap [23, 24]. A higher than normal PCO_2 gap (>6 mmHg) should encourage one to increase cardiac output and thus DO_2 with the aim of restoring, at least partly, adequate hemodynamic conditions. A normal or low PCO_2 gap should rather discourage any attempt to increase cardiac output [24].

Third, $ScvO_2$ targets should be individualized. As for many variables, one size does not fit all and chasing a $ScvO_2$ of 70–75% in all patients is likely to result in excessive therapy. The $ScvO_2$ should be integrated with other markers of tissue hypoperfusion and, whenever possible, the other determinants of $ScvO_2$ should be simultaneously measured (including cardiac output).

17.6 Conclusion

The vast majority of patients with septic shock are equipped with a CVC at least for administration of fluids and catecholamines. In this way, $ScvO_2$ can be easily obtained by blood sampling. The use of a fiberoptic probe allowing continuous monitoring of $ScvO_2$ is expensive and has no advantages over intermittent blood sampling. Knowledge of $ScvO_2$ at the initial phase of septic shock can help the clinician to better understand a patient's hemodynamic picture in order to hopefully make the appropriate therapeutic decision. However, hemodynamic resuscitation should not be based solely on $ScvO_2$ since there are: 1) potential limitations due to the fact that $ScvO_2$ and change in $ScvO_2$ do not always reflect SvO_2 and change in SvO_2; and 2) situations where its interpretation cannot be straightforward (e.g., for values within the so-called normal range). In any case, rational use of $ScvO_2$ requires its integration in a personalized and multimodal approach including other important hemodynamic and metabolic variables such as arterial blood pressure, cardiac output, lactate, PCO_2 gap and peripheral perfusion markers.

References

1. Rivers E, Nguyen B, Havstad S, et al. Early goal-directed therapy in the treatment of severe sepsis and septic shock. N Engl J Med. 2001;345:1368–77.
2. Dellinger RP, Carlet JM, Masur H, et al. Surviving Sepsis Campaign guidelines for management of severe sepsis and septic shock. Crit Care Med. 2004;32:858–73.
3. Yealy DM, Kellum JA, Huang DT, et al. A randomized trial of protocol-based care for early septic shock. N Engl J Med. 2014;370:1683–93.
4. Peake SL, Delaney A, Bailey M, et al. Goal-directed resuscitation for patients with early septic shock. N Engl J Med. 2014;371:1496–506.
5. Mouncey PR, Osborn TM, Power GS, et al. Trial of early, goal-directed resuscitation for septic shock. N Engl J Med. 2015;372:1301–11.
6. Rowan KM, Angus DC, Bailey M, et al. Early, goal-directed therapy for septic shock - a patient-level meta-analysis. N Engl J Med. 2017;376:2223–34.
7. Rhodes A, Evans LE, Alhazzani W, et al. Surviving sepsis campaign: international guidelines for management of sepsis and septic shock: 2016. Intensive Care Med. 2017;43:304–77.
8. De Backer D, Vincent JL. Early goal-directed therapy: do we have a definitive answer? Intensive Care Med. 2016;42:1048–50.
9. Kasnitz P, Druger GL, Yorra F, Simmons DH. Mixed venous oxygen tension and hyperlactatemia. JAMA. 1976;236:570–4.
10. Schlichtig R, Cowden WL, Chaitman BR. Tolerance of unusually low mixed venous oxygen saturation. Adaptations in the chronic low cardiac output syndrome. Am J Med. 1986;80:813–8.
11. Vincent JL, De Backer D. Circulatory shock. N Engl J Med. 2013;369:1726–34.
12. Chawla LS, Zia H, Gutierrez G, Katz NM, Seneff MG, Shah M. Lack of equivalence between central and mixed venous oxygen saturation. Chest. 2004;126:1891–6.

13. Reinhart K, Kuhn HJ, Hartog C, Bredle DL. Continuous central venous and pulmonary artery oxygen saturation monitoring in the critically ill. Intensive Care Med. 2004;30:1572–8.
14. Dueck MH, Klimek M, Appenrodt S, Weigand C, Boerner U. Trends but not individual values of central venous oxygen saturation agree with mixed venous oxygen saturation during varying hemodynamic conditions. Anesthesiology. 2005;103:249–57.
15. Varpula M, Karlsson S, Ruokonen E, Pettilä V. Mixed venous oxygen saturation cannot be estimated by central venous oxygen saturation in septic shock. Intensive Care Med. 2006;32:1336–43.
16. Gutierrez G, Comignani P, Huespe L, et al. Central venous to mixed venous blood oxygen and lactate gradients are associated with outcome in critically ill patients. Intensive Care Med. 2008;34:1662–8.
17. van Beest PA, van Ingen J, Boerma EC, et al. No agreement of mixed venous and central venous saturation in sepsis, independent of sepsis origin. Crit Care. 2010;14:R219.
18. De Backer D, Creteur J, Noordally O, Smail N, Gulbis B, Vincent JL. Does hepato-splanchnic VO_2/DO_2 dependency exist in critically ill septic patients? Am J Respir Crit Care Med. 1998;157:1219–25.
19. Boulain T, Garot D, Vignon P, et al. Prevalence of low central venous oxygen saturation in the first hours of intensive care unit admission and associated mortality in septic shock patients: a prospective multicentre study. Crit Care. 2014;18:609.
20. Pope JV, Jones AE, Gaieski DF, Arnold RC, Trzeciak S, Shapiro NI. Multi-center study of central venous oxygen saturation ($ScvO_2$) as a predictor of mortality in patients with sepsis. Ann Emerg Med. 2010;55:40–6.
21. Textoris J, Fouché L, Wiramus S, et al. High central venous oxygen saturation in the latter stages of septic shock is associated with increased mortality. Crit Care. 2011;15:R176.
22. Monnet X, Julien F, Ait-Hamou N, et al. Lactate and veno-arterial carbon dioxide difference/arterial-venous oxygen difference ratio, but not central venous oxygen saturation, predict increase in oxygen consumption in fluid responders. Crit Care Med. 2013;41:1412–20.
23. Cecconi M, De Backer D, Antonelli M, et al. Consensus on circulatory shock and hemodynamic monitoring. Task force of the European Society of Intensive Care Medicine. Intensive Care Med. 2014;40:1795–815.
24. Teboul JL, Saugel B, Cecconi M, et al. Less invasive hemodynamic monitoring in critically ill patients. Intensive Care Med. 2016;42:1350–9.

Perioperative Hemodynamic Monitoring: MERCI to Predict Economic Impact

18

F. Michard and G. Manecke

18.1 Introduction

Most hemodynamic monitoring techniques have an associated cost. Although difficult to quantify, the cost of their implementation may be significant, particularly for techniques requiring prolonged high-level training, such as echocardiography. These costs, or upfront investments, may be an obstacle to hospital adoption. Importantly, a fair evaluation of the return on investment must take into account the potential savings associated with a reduction in postoperative complications and hospital length of stay.

18.2 Cost of Postoperative Complications

The cost of postoperative complications is not easy to assess precisely for several reasons. First, in many countries, there are no reliable clinical databases where clearly defined postoperative complications are collected prospectively. Second, in countries using the diagnosis-related group (DRG) billing method, two patients with the same comorbidities, undergoing the same surgery and spending the same number of days in the hospital, may be charged the same amount even if they develop complications that differ in terms of real diagnosis (e.g., abdominal computed tomography [CT] scan vs. bacterial sample) and treatment costs (e.g., reintervention vs. antibiotics). Third, even when reliable complication data are available, for example from the National Surgical Quality Improvement Program (NSQIP) database in the USA, patients often develop several complications at the same time. When this is the case, it is challenging, when

F. Michard (✉)
MiCo, Denens, Switzerland
e-mail: frederic.michard@bluewin.ch

G. Manecke
Department of Anesthesiology, UCSD Medical Center, San Diego, CA, USA

J.-L. Vincent (ed.), *Annual Update in Intensive Care and Emergency Medicine 2019*, Annual Update in Intensive Care and Emergency Medicine,
https://doi.org/10.1007/978-3-030-06067-1_18

Table 18.1 Extra costs associated with postoperative complications in studies including >1000 surgical patients

Study	Population, n	Extra-costs/patient
Michard et al. 2015 [5]	204,680	$11,824
Manecke et al. 2014 [4]	75,140	$29,876
Eappen et al. 2013 [3]	34,256	$22,398
Vonlanthen et al. 2011 [2]	1200	$34,446
Dimik et al. 2006 [1]	1008	$10,178
Weighted average in $US		$17,338
Weighted average in € (exchange rate from July 28, 2018)		€14,873

not impossible, to determine which proportion of the increase in length of stay and related costs is associated with each specific complication. To bypass this limitation, several studies [1–5] did not try to determine the cost of individual complications but looked at surgical populations in a dichotomous way with patients who did not develop any complications on one side, and patients who developed one or more complications on the other. These studies enable an estimation of the average extra costs associated with the development of one or more complications for a given surgical population. Studies that have included >1000 patients are summarized in Table 18.1. The average cost difference between a patient with one or more complications and a patient without any complication is around $17,000 or €15,000.

18.3 Cost of Hemodynamic Monitoring Systems

The cost of monitoring to achieve hemodynamic optimization is highly variable, not only from one method to another, but also from one country to another, depending on reimbursement policies. For example, if the operating room is already equipped with bedside monitors that automatically calculate and continuously display the arterial pulse pressure variation (PPV), using this variable to individualize intraoperative fluid management will not induce any additional equipment costs, although there may be some costs of training and education of personnel. In contrast, the purchase of disposable sensors (e.g., for pulse contour analysis or esophageal Doppler, the most commonly used techniques for hemodynamic optimization) or of an ultrasound machine will result in added equipment costs that are usually easy to quantify. The cost of hemodynamic monitors (the box with a display) is also highly variable from one product to the other, and some companies offer sensor connectivity to multiparameter bedside monitors via a module, so that a stand-alone hemodynamic monitor is not necessary. Rentals, per-usage plans, and unlimited usage plans are also available from some companies.

18.4 Can We Estimate what Investment Is Justified?

The estimation of the return on investment is possible as soon as the clinical benefits are established and quantified. Pulse contour methods and the esophageal Doppler are the preferred monitoring choices of anesthesiologists for hemodynamic

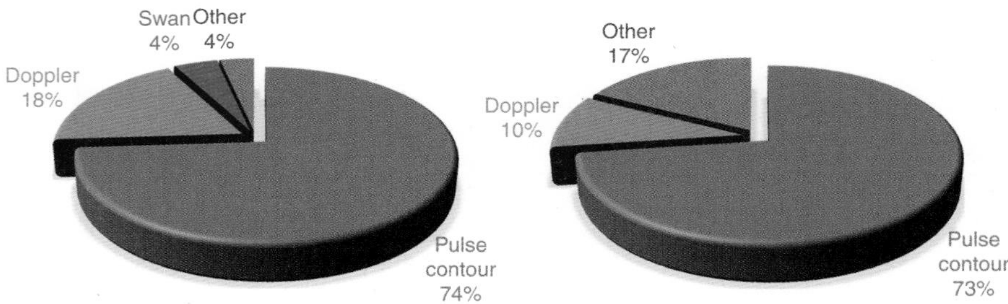

Fig. 18.1 Hemodynamic monitoring techniques used during non-cardiac surgery in two large multinational studies. Left: EuSOS [6] published in 2012; right: RELIEF [7] published in 2018

optimization in major non-cardiac surgical procedures [6, 7] (Fig. 18.1). Many studies and meta-analyses have suggested that implementation of these techniques, with well-defined hemodynamic objectives, is useful to decrease the proportion of high-risk surgical patients who develop one or more postoperative complications, aka postoperative morbidity. In four highly cited meta-analyses [8–11], the reduction in postoperative morbidity ranged from 23 to 57% (Table 18.2). However, it is important to acknowledge that (1) most studies done in patients who were part of enhanced recovery after surgery (ERAS) programs failed to show a similar benefit [12]; and (2) studies investigating the use of non-invasive techniques in lower risk patients have also been disappointing [13, 14].

Table 18.2 Reduction rate of postoperative morbidity with perioperative hemodynamic optimization in four highly cited meta-analyses

Meta-analysis	Number of studies & patients	Relative reduction in morbidity (%)
Hamilton et al. 2011 [8]	29 & 4805	57
Grocott et al. 2013 [9]	31 & 5292	32
Pearse et al. 2014 [10]	22 & 3024	23
Michard et al. 2017[a] [11]	19 & 2159	54

[a]Uncalibrated pulse contour techniques only

The 'MERCI' equation [15] enables an easy estimation of the possible Investment (I) to implement hemodynamic monitoring at no net costs (Fig. 18.2). It takes into account the current Morbidity rate (M), the Expected Reduction (ER) in postoperative morbidity, and the current cost (C) of complications:

$$\mathrm{M} \times \mathrm{ER} \times \mathrm{C} = \mathrm{I}$$

If the morbidity rate after colorectal surgery is 25% (M = 25%), the expected reduction in postoperative morbidity is 23% (ER = 23%), and the average cost of complications per patient is $17,000 (Table 18.1), the investment to implement hemodynamic monitoring at no net cost is $978/patient:

$$0.25 \times 0.23 \times \$17{,}000 = \$978$$

If the actual cost of the monitoring is greater than $978/patient, the monitoring cost above $978/patient would represent new net cost to the health system. If the

M x ER x C = I

M = Morbidity rate % ER = Expected Reduction % C = Cost of complications / patient **I = Investment/patient**

Fig. 18.2 The MERCI equation

cost of monitoring is less than \$978/patient, the difference would be savings to the health system. This is just an example using the expected reduction in morbidity of 23% from the meta-analysis by Pearse et al. [10] published in the JAMA (Table 18.2). If the baseline morbidity rate and cost of complications are lower and the clinical impact of hemodynamic monitoring is not as significant, then the investment, or 'break even point' will logically be lower as well. For example, if the morbidity rate after femur and hip fracture repair is only 15%, the expected reduction in postoperative morbidity is only 10%, and the average cost of complications in this specific population is only \$5400 [5], then the investment to implement hemodynamic monitoring at no net cost is only \$81/patient:

$$0.15 \times 0.10 \times \$5,400 = \$81$$

In this example, if the cost of implementing the monitoring is greater than \$81/patient, the cost above \$81/patient would represent new net cost to the health system. It is clear that the greater the incidence and cost of complications, the greater the cost of monitoring can be while maintaining either net cost savings or no net cost ('break even').

In summary, the MERCI equation has been created to help any given hospital to predict the economic impact of perioperative hemodynamic monitoring from its own morbidity rates and own costs of complications [15].

Several studies have used the MERCI equation to predict the economic impact of hemodynamic monitoring in large populations of patients undergoing major non-cardiac surgery. A first study [4] including >75,000 patients from >200 US academic hospitals reported a possible investment of around \$750/patient. This means that if the cost of hemodynamic monitoring is around \$300/patient (classical cost in the USA, including the amortization of the monitor), the hospital will save around \$450/patient. A larger and more recent study (>200,000 patients from >500 academic and non-academic hospitals in the USA) reported a possible investment around \$1000/patient, suggesting, in addition to the clinical benefits, potential savings around \$700/patient [5]. A French study [16], including 2388 patients from three hospitals, predicted savings around 600-€1000/patient for major abdominal, vascular, orthopedic, urologic and gynecologic procedures.

Two other simulation studies modelled the potential impact of hemodynamic monitoring on quality-adjusted life years (QALYs) to assess its cost-effectiveness. In the first study [17], done with Swedish financial data and focusing on elderly hip fracture patients, hemodynamic monitoring was less costly (−€1882/patient) and provided more QALYs than standard management in 96.5% of the simulations. In the second study [18], done with UK data and focusing on high-risk patients, hemodynamic monitoring decreased costs (−£2135/patient) and prolonged QALYs by almost 10 months.

18.5 Economic Impact in Real Life

Studies based on the MERCI equation [4, 5, 16] or simulation models [17, 18] can only predict or project the economic impact of hemodynamic monitoring. It is important to support such projections, by determining what has happened in hospitals where hemodynamic optimization was implemented in 'real life'.

Two old studies [19, 20] done in the UK compared the cost of patients who were managed with a hemodynamic monitoring tool to the cost of patients from a standard management group. Both studies showed a significant reduction in costs in the hemodynamic monitoring group, ranging between £1259 [19] and £3467/patient [20]. Of note, these studies were done >20 years ago when the Swan-Ganz catheter was the only option for advanced monitoring for hemodynamic optimization of non-cardiac surgical patients. Therefore, these results may not be applicable to current monitoring and billing practices.

More recent studies done with a pulse contour technique have reported savings ranging from zero in China [21] to more than $3500/patient in the USA [22]. The largest economic evaluation published so far (>700 patients), done in the UK, also with a pulse contour technique, showed net savings of around £400/patient [23].

In addition, it is important to note that the reduction in postoperative morbidity is often associated with a reduction in hospital length of stay. When this is the case, the increase in the number of free beds may allow a boost in surgical activity, with the opportunity for increased productivity, decreased wait times for patients, and increased revenue (depending on the country and health system). The opportunities generated by decreased length of stay and the associated available beds can be particularly advantageous to busy, private hospitals. The opportunities may also help large facilities that have available operating room capacity but limited bed availability address a surgical backlog with long waiting times.

18.6 Hospital Savings Versus Profits

When patients develop complications, hospital costs are higher, but reimbursements are higher too. Therefore, it is important to look at the impact of hemodynamic monitoring on hospital profitability (reimbursements–costs) and margin (profitability expressed as a percentage) since they may end up being the main drivers for adoption by the hospital administration.

A 2006 US study from Dimick et al. [1] reported hospital costs for surgery on average $10,178 higher in case of complications, whereas reimbursements were only $7645 higher. As a result, the profit dropped from $3288 to $755 and the margin from 23 to 3% in patients who developed one or more complication. A more recent study [24] from Flynn et al., focusing on patients undergoing open colectomy, showed a decrease in profit by more than $12,000 when patients developed postoperative complications. Payers are currently much less likely to pay for the care of complications than they were in the past. Thus, these studies suggest that, at least in the USA, hospitals have real financial incentives to help clinicians improve quality of surgical and perioperative care.

18.7 Conclusion

Most hemodynamic monitoring techniques, beyond standard monitors such as electrocardiogram (EKG) and non-invasive blood pressure cuff, have added cost. This cost, often relatively minor for an intensive care unit, may double or triple the average cost of anesthesia. Therefore, in the operating room, it is important to carefully select patients who may benefit from hemodynamic optimization, i.e., patients with comorbidities and/or undergoing major procedures with significant blood loss [25]. With the MERCI equation, it is easy to predict the return on investment, and hence to kick off a constructive discussion between clinicians, medical technology companies and hospital administration.

References

1. Dimick JB, Weeks WB, Karia RJ. Who pays for poor surgical quality? Building a business case for quality improvement. J Am Coll Surg. 2006;202:933–7.
2. Vonlanthen R, Slankamenac K, Breitenstein S, et al. The impact of complications on costs of major surgical procedures: a cost analysis of 1200 patients. Ann Surg. 2011;254:907–13.
3. Eappen S, Lane BH, Rosenberg B, et al. Relationship between occurrence of surgical complications and hospital finances. JAMA. 2013;309:1599–606.
4. Manecke G, Asemota A, Michard F. Tackling the economic burden of postsurgical complications: would goal directed fluid therapy help? Crit Care. 2014;18:566.
5. Michard F, Mountford WK, Krukas MR, et al. Potential return on investment for implementation of perioperative goal-directed fluid therapy in major surgery: a nationwide database study. Perioper Med. 2015;4:11.
6. Ahmad T, Beilstein CM, Aldecoa C, et al. Variation in haemodynamic monitoring for major surgery in European nations: secondary analysis of the EuSOS dataset. Perioper Med. 2015;4:8.
7. Myles PS, Bellomo R, Corcoran T, et al. Restrictive versus liberal fluid therapy for major abdominal surgery. N Engl J Med. 2018;378:2263–74.
8. Hamilton MA, Cecconi M, Rhodes A. A systematic review and meta-analysis on the use of preemptive hemodynamic intervention to improve postoperative outcomes in moderate and high-risk surgical patients. Anesth Analg. 2011;112:1392–402.
9. Grocott MPW, Dushianthan A, Hamilton MA, et al. Perioperative increase in global blood flow to explicit defined goals and outcomes after surgery: a Cochrane systematic review. Br J Anaesth. 2013;111:535–48.

10. Pearse RM, Harrison DA, MacDonald N, et al. Effect of a perioperative, cardiac output-guided hemodynamic therapy algorithm on outcomes following major gastrointestinal surgery: a randomized clinical trial and systematic review. JAMA. 2014;311:2181–90.
11. Michard F, Giglio MT, Brienza N. Perioperative goal-directed therapy with uncalibrated pulse contour methods: impact on fluid management and postoperative outcome. Br J Anaesth. 2017;119:22–30.
12. Joshi GP, Kehlet H. CON: perioperative goal-directed fluid therapy is an essential element of an enhanced recovery protocol? Anesth Analg. 2016;122:1261–3.
13. Pestana D, Espinosa E, Eden A, et al. Perioperative goal-directed hemodynamic optimization using noninvasive cardiac output monitoring in major abdominal surgery: a prospective, randomized, multicenter, pragmatic trial: POEMAS Study (PeriOperative goal-directed therapy in Major Abdominal Surgery). Anesth Analg. 2014;119:579–87.
14. Stens J, Hering JP, van der Hoeven CWP, et al. The added value of cardiac index and pulse pressure variation monitoring to mean arterial pressure-guided volume therapy in moderate-risk abdominal surgery (COGUIDE): a pragmatic multicenter randomised controlled trial. Anaesthesia. 2017;72:1078–87.
15. Michard F. MERCI for improving quality of surgical care at no cost. World J Surg. 2016;40:3095–6.
16. Landais A, Morel M, Goldstein J, et al. Evaluation of financial burdens following complications after major surgery in France: potential returns after perioperative goal directed therapy. Anaesth Crit Care Pain Med. 2017;36:151–5.
17. Bartha E, Davidson T, Hommel A, et al. Cost-effectiveness analysis of goal-directed hemodynamic treatment of elderly hip fracture patients: before clinical research starts. Anesthesiology. 2012;117:519–30.
18. Ebm C, Cecconi M, Sutton L. A cost-effectiveness analysis of postoperative goal directed therapy for high-risk surgical patients. Crit Care Med. 2014;42:1194–203.
19. Boyd O, Grounds M, Bennett ED. A randomized clinical trial of the effect of deliberate perioperative increase of oxygen delivery on mortality in high-risk surgical patients. JAMA. 1993;270:2699–707.
20. Wilson J, Woods I, Fawcett J, et al. Reducing the risk of major elective surgery: randomised controlled trial of preoperative optimisation of oxygen delivery. BMJ. 1999;318:1099–103.
21. Jin J, Min S, Liu D, et al. Clinical and economic impact of goal-directed fluid therapy during elective gastrointestinal surgery. Perioper Med. 2018;7:22.
22. Hand WR, Stoll WD, McEvoy MD, et al. Intraoperative goal-directed hemodynamic management in free tissue transfer for head and neck cancer. Head Neck. 2016;38:E1974–80.
23. Sadique Z, Harrison DA, Grieve R, et al. Cost-effectiveness of a cardiac output-guided haemodynamic therapy algorithm in high-risk patients undergoing major gastrointestinal surgery. Perioper Med. 2015;4:13.
24. Flynn DN, Speck RM, Mahmoud NN, et al. The impact of complications following open colectomy on hospital finances: a retrospective cohort study. Perioper Med. 2014;3:1.
25. Vincent JL, Pelosi P, Pearse R, et al. Perioperative cardiovascular monitoring of high-risk patients: a consensus of 12. Crit Care. 2015;19:224.

The Pulmonary Artery Catheter in the Management of the High-Risk Surgical Patient

19

M. Heringlake, S. Brandt, and C. Schmidt

19.1 Introduction

The introduction of the pulmonary artery catheter (PAC) into clinical practice almost 50 years ago was a landmark for the treatment of critically ill and high-risk surgical patients as well as the future development of critical care medicine [1]. Hemodynamic measurements which—at that time—were restricted to cardiology labs and based on the use of expensive dyes and time consuming measurements, could now easily be performed at the bedside on the intensive care unit (ICU) and in the operating room (OR). Thus it was not astonishing that, within a few years, the PAC became a standard tool for hemodynamic monitoring in patients during critical illness conditions and the tool of choice for managing perioperative hemodynamic optimization in high-risk patients.

Since the beginning of this century, enthusiasm for the PAC has decreased markedly. This may be related to three developments: the evolution of critical care echocardiography [2]; the development of less invasive, alternative hemodynamic monitoring tools [3]; and, probably the most important aspect, 'negative publicity' [4]. The latter phenomenon was primarily triggered by the results of the observational SUPPORT trial [5], suggesting increased mortality in critical care patients monitored with a PAC. The results of multiple randomized studies published in subsequent years clearly refuted this hypothesis [6, 7], but these studies (as well as a large multicenter trial of high-risk surgical patients [8] and another trial in patients with decompensated heart failure [9]) did not reveal a benefit of using a PAC. Thus more and more clinicians refrained from using this monitoring modality.

Interestingly, although PAC use has declined tremendously in many clinical fields, it is still the standard extended monitoring system in many patients

M. Heringlake (✉) · S. Brandt · C. Schmidt
Department of Anesthesiology and Intensive Care Medicine,
University of Lübeck, Lübeck, Germany
e-mail: Heringlake@t-online.de

J.-L. Vincent (ed.), *Annual Update in Intensive Care and Emergency Medicine 2019*, Annual Update in Intensive Care and Emergency Medicine,
https://doi.org/10.1007/978-3-030-06067-1_19

undergoing cardiac surgery [10], is increasingly used in patients with severe heart failure [11] and is recommended by recent guidelines [12].

In this chapter, we describe the available evidence on PAC use for management of the high risk surgical (cardiac as well as non-cardiac) patient, relate these findings to alternative concepts in this setting, and provide some perspectives on future developments of this monitoring modality.

19.2 PAC Monitoring in the High-Risk Surgical Patient: The History

Immediately after clinical introduction of the PAC, Shoemaker and colleagues performed several observational studies in high-risk surgical and trauma patients revealing the pivotal role of an adequate oxygen balance for achieving good clinical outcomes, and that a mismatch between oxygen delivery and demand was associated with increased morbidity and mortality [13]. Subsequently they developed a therapeutic concept of optimizing oxygen balance by increasing cardiac index (using fluids and inotropes) as well as oxygen content of the blood to reach the hemodynamic goals achieved in the surviving patients, and indeed observed a significant reduction in mortality [14]. Furthermore (but later largely ignored by the critical care community), they found that this concept of hemodynamic optimization was only effective if applied *before* severe organ dysfunction had occurred [14].

Since the suggested hemodynamic goals were higher than those typically observed in an unstressed patient at rest, they unfortunately used the misnomer "supranormal" for this goal-directed optimization approach, although—using typical hemoglobin targets at that time—this "supranormal" approach would have resulted in a mixed venous oxygen saturation (SvO_2) within the normal range (Fig. 19.1). This suggests,

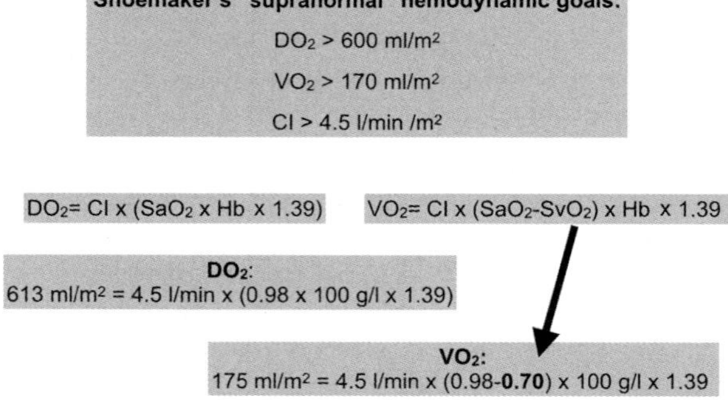

Fig. 19.1 Shoemaker's "supranormal" hemodynamic goals are reflective of a 'normal' mixed venous oxygen saturation. Calculation of oxygen delivery (DO_2) and consumption (VO_2) based on cardiac index (CI) and hemoglobin (Hb) levels observed in surviving high-risk surgical patients [13] reveals that Shoemaker's seemingly "supranormal" goals were associated with a 'normal' mixed venous oxygen saturation (SvO_2) of 70%

that the apparently "supranormal" hemodynamic goals were reflective of a 'normal' postsurgical stress response, which is typically associated with a higher than normal cardiac index to match the increased metabolic needs in this situation.

Following the landmark studies by Shoemaker et al. [13, 14], several monocenter studies confirmed their findings [15, 16]. Of note, one of the larger studies showed that the outcome benefit of goal-directed optimization was even detectable years after surgery [17]. Unfortunately, an attempt to validate the concept in a large multicenter trial failed and, with the exception of a trend towards improved renal function, did not reveal a substantial effect on outcomes [8]. However, this study has frequently been criticized because only a minority of patients reached the hemodynamic goals before ICU admission and no information on treatment was provided.

19.3 What Is the Difference Between Other Monitoring Modalities and the PAC?

In contrast to other monitoring modalities, the PAC as a right heart catheter does not only allow measurement of cardiac index (CI) and stroke volume index (SVI), but also SvO_2, pulmonary artery and right ventricular (RV) pressures, RV ejection fraction, and RV end-diastolic volume index (RVEDVI).

Modern fiberoptic catheters enable SvO_2 and pressures to be displayed continuously while CI is determined by semi-continuous thermodilution. Entering heart rate from the bedside monitor and using a fast-response thermistor (capable of detecting individual beats within the thermodilution signal) additionally allows semi-continuous determination of RV ejection fraction and RVEDVI.

Thus, a modern PAC gives instantaneous information on more hemodynamic variables than any other commercially available monitoring device. Additionally, with the exception of arterial oxygen content, any information necessary to assess oxygen balance is almost continuously available; a clear difference, especially compared to transpulmonary thermodilution monitors that need to be calibrated intermittently to get reliable cardiac output data [18].

While determination of cardiac output and stroke volume can—more or less reliably—be performed either with uncalibrated pulse contour analysis systems, transpulmonary thermodilution or echocardiography, two important features distinguish the PAC from other hemodynamic devices: the capability of assessing cardiopulmonary interactions and right heart function as well as the determination of SvO_2.

It is increasingly recognized that right heart dysfunction and/or pulmonary arterial hypertension may not only be encountered in patients with heart failure [19] and after cardiac surgery [20] but also in patients with chronic obstructive lung disease (COPD) [21] and acute lung disease [22]. Additionally, changes in pulmonary mechanics induced by mechanical ventilation may have relevant implications on pulmonary vascular resistance and right ventricular afterload [23].

While it is obvious that primarily left sided monitoring (with the notable exception of falsely positive increases in dynamic preload variables upon right heart failure [24]) cannot give any useful information on right heart function, echocardiography has been claimed to be a less invasive modality to determine pulmonary artery pressure. Unfortunately, determination of pulmonary artery pressure is only feasible in two-thirds of patients due to lack of tricuspid regurgitation; additionally, echocardiographic determinations have been reported to be rather imprecise, and are of course not available on a continuous basis [25]. In contrast, the PAC allows continuous assessment of cardiopulmonary interactions and right heart function. Additionally, the ratio of pulmonary artery occlusion pressure (PAOP) to central venous pressure (CVP) may help better understand the underlying pathology of an individual patient and help quantify right heart dysfunction.

In recent years, central venous oxygen saturation ($ScvO_2$) has gained attention as a possible substitute for SvO_2 to assess systemic oxygen balance. Unfortunately, large differences between $ScvO_2$ and SvO_2 have been observed in patients undergoing cardiac surgery [26] and in patients with septic shock [27], possibly related to increased oxygen extraction of the splanchnic region during hemodynamic compromise [26, 28]. Thus a 'normal' $ScvO_2$ does not rule out a significantly depressed SvO_2 in these situations and assessing systemic oxygen balance by $ScvO_2$ may become unreliable. Of note, absolute differences of more than 5/10% were observed in more than 50/25% of cardiac surgical patients, respectively [28]. This observation has important clinical implications.

In line with the pivotal findings from Shoemaker and colleagues [13], Holm and coworkers showed that a SvO_2 <60% on ICU admission after cardiac surgery was associated with a high mortality [29]. Interestingly, patients presenting with a SvO_2 in the range of 60–70% had a mortality rate of around 1%, whereas patients with SvO_2 values between 55–60% and 50–55% had mortality rates of 5 and 7%, respectively. This finding suggests that even minor differences in SvO_2 may have relevant impact on outcomes and that, if venous oxygen saturation is to be used for hemodynamic optimization, SvO_2 is clearly superior to $ScvO_2$ as a goal.

19.4 Is There Any Evidence to Support Use of a PAC Instead of (or in Addition to) Alternative Monitoring Modalities in High-Risk Surgical Patients?

Some years ago, Hamilton and coworkers performed a detailed systematic analysis on the effects of goal-directed hemodynamic optimization in moderate and high-risk surgical patients and—based on the evidence available in 2011—showed that, while multiple monitoring technologies were effective in reducing complications, only the use of a PAC was associated with a reduction in mortality, if used to achieve "supranormal" hemodynamics [30]. Interestingly, Gurgel and do Nascimento independently came to the conclusion that in high-risk surgical patients without preoperative evidence of organ dysfunction, the use of the PAC and DO_2 and VO_2 reduced postoperative mortality and morbidity [31]. Additionally they noted a proportional relationship between the level of perioperative risk and the benefit of hemodynamic control.

These findings have been questioned because some of the high-risk studies employing the PAC dated back to the early period after Shoemaker's initial studies [14–16] and the mortality rates for comparable surgeries have decreased considerably since then. However, multiple observational studies have shown that, especially in the increasing population of patients with heart failure, many standard surgical procedures are still associated with substantial mortality rates [32]. Taking into account the classic definition of heart failure as the inability of the heart to generate a sufficient blood flow to adequately meet the metabolic needs of the tissues, monitoring such patients with a PAC and aiming for optimization of oxygen balance is more than reasonable.

In line with these assumptions, recent evidence, especially in patients with heart failure and patients undergoing cardiac surgery, suggests that hemodynamic monitoring with a PAC may be associated with improved outcomes. Sotomi et al. observed significantly improved 30-day mortality in patients monitored with a PAC during inotropic treatment of an acute heart failure syndrome associated with hypotension in a propensity matched cohort of 1000 patients from the ATTEND register [33]. In a registry study of more than 116,000 cardiac surgical patients, Brovman and coworkers showed that the use of the PAC was associated with significantly fewer transfusions and a trend ($p = 0.086$) towards a reduction in mortality [34]. Interestingly, the authors observed that use of a PAC had steadily increased between 2010 and 2014 from 25% to almost 40%. Comparably, Shaw and coworkers recently showed that the use of the PAC was associated with a significant reduction in cardiopulmonary and bleeding complications in a propensity matched cohort of more than 6000 patients [35].

These positive findings contrast sharply with the sparse data available on the use of transpulmonary thermodilution technology in high-risk surgical patients. Despite being in clinical use for more than 20 years, the effectiveness of goal-directed hemodynamic optimization using this modality has only been tested in a handful of studies. Goepfert and coworkers showed a reduction in catecholamine use and duration of mechanical ventilation as well as a shorter time to fitness for discharge in a partially retrospective analysis of 80 cardiac surgical patients [36]. However, the study was clearly limited by the use of a historical control group. In another study, in 100 cardiac surgical patients, these authors analyzed the effects of a combined approach, using dynamic preload variables to individually determine the optimal global end-diastolic volume and to maintain this fluid status perioperatively, and observed a significant reduction in postoperative complications [37]. Unfortunately, it is hard to imagine that this complex approach may be transferred into routine clinical practice.

In contrast to the positive signals derived from these studies in cardiac surgical patients, a study in 180 non-cardiac high-risk surgical patients failed to show any benefit of hemodynamic optimization based on a transpulmonary thermodilution algorithm in comparison with best practice standard therapy [38]. Of note, a recent comparison study revealed no differences in global end-diastolic volume determined by the transpulmonary thermodilution technique in patients with severe aortic stenosis and those with dilated cardiomyopathy despite a marked difference in biplanar left ventricular (LV) levocardiography [39]. This raises questions as to whether the volumetric variables derived from transpulmonary thermodilution are indeed reflective of a physiological substrate.

In contrast to the transpulmonary thermodilution technology, many studies employing calibrated as well as uncalibrated pulse contour cardiac output and esophageal Doppler systems for goal-directed hemodynamic optimization are available, often showing a benefit in terms of a reduction in morbidity [40, 41]. However, the largest of these trials, the OPTIMISE study [42], failed to show a significant effect of stroke volume and DO_2 optimization on a combined endpoint of complications or death.

In addition to transpulmonary thermodilution, pulse contour and esophageal Doppler devices, echocardiography is another monitoring modality that has been repeatedly suggested to be superior to the PAC for assessing hemodynamics and guiding hemodynamic resuscitation [2]. Interestingly, despite the role of echocardiography as a diagnostic tool and the fact that it, in many situations, adds important complementary information to the data derived from extended monitoring, the effects of goal-directed hemodynamic optimization using echocardiography on outcomes have never been tested in a randomized trial in high-risk surgical patients [2].

19.5 Limitations and Risks

Like any other technology, the PAC has technical and clinical limitations that need to be taken into account for appropriate use. One important aspect is related to the potentially confounding effect of intracardiac shunts, such as atrial or ventricular septal defects, which may influence the thermodilution signal and (in case of a left-to-right shunt) may lead to overestimation of cardiac output as well as (true) SvO_2. Similarly, a high degree of tricuspid regurgitation may lead to erroneous measurements and usually underestimation of cardiac output measurements [43]. However, in this situation, SvO_2 is still valid and may still be used to assess oxygen balance.

The device specific risks of the PAC in a recent cohort (0.3% severe complications, 0.1% attributable mortality) [44] are lower than the risks that have been contemporarily reported, e.g., for transesophageal echocardiography [45]. Nonetheless, atrial and ventricular premature beats as well as sustained arrhythmias may be induced during introduction of a PAC. Consequently, close observation as well as experience in the adequate management of rhythm disturbances is pivotal, especially in patients with myocardial ischemia and aortic stenosis.

19.6 Perspectives

As a consequence of the controversies about the PAC after the SUPPORT trial [5], little effort has been made by the industry to further develop this technology. However, applications already implemented in other monitoring modalities, e.g., pulse contour analysis, could easily be integrated into a PAC bedside monitor. This approach might allow an autocalibrating pulse contour stroke volume monitor to be created for the low pressure system that most likely will be less influenced by changes in vascular tone than arterial pulse contour devices. Additionally, with intelligent software solutions, safety features such as automated pressure curve analyses could be implemented to determine whether spontaneous wedging has occurred. Consequently, there are plenty of opportunities to further improve this technology in the near future.

However, one important feature to obtain additional information from the PAC is already available and has been reported by colleagues at the Montreal Heart Institute. Using a special PAC with an additional RV pressure port, they showed that direct pressure monitoring of the RV pressure curve allows immediate determination of RV function and, in combination with pulmonary artery pressure measurements, detection of dynamic RV outflow tract obstruction, a phenomenon which, comparable to the left side of the heart, may be observed during high dose inotrope treatment [46].

19.7 Conclusion

Based on multiple meta-analyses [32, 33], the PAC is still the only monitoring device that, if appropriately used within a hemodynamic protocol aiming to normalize and to maintain systemic oxygen balance and thereby tissue oxygenation perioperatively, has ever been shown to improve mortality in high-risk surgical patients. Taking into account the substantial mortality risk still present in various kinds of surgery and in patients with heart failure, any reluctance to use this tool and to favor seemingly less- or non-invasive technologies, such as calibrated or non-calibrated pulse contour cardiac output devices, in high-risk patients is hard to justify. However, although not directly supported by scientific evidence, the complementary use of echocardiography seems highly reasonable.

References

1. Swan HJC, Ganz W, Forrester J, et al. Catheterization of the heart in man with the use of a flow directed balloon catheter. N Engl J Med. 1970;283:447–51.
2. Sing K, Mayo P. Critical care echocardiography and outcomes in the critically ill. Curr Opin Crit Care. 2018;24:316–21.
3. Thiele RH, Bartels K, Gan TJ. Cardiac output monitoring: a contemporary assessment and review. Crit Care Med. 2015;43:177–85.
4. Marik PE. Obituary: pulmonary artery catheter 1970 to 2013. Ann Intensive Care. 2013;3:38.
5. Connors AF Jr, Speroff T, Dawson NV, et al. The effectiveness of right heart catheterization in the initial care of critically ill patients. JAMA. 1996;276:889–97.
6. Harvey S, Harrison DA, Singer M, et al. Assessment of the clinical effectiveness of pulmonary artery catheters in management of patients in intensive care (PAC-Man): a randomised controlled trial. Lancet. 2005;366:472–7.

7. Wheeler AP, Bernard GR, Thompson BT, et al. Pulmonary-artery versus central venous catheter to guide treatment of acute lung injury. National Heart, Lung, and Blood Institute Acute Respiratory Distress Syndrome (ARDS) Clinical Trials Network. N Engl J Med. 2006;354:2213–24.
8. Sandham JD, Hull RD, Brant RF, et al. A randomized, controlled trial of the use of pulmonary-artery catheters in high-risk surgical patients. N Engl J Med. 2003;348:5–14.
9. Binanay C, Califf RM, Hasselblad V, et al. Evaluation study of Congestive heart failure and pulmonary artery catheterization effectiveness: the ESCAPE trial. JAMA. 2005;294:1625–33.
10. Kastrup M, Carl M, Spies C, Sander M, Markewitz A, Schirmer U. Clinical impact of the publication of S3 guidelines for intensive care in cardiac surgery patients in Germany: results from a postal survey. Acta Anaesthesiol Scand. 2013;57:206–13.
11. Ikuta KM, Wang Y, Robinson A, Ahmad T, Krumholz HM, Desai NR. National trends in use and outcomes of pulmonary artery catheters among medicare beneficiaries, 1999–2013. JAMA Cardiol. 2017;2:908–13.
12. Habicher M, Zajonz T, Heringlake M, et al. S3 guidelines on intensive medical care of cardiac surgery patients: Hemodynamic monitoring and cardiovascular system-an update. Anaesthesist. 2018;67:375–9.
13. Bland RD, Shoemaker WW, Abraham E, et al. Hemodynamic and oxygen transport patterns in surviving and nonsurviving postoperative patients. Crit Care Med. 1985;13:85–90.
14. Shoemaker WC, Appel PI, Kram HB, et al. Prospective trial of supranormal values of survivors as therapeutic goals in high-risk surgical patients. Chest. 1988;94:1176–86.
15. Boyd O, Grounds RM, Bennett ED. A randomized clinical trial of the effect of deliberate perioperative increase of oxygen delivery on mortality in high-risk surgical patients. JAMA. 1993;270:2699–707.
16. Wilson J, Woods I, Fawcett J, Whall R, Dibb W, Morris C, McManus E. Reducing the risk of major elective surgery: randomised controlled trial of preoperative optimisation of oxygen delivery. BMJ. 1999;318:1099–103.
17. Rhodes A, Cecconi M, Hamilton M, et al. Goal-directed therapy in high-risk surgical patients: a15-year follow-up study. Intensive Care Med. 2010;36:1327–32.
18. Monnet X, Teboul JL. Transpulmonary thermodilution: advantages and limits. Crit Care. 2017;21:147.
19. Thenappan T, Gomberg-Maitland M. Epidemiology of pulmonary hypertension and right ventricular failure in left heart failure. Curr Heart Fail Rep. 2014;4:428–35.
20. Bootsma IT, de Lange F, Koopmans M, et al. Right ventricular function after cardiac surgery is a strong independent predictor for long-term mortality. J Cardiothorac Vasc Anesth. 2017;31:1656–62.
21. Tannus-Silva DG, Rabahi MF. State of the art review of the right ventricle in COPD patients: it is time to look closer. Lung. 2017;195:9–17.
22. Repessé X, Charron C, Vieillard-Baron A. Acute cor pulmonale in ARDS: rationale for protecting the right ventricle. Chest. 2015;147:259–65.
23. Pinsky MR. The right ventricle: interaction with the pulmonary circulation. Crit Care. 2016;20:266.
24. Mahjoub Y, Pila C, Friggeri A, et al. Assessing fluid responsiveness in critically ill patients: false-positive pulse pressure variation is detected by Doppler echocardiographic evaluation of the right ventricle. Crit Care Med. 2009;37:2570–5.
25. Soliman D, Bolliger D, Skarvan K, et al. Intra-operative assessment of pulmonary artery pressure by echocardiography. Anaesthesia. 2015;70:264–71.
26. Sander M, Spies CD, Foer A, et al. Agreement of central venous saturation and mixed venous saturation in cardiac surgery patients. Intensive Care Med. 2007;33:1719–25.
27. Varpula M, Karlsson S, Ruokonen E, et al. Mixed venous oxygen saturation cannot be estimated by central venous oxygen saturation in septic shock. Intensive Care Med. 2006;32:1336–43.
28. Lorentzen AG, Lindskov C, Sloth E, Jakobson CJ. Central venous oxygen saturation cannot replace mixed venous saturation in patients undergoing cardiac surgery. J Cardiothorac Vasc Anesth. 2008;22:853–7.

29. Holm J, Håkanson E, Vánky F, Svedjeholm R. Mixed venous oxygen saturation predicts short- and long-term outcome after coronary artery bypass grafting surgery: a retrospective cohort analysis. Br J Anaesth. 2011;107:344–50.
30. Hamilton MA, Cecconi M, Rhodes A. A systematic review and meta-analysis on the use of preemptive hemodynamicintervention to improve postoperative outcomes in moderate and high-risk surgical patients. Anesth Analg. 2011;112:1392–402.
31. Gurgel ST, do Nascimento P Jr. Maintaining tissue perfusion in high-risk surgical patients: a systematic review of randomized clinical trials. Anesth Analg. 2011;112:1384–13.
32. Hammill BG, Curtis LH, Bennett-Guerrero E, et al. Impact of heart failure on patients undergoing major noncardiac surgery. Anesthesiology. 2008;108:559–67.
33. Sotomi Y, Sato N, Kajimoto K, et al. Impact of pulmonary artery catheter on outcome in patients with acute heart failure syndromes with hypotension or receiving inotropes: from the ATTEND Registry. Int J Cardiol. 2014;172:165–72.
34. Brovman EY, Gabriel RA, Dutton RP, Urman RD. Pulmonary artery catheter use during Cardiac Surgery in the United States 2010 to 2014. J Cardiothorac Vasc Anaesth. 2016;30:579–84.
35. Shaw A, Mythen MG, Shooks D, Hayashida D, Zhang X, Munson SH. Pulmonary artery catheter (PAC) use is associated with improved clinical outcomes after adult cardiac surgery. Crit Care. 2017;21(Suppl 1):P103.
36. Göpfert MS, Reuter DA, Akyol D, Lamm P, Kilger E, Goetz AE. Goal-directed fluid management reduces vasopressor and catecholamine use in cardiac surgery patients. Intensive Care Med. 2007;33:96–103.
37. Goepfert MS, Richter HP, Zu Eulenburg C, et al. Individually optimized hemodynamic therapy reduces complications and length of stay in the intensive care unit: a prospective, randomized controlled trial. Anesthesiology. 2013;119:824–36.
38. Schmid S, Kapfer B, Heim M, et al. Algorithm-guided goal-directed haemodynamic therapy does not improve renal function after major abdominal surgery compared to good standard clinical care: a prospective randomised trial. Crit Care. 2016;20:50.
39. Hilty MP, Franzen DP, Wyss C, Biaggi P, Maggiorini M. Validation of transpulmonary thermodilution variables in hemodynamically stable patients with heart diseases. Ann Intensive Care. 2017;7:86.
40. Michard F, Giglio MT, Brienza N. Perioperative goal-directed therapy with uncalibrated pulse contour methods: impact on fluid management and postoperative outcome. Br J Anaesth. 2017;119:22–30.
41. Grocott MP, Dushianthan A, Hamilton MA, Mythen MG, Harrison D, Rowan K. Perioperative increase in global blood flow to explicit defined goals and outcomes following surgery. Cochrane Database Syst Rev. 2012;11:CD004082.
42. Pearse RM, Harrison DA, MacDonald N, et al. Effect of a perioperative, cardiac output-guided hemodynamic therapy algorithm on outcomes following major gastrointestinal surgery: a randomized clinical trial and systematic review. JAMA. 2014;311:2181–90.
43. Balik M, Pachl J, Hendl J. Effect of the degree of tricuspid regurgitation on cardiac output measurements by thermodilution. Intensive Care Med. 2002;28:1117–21.
44. Bossert T, Gummert JF, Bittner HB, et al. Swan-Ganz catheter-induced severe Complications in cardiac surgery: right ventricular perforation, knotting, and rupture of a pulmonary artery. J Card Surg. 2006;21:292–5.
45. Piercy M, Mcniconl L, Dinh DT, et al. Major Complications related to the use of transesophageal echocardiography in cardiac surgery. J Cardiothorac Vasc Anesth. 2009;23:62–5.
46. Denault AY, Haddad F, Jacobsohn E, Deschamps A. Perioperative right ventricular dysfunction. Curr Opin Anaesthesiol. 2013;26:71–81.

Part VIII

Fluid Issues

Resuscitation Fluid Choices to Preserve the Endothelial Glycocalyx

20

E. M. Milford and M. C. Reade

20.1 Introduction

Despite decades of intense pre-clinical and clinical research there is still much uncertainty regarding the volume-expanding efficacy of different fluid resuscitation strategies across a range of disease states, particularly for the critically ill [1]. New concepts in vascular permeability promise to change the way we approach fluid resuscitation and ultimately lead to improvements in its efficacy. Central to these new concepts is the endothelial glycocalyx, which lines the luminal aspect of the vascular endothelium. Knowledge of the endothelial glycocalyx has permitted revision of the classic Starling principle to one that better explains the observed flux of fluid across the endothelial barrier [2].

This new model of endothelial permeability largely explains the difference in the predicted (1:3–1:5) versus the observed (approximately 1:1.3–1:1.4) ratio of colloid to crystalloid required to achieve similar hemodynamic end-points in clinical trials [1]. It also explains why the infusion of an iso-oncotic colloid fluid will not reverse existing interstitial edema [3], and may in some situations result in less volume expansion and greater tissue edema than a crystalloid in critically ill patients [4]. The volume expanding effects of infused fluids also differ depending on the rate of infusion, the degree of vasoconstriction, the integrity of the endothelial glycocalyx

E. M. Milford (✉)
Intensive Care Medicine, 2nd General Health Battalion, Australian Army, Brisbane, QLD, Australia

Faculty of Medicine, The University of Queensland, Herston, QLD, Australia
e-mail: elissa.milford@defence.gov.au

M. C. Reade
Faculty of Medicine, The University of Queensland and Australian Defence Force Joint Health Command, Brisbane, QLD, Australia

Clinical Services, 2nd General Health Battalion, Australian Army, Brisbane, QLD, Australia

J.-L. Vincent (ed.), *Annual Update in Intensive Care and Emergency Medicine 2019*, Annual Update in Intensive Care and Emergency Medicine,
https://doi.org/10.1007/978-3-030-06067-1_20

and the volume status. Because of this, the effectiveness of fluid resuscitation is said to be context-sensitive.

Damage to the endothelial glycocalyx, termed shedding, occurs in a number of critical illnesses, including sepsis and severe trauma, and the degree of shedding is associated with poor outcomes [5]. It is likely, but not yet proven, that protecting and restoring the endothelial glycocalyx in these conditions will improve outcomes. Several pharmacologic therapies are under investigation, but these are in the pre-clinical phase of development and there is not yet enough evidence to support their clinical use [6]. However, there is growing evidence that commonly used resuscitation fluids protect and restore the endothelial glycocalyx and modulate endothelial permeability, but differ in their ability to do so. It is therefore important that, when choosing resuscitation fluids for particular patients, clinicians consider factors additional to oncotic properties, including ability to protect and repair the endothelial glycocalyx.

20.2 The Endothelial Glycocalyx

The endothelial glycocalyx consists of a scaffolding network of proteoglycans, predominantly the transmembrane bound syndecan and the membrane bound glypican. Bound to these are five types of glycosoaminoglycan side chains, predominantly heparan sulfate, with chondroitin sulfate and hyaluronan less abundant [7]. Glycoproteins are also attached to the endothelium. These are diverse in function and include the cell adhesion molecules, receptors in intercellular signaling and receptors involved in fibrinolysis and coagulation. Incorporated into the scaffolding network are numerous endothelial and plasma-derived soluble molecules [7] (Fig. 20.1).

The endothelial glycocalyx is a key regulator of endothelial function. Most is known about its role in regulating vascular permeability, but it is also integral to cell-vessel wall interactions, blood rheology, mechanotransduction, inflammation,

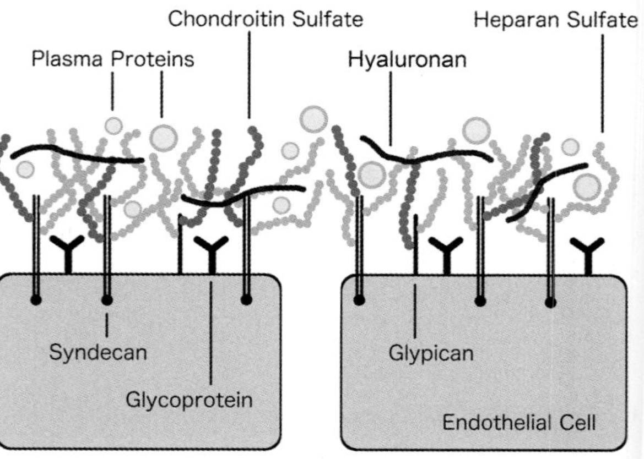

Fig. 20.1 The structure of the endothelial glycocalyx

coagulation and fibrinolysis [7]. The fragile structure and small dimensions of the endothelial glycocalyx make it difficult to detect and quantify. Experimentally, the endothelial glycocalyx can be directly visualized by a number of techniques including electron microscopy, intravital microscopy, comparison of the volumes of distribution of endothelial glycocalyx permeable and non-permeable tracers, confocal microscopy, and immunohistochemical staining [8]. These techniques are all invasive and not suitable for repeated measurements, if at all, in clinical applications.

For clinical purposes, detecting endothelial glycocalyx breakdown products in plasma or serum has been widely used in a research context, but is not yet routinely available for clinical practice, and indeed the clinical significance of elevated levels has not been validated. The most commonly measured is syndecan-1 (SDC-1), the main structural backbone of the endothelial glycocalyx [7]. Heparan sulfate, chondroitin sulfate and hyaluronan have also been used to detect endothelial glycocalyx damage [8]. Alternatively, visualization with a side-stream dark field (SDF) camera or its predecessor orthogonal polarization spectral imaging (OPS) has been used to detect endothelial glycocalyx thickness in the nail fold or oral mucosa in a clinical research context. These cameras estimate endothelial glycocalyx thickness based on the speed and deformation of passing red blood cells (RBCs) and leukocytes [8].

Loss of the endothelial glycocalyx, or glycocalyx shedding, occurs commonly in a number of diseases including trauma and sepsis, and has been associated with poor patient outcomes [5]. However, it is unclear whether endothelial glycocalyx shedding is simply a marker of disease severity or if it contributes directly to poor outcomes. There are a number of biologically plausible pathways whereby endothelial glycocalyx shedding could cause harmful effects, but no clinical study has attempted to restore the endothelial glycocalyx, and in animal studies there are no data on outcomes after restoration [9].

Mirroring the diverse range of conditions that are associated with endothelial glycocalyx shedding is the diverse range of mediators known to cause shedding. These include, but are not limited to, tumor necrosis factor (TNF)-α, reactive oxygen species (ROS), heparanase, hypoperfusion, hyperglycemia, bacterial toxins and growth factors [10]. The final common pathway for many initiators of shedding is the activation of proteases that cleave endothelial glycocalyx components from the cell surface [10].

20.3 Role in Regulating Vascular Permeability: The Revised Starling Principle

The movement of fluid across the endothelium has, until recently, been explained by the classical Starling principle, which describes the filtration rate as being a function of two opposing forces—hydrostatic pressure and osmotic pressure—across the vessel wall [11]:

$$\mathrm{Jv/A} = \mathrm{L_p}\left[\left(\mathrm{P_c} - \mathrm{P_i}\right) - \sigma\left(\Pi_c - \Pi_i\right)\right]$$

where Jv/A is the outward filtration force for a given area, L_p is the membrane hydraulic conductivity, P_c is the luminal hydrostatic pressure, P_i is the interstitial hydrostatic pressure, σ is the macromolecule reflection coefficient of the membrane, Π_c is the luminal osmotic pressure and Π_i is the interstitial osmotic pressure.

When Starling first described his theory in 1896 [11], the model was consistent with experimental data available at the time. However, in recent years, modern technology has enabled the observation of a number of contradictions to the classic equation. Specifically, there is no venous reabsorption of fluid, transcapillary flow rate is lower than predicted, and the interstitial protein concentration has a minimal effect on fluid flux [2]. This has led to four major modifications to the Starling model, with the endothelial glycocalyx central to these modifications.

20.3.1 No Absorption in the Steady State

Starling theorized that after being filtered out from the arterial end of a capillary (the segment under high $P_{c)}$, fluid was then reabsorbed at the venous end (the segment under low P_c). However, experiments have found that while there is an initial transient response where fluid is absorbed after a sudden decrease in P_c, this rapidly changes back to outward filtration, even at the venous end of the capillary. This transient absorption phase lasts approximately 15–30 min in humans following acute hemorrhage, allowing the absorption, or 'auto-resuscitation', of approximately 0.5 L of interstitial fluid [2, 12]. However, in the steady state, no absorption is seen along the entire length of most capillaries, regardless of the P_c (the "no absorption rule") [2, 12]. Instead, fluid is removed from the interstitium via the lymphatic system [12]. Only in certain unique organs, notably those of the renal, intestinal and lymphatic systems, is absorption seen in the steady state due to mechanisms that maintain a low Π_i and a raised P_i [2].

The no absorption rule explains why the intravenous administration of iso- or hyper-oncotic colloid fluids will not reverse existing interstitial edema [3], and is due to the inverse relationship between capillary filtration rate and the interstitial protein concentration gradient adjacent to the vessel wall. After the initial drop in P_c, the balance of forces directs fluid inwards into the vessel lumen. This movement of fluid concentrates the interstitial proteins, increasing Π_i, which opposes the absorption force inwards. Eventually, a new steady state is reached, at which point the balance of forces always results in outward filtration [2].

20.3.2 The Sub-glycocalyx Space

Starling's original theory assumes that Π_i is substantially lower than Π_c. This is not correct. The interstitium is packed with proteins due to the physiological extravasation of plasma proteins, possibly through large pores located in the venular segments of capillaries, which results in Π_i approaching Π_c [2, 4]. But solving the original equation with the measured Π_i and Π_c values predicts a much higher

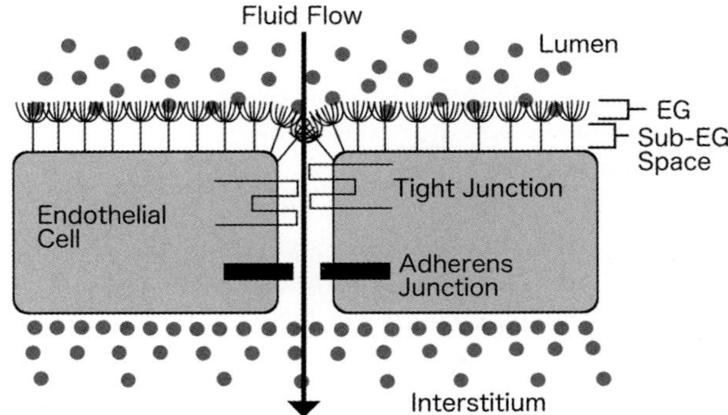

Fig. 20.2 The sub-glycocalyx space. EG: endothelial glycocalyx

filtration rate than that measured experimentally [13]. Furthermore, modifying Π_i experimentally only has a minor impact on filtration rate [2].

The discrepancies between predicted and measured filtration rates are resolved by revising the Starling equation and replacing Π_i with the osmotic pressure in a small protein-free zone between the endothelial glycocalyx and the endothelial cells [2] (Fig. 20.2). That is:

$$Jv / A = L_p\left[\left(P_c - P_i\right) - \sigma\left(\Pi_c - \Pi_g\right)\right]$$

where Π_g is the sub-glycocalyx osmotic pressure. As the osmotic pressure counteracting Π_c is Π_g, and not Π_i, changes in Π_i will have little impact on the filtration rate, as has been observed [2]. Π_g is almost negligible in comparison to Π_c, so the osmotic pressure gradient approaches Π_c.

The sub-glycocalyx space is maintained protein-free by the constant outward filtration of fluid as explained by the no absorption rule and the plasma protein filtering effect of an intact endothelial glycocalyx. The resulting ultra filtrate flows through the sub-glycocalyx space, and then out through the intercellular clefts via breaks in the tight junction strands [2]. Due to their narrow width, the velocity in the breaks is high even at low filtration rates, which prevents movement of interstitial protein back into the sub-glycocalyx space [2].

20.3.3 The Endothelial Glycocalyx Is a Determinant of Hydraulic Conductivity

The endothelial glycocalyx is also an important determinant of hydraulic conductivity. Hydraulic conductivity (L_p) is the change in filtration rate for a given change in transendothelial pressure, and can be thought of as the ease with which water passes across the vessel wall. Far from being a static variable, L_p is dynamically influenced by the endothelial glycocalyx and the endothelium. The endothelial glycocalyx reduces L_p by mechanically resisting fluid flow [2, 4]. It also affects L_p by mechanotransducing shear force to the underlying endothelial cells, which respond to increased shear stress by releasing nitric oxide (NO) and altering junctional proteins resulting in an increase in L_p [14]. This process is physiologically relevant when meeting the increased demand for metabolic substrates to skeletal muscle during exercise, but the relevance in a critically unwell patient, where in most cases the endothelial glycocalyx is degraded and the shear stress is low, remains to be seen.

Endothelial cells have a significant role in regulating L_p. The tight and adherens junctions contribute to the high hydraulic resistance of the intercellular space. Breakdown of these junctions occurs in response to a variety of mediators, such as vascular endothelial growth factors (VEGF) and cytokines, increasing L_p [15]. In addition, apoptosis, mitosis and transcellular pathways, such as aquaporins, may contribute to increased L_p depending on the vascular bed and the prevailing pathophysiological conditions [15]. The trans- and para-cellular pathways that mediate endothelial permeability to fluid, solutes and cells in a number of disease processes are complex and not completely understood, and are reviewed elsewhere [15].

20.3.4 The Modified Starling Model Is Non-linear at Low Filtration Rates

The effect of capillary hydrostatic pressure, P_c, on filtration rate is more complex than previously thought. The original and modified Starling equations both describe the relationship between Jv/A and P_c as linear, when the other variables are constant. This relationship is described by the linear equation:

$$Jv / A = L_p P_c + \left[L_p \left(-P_i - \sigma \Pi_c + \sigma \Pi_{g/i} \right) \right]$$

However, due to the no absorption rule, at low values of Jv/A in the steady state the flow rate only approaches zero, never actually reaching zero or becoming negative. This results in an asymptotic curve at low values of Jv/A and a linear curve at higher values. Woodcock and Woodcock [16] have described the inflection point as the J-point, and theorized that at P_c values below the J-point both crystalloids and colloids will have almost the same volume expanding effects due to the filtration rate of both being near zero. The x-intercept, that is, P_c when Jv/A is zero (or rather what it would be if the curve was linear at a Jv/A of zero), approximates the J-point, and is given by:

$$\text{J-point} = P_i + \sigma \Pi_c - \sigma \Pi_{g/i}$$

Increasing P_i or Π_c will shift the J-point to the right, whereas increasing $\Pi_{g/i}$ will have the opposite effect (Fig. 20.3). Contextualizing this clinically, a right shift in the J-point is advantageous for increasing intravascular volume—more fluid can be infused (and crystalloid or colloid will have similar volume expanding effects) before the hydrostatic pressure threshold for movement of fluid interstitially is reached; whereas a shift to the left is deleterious for volume expansion—fluid will move interstitially at a lower P_c and hence lower intravascular volume. An increase

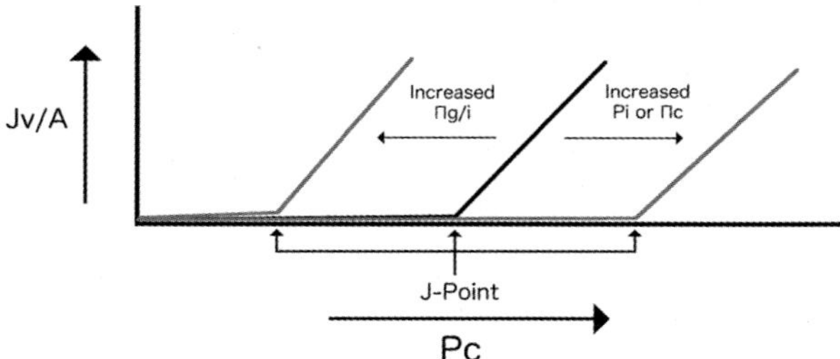

Fig. 20.3 The relationship between capillary lumen hydrostatic pressure (P_c) and the outward filtration force for a given area (Jv/A) showing the J-point, below which both crystalloids and colloids have almost the same volume expanding effect. P_i interstitial hydrostatic pressure, Π_c, luminal osmotic pressure, Π_i interstitial osmotic pressure, Π_g sub-glycocalyx osmotic pressure

in P_i is usually due to edema formation, which is not desirable, so the best way to achieve a right shift is to increase Π_c and avoid increases in $\Pi_{g/i}$.

In an intact endothelial glycocalyx, Π_g is negligible, and the colloid particles in an infused colloid fluid remain in the intravascular space due to the filtration effect of the endothelial glycocalyx. This results in either no change or a rightward shift of the J-point, a low filtration rate, and sustained plasma volume expansion from the infused fluid. Whether a colloid compared to a crystalloid results in greater volume expansion in this context depends on the P_c. If the P_c is below the J-point, then as the filtration rate is near zero, both crystalloids and colloids will have a similar volume expanding effect. If the P_c is above the J-point, then colloids will persist in the intravascular space for longer than crystalloids.

While there is currently no way to measure P_c at the bedside (there is a poor correlation between measurable macrocirculatory parameters such as blood pressure and those of the microcirculation [17]), there are indications that in healthy volunteers, the J-point does appear to approximate the P_c in what is regarded as normovolemia. When 900 mL of blood was removed from normotensive human volunteers, the volume of crystalloid required to restore normovolemia was estimated to be somewhere between one and two times the hemorrhaged volume [18], depending on the rate of replacement. By comparison, in experiments where crystalloid was infused to achieve hypervolemia, as little as 17 ± 10% was found to remain intravascularly [19].

In contrast, if the endothelial glycocalyx is damaged, the J-point is shifted to the left due to the higher Π_i replacing Π_g [20], and the plasma expanding efficacy of any infused fluid is reduced (that is, the outward filtration rate will be above zero at a lower plasma volume). Paradoxically, while it might initially seem that in this context (with the P_c being more likely to be above the J-point) a colloid fluid would persist in the intravascular space longer than a crystalloid, this is not necessarily the case as the colloid particles are free to move interstitially, further increasing Π_i and worsening the leftward shift [20]. Endothelial glycocalyx shedding also decreases σ, making the J-point more dependent on P_i and less dependent on the osmotic pressure difference.

This concept has been demonstrated experimentally by Jacob et al. [4] who measured perfusion pressure (approximating P_c) and transudate flow (approximating Jv/A) in *ex vivo* guinea pig hearts. The P_c of the estimated J-point after a crystalloid infusion was approximately 10 cmH_2O, and this was the same before and after enzymatically degrading the endothelial glycocalyx (although the protein-free perfusate likely resulted in endothelial glycocalyx shedding prior to the enzymatic degradation). The positive J-point was likely caused by the increased P_i from fluid movement interstitially. After a colloid infusion, this point was 0 cmH_2O in an intact endothelial glycocalyx, but was reduced to −12 cmH_2O after enzymatic degradation—the interstitium was essentially 'sucking' fluid from the intravascular space. The negative J-point was likely due to the increased Π_i from the movement of colloid particles interstitially. In a similar study there were similar levels of tissue edema after infusing a colloid compared to a crystalloid through endothelial glycocalyx denuded vessels [20]. And in another, the increase in Π_i resulted in an increase in the filtration rate of subsequent fluid infusions [21].

20.3.5 Additional Theoretical Considerations

Vasoconstriction and vasodilation via exogenous or endogenous mechanisms also affect P_c and the filtration rate but in a somewhat unpredictable fashion, as these are dependent on the balance of constriction/dilation in the venules and arterioles [17]. In addition, an increased rate of intravenous fluid infusion should, theoretically, lead to increased fluid extravasation from a transient increase in P_c, but the experimental data are not conclusive. The relationship between rapid fluid infusion rate, P_c, filtration rate and poor clinical outcomes is therefore still poorly understood. Furthermore, the permeability of the intact, or partially intact, endothelial glycocalyx to macromolecules such as albumin and semisynthetic colloids also increases with increasing P_c, adding additional complexity to the relationship between P_i and P_c [17].

20.4 Clinical Implications of the Revised Starling Model

Methods for measuring endothelial glycocalyx status clinically are not yet routinely available outside of a research context and have unvalidated clinical significance. However, overwhelming pre-clinical and clinical evidence suggests that the endothelial glycocalyx is likely to be damaged in critically unwell patients [5]. Infusing an iso-oncotic colloid into these patients will have a similar volume expanding effect to a crystalloid fluid. How similar will depend on the degree of endothelial glycocalyx shedding, the endothelial glycocalyx permeability, the patient's pre-infusion volume status, the infusion rate, and the degree of vasoconstriction, and is difficult to predict clinically due to the complexity of the interactions between the variables involved. This could explain why in large clinical trials of critically unwell patients the volume expanding effects of colloids compared to crystalloids are much less than predicted. For example, in the Crystalloid versus

Hydroxyethyl Starch Trial (CHEST) [22] and the Saline versus Albumin Fluid Evaluation (SAFE) [23] clinical trials, the observed ratio of colloid to crystalloid to achieve the same hemodynamic resuscitation end-points was 1:1.3 and 1:1.4 respectively, which is markedly different to the ratio of 1:3–1:5 predicted by the classical Starling principle [1].

Using an iso-oncotic colloid for a potential, even if only marginally, greater volume expanding effect is not without risk. Infusing a colloid solution into a patient with a degraded endothelial glycocalyx comes at the expense of interstitial protein accumulation resulting in tissue edema to levels similar to that seen in crystalloid infusions [4]. Paradoxically, in some cases tissue edema could actually be higher and volume expansion lower after an infusion of colloids compared to a crystalloid infusion [4]. In addition, the use of semisynthetic colloids may have deleterious consequences (e.g., allergy, coagulopathy) beyond causing edema [1], and they appear to extravasate faster than albumin [20]. Furthermore, due to the no absorption rule, a colloid infusion cannot reverse existing interstitial edema regardless of the integrity of the endothelial glycocalyx.

All of these considerations could explain why, despite the slightly greater volume expansion properties, overall there have not been any significant mortality benefits from using a colloid over a crystalloid in clinical trials [1]. The volume expansion effect may be so marginal as to make no difference in outcomes, or the deleterious effects may counteract any advantage from greater volume expansion.

20.5 Fluids that Preserve the Glycocalyx

The preceding discussion has focused on the differential resuscitation effects of crystalloid and colloid according to the prevailing state of the endothelial glycocalyx, finding physiological rationale for the absence of evidence for superiority of one over the other. However, some colloids do appear to be markedly superior as resuscitation fluids. In hemorrhagic shock, for example, resuscitation with higher ratios of plasma seems to result in lower mortality than crystalloid [24], despite there being seemingly little advantage in terms of preservation of coagulation factors [25]. The explanation may lie not with the Starling equation but rather that certain colloids act to preserve the endothelial glycocalyx.

As there have been no clinical trials that have directly sought to assess whether restoring or protecting the endothelial glycocalyx changes clinical outcomes, the rationale for preserving the endothelial glycocalyx is based on observational and pre-clinical *in vitro* and *in vivo* data. Taken together, these data suggest that the early repair of the endothelial glycocalyx might improve the systemic inflammatory response, coagulopathy and volume responsiveness following a systemic ischemic or inflammatory stimulus such as severe sepsis or major trauma. The timeframe for the endothelial glycocalyx to repair itself clinically without any intervention is not clear, but data from a rat model and human endothelial cell culture experiments suggest that following the cessation of the shedding stimulus, it takes 5–7 days to restore the glycocalyx to baseline [26]. There is therefore a window in this relatively long timeframe for an intervention to stimulate earlier repair. There is growing evidence that commonly used resuscitation fluids have differing abilities to protect and restore the endothelial glycocalyx.

20.5.1 Albumin

A low-protein environment has long been recognized to cause a rapid breakdown, or shedding, of the endothelial glycocalyx [27]. This phenomena is independent of the effect on osmotic pressure, as, for the same intravascular osmotic pressure, plasma and albumin are more effective than semisynthetic colloids such as hydroxyethyl starch (HES) at preserving and restoring the endothelial glycocalyx, reducing vascular permeability, and reducing platelet and leukocyte adhesion in pre-clinical studies [4, 20, 28, 29]. The mechanism of the superior 'sealing effect' of albumin and plasma is still not entirely clear and has been termed the "colloid osmotic pressure paradox".

Initially, it was thought that perfusing the endothelium with a protein-free solution collapsed the endothelial glycocalyx due to washout of its integrated proteins. However, immunohistochemical staining and electron microscopy have revealed that a low-protein environment causes a complete absence, rather than collapse, of the endothelial glycocalyx [27]. This appears to be caused by matrix metalloproteinase (MMP) cleavage of the endothelial glycocalyx components from the underlying endothelium [27]. The protective effect of protein might be mediated by a protein bound substance that inhibits MMP cleavage of the endothelial glycocalyx, such as the lipid mediator sphingosine 1-phosphate (S1P). In *in vitro* experiments, activation of the $S1P_1$ receptor inhibits MMPs, preventing endothelial glycocalyx shedding [27, 28], while at the same time the endothelial glycocalyx is restored by the mobilization of intracellular pools of glycocalyx components via golgi-mediated translocation [4]. RBCs, followed by platelets, are the major source of S1P in the body [30]. Plasma proteins, predominantly high-density lipoprotein (HDL) and albumin, facilitate the release of S1P from these sources [30]. In the absence of albumin, up to 25 times less S1P is released from RBCs [28]. Whether S1P is the only mediator responsible for the colloid osmotic pressure paradox is not known, nor is it known whether agonizing the $S1P_1$ receptor has any clinically relevant effect on the endothelial glycocalyx *in vivo*.

It is unclear whether the infusion of albumin *in vivo* has the same endothelial glycocalyx restoration effect as that seen *in vitro*. Animal studies have yielded conflicting results—in a mouse model of hemorrhage where fresh frozen plasma (FFP) attenuated the increase in vascular permeability, human albumin had almost no effect [31], whereas in a rat model of hemorrhage, albumin restored the glycocalyx thickness to 81 ± 31% of the baseline, compared to the full restoration achieved by FFP, but better than the 42 ± 21% of that from 0.9% saline [32]. Permeability in this study was restored to baseline after both FFP and albumin infusion. Furthermore, in clinical trials, there is only a narrow, if any, survival benefit of using albumin as a resuscitation fluid, although there is weak evidence that there may be an advantage of albumin in septic patients [1]. There are also concerns about the safety of albumin in traumatic brain injury (TBI), although a recent study has suggested that the harm in this patient population might actually be caused by the hypotonicity of the carrier fluid, not by the albumin itself [1].

There are a number of possible explanations for these contradictory data. It could be that albumin restores the endothelial glycocalyx, but this restoration does not change clinical outcomes. It could also be that circulating albumin levels are required to drop below a critical level before supplementation has any clinically significant effect. Or, it could be that it is not albumin itself that is a mediator of endothelial glycocalyx repair, but rather another mediator contained in the albumin solution, such as S1P. Supporting this hypothesis is a study in which albumin exposed to RBCs for 20 min or a solution without albumin but containing S1P maintained normal vessel permeability in rat microvessels, but albumin not conditioned by RBCs did not, nor did Ringer's solution that was conditioned to RBCs [28]. Commercially available sources of albumin for pre-clinical research use, such as fetal calf serum and bovine serum albumin, contain physiologically active levels of S1P [28], which may account for their efficacy in protecting and restoring the endothelial glycocalyx in *in vitro* experiments. The levels of S1P in human albumin manufactured for clinical purposes have not been reported, and the albumin used in the aforementioned studies was not analyzed for any other potential mediators. Differing levels of these mediators could account for the difference in observed effects. Artificially S1P-enriched human albumin would be an attractive solution for trials in human resuscitation.

20.5.2 Fresh Frozen Plasma

The evidence for the endothelial glycocalyx-restoring properties of FFP is more compelling. In cell culture and animal models of endothelial glycocalyx injury, FFP consistently attenuates glycocalyx shedding and the associated increase in vascular permeability and leukocyte adhesion, and in animal models it also attenuates acute lung injury and gut inflammation following hemorrhagic shock [29]. In a clinical study of 33 non-bleeding critically-ill patients given 12 mL/kg FFP as pre-procedure prophylaxis, SDC-1 blood levels were significantly lower following the administration off FFP, indicating that FFP had reduced the degree of endothelial glycocalyx shedding [9]. FFP starts repairing the endothelial glycocalyx within 1 h, and this appears to be mediated via not only the cessation of ongoing shedding, but also by up-regulation of endothelial glycocalyx component production. Hemorrhagic shock reduces the expression of SDC-1 mRNA, and resuscitation with crystalloid reduces this expression even further, while FFP returns SDC-1 mRNA expression back to baseline [33].

The increase in endothelial glycocalyx production by FFP could confound the clinical detection of glycocalyx shedding with blood levels of glycocalyx components. In a rat model of hemorrhage and TBI, SDC-1 blood levels at 23 h were higher in the FFP resuscitated group compared to the 0.9% saline resuscitated group, suggesting higher levels of endothelial glycocalyx shedding in the FFP group [34]. The authors suggested the low levels of SDC-1 at 23 h actually most likely reflected a reduction in endothelial glycocalyx production in the saline group, not a reduction in endothelial glycocalyx shedding.

The mechanism by which FFP restores the endothelial glycocalyx, reduces endothelial permeability, and attenuates early inflammation is not clear. It is not known if the same mediator is responsible for the endothelial glycocalyx repairing properties of both FFP and albumin. Similar to albumin, the pre- and post-transfusion levels of S1P in FFP approved for clinical use have not been measured. In addition, FFP's effects are pleiotropic: for instance it also repairs the endothelial adherens junction, which would account for some of the improvement in permeability [35]. This is not surprising given that plasma contains over 1000 proteins and numerous soluble mediators [36]. S1P in FFP may play an important role in preserving and restoring the endothelial glycocalyx, but so may other mediators of protease activity such as TIMP3 (tissue inhibitor of metalloproteinase 3) [37] or ADAMTS13 (a disintegrin and metalloproteinase with a thrombospondin type 1 motif, member 13) [9]. However, there is as yet less evidence for these mediators in the pathogenesis of endothelial glycocalyx shedding than S1P.

The components of FFP that repair the endothelial glycocalyx may also be present in plasma-derived products such as prothrombin complex concentrate (PCC). Pati et al. demonstrated that in a mouse model of hemorrhagic shock, PCC attenuated the increase in vascular permeability with equal efficacy as FFP [31]. Interestingly, the PCC was not as effective as FFP in an endothelial cell culture model [31]. It may be that multiple components of plasma are required to act synergistically to mediate their restorative effects. This study did not measure the endothelial glycocalyx, so it can only be speculated that the permeability reducing effect was mediated via glycocalyx restoration. Lyophilized and spray-dried plasma also appear to have the same endothelial protective properties as FFP [9].

Other variations in the processing and storage of FFP may not preserve its endothelial glycocalyx repairing properties, and as it is not known what mediates these properties it is difficult to predict how these may differ with different processes. For example, the protective effects of FFP are substantially diminished by post-thaw storage at 4 °C for 5 days [9]. Furthermore, the timing of resuscitation could also be important. In a cell culture model, resuscitation with plasma immediately following injury restored the endothelial glycocalyx and vessel permeability, whereas resuscitation with plasma at 3 h following injury had no protective effect [38].

Clinically, there is evidence that the infusion of FFP, particularly in traumatic hemorrhage, decreases early deaths, particularly when the plasma is administered early [39]. In the PAMPer trial, a 564 patient multicenter randomized controlled trial (RCT) of pre-hospital administration of FFP compared to standard care (no FFP pre-hospital), 30-day mortality was lower in the group that received pre-hospital FFP (23.2% vs. 33.0%) [39]. The improvement in mortality occurred early; there was separation in the survival curve after only 3 h following randomization [39]. FFP's beneficial effects were independent of any attenuation of coagulopathy [40], and it could be speculated that it may instead, at least in part, have been mediated by endothelial protection.

There has historically been a reluctance to use FFP due to concern about the risk of adverse events, such as transfusion-associated acute lung injury and allergic transfusion reactions [41]. However, a variety of strategies to reduce these risks, such as using male only donor plasma and leukoreduction, have resulted in a safer product [41]. Recent RCTs have found no increased incidence of major complications including multiorgan failure, acute lung injury or sepsis with the use of FFP, and only a low incidence of minor transfusion-related reactions in patients who receive FFP [24, 39]. Interestingly, in a pilot study of 44 bleeding patients undergoing surgery for thoracic aorta dissection, patients randomized to OctaplasLG had significantly lower SDC-1 and sVE-cadherin levels (a marker of endothelial cell intercellular junction integrity) compared to patients given standard FFP [42]. OctaplasLG is a pathogen-reduced product derived from approximately 1000 plasma donations with standardized concentrations of clotting factors, and is free from damage-associated molecular patterns, cytokines, cell debris and microparticles due to several stages of microfiltration. The removal of these particles could result in a product that has fewer adverse effects, but is also more effective at restoring the endothelial glycocalyx than standard FFP. Potentially, isolating the endothelial glycocalyx protective mediator among FFP's thousand or so proteins and soluble mediators could prove to be the most effective and safest therapy for protecting the endothelial glycocalyx.

20.5.3 Red Blood Cells

Packed RBCs (PRBCs) could, theoretically, have an endothelial glycocalyx protective effect due to their role as a source of S1P. RBCs, followed by platelets, are the major source of S1P in the body; S1P is rapidly removed from the circulation, so circulating RBCs and platelets may be integral in maintaining sufficient plasma levels [30]. A study of individually perfused rat microvessels supports this hypothesis. Albumin exposed to PRBCs for 20 min or a solution without albumin but containing S1P maintained normal vessel permeability, but albumin not conditioned by PRBCs did not [28].

However, PRBCs transfused systemically do not appear to be protective of the endothelial glycocalyx. In a rat hemorrhagic shock model, resuscitation with fresh whole blood or unwashed PRBCs, but not with washed PRBCs or lactated Ringers, increased endothelial glycocalyx thickness and reduced vascular permeability, suggesting that the residual plasma in the unwashed PRBCs is responsible for the endothelial protective effect, and not the PRBCs themselves [43]. The equivalent of approximately 4 units of blood product was transfused to each animal in this study. It could be that there were enough circulating endogenous RBCs in these animals to keep S1P levels above a critical level, so supplementation did not achieve any noticeable effect. If this were the case, then this has consequences for patients who receive massive blood transfusions where their entire circulating blood volume is replaced with exogenous blood products. For these patients, the S1P content of transfused blood products could be of great clinical significance.

Notably, aged PRBC units contain less S1P than fresh units [44]. There is high quality evidence that transfusion of fresher PRBCs does not improve patient outcomes [45]. However, the large trials that have addressed this question did not consider PRBCs towards the end of their 42-day shelf life, but were instead pragmatic responses to the emerging clinical tendency to transfuse the freshest available PRBCs in preference to units with a median age of around 20 days [45]. In addition, these trials did not specifically look at massive transfusion, and it is possible that the age of PRBCs matters in this population, but not in those who receive a small number of PRBC units.

20.5.4 Platelets

There is growing evidence that the transfusion of platelets early following hemorrhagic shock improves patient outcomes. Most recently, a sub-study of the Pragmatic, Randomized Optimal Platelet and Plasma Ratios (PROPPR) trial analyzed the 261 patients in the trial who only received the first cooler of blood products, and therefore either did or did not receive platelets along with their PRBC resuscitation. Patients who received platelets had significantly lower 24-h (5.8% vs. 16.9%) and 30-day mortality (9.5% vs. 20.2%) [46]. While there are inherent limitations with such a sub-study, this finding is consistent with previous observational studies that have suggested that increased plasma and platelet to PRBC ratios improve outcomes in bleeding trauma patients [47].

Almost certainly some of the mortality benefit from platelet transfusion would be attributed to an improvement in hemostasis. However, it is also possible that the endothelial protective effects of platelets also play a role in improving outcomes. Platelets release cytokines and growth factors that preserve the integrity of the endothelial intercellular junction and thereby maintain a low vascular permeability [48]. Platelets are also a source of S1P [30], so it is possible that S1P plays a role in maintaining a low vascular permeability by protecting the endothelial glycocalyx; however the effect of transfused platelets on the endothelial glycocalyx specifically has not yet been studied.

Similar to plasma and PRBCs, the processing and storage conditions of platelets affect their ability to preserve vascular permeability. Washed platelets stored for 5 days, compared to one, have approximately 50% lower levels of S1P [49] and increase vascular permeability both *in vitro* and *in vivo* [48]. There is also significant inter-donor variability in the ability of transfused platelets to preserve endothelial permeability. In addition, washed platelets stored at 4 °C (cold stored), compared to standard storage at room temperature (22 °C), were more effective at preserving endothelial permeability in both *in vitro* and *in vivo* models [50].

20.5.5 Crystalloids and Artificial Colloids

Crystalloids have no ability to restore the endothelial glycocalyx [4, 9], although they may differ in their effects on L_p (hydraulic conductivity) primarily through the effects of calcium on endothelial cells [4]. Artificial colloids do have some protective and restorative properties through an unknown mechanism, but they are inferior to albumin and FFP in this regard. This has been demonstrated in *in vivo* and *ex vivo* animal studies of endothelial glycocalyx injury, in which HES was marginally more effective than crystalloid at restoring the endothelial glycocalyx and reducing the corresponding increase in vascular permeability, but significantly inferior to albumin and FFP [9, 20].

However, the protective effect of HES seen in pre-clinical studies does not appear to translate clinically. In clinical trials of sepsis and off-pump coronary bypass graft surgery, which both caused a significant elevation in blood concentration of SDC-1, indicating glycocalyx shedding, there was no difference in blood concentrations of SDC-1 in patients resuscitated with HES compared to those resuscitated with a crystalloid [51, 52]. In addition, large randomized clinical trials of HES in critically ill patients have found no benefit to using HES over a crystalloid, instead finding that HES is associated with the increased use of blood products and the development of acute kidney injury [1]. There is little evidence about the effects of other types of artificial colloids on the endothelial glycocalyx.

20.6 Conclusion

Until fairly recently, the theoretical advantages of one type of resuscitation fluid over another have been based on a now outdated understanding of vascular permeability. Colloid fluids were considered superior to crystalloids due to their theorized greater retention within the intravascular space, but clinical trial data have neither supported this nor convincingly demonstrated a mortality or efficacy benefit from any one fluid type over another [1]. These observations are clarified by the revised Starling equation, which explains the similar volume expanding and interstitial edema forming properties of crystalloid and colloid fluids when the endothelial glycocalyx is shed and the hydrostatic pressure is low in critically ill patients, as well as other considerations, such as the effects of colloid accumulation in the interstitial space. Future research into fluid resuscitation will benefit from an updated understanding of the determinants of vascular permeability, and perhaps most promising is the identification of the endothelial glycocalyx as a possible therapeutic target. Resuscitation fluids differ in their ability to protect and restore the endothelial glycocalyx. While FFP has been identified as the most effective, further work is needed to establish the mechanisms, and to determine whether glycocalyx repair improves clinical outcomes. A fluid resuscitation strategy that protects and repairs the endothelial glycocalyx may prove to be the most effective.

References

1. Finfer S, Myburgh J, Bellomo R. Intravenous fluid therapy in critically ill adults. Nat Rev Nephrol. 2018;14:541–57.
2. Levick JR, Michel CC. Microvascular fluid exchange and the revised Starling principle. Cardiovasc Res. 2010;87:198–210.

3. van der Heijden M, Verheij J, van Nieuw Amerongen GP, Groeneveld AB. Crystalloid or colloid fluid loading and pulmonary permeability, edema, and injury in septic and nonseptic critically ill patients with hypovolemia. Crit Care Med. 2009;37:1275–81.
4. Jacob M, Bruegger D, Rehm M, et al. The endothelial glycocalyx affords compatibility of Starling's principle and high cardiac interstitial albumin levels. Cardiovasc Res. 2007;73:575–86.
5. Johansson P, Stensballe J, Ostrowski S. Shock induced endotheliopathy (SHINE) in acute critical illness - a unifying pathophysiologic mechanism. Crit Care. 2017;21:25.
6. Schott U, Solomon C, Fries D, Bentzer P. The endothelial glycocalyx and its disruption, protection and regeneration: a narrative review. Scand J Trauma Resusc Emerg Med. 2016;24:48.
7. Reitsma S, Slaaf DW, Vink H, van Zandvoort MA, oude Egbrink MG. The endothelial glycocalyx: composition, functions, and visualization. Pflug Arch. 2007;454:345–59.
8. Lekakis J, Abraham P, Balbarini A, et al. Methods for evaluating endothelial function: a position statement from the European Society of Cardiology Working Group on peripheral circulation. Eur J Cardiovasc Prev Rehabil. 2011;18:775–89.
9. Straat M, Muller MC, Meijers JC, et al. Effect of transfusion of fresh frozen plasma on parameters of endothelial condition and inflammatory status in non-bleeding critically ill patients: a prospective substudy of a randomized trial. Crit Care. 2015;19:163.
10. Nam EJ, Park PW. Shedding of cell membrane-bound proteoglycans. Methods Mol Biol. 2012;836:291–305.
11. Starling EH. On the absorption of fluids from the connective tissue spaces. J Physiol. 1896;19:312–26.
12. Levick JR. Revision of the Starling principle: new views of tissue fluid balance. J Physiol. 2004;557(Pt 3):704.
13. Levick JR. Capillary filtration-absorption balance reconsidered in light of dynamic extravascular factors. Exp Physiol. 1991;76:825–57.
14. Yen WY, Cai B, Yang JL, et al. Endothelial surface glycocalyx can regulate flow-induced nitric oxide production in microvessels in vivo. PLoS One. 2015;10:e0117133.
15. Trani M, Dejana E. New insights in the control of vascular permeability: vascular endothelial-cadherin and other players. Curr Opin Hematol. 2015;22:267–72.
16. Woodcock TE, Woodcock TM. Revised Starling equation and the glycocalyx model of transvascular fluid exchange: an improved paradigm for prescribing intravenous fluid therapy. Br J Anaesth. 2012;108:384–94.
17. Tatara T. Context-sensitive fluid therapy in critical illness. J Intensive Care. 2016;4:20.
18. Hahn RG. Fluid therapy in uncontrolled hemorrhage--what experimental models have taught us. Acta Anaesthesiol Scand. 2013;57:16–28.
19. Jacob M, Chappell D, Hofmann-Kiefer K, et al. The intravascular volume effect of Ringer's lactate is below 20%: a prospective study in humans. Crit Care. 2012;16:R86.
20. Jacob M, Bruegger D, Rehm M, Welsch U, Conzen P, Becker BF. Contrasting effects of colloid and crystalloid resuscitation fluids on cardiac vascular permeability. Anesthesiology. 2006;104:1223–31.
21. Borup T, Hahn RG, Holte K, Ravn L, Kehlet H. Intra-operative colloid administration increases the clearance of a post-operative fluid load. Acta Anaesthesiol Scand. 2009;53:311–7.
22. Myburgh JA, Finfer S, Bellomo R, et al. Hydroxyethyl starch or saline for fluid resuscitation in intensive care. N Engl J Med. 2012;367:1901–11.
23. Finfer S, Bellomo R, Boyce N, et al. A comparison of albumin and saline for fluid resuscitation in the intensive care unit. N Engl J Med. 2004;350:2247–56.
24. Holcomb JB, Tilley BC, Baraniuk S, et al. Transfusion of plasma, platelets, and red blood cells in a 1:1:1 vs a 1:1:2 ratio and mortality in patients with severe trauma: the PROPPR randomized clinical trial. JAMA. 2015;313:471–82.
25. Khan S, Brohi K, Chana M, et al. Hemostatic resuscitation is neither hemostatic nor resuscitative in trauma hemorrhage. J Trauma Acute Care Surg. 2014;76:561–7.
26. Potter DR, Jiang J, Damiano ER. The recovery time course of the endothelial cell glycocalyx in vivo and its implications in vitro. Circ Res. 2009;104:1318–25.

27. Zeng Y, Adamson RH, Curry FRE, Tarbell JM. Sphingosine-1-phosphate protects endothelial glycocalyx by inhibiting syndecan-1 shedding. Am J Physiol Heart Circ Physiol. 2014;306:H363–72.
28. Adamson RH, Clark JF, Radeva M, Kheirolomoom A, Ferrara KW, Curry FE. Albumin modulates S1P delivery from red blood cells in perfused microvessels: mechanism of the protein effect. Am J Physiol Heart Circ Physiol. 2014;306:H1011–7.
29. Barelli S, Alberio L. The role of plasma transfusion in massive bleeding: protecting the endothelial glycocalyx? Front Med. 2018;5:91.
30. Ksiazek M, Chacinska M, Chabowski A, Baranowski M. Sources, metabolism, and regulation of circulating sphingosine-1-phosphate. J Lipid Res. 2015;56:1271–81.
31. Pati S, Potter DR, Baimukanova G, Farrel DH, Holcomb JB, Schreiber MA. Modulating the endotheliopathy of trauma: factor concentrate versus fresh frozen plasma. J Trauma Acute Care Surg. 2016;80:576–85.
32. Torres LN, Chung KK, Salgado CL, Dubick MA, Torres Filho IP. Low-volume resuscitation with normal saline is associated with microvascular endothelial dysfunction after hemorrhage in rats, compared to colloids and balanced crystalloids. Crit Care. 2017;21:160.
33. Kozar RA, Peng ZL, Zhang RZ, et al. Plasma restoration of endothelial glycocalyx in a rodent model of hemorrhagic shock. Anesth Analg. 2011;112:1289–95.
34. Genet GF, Bentzer P, Ostrowski SR, Johansson PI. Resuscitation with pooled and pathogen-reduced plasma attenuates the increase in brain water content following traumatic brain injury and hemorrhagic shock in rats. J Neurotrauma. 2017;34:1054–62.
35. Haywood-Watson RJ, Holcomb JB, Gonzalez EA, et al. Modulation of syndecan-1 shedding after hemorrhagic shock and resuscitation. PLoS One. 2011;6:e23530.
36. Schenk S, Schoenhals GJ, de Souza G, Mann M. A high confidence, manually validated human blood plasma protein reference set. BMC Med Genet. 2008;1:41.
37. Kozar RA, Pati S. Syndecan-1 restitution by plasma after hemorrhagic shock. J Trauma Acute Care Surg. 2015;78(6 Suppl 1):S83–6.
38. Diebel LN, Martin JV, Liberati DM. Microfluidics: a high-throughput system for the assessment of the endotheliopathy of trauma and the effect of timing of plasma administration on ameliorating shock-associated endothelial dysfunction. J Trauma Acute Care Surg. 2018;84: 575–82.
39. Sperry JL, Guyette FX, Brown JB, et al. Prehospital plasma during air medical transport in trauma patients at risk for hemorrhagic shock. N Engl J Med. 2018;379:315–26.
40. Brown LM, Aro SO, Cohen MJ, et al. A high fresh frozen plasma: packed red blood cell transfusion ratio decreases mortality in all massively transfused trauma patients regardless of admission international normalized ratio. J Trauma. 2011;71(2 Suppl 3):S358–63.
41. Pandey S, Vyas GN. Adverse effects of plasma transfusion. Transfusion. 2012;52(Suppl 1):65S–79S.
42. Stensballe J, Ulrich AG, Nilsson JC, et al. Resuscitation of endotheliopathy and bleeding in thoracic aortic dissections: the VIPER-OCTA randomized clinical pilot trial. Anesth Analg. 2018;127:920–7.
43. Torres LN, Sondeen JL, Dubick MA, Filho IT. Systemic and microvascular effects of resuscitation with blood products after severe hemorrhage in rats. J Trauma Acute Care Surg. 2014;77:716–23.
44. Selim S, Sunkara M, Salous AK, et al. Plasma levels of sphingosine 1-phosphate are strongly correlated with haematocrit, but variably restored by red blood cell transfusions. Clin Sci. 2011;121:565–72.
45. McQuilten ZK, French CJ, Nichol A, Higgins A, Cooper DJ. Effect of age of red cells for transfusion on patient outcomes: a systematic review and meta-analysis. Transfus Med Rev. 2018;32:77–88.
46. Cardenas JC, Zhang X, Fox EE, et al. Platelet transfusions improve hemostasis and survival in a substudy of the prospective, randomized PROPPR trial. Blood Adv. 2018;2:1696–704.
47. Holcomb JB, Zarzabal LA, Michalek JE, et al. Increased platelet:RBC ratios are associated with improved survival after massive transfusion. J Trauma. 2011;71(2 Suppl 3):S318–28.

48. Baimukanova G, Miyazawa B, Potter DR, et al. Platelets regulate vascular endothelial stability: assessing the storage lesion and donor variability of apheresis platelets. Transfusion. 2016;56(Suppl 1):S65–75.
49. Pienimaeki-Roemer A, Ruebsaamen K, Boettcher A, et al. Stored platelets alter glycerophospholipid and sphingolipid species, which are differentially transferred to newly released extracellular vesicles. Transfusion. 2013;53:612–26.
50. Baimukanova G, Miyazawa B, Potter DR, et al. The effects of 22 degrees C and 4 degrees C storage of platelets on vascular endothelial integrity and function. Transfusion. 2016;56(Suppl 1):S52–64.
51. Muller RB, Ostrowski SR, Haase N, Wetterslev J, Perner A, Johansson PI. Markers of endothelial damage and coagulation impairment in patients with severe sepsis resuscitated with hydroxyethyl starch 130/0.42 vs ringer acetate. J Crit Care. 2016;32:16–20.
52. Kim TK, Nam K, Cho YJ, et al. Microvascular reactivity and endothelial glycocalyx degradation when administering hydroxyethyl starch or crystalloid during off-pump coronary artery bypass graft surgery: a randomised trial. Anaesthesia. 2017;72:204–13.

21 Should Albumin be the Colloid of Choice for Fluid Resuscitation in Hypovolemic Patients?

J. Montomoli, A. Donati, and C. Ince

21.1 Introduction

Hemodynamic management represents a major therapeutic challenge in critical care and emergency medicine. It plays a key role during the entire healing process of a patient from hospital admission to discharge. Within hemodynamic stabilization, resuscitation is one of the major indications for fluid administration and is often a life-saving therapy that has to be administered as soon as possible, with the right dose and rate, and choosing the right types of fluid. Unfortunately, these pillars of fluid therapy are not supported by consistent and solid evidence in the scientific literature. The agreement on the right fluid for the right patient is a mantra that is still a source of debate. However, after the restriction of hydroxyethyl starch (HES) use in critically ill patients issued by the European Medicine Agency (EMA) and the Food and Drug Administration (FDA) in 2013, crystalloids now dominate resuscitation fluids in hypovolemia although recent evidence has demonstrated increased mortality in critically ill patients receiving 0.9% NaCl (normal saline)—by far, one of the most used crystalloids [1].

J. Montomoli
Anesthesia and Intensive Care, Department of Biomedical Sciences and Public Health, Università Politecnica delle Marche, Ancona, Italy

Department of Intensive Care, Erasmus MC, University Medical Center Rotterdam, Rotterdam, The Netherlands

A. Donati
Anesthesia and Intensive Care, Department of Biomedical Sciences and Public Health, Università Politecnica delle Marche, Ancona, Italy

C. Ince (✉)
Department of Intensive Care, Erasmus MC, University Medical Center Rotterdam, Rotterdam, The Netherlands
e-mail: c.ince@erasmusmc.nl

J.-L. Vincent (ed.), *Annual Update in Intensive Care and Emergency Medicine 2019*, Annual Update in Intensive Care and Emergency Medicine,
https://doi.org/10.1007/978-3-030-06067-1_21

Among colloid solutions, albumin is the most used in clinical practice and in recent years its administration has been promoted mainly in septic patients [2]. Albumin is the main determinant of plasma oncotic pressure in healthy individuals and has, therefore, been recommended for treating hypovolemia [3]. However, current practice in critical care is more focused on replenishing albumin to physiological levels instead of using it for hemodynamic normalization during hypovolemia in the manner synthetic colloids are used. In addition to its use as a plasma expander, the structure of albumin confers other functions, so called non-oncotic or pleiotropic properties, which include binding and transporting endogenous and exogenous substances, antioxidant function, regulating immunomodulatory and anti-inflammatory activity, and contributing to acid-base regulation and endothelial stabilization [3].

Historically, a major boost to our knowledge on albumin occurred when the USA entered World War II [4]. As the need for a stable substitute for whole blood to treat hemorrhagic shock on the battlefield arose, the Harvard Physical Laboratory undertook preparation of serum albumin for this purpose. Since then an impressive amount of literature has been produced about albumin and its use in the clinical setting. At present, the major clinical indications for albumin administration are treatment or prevention of clinical complications associated with extreme effective hypovolemia in patients with liver cirrhosis and fluid resuscitation in critically ill patients, especially when crystalloids or artificial colloids are not effective or contraindicated [5].

The purpose of this chapter is to discuss the administration of albumin as a colloid to treat hypovolemia in comparison to other fluid types. In this context, we looked into the existing literature to evaluate whether the potential benefits of albumin have been supported by experimental findings.

21.2 Hypovolemia and the Hemodynamic Rationale for Its Treatment

Hypovolemia is a condition defined as a reduction in the intravascular volume that is effectively perfusing the tissues, usually called the effective circulating volume. Such a reduction may be caused by either an absolute drop in the total circulating volume related to blood loss (hemorrhage) or plasma loss (gastrointestinal, renal, cutaneous, extravasation into interstitial tissues) or by an inadequate distribution of blood volume between the central and peripheral compartments (venodilatation). Moreover, the onset of hypovolemia may be acute or develop gradually. Reductions in effective circulating volume result in decreased venous return, cardiac output and blood pressure. All these modifications activate a sympathetic response that essentially aims to correct previous modifications and prioritize blood flow to vital organs. Consequently, an increase in sympathetic tone determines changes in a patient's vital signs that are usually detected by clinicians as tachycardia, increased diastolic blood pressure, impaired capillary refill and tachypnea. Additional mechanisms mainly mediated by hormones are activated to restore the effective circulating volume over a medium-term and will not be described.

21.2.1 Hypovolemic Shock

Shock is a life-threating condition that develops when there is a relative insufficiency of intracellular energy production with respect to demand with consequent tissue dysoxia, disregarding the anatomo-physiological impairment that causes this condition. In critical care, shock is most often caused by a decrease in effective blood flow and oxygen delivery to tissues and, therefore, defined as circulatory shock. Based on the pathophysiological mechanism that leads to circulatory shock, four types of shock—not necessarily exclusive—can be identified: hypovolemic, cardiogenic, obstructive and distributive [6]. Hemodilution may be considered to constitute another type of shock. For a long time, a systolic blood pressure <90 mmHg has been considered a cardinal sign of shock. However, in recent years, the diagnosis of shock has moved towards systemic and organ-specific signs of tissue dysoxia [7]. A concentration of blood lactate >2 mEq/L is considered the most important marker of circulatory shock [6]. However, it has been shown that even values between 1.5 and 2.0 mEq/L are associated with increased mortality [6]. Other clues of shock are what Vincent and colleagues have previously described as "windows", through which we can see the effects of the altered tissue perfusion [6]. These "windows" provide us with surrogates of shock including the conditions of the skin, the kidneys and the brain, namely showing mottled skin and slow capillary refill (>2 s), oliguria (<0.5 mL/kg/h) and altered mental status (Glasgow Coma Scale [GCS] <15), respectively. All the previous organ-specific signs stem from a common feature found in all types of circulatory shock that consists of the impairment of the microcirculation. Based on this factor, sublingual microcirculation monitoring has the potential to provide a fairly objective "window" to evaluate real-time microcirculatory impairment associated with hypovolemia [8]. Despite the improvement of image quality in the last decade, current equipment is still not suitable for routine clinical use but it has been used widely for research with consistent and relevant findings [9]. Hopefully, in the coming years, breakthrough technologies and supportive clinical trials will help to bring sublingual microcirculation monitoring into clinical practice.

21.2.2 Fluid Resuscitation

According to the physiopathology of hypovolemic shock, the "VIP" (Ventilate, Infuse, Pump) therapeutic approach introduced by Dr. Weil in 1969 is still fundamental [10]. Most recently, the concept of fluid therapy has been expanded according to the clinical course of circulatory shock and more accurate fluid stewardship has been proposed mainly consisting of four phases: resuscitation, optimization, stabilization, and de-escalation [11]. Fluid resuscitation should be started as soon as possible with the least negative impact on blood homeostasis. The effectiveness of treatment requires a fluid able to produce a predictable and sustained increase in the intravascular compartment without detrimental effects on the endothelium, to be completely eliminated without tissue accumulation, and possibly to be cost-effective in terms of outcomes. No such 'physiological' resuscitation fluid exists at the moment and all choices of fluid therapy carry risks. Moreover, in addition to the choice of which type of fluid to use, further issues need to be addressed during the resuscitation phase, such as the target to reach, the best dose, the duration and the rate of infusion. Finally, assessment of fluid responsiveness using dynamic variables and continuous or intermittent evaluation of cardiac output, cardiac function and preload are essential to monitor the impact of therapeutic interventions and to avoid severe hemodilution and fluid overload [7].

Fluid solutions are roughly classified as colloids and crystalloids. According to the classic Starling model, colloid solutions should have the advantage of reducing the total amount of fluid needed to improve hemodynamics and systemic perfusion by increasing intravascular oncotic pressure. However, experiments using volume kinetics models have shown little or no advantages from colloids in terms of fluid expansion in conditions with low capillary pressure such as hypovolemia and sepsis [11]. Nevertheless, when clear hemodynamic endpoints are targeted during fluid resuscitation in septic patients, substantially less volume of colloids than crystalloids is required [12]. A biological explanation lies in the active role of the endothelium and the glycocalyx layer on regulating capillary permeability [13]. However, conditions characterized by sustained systemic inflammation but also persistently high rates of fluid infusion alter capillary permeability and may determine a state of globally increased permeability perpetuating fluid accumulation [11].

21.3 Human Serum Albumin: Oncotic and Non-Oncotic Properties

Although albumin is often considered as an intravascular protein, it is predominantly an interstitial protein with a concentration of about 20 g/L (total mass 160 g) and partially tissue-bound and, therefore, unavailable for circulation [3]. Albumin plasma concentration is approximately 45 g/L in healthy individuals with an intravascular mass of 120 g and it circulates across the capillary wall with a transcapillary escape rate of 5% per hour leading to a circulation half-life of 16 h [3]. In the 28–36 days between synthesis and degradation, it is roughly estimated that one albumin molecule makes 15,000 passes through the circulation. Albumin is not stored in the liver and there is no reserve for rapid release if required. Under physiological conditions, only 20–30% of hepatocytes produce albumin and its synthesis can be increased on demand by 200–300% [3]. Plasma albumin levels may fall during periods of stress, trauma or sepsis despite its long half-life resulting from accelerated redistribution from the intravascular space and increased catabolism.

21.3.1 Oncotic Pressure and Albumin

Albumin is responsible for approximately 80% of plasma oncotic pressure and one of the prime factors stimulating its synthesis is indeed oncotic pressure [3]. Two thirds of albumin-related oncotic pressure are attributed to its molecular weight of

66.5 kDa, which is less than half that of a gamma globulin (160 kDa) with an estimated osmotic activity per gram about 2.3 times higher than globulins. The other one third comes from the high negative charge carried by albumin at physiological pH, which holds sodium ions in its field without binding them, leading to a further increase in the intrinsic osmotic activity of albumin (Gibbs-Donnan effect). Notably, albumin is also the predominant protein in the interstitium and contributes to the interstitial oncotic pressure. Therefore, the colloid osmotic gradient across the capillary membrane is a more relevant determinant of fluid shift from and towards the interstitium, than its absolute plasma concentration. Moreover, the oncotic pressure difference pertinent to fluid homeostasis is not built up between the intravascular and the interstitial tissue spaces, but within a small protein-free zone beneath the glycocalyx surface layer. As a consequence, the prevailing oncotic gradient opposing fluid filtration originates from the sub-glycocalyx space and replaces the classical Starling model. Moreover, only a small amount of fluid from the interstitial space enters the circulation through a small number of large pores while the great majority of the interstitial fluid returns to the circulation as lymph fluid [13]. Albumin solutions most commonly used in clinical practice have concentrations of 5% or 20%, which represent approximately 1.2 and 5-times the physiological concentration in the plasma. At the highest concentration, albumin exerts 75–113 mmHg of oncotic pressure, justifying its use as plasma expander. In comparison to albumin 20%, all artificial colloids are provided at a lower concentration; HES and gelatins but not dextran 40 are characterized by a lower contribution to plasma oncotic pressure, and gelatins and dextran but not HES have a lower molecular weight.

21.3.2 Non-oncotic Properties of Albumin

During the past decade, better understanding of the structure of albumin and its functions has led to the concept that albumin, in addition to its oncotic function, has multifunctional properties ranging from immune regulation and endothelial stabilization to being a molecule that works in the intracellular compartment to modify several key pathophysiological mechanisms [3]. Among the various pleiotropic functions of albumin, one of the most relevant for its use during fluid resuscitation regards its capacity to bind to endothelium via the glycocalyx, despite both possessing a negative charge. Thus, albumin may increase glycocalyx stability, hinder its degradation, and, consequently, alter the permeability of these layers to macromolecules and other solutes and reduce vascular permeability [3]. By contrast, the systemic inflammation and oxidative stress present in critically ill patients induce and promote endothelial dysfunction. Apart from its direct role on endothelium preservation, albumin also acts as a major and predominant antioxidant exerting a glutathione-linked thiol peroxidase activity that contributes to modulate inflammation, reduce oxidative damage, and interfere in neutrophil adhesion with the beneficial effect of stabilizing the endothelium [3]. Interestingly, the protective effect of albumin on endothelial dysfunction was shown in endotoxemic mice receiving 4%

albumin, but not in those treated with 20% albumin or normal saline solution, suggesting a dose-dependent effect [14, 15]. Poorly understood properties of albumin include its anticoagulant and antithrombotic functions that seem partly related to its ability to bind nitric oxide (NO) in position Cys-34 but also associated with the neutralization of factor Xa and the inhibition of platelet-activating factors [3]. At the same time, there is no evidence of an increased risk of bleeding associated with albumin administration. Therefore, given the tendency of crystalloids to induce a moderate hypercoagulable state with a 10–30% hemodilution [16], the increased tendency of bleeding described with HES [17], and frequent coagulation disorders present in critically ill patients, the hemostatic effect displayed by albumin may be beneficial.

21.4 History of Fluid Management in Recent Decades

21.4.1 The Albumin Fall

There has been considerable debate over the last 30 years or more in relation to the best type of fluid to use for fluid resuscitation. In order to better understand the actual situation it is worthwhile to summarize the events. Despite the development of synthetic plasma expanders (dextrans, gelatins and starches) from the 1950s onwards, albumin retained its status as the plasma expander of choice well into the 1990s. Inconsistent evidence on its efficacy, relative or otherwise, and even scientific fraud regarding its safety [18] did not impact on this status. Its safety from pathogen submission appeared high, with only one incident, due to a breakdown in good manufacturing practice, reported in 50 years. Albumin's status appeared unquestioned until, in 1998, the publication of a meta-analysis from the Cochrane collaboration claimed an increase in mortality by 6% when using albumin across a series of randomized controlled trials (RCTs) over a 40-year period [19]. The consequences of those findings had a dramatic impact on albumin use, especially in the UK where use of albumin decreased by 40–45% in the six months after publication [20]. Subsequent meta-analyses of trials using more modern albumin preparations [21], as well as pharmacovigilance data of adverse events associated with albumin administration did not confirm the Cochrane meta-analysis findings [22]. In 2004, a large RCT in Australia and nearby countries compared 4% albumin and normal saline in a large and heterogeneous population of intensive care patients. The designated endpoint was mortality and the results showed equivalent outcomes between the two therapies, giving some comfort to each side of the albumin debate: albumin appeared safe but no better in therapeutic effect than normal saline [23]. Subsequent to this study, albumin use has increased, but has not recovered to previous levels. Moreover, from the end of the 1990s, albumin's position in the therapeutic armamentarium was challenged by cheaper synthetic colloids, particularly 'third generation' HES preparations. However, another turning point in the history of fluid therapy was approaching.

21.4.2 The 'HES Ban': Do Hemodynamics Matter?

Between 2008 and 2012, the results from five RCTs comparing colloid versus crystalloid use during fluid resuscitation in critically ill patients were published [17, 24–27]. Three of the five trials (VISEP, CHEST, and 6S) showed that HES was associated with worse patient prognosis and increased recourse to renal replacement therapy (RRT), although no objective criteria were implemented for its use [17, 24, 25]. Ninety-day mortality was higher in the HES group than in the crystalloid group in two studies [24, 25]; however, in one study the difference was not statistically significant [24]. Among the HES group, a 1.5-fold increased risk of bleeding was reported in the 6S trial [17] and more adverse events were reported with HES in the CHEST study [25]. In the other two studies, the FIRST trial compared resuscitation in patients with either blunt or penetrating trauma and described similar mortality in the two groups, with an increased risk of renal injury but not RRT in the saline group [26]. The CRYSTMAS study reported a lower fluid volume administered in the HES group than in the crystalloid group to reach hemodynamic stability [27], a finding also supported by the VISEP study [24]. However, the HES group required significantly more blood products than the crystalloid group in two studies [25, 26]. In June 2013, based on a review of existing studies, both the EMA and the FDA took the initiative to strongly discourage use of HES, respectively suspending marketing and issuing a 'black box' warning. In October 2018, a reassessment of the previous decision was performed in consideration of the recently published CRISTAL trial in which colloids (HES, gelatins and albumin) were compared to crystalloids among patients with hypovolemic shock. The results showed a significantly lower fluid volume administered to the colloid group associated with better survival and no increased risk in terms of kidney failure compared to crystalloids [28]. Moreover, 90-day mortality was significantly lower among patients receiving HES than in patients treated with crystalloids only. The EMA revised its original recommendation and allowed use of HES for resuscitation in patients with severe hypovolemia but required extended monitoring of kidney function. As a consequence, the use of HES has decreased substantially across Europe, although it continues to be used widely in Asia. Despite the decision of the EMA and the FDA, the debate on which type of fluid to use in the resuscitation phase is still open [29–31]. On one side, supporters of the 'HES-ban' rely on the high quality and strong results from RCTs [30], but on the other side, major concerns are raised against the decision of the regulatory agencies because of the lack of need of fluid resuscitation at the time of randomization for patients in the studies showing a negative impact of HES as well as impropriety in data handling [29, 31]. Indeed, baseline hemodynamic variables of patients enrolled in the CRISTAL and FIRST trials described study populations with systemic hemodynamic impairment at the time of randomization that was unlikely in the other studies (Table 21.1). Compared with the other studies, patients enrolled in the CRISTAL and in the FIRST study had, approximately, a mean arterial pressure (MAP) 10 mmHg lower and a central venous pressure (CVP) from 1–3 to 4–6 mmHg lower. The lactate concentration and the heart rate were higher in FIRST than in all the other trials (Table 21.1). Moreover, only the CRISTAL trial

Table 21.1 Comparison of descriptive data from the study populations of the main randomized clinical trials comparing colloids versus crystalloids in fluid resuscitation

		Hemodynamic				Laboratory	Organ dysfunction	Fluids before randomization[a]			
								Crystalloids		Colloids	
	No.	HR (beats/min)	MAP[b] (mmHg)	CVP (mmHg)	UO (mL/h)	Lactate (mmol/L)	SOFA	%	mL	%	mL
SAFE [23]											
Albumin 4%	3497	91 ± 24	78 ± 16	9 ± 5	90 ± 132	NA	NA	NA	NA	NA	NA
NS	3500	92 ± 24	78 ± 16	9 ± 5	95 ± 161	NA	NA	NA	NA	NA	NA
ALBIOS [42]											
Albumin 20%	903	105 ± 22	74 ± 16	10 ± 5	50 [20–100]	2.3 [1.4–4.2]	8 [6–10]	NA	NA	50%	NA
Crystalloid	907	106 ± 20	73 ± 15	10 ± 5	50 [25–100]	2.5 [1.6–4.3]	8 [5–10]	NA	NA	53%	NA
CRISTAL [28]											
Colloid	1414	105 [86–123]	65 [56–79]	7 [5–11]	40 [20–70]	2.3 [1.3–3.8]	8 [5–11]	37%	1000 [500–1000]	41%	1000 [500–2000]
Crystalloid	1443	105 [88–121]	66 [56–80]	8 [4–11]	40 [20–60]	2.4 [1.4–4.5]	8 [5–11]	28%	650 [500–1000]	48%	1000 [500–2000]
FIRST[c] [26]											
Overall	109	115	67 ± 21	6 ± 4	NA	4.9 ± 3.4	NA	92%	1881 [1100–2250]	NA	NA
6S [17]											
$HES_{130/0.42}$	398	NA	NA	10 [7–13]	NA	2.0 [1.3–3.5]	7 [5–9]	NA	NA	42%	700 [500–1000]
Ringer's acetate	400	NA	NA	10 [8–13]	NA	2.1 [1.4–3.7]	7 [5–9]	NA	NA	42%	500 [500–1000]
VISEP [24]											
$HES_{200/0.5}$	262	103 [90–118]	75 [67–85]	12 [8–15]	NA	2.2 [1.5–3.8]	NA	82%	2000 [1000–3500]	59%	979 [500–1000]
Ringer's lactate	275	104 [90–117]	75 [68–85]	12 [8–15]	NA	2.2 [1.5–4.3]	NA	59%	2000 [1000–3600]	58%	725 [500–1000]
CHEST [25]											
$HES_{130/0.4}$	3315	89 ± 24	74 ± 15	10 ± 5	NA	2.1 ± 2.0	NA	NA	NA	15%	NA
NS	3336	89 ± 23	74 ± 15	9 ± 5	NA	2.0 ± 1.5	NA	NA	NA	15%	NA

Estimates are reported as mean ± SD, median [IQR], n (%). *CVP* central venous pressure, *HR* heart rate, *HES* hydroxyethyl starch, *IQR* interquartile range, *NA* not available, *NS* normal saline, *UO* urinary output, *SOFA* Sequential Organ Failure Assessment, *SD* standard deviation

[a]Fluids administered in the 24 h prior to randomization in the 6S and in the ALBIOS and in the 12 h before randomization in the VISEP and before admission to the ICU in the CRISTAL

[b]MAP and IQR for the CRYSTAL study are computed as systolic pressure + (2*diastolic pressure)/3

[c]Data were kindly provided by Prof James. Blood administered before randomization was on average 103 mL

included patients with no fluids for resuscitation prior to randomization during their ICU stay and reported the amount of fluid received by patients in the 12 h before ICU admission whereas other studies (not all) reported a fluid volume administered before randomization in the ICU that ranged in average from 500 to 1000 mL just of colloids excluding crystalloids in approximately 50% of the patients (Table 21.1). In the VISEP study, it is noteworthy that the dose limit for HES (20 mL/kg/day) was exceeded by more than 10% on at least 1 day in 100 of 262 patients in the HES group with a median cumulative dose of 70 mL/kg [24]. Unfortunately, other variables describing the hemodynamic status are available for comparison in the published material only for the CRISTAL trial [31]. Obviously the impact of findings provided by the described RCTs and the initiative taken by the EMA and FDA had a dramatic impact on the type of fluid used in clinical practice [32]. Data from 84 ICUs in 17 countries showed that the proportion of patients that received crystalloids for fluid resuscitation was 43% in 2007 and 72% in 2014. Correspondingly, the use of colloids decreased from 62% to 31% in the same period. Among fluid resuscitation using colloids, the proportion of events in which albumin was administered increased from 38% in 2007 to 87% in 2014 resulting in a decrease of HES and gelatin from 35% and 26% in 2007 to 7% and 5% in 2014, respectively [32]. This worrying reaction to these trials led to concerns being voiced in an open letter by European Societies of Anesthesiology who argued for continued availability of HES for the treatment of hypovolemia [33]. Currently, despite the open debate and the ongoing production of opinion papers and reviews on fluid management including the discussion about which fluid should be used, the restrictions decided by the EMA and initial evidence from a RCT about the harmful effects of normal saline 0.9% [1] limit the choice to either balanced crystalloid solutions or albumin.

21.5 Current Indications for Albumin Use in Clinical Settings

Albumin is used for different indications in clinical practice, although its efficacy is not always supported by evidence. Hepatology is the field where international guidelines recommend albumin administration for specific indications, because its efficacy has been documented by RCTs and meta-analyses. The main indications in cirrhotic patients are based on albumin's capacity to act as a plasma-expander and the aim to treat or prevent clinical complications all characterized by extreme effective hypovolemia, such as preventing post-paracentesis circulatory dysfunction and renal failure induced by spontaneous bacterial peritonitis [34]. Similarly, albumin is indicated, in association with vasoconstrictors, to treat hepatorenal syndrome [34]. Finally, although using albumin to correct hypoalbuminemia is an inappropriate indication, two recently published multicenter RCTs examining effectiveness of long-term albumin administration among patients with liver cirrhosis and persistent uncomplicated ascites provided new findings for discussion [35, 36]. Indeed, Caraceni et al., using a protocol with more frequent administration of albumin (human albumin 40 g twice weekly for 2 weeks, and then 40 g weekly), were able to significantly increase albumin concentration in the treatment group compared to a standard medical treatment group with concomitant improvement in survival [35]. In a similar study by Solà and colleagues, both groups (placebo or albumin 40 g/15 days plus midodrine 15–30 mg/day) increased albumin concentration in a similar manner and there was no difference in the development of complications among the two groups [36]. Hopefully, the upcoming PRECIOSA trial will provide conclusive evidence on the topic (ClinicalTrials.gov Identifier: NCT03451292).

Apart from hepatology, there is no other specialty where indications for albumin administration have such strong recommendations. In intensive care, albumin has been used for many decades in a large number of conditions during fluid resuscitation or in acute clinical situations associated with hypoproteinemia. In the most recent guidelines of the Surviving Sepsis Campaign, there is a weak recommendation for albumin use in addition to crystalloids for initial resuscitation and subsequent intravascular volume replacement in patients with sepsis and septic shock when patients require substantial amounts of crystalloids [37]. Other licensed indications for albumin administration, such as in burns and hypoalbuminemia, were not supported by meta-analyses [38]. Existing studies examining the appropriateness of albumin prescription showed that albumin orders for an indication not supported by clinical evidence range from 40% to more than 90% but may improve with the implementation of internal practice guidelines [39, 40].

21.6 Evidence on Efficacy of Albumin Administration for the Treatment of Hypovolemia

Several meta-analyses have been published regarding albumin administration in critically ill patients since 1998 when the Cochrane meta-analyses reported higher mortality in patients receiving albumin [19]. The most common conclusion is that, except for patients with brain injury, albumin solutions as part of fluid expansion and resuscitation for critically ill patients seem to be safe with a potential positive effect in patients with severe sepsis. However, although meta-analyses may benefit from pooled data and robust estimates, the downside is that evidence comes from largely heterogeneous populations and interpretation is difficult from a physiological perspective. In the present section, we examine whether existing studies support the hypothetical advantages of albumin administration in the resuscitation phase mentioned previously.

To our knowledge, only four RCTs have been published examining albumin administration in critically ill patients and none had hemodynamic endpoints [23, 28, 41, 42]. Among the four previous studies, the SAFE study was the only one specifically assessing the role of albumin versus 0.9% NaCl in the context of fluid resuscitation in critically ill patients [23] while the CRISTAL trial included albumin among other colloids in the treatment group [28]. The two remaining studies had, as the primary aim, replenishment of albumin [41, 42]. Unfortunately, hemodynamic data about patients treated with albumin were available only in the SAFE and in the ALBIOS trial [23, 42] (Fig. 21.1). Because of heterogeneity in inclusion criteria and different study aims, possible differences regarding baseline hemodynamic status of the study populations should be examined. Indeed, patients included in the SAFE and in the ALBIOS studies had similar or lower heart rate, higher CVP, higher MAP and greater urinary output than patients in the FIRST and in the CRISTAL studies (Table 21.1). Such differences could, again, suggest non-hypovolemic populations at time of randomization in the two studies investigating albumin administration. Of note, requirement for fluid resuscitation was not among the inclusion criteria of the ALBIOS study [42].

Compared with crystalloids, albumin should have been associated with a more efficient volume expanding effect. However, the ratio of the volume of albumin to the volume of crystalloids administered in the SAFE (first 4 days) and in the ALBIOS (first 7 days) studies was lower than expected being, respectively, 1:1.4 and 1:1 [23, 42]. On day 1, the albumin to crystalloid ratio was 1:1.3 in SAFE and 1:1 in ALBIOS. The reported differences between the two studies could be related to the degree of impairment of capillary permeability being less severe in patients included in the SAFE study than in the ALBIOS study.

The HES to 0.9% NaCl ratio reported in the CRYSTMAS study examining the hemodynamic efficacy of 6% HES in patients with severe sepsis was 1:1.2 for the volume necessary to reach hemodynamic stability and 1:1 over the entire study period [27]. Looking at the hemodynamic trends in the two studies, albumin administration was associated with a higher CVP (11.2 ± 4.8 vs. 10.0 ± 4.5 mmHg, $p < 0.001$) and lower heart rate (88.0 ± 20.2 vs. 89.7 ± 20.8 beats/min, $p < 0.001$) on the first day of treatment in SAFE, although the absolute difference was small (Fig. 21.1). In ALBIOS, over the first 7 days after randomization, patients in the albumin arm experienced lower heart rate, higher CVP, higher MAP and a shorter duration of vasopressor therapy. However, differences in the parameters were small and mostly attributable to changes occurring in the 6 h after randomization and normalized afterwards suggesting a role of albumin as a fluid expander limited to the first hours after administration. Interestingly, similar to what has been pointed out for some of the RCTs looking at HES, patients randomized to albumin received more red blood cells (RBCs) both in the SAFE and in the ALBIOS studies than patients assigned to the crystalloid group. Only a trend in serum lactate was reported in the ALBIOS trial, being in general 0.1 mmol/L lower in the albumin group.

Regarding clinical endpoints, there was no improvement in terms of 28-day mortality for the albumin group in the SAFE and in the ALBIOS studies. The subanalysis of the CRISTAL study comparing albumin with normal saline did not show significant differences among the groups for 28- or 90-day mortality, although suggested a superior effect for HES (relative risk 0.79; 95% confidence interval (CI): 0.66–0.95) over albumin (relative risk 1.02; 95% CI: 0.69–1.50) on 90-day mortality [28]. However, patients randomized to albumin were markedly fewer than those randomized to HES, potentially introducing unequal distribution of confounding factors. In the SAFE trial, albumin administration had a tendency towards a beneficial effect on 28-day survival among septic patients but an opposite effect in trauma patients with brain injury [23]. According to the results published by Semler et al. in 2018, septic patients showed a 30-day in-hospital mortality of 25.2% when

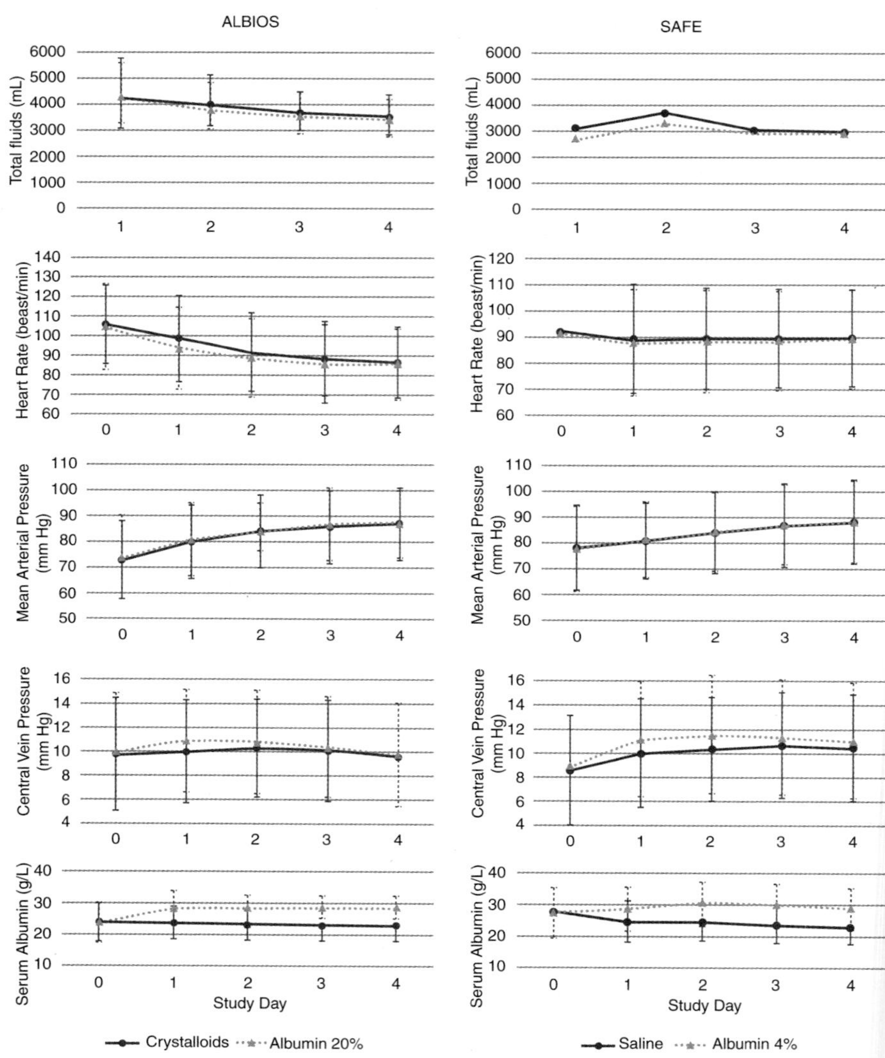

Fig. 21.1 Trends in hemodynamic parameters and serum albumin concentrations in the first 4 days of the ALBIOS trial [42] and the SAFE trial [23]. The figure shows that in both trials, patients were unlikely to be hypovolemic at baseline (mean arterial pressure >70 mmHg and central venous pressure >8 mmHg). Total fluids in the ALBIOS trial were reported as median and interquartile range while for the SAFE trial were computed as the sum of the means of all types of administered fluids (resuscitation fluid, maintenance fluid, packed red blood cells) provided in the published manuscripts. Therefore, it was not possible to provide error bars. Hemodynamic parameters and serum albumin are reported as mean and standard deviation for both trials. Data were extracted from the supplement material Tables S3 and S4 of the ALBIOS trial and from Table 2 of the SAFE trial

randomized to balanced crystalloids compared to 29.4% with 0.9% NaCl (adjusted odds ratio 0.80; 95% CI: 0.67–0.97) [1]. These findings provide the rationale to reconsider the results of the SAFE trial not because of the beneficial effect of albumin but the detrimental effect of saline. Consistent with this, findings from the ALBIOS trial published in 2014 showed no improvement in mortality among septic patients treated with albumin compared to crystalloids [42]. But in a subanalysis considering only patients with septic shock, albumin was associated with better 28-day mortality (relative risk 0.87, 95% CI: 0.77–0.99) but there were no analyses stratified by the type of crystalloid administered. However, data comparing fluid expanding effects among albumin and other colloids during fluid resuscitation are lacking. Unfortunately, based on data available from existing studies it is not possible to examine whether the studies supported speculated non-oncotic properties of albumin. Moreover, an observational study in patients undergoing cardiac surgery suggested a dose-dependent risk of acute kidney injury associated with albumin administration and not with 6% HES [43].

In conclusion, there is a lack of knowledge about the best strategy for albumin administration: bolus versus continuous infusion, high versus low rate of infusion, albumin concentration, and types of target (hemodynamic vs. serum concentration). The infusion rate issue will be addressed by the AIR trial (ClinicalTrials.gov Identifier: NCT02728921) among patients following non-emergent major abdominal surgery. However, although the trial was concluded in November 2016, no results are available yet. Future studies should take into consideration albumin administration modalities in the study design. Of note, we decided not to discuss recombinant human albumin due to the lack of evidence in clinical use. However, in view of the therapeutic limitations of human albumin described in this chapter, recombinant albumin dimers (molecular weight 130 kDa) appear a promising plasma expander in the presence of severe capillary leakage [44].

21.7 Concerns Raised About Commercial Albumin Solutions

Currently available albumin solutions are developed using various techniques, such that there is worldwide variation between manufacturers in terms of manufacturing standards, use of stabilizers, protein content and composition, binding capacity, metal ion content, antioxidant properties, charge, capacity to bind drugs, and so forth. Unfortunately, there are few data available about the compositions of the different albumin solutions and whether or how this may impact on its clinical effects. Interestingly, although we have demonstrated that the rationale for albumin administration in critically ill patients is not exclusively associated with its oncotic properties, the FDA does not require clinical efficacy data for commercialization of albumin products. Indeed, the FDA only requires at least 95% of the total protein in the final product to be albumin and assumes albumin has a well-established safety and efficacy profile because of extensive clinical experience with the product.

Therefore, no new clinical efficacy data are required for the approval of new therapeutic albumin (natural source) products since the mechanism of action of therapeutic albumin in support of colloid osmotic pressure is well understood and albumin products are purified using well-established and consistent manufacturing methods [45]. There are some concerns that arise from the above considerations. First, several methods have been validated and applied for manufacturing albumin and those methods may be associated with different adverse event patterns [46] or have different impact on albumin degradation and, consequently, on its properties. Albumin solutions are available in various formulations with different concentrations and differences in electrolyte composition of the 'solvent' employed have been reported [47]. Large and potentially clinically significant differences in albumin oxidative status were reported in commercial albumin solutions compared with albumin from healthy individuals, between manufacturers, and even between batches produced by a single manufacturer [48, 49]. Finally, commercial albumin solutions have been found to have a potential immunosuppressive role *in vitro* [50].

21.8 Conclusion

To summarize, from a theoretical point of view albumin may, due to a range of characteristics, be considered the fluid of choice to treat hypovolemia in critically ill patients. However, the advantages of albumin as a plasma expander compared with crystalloids seem to be correlated with the capillary permeability, being maximum in healthy individuals and decreasing according to the disease severity of patients. Existing evidence does not suggest a clear superiority of albumin in comparison with other colloids, reporting similar albumin to crystalloid volume ratios and similar increased requirement of RBC administration. Analyses of commercial solutions have raised concerns about the capacity of albumin to carry out pleiotropic functions promoted as beneficial, especially in septic patients. The present review highlights the need for future studies with well-defined inclusion criteria able to guarantee the enrollment of hypovolemic patients and to limit fluid administration before randomization, a fluid resuscitation phase driven by hemodynamic targets, and endpoints able to evaluate possible benefit associated with non-oncotic properties of albumin.

References

1. Semler MW, Self WH, Wanderer JP, et al. Balanced crystalloids versus saline in critically ill adults. N Engl J Med. 2018;378:829–39.
2. Vincent JL, De Backer D, Wiedermann CJ. Fluid management in sepsis: the potential beneficial effects of albumin. J Crit Care. 2016;35:161–7.
3. Fanali G, di Masi A, Trezza V, et al. Human serum albumin: from bench to bedside. Mol Asp Med. 2012;33:209–90.
4. Kendrick DB. The blood program. 1962. Available at: http://history.amedd.army.mil/booksdocs/wwii/actvsurgconvoli/CH06.htm. Accessed 15 Aug 2018.

5. Caraceni P, Domenicali M, Tovoli A, et al. Clinical indications for the albumin use: still a controversial issue. Eur J Intern Med. 2013;24:721–8.
6. Vincent JL, Ince C, Bakker J. Clinical review: circulatory shock—an update: a tribute to Professor Max Harry Weil. Crit Care. 2012;16:239.
7. Cecconi M, De Backer D, Antonelli M, et al. Consensus on circulatory shock and hemodynamic monitoring. Task force of the European Society of Intensive Care Medicine. Intensive Care Med. 2014;40:1795–815.
8. Ince C. The rationale for microcirculatory guided fluid therapy. Curr Opin Crit Care. 2014;20:301–8.
9. Ince C. Hemodynamic coherence and the rationale for monitoring the microcirculation. Crit Care Lond Engl. 2015;19(Suppl 3):S8.
10. Weil MH. The "VIP" approach to the bedside management of shock. JAMA. 1969;207:337.
11. Malbrain MLNG, Van Regenmortel N, Saugel B, et al. Principles of fluid management and stewardship in septic shock: it is time to consider the four D's and the four phases of fluid therapy. Ann Intensive Care. 2018;8:66.
12. Dubin A, Pozo MO, Casabella CA, et al. Comparison of 6% hydroxyethyl starch 130/0.4 and saline solution for resuscitation of the microcirculation during the early goal-directed therapy of septic patients. J Crit Care. 2010;25:659.e1–8.
13. Woodcock TE, Woodcock TM. Revised Starling equation and the glycocalyx model of transvascular fluid exchange: an improved paradigm for prescribing intravenous fluid therapy. Br J Anaesth. 2012;108:384–94.
14. Kremer H, Baron-Menguy C, Tesse A, et al. Human serum albumin improves endothelial dysfunction and survival during experimental endotoxemia: concentration-dependent properties. Crit Care Med. 2011;39:1414–22.
15. Damiani E, Ince C, Orlando F, et al. Effects of the infusion of 4% or 20% human serum albumin on the skeletal muscle microcirculation in endotoxemic rats. PLoS One. 2016;11:e0151005.
16. Hahn RG. Adverse effects of crystalloid and colloid fluids. Anaesthesiol Intensive Ther. 2014;49:303–8.
17. Perner A, Haase N, Guttormsen AB, et al. Hydroxyethyl starch 130/0.42 versus Ringer's acetate in severe sepsis. N Engl J Med. 2012;367:124–34.
18. Wise J. Boldt: the great pretender. BMJ. 2013;346:f1738.
19. Cochrane Injuries Group Albumin Reviewers. Human albumin administration in critically ill patients: systematic review of randomised controlled trials. BMJ. 1998;317:235–40.
20. Roberts I, Edwards P, McLelland B, et al. More on albumin. BMJ. 1999;318:1214.
21. Wilkes MM, Navickis RJ. Patient survival after human albumin administration. A meta-analysis of randomized, controlled trials. Ann Intern Med. 2001;135:149–64.
22. Vincent JL, Wilkes MM, Navickis RJ. Safety of human albumin—serious adverse events reported worldwide in 1998–2000. Br J Anaesth. 2003;91:625–30.
23. Finfer S, Bellomo R, Boyce N, et al. A comparison of albumin and saline for fluid resuscitation in the intensive care unit. N Engl J Med. 2004;350:2247–56.
24. Brunkhorst FM, Engel C, Bloos F, et al. Intensive insulin therapy and pentastarch resuscitation in severe sepsis. N Engl J Med. 2008;358:125–39.
25. Myburgh JA, Finfer S, Bellomo R, et al. Hydroxyethyl starch or saline for fluid resuscitation in intensive care. N Engl J Med. 2012;367:1901–11.
26. James MFM, Michell WL, Joubert IA, et al. Resuscitation with hydroxyethyl starch improves renal function and lactate clearance in penetrating trauma in a randomized controlled study: the FIRST trial (Fluids in Resuscitation of Severe Trauma). Br J Anaesth. 2011;107:693–702.
27. Guidet B, Martinet O, Boulain T, et al. Assessment of hemodynamic efficacy and safety of 6% hydroxyethylstarch 130/0.4 vs. 0.9% NaCl fluid replacement in patients with severe sepsis: the CRYSTMAS study. Crit Care Lond Engl. 2012;16:R94.
28. Annane D, Siami S, Jaber S, et al. Effects of fluid resuscitation with colloids vs crystalloids on mortality in critically ill patients presenting with hypovolemic shock: the CRISTAL randomized trial. JAMA. 2013;310:1809–17.

29. Can I, Thomas WLS. Even normal saline is harmful if used wrongly, so why did EMA single out hydroxyethyl starch? 2018. Available at: https://blogs.bmj.com/bmj/2018/05/11/even-normal-saline-is-harmful-if-used-wrongly-so-why-did-ema-single-out-hydroxyethyl-starch/. Accessed 6 June 2018.
30. Wiedermann CJ, Bellomo R, Perner A. Is the literature inconclusive about the harm from HES? No. Intensive Care Med. 2017;43:1523–5.
31. Doshi P. EMA recommendation on hydroxyethyl starch solutions obscured controversy. BMJ. 2018;360:k1287.
32. Hammond NE, Taylor C, Finfer S, et al. Patterns of intravenous fluid resuscitation use in adult intensive care patients between 2007 and 2014: an international cross-sectional study. PLoS One. 2017;12:e0176292.
33. Zwissler B. Open letter to the European Commission: marketing authorization of colloid solutions containing hydroxyethyl starch (HES). 2018. Available at: https://www.dgai.de/aktuelles/464. Accessed 3 Nov 2018.
34. Angeli P, Bernardi M, Villanueva C, et al. EASL Clinical Practice Guidelines for the management of patients with decompensated cirrhosis. J Hepatol. 2018;69:406–60.
35. Caraceni P, Riggio O, Angeli P, et al. Long-term albumin administration in decompensated cirrhosis (ANSWER): an open-label randomised trial. Lancet. 2018;391:2417–29.
36. Solà E, Solé C, Simón-Talero M, et al. Midodrine and albumin for prevention of complications of cirrhosis in patients in the waiting list for liver transplantation. A randomized, multicenter, double-blind, placebo-controlled trial. J Hepatol. 2017;66:S11.
37. Rhodes A, Evans LE, Alhazzani W, et al. Surviving sepsis campaign: international guidelines for management of sepsis and septic shock. Crit Care Med. 2017;45:486–552.
38. Roberts I, Blackhall K, Alderson P, et al. Human albumin solution for resuscitation and volume expansion in critically ill patients. Cochrane Database Syst Rev. 2011;2011:CD001208.
39. Laki B, Taghizadeh-Ghehi M, Assarian M, et al. Effect of hospital-wide interventions to optimize albumin use in a tertiary hospital. J Clin Pharm Ther. 2017;42:704–9.
40. Tarin R, Sanchez A, Santos R, et al. Costs related to inappropriate use of albumin in Spain. Ann Pharmacother. 2000;34:1198–205.
41. Dubois M-J, Orellana-Jimenez C, Melot C, et al. Albumin administration improves organ function in critically ill hypoalbuminemic patients: a prospective, randomized, controlled, pilot study. Crit Care Med. 2006;34:2536–40.
42. Caironi P, Tognoni G, Masson S, et al. Albumin replacement in patients with severe sepsis or septic shock. N Engl J Med. 2014;370:1412–21.
43. Frenette AJ, Bouchard J, Bernier P, et al. Albumin administration is associated with acute kidney injury in cardiac surgery: a propensity score analysis. Crit Care. 2014;18:602.
44. Taguchi K, Giam Chuang VT, Maruyama T, Otagiri M. Pharmaceutical aspects of the recombinant human serum albumin dimer: structural characteristics, biological properties, and medical applications. J Pharm Sci. 2012;101:3033–46.
45. Woodcock J, Griffin J, Behrman R, et al. The FDA's assessment of follow-on protein products: a historical perspective. Nat Rev Drug Discov. 2007;6:437–42.
46. Che Y, Wilson FJ, Bertolini J, et al. Impact of manufacturing improvements on clinical safety of albumin: Australian pharmacovigilance data for 1988–2005. Crit Care Resusc. 2006;8:334–8.
47. Lai AT, Zeller MP, Millen T, et al. Chloride and other electrolyte concentrations in commonly available 5% albumin products. Crit Care Med. 2018;46:e326–9.
48. Bar-Or D, Bar-Or R, Rael LT, et al. Heterogeneity and oxidation status of commercial human albumin preparations in clinical use. Crit Care Med. 2005;33:1638–41.
49. Plantier J-L, Duretz V, Devos V, et al. Comparison of antioxidant properties of different therapeutic albumin preparations. Biologicals. 2016;44:226–33.
50. Bar-Or D, Thomas GW, Bar-Or R, et al. Commercial human albumin preparations for clinical use are immunosuppressive in vitro. Crit Care Med. 2006;34:1707–12.

What the Intensive Care Physician Should Know About the Transurethral Resection Syndrome

22

R. G. Hahn

22.1 Introduction

The transurethral (TUR) syndrome is caused by absorption of fluid used to irrigate the operating field during endoscopic surgery. The intensivist and the anesthetic team should be able to successfully master this complication, which has good prognosis if diagnosed and treated early. Parts of the pathophysiology and the best treatment of the TUR syndrome have not been clarified until recently.

22.2 History, Surgeries and Types of Absorption

Endoscopic monopolar electroresection for resection of benign prostatic enlargement was pioneered by American urologists in the 1930s. About 10 years later, Creevy [1] described a hemolytic syndrome with kidney failure that could be related to the sterile water used for irrigation of the bladder. From the early 1950s and onward, various non-electrolyte solutes, such as glycine, glucose, mannitol, and sorbitol, were added to the irrigating fluid to avoid this hemolysis. However, the iatrogenic complication continued to cause trouble, despite the absence of hemolysis. The first clinical description of the TUR syndrome, as we know it today, was published in 1956 by Harrison et al. [2]. They suggested that the syndrome was caused by absorption of at least 3 L of irrigating solution, and they estimated the incidence of the complication to be 10% of the prostatic resections performed.

During the 1970s, the view of the TUR syndrome was that it was essentially a yes/no complication, almost like an allergic reaction. Later research, using methods to quantify fluid absorption, associated an increasing number and severity of

R. G. Hahn (✉)
Research Unit, Södertälje Hospital, Södertälje, Sweden

Karolinska Institutet at Danderyds Hospital (KIDS), Stockholm, Sweden
e-mail: r.hahn@telia.com

J.-L. Vincent (ed.), *Annual Update in Intensive Care and Emergency Medicine 2019*, Annual Update in Intensive Care and Emergency Medicine,
https://doi.org/10.1007/978-3-030-06067-1_22

symptoms with a gradual increase in the amount of absorbed fluid [3]. This fluid can be absorbed in two ways. The most common route is by direct inflow to the periprostatic veins, which then requires a fluid pressure that exceeds the venous pressure ('intravascular absorption'). More rarely, fluid enters the body through instrument-induced perforations of the prostatic capsule of the bladder, which cause large amounts of irrigating fluid to be deposited in potential periprostatic tissue spaces ('extravascular absorption') [3, 4]. From there, the fluid slowly diffuses throughout the body fluid compartments.

Fluid absorption can occur during all operations where irrigation of an operating field is combined with electrocautery, with the best known being transurethral resection of the prostate (TURP). Since the late 1980s, transcervical resection of the endometrium (TCRE) has become a common surgical approach to alleviate menstrual bleeding causing anemia, and the TUR syndrome can also occur in these patients [5–7]. One difference from TURP is that perforations during TCRE commonly result in deposition of irrigating fluid in the intra-abdominal cavity.

Most studies of fluid absorption deal with the use of electrolyte-free irrigating fluids and most were published in urology journals at the end of the past decade. The clinical scenario has changed in recent years, as the introduction of the bipolar resection technique allows the use of electrolyte-containing irrigating solutions, most commonly isotonic saline [8]. Perhaps half of the endoscopic resections performed in Europe today are performed with the bipolar irrigation technique.

22.3 Symptoms

Absorption of up to 1 L of irrigating fluid, such as 1.5% glycine, does not have untoward consequences, whereas uptake of between 1 and 2 L results in increased postoperative incidence of nausea, vomiting, bradycardia and arterial hypotension. The risk of these symptoms increases sevenfold when compared to when 0–300 mL is absorbed [3]. Absorption of more than 2 L may further be followed by depressed consciousness, dizziness and confusion. Rapid absorption often causes restlessness on the operating table and, more rarely, overt pulmonary edema [9].

The cut-off for the full-fledged TUR syndrome in men is when more than 3 L of fluid is absorbed. The patient may undergo a transient phase of hypertension that, typically, suddenly changes into a hypotensive state. The other chief symptoms are confusion, depressed or loss of consciousness and oliguria [3]. However, the full-fledged TUR syndrome may also present as a sudden cardiac arrest on the operating table that is preceded by only scant warning signs, if any [10, 11].

Extravascular absorption is characterized by a swollen abdomen and a delayed onset of symptoms, where arterial hypotension is prominent [3].

The likelihood of occurrence of nausea and depressed consciousness is lower for 3% mannitol than for 1.5% glycine, but the incidence of circulatory symptoms is similar [12]. Reliable comparative data for sorbitol solutions are scarce, particularly for large-scale absorption [13].

Visual disturbance, which may proceed to transient blindness, is a symptom peculiar to glycine absorption [14, 15] and sometimes occurs in response to only a few hundred milliliters of this fluid [16]. This complication might be frightening but the condition resolves spontaneously within 24 h.

Symptoms from absorption of electrolyte-containing solutions consist of agitation, shortness of breath, a sense of being swollen, and other signs associated with volume overload [8, 17]. Only a few studies report actual measurements of saline absorption and compare them with symptoms.

Mild forms of the TUR syndrome are often overlooked and interpreted as being due to anesthesia, old age or medication. The mild forms typically appear in the postoperative unit 30–60 min after the surgery ends. More severe forms of the syndrome become apparent during the surgery and the symptoms become more severe during the postoperative period.

22.3.1 Pathophysiology of Neurological Symptoms

Absorption of electrolyte-free irrigating fluid induces acute hyponatremia, which is crucial to the symptomatology. If measured at the end of surgery, 2 L of irrigating fluid depresses plasma sodium by 10–12 mmol/L in men [18] (Fig. 22.1a) and by almost 20 mmol/L in women [20]. Rapid absorption induces a greater decrease. Plasma sodium <130 mmol/L is usually symptomatic and is associated with dizziness, lethargy and confusion. The clinical picture becomes aggravated if plasma sodium falls <120 mmol/L, and it might then also include epileptic seizures [21, 22]. Hyponatremia causes brain edema, which might cause death 6–8 h after the surgery.

Irrigating fluid also causes hypo-osmolality, as the fluids (except mannitol 5%) are hypo-osmolar. The reduction in osmolality is typically in the range of 10–15 mosmol/kg in cases of large-scale absorption. A greater depression of serum osmolality worsens the symptomatology.

The metabolism of glycine is troublesome in about 10% of humans. In these patients, even a moderate load of this amino acid (about 1 L of 1.5% glycine solution) causes hyperammonemia, which clearly aggravates any hyponatremia-induced nausea and dizziness [15, 23, 24].

22.3.2 Pathophysiology of Circulatory Symptoms

The origin of the cardiovascular complications of fluid absorption and their treatment has long been controversial. Intravascular fluid absorption causes an acute rise in central venous pressure (CVP), at 2–3 mmHg for absorption of 500 mL over 10 min [25], while cardiac output can increase or decrease. The transient hypertensive phase, which may be seen in patients with minor blood loss, can be explained by the marked hypervolemia that prevails at the time [15]. However, the transition into a hypotensive state has been difficult to understand.

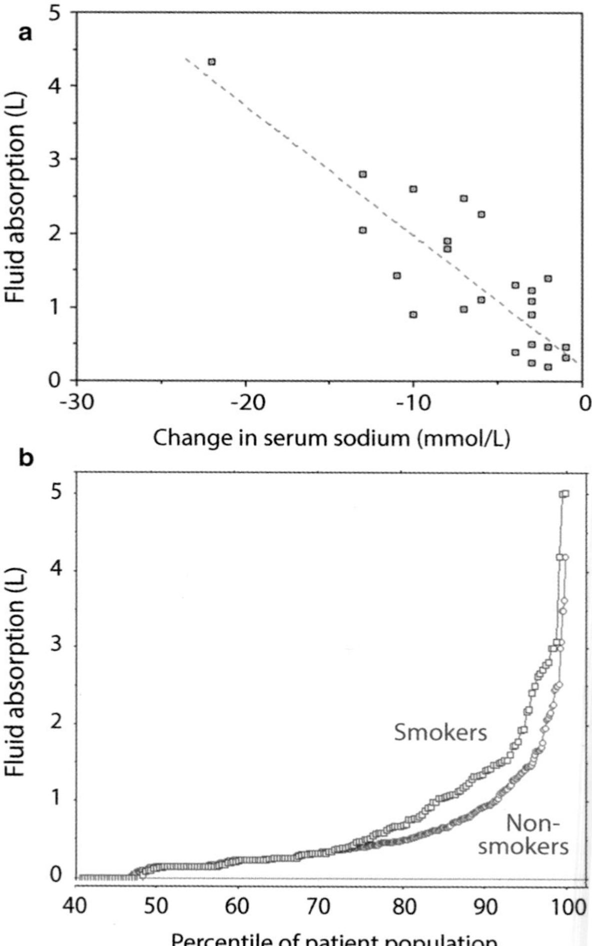

Fig. 22.1 (**a**) Decrease in serum sodium at the end of transurethral resection of the prostate (TURP), when various volumes of 1.5% glycine had been absorbed. The volume of irrigant absorbed was measured volumetrically after correction for admixture with blood in the fluid returns. Data stem from clinical trials of irrigating fluid containing 1% ethanol as a marker of absorption. (**b**) Fluid absorption is larger in smokers and past smokers than in those who have never smoked. Data from 1034 patients where fluid absorption was quantified by the ethanol method [19]. Overall, half of the patients showed absorption and about 10% absorbed a volume >1 L

The modern view is that the hypotensive phase is the result of paradoxical hypovolemia, which arises because electrolyte-free irrigating fluids induce osmotic diuresis and also (except mannitol 5%) enter the cells. Ninety minutes after an absorption event, the entire inflicted hyponatremia appears to be due to natriuresis alone [26]. Experiments in pigs showed, based on volume kinetic analysis, that diffusion of fluid into the cells results in a flow of fluid from the plasma to the interstitium that is not balanced by a return flow back to the plasma. The brisk osmotic diuresis and the lack of back-flow both contribute to the development of hypovolemic hypotension [27]. Recent microcirculatory studies suggest that 'back-flow' from the interstitium is transmitted via the lymphatics [28]; therefore, we may assume that the normal lymphatic flow is interrupted in this syndrome.

Absorption of electrolyte-containing irrigating fluid does not induce hyponatremia. Here, the problem is the volume overload that results in cardiovascular strain and pulmonary edema. Other issues are the same as those reported when saline is used as an infusion fluid, namely metabolic acidosis and impaired kidney function. As with electrolyte-free fluids, rapid absorption far in excess of 3 L disrupts the cytoarchitecture of the tissues, which is most crucial to heart function. Electrocardiographic changes occur, and death might ensue [29].

The literature contains many Case Reports with fatal outcomes [30–33]. If cardiac arrest does not occur on the operating table [10, 11], poor outcome is most commonly associated with a 'doctor's delay' in treatment. Mortality of the severe TUR syndrome is estimated at 25% [34]. The cause of death is either cardiovascular collapse or brain herniation.

22.4 Incidence

Prospective studies in the 1980s and 1990s showed that fluid absorption large enough to cause symptoms (>1 L) occurred in approximately 2–10% of the TURPs performed [12, 13, 35], although both higher and lower figures have been published. Absorption often occurs very rapidly once it is initiated (0.5–2 L per 10 min). The full-fledged TUR syndrome, requiring intensive care, is usually reported to occur in a range of 1/300–1/500 of TURP cases. Data from the present millennium are lacking.

Many authors have claimed that the TUR syndrome has disappeared with the use of the bipolar resection techniques because hyponatremia no longer occurs. However, measurements with tracers suggest that absorption is just as common as with electrolyte-free irrigating fluids [8, 36, 37], although the symptoms are not as severe.

Fluid absorption in TCRE is in the range of that reported for TURP [5, 7], although the incidence is believed to have decreased with the use of better resection instruments and monitoring. Menstruating women are more prone than men to develop brain injury in response to hyponatremia [38], making fluid absorption a more serious issue. Istre et al. [20] used computed tomography (CT) scans to demonstrate brain edema in TCRE patients after absorption of as little as 1 L of 1.5% glycine.

22.5 Monitoring

Spinal anesthesia is traditionally recommended for endoscopic operations because the earliest signs of the TUR syndrome (restlessness, nausea and a sensation of being swollen) can be detected during the actual surgery.

Measuring plasma sodium is the most popular way to confirm or refute that fluid absorption has occurred. This is usually done at the end of surgery. No practice of bedside monitoring with repeated measurements of plasma sodium has been adopted, which is probably due to the effort involved and the invasive nature of the test.

The use of saline for irrigation with the bipolar resection technique precludes the use of plasma sodium for this purpose. However, large-scale absorption of saline can be quantified by measuring plasma chloride, which is abundant in isotonic saline [17].

Several types of perioperative monitoring have been developed. The most widely used is volumetric fluid balance, which means that all fluids used are compared with the volumes recovered [25]. This method is fairly accurate during TCRE, whereas the results during TURP are more easily confused by spillage on the floor and admixture of the irrigating fluid returns with blood. Automatic systems for calculation of the volumetric balance during TCRE are commercially available.

Placing the patient's bed on an electronic scale during surgery has also been used [13]. This allows immediate detection of fluid absorption, but useful results can be obtained only when the bladder has been emptied.

Ethanol monitoring relies on the addition of ethanol to a concentration of 1% in the irrigating fluid and repeated measurements of the ethanol concentration in the patient's exhaled breath during surgery. This method was evaluated in clinical trials in the late 1980s and was found to be reliable during TURP [18, 39] and TCRE [7]; it can be used during spinal as well as general anesthesia. As for serum sodium, different patterns are found for the intra- and extravascular absorption types. The recommendation is to alert the surgeon to any ongoing absorption when 1 L has been taken up, and to conclude the operation (if possible) when 2 L has been absorbed [35]. Automatic systems for ethanol monitoring have been developed, but have not reached the market [40].

Both the anesthetist and the surgeon need to agree upon a monitoring approach. Historically, anesthetists have been interested and have understood the value of monitoring, while, at least in urology, most surgeons have resisted this use. The reason is that urologists regard fluid absorption as evidence of poor surgical skill, a 'beginner's' problem. Even without measuring fluid absorption, it is common to state that this complication does not exist at their particular institution.

22.6 Precautions

Fluid absorption is more common during lengthy surgery and typically arises when a temporary increase occurs in surgical bleeding [25, 35]. As a precaution, an operating time of less than 1 h is recommended.

Keeping the fluid pressure low limits or even prevents intravascular, but not extravascular, absorption, which is a fact used in continuous-flow and low-pressure irrigation systems. The problem with continuous-flow systems is that the pressure might suddenly become high if a blood clot prevents free outflow from the bladder. Therefore, a low pressure and absence of fluid absorption may not be guaranteed at all times.

Smoking is a patient factor that has been associated with greater absorption [19] (Fig. 22.1b). The reason is unclear but could possibly be related to hypertrophy of the prostatic veins.

Lowering the fluid bag to 60 cm above the operating table has been used to control absorption since the 1970s. The effectiveness of this precaution depends on which fluid pressure the surgeon is accustomed to using. This pressure is usually much lower than the one allowed by the height of the fluid bag.

Several surgical techniques have been developed to replace TURP and TCRE, often with the outspoken goal of limiting fluid absorption. One such technique is vaporization. Although the alternatives may reduce absorption, they have not abolished this complication [36].

22.7 Treatment

Hypertension and difficulties in breathing during surgery should only be treated by lowering the legs from the stirrups, since these problems are most likely transient. Within 10–15 min after the end of surgery, the typical scene is that of bradycardia and arterial hypotension [15]. Treatment consists of a bolus of colloid fluid and, if insufficient, in infusion of a vasopressor. Intravenous calcium is also warranted, due to the dilution effect of the absorbed fluid.

An infusion of 100 mL of hypertonic saline (3–7.5%) should be initiated. Hypertonic saline might cause demyelination if given rapidly in chronic hyponatremia, while there is no evidence of this problem in acute hyponatremia [22, 41]. Therefore, giving the hypertonic fluid as a bolus infusion is not contraindicated. The saline withdraws fluid from the cells, increases the blood volume, and restores urinary excretion [42]. Correction of plasma sodium should stop when the concentration reaches 130 mmol/L.

In addition, only supportive means are indicated, such as antiemetics in case of nausea and mechanical ventilation if the patient becomes unconscious.

With no other evidence than logic, urological textbooks often recommend furosemide as the only treatment. The hyponatremia is assumed to be due to dilution alone, which is not true, and the blood volume is assumed to be increased, which is only the case during the actual period of absorption. Therefore, diuretics should be avoided in the initial phase. Early treatment with furosemide aggravates the hypotension [43], which is probably due to the osmotic diuresis, which is accompanied by marked loss of sodium ions, as well as the intracellular uptake of water. Hence, the body has a high content of water but the water is allocated to the wrong compartment. The content of extracellular electrolytes is reduced and, therefore, the plasma volume is on the low side. Hence, diuretics should be postponed until the hemodynamic situation is stable and treatment with hypertonic saline has been initiated.

The optimal treatment of overload with electrolyte-containing irrigating fluid is still poorly understood but should rely on alleviating the circulatory strain with diuretics and perhaps with a vasodilator. The latter type of drug should not be used when the absorbed irrigating fluid is devoid of electrolytes.

22.8 Conclusion

The risk of fluid absorption is an inherent danger in endoscopic surgeries where electrocutting is performed. More than 1 L of fluid presents a risk of causing symptoms and >3 L causes a more severe clinical picture (the TUR syndrome). Electrolyte-free irrigating fluids, which are used with monopolar electrocutting, cause a brisk osmotic diuresis and also enter the cells, thereby causing paradoxical hypovolemia with arterial hypotension that might be life-threatening. Treatment with a vasopressor and plasma volume expansion is more crucial than treatment with diuretics, which may be used only in the presence of stable hemodynamics. The second treatment consists of hypertonic saline, which does not need to be given slowly, to combat cerebral edema.

Absorption of the saline used with bipolar electrocutting is difficult to confirm since hyponatremia does not develop. The TUR syndrome is then less severe. Symptoms are limited to cardiovascular overload, but the cytoarchitecture of the heart and other organs might still be damaged due to distention by absorbed fluid.

References

1. Creevy CD. Hemolytic reactions during transurethral prostatic resection. J Urol. 1947;58:125–31.
2. Harrison RH, Boren JS, Robison JR. Dilutional hyponatremic shock: another concept of the transurethral prostatic resection reaction. J Urol. 1956;75:95–110.
3. Olsson J, Nilsson A, Hahn RG. Symptoms of the transurethral resection syndrome using glycine as the irrigant. J Urol. 1995;154:123–8.
4. Conger KB, Karafin L. A study of irrigating medium extravasation during transurethral surgery. J Urol. 1957;78:633–43.
5. Istre O, Skajaa K, Schoensbye A, Forman A. Changes in serum electrolytes after transcervical resection of the endometrium and submucous fibroids with the use of glycine 1.5% for uterine irrigation. Obstet Gynecol. 1992;80:218–22.
6. McSwiney M, Myatt J, Hargreaves M. Transcervical endometrial resection syndrome. Anaesthesia. 1995;50:254–8.
7. Olsson J, Hahn RG. Ethanol monitoring of irrigating fluid absorption in transcervical resection of the endometrium. Acta Anaesthesiol Scand. 1995;39:252–8.
8. Hermanns T, Fankhauser CD, Hefermehl LJ, et al. Prospective evaluation of irrigating fluid absorption during pure transurethral bipolar plasma vaporisation of the prostate using expired-breath ethanol measurements. BJU Int. 2013;112:647–54.
9. Sellevold O, Breivik H, Tveter K. Changes in oncotic pressure, osmolality and electrolytes following transurethral resection of the prostate using glycine as irrigating solution. Scand J Urol Nephrol. 1983;17:31–6.
10. Charlton AJ. Cardiac arrest during transurethral prostatectomy after absorption of 1.5% glycine. Anaesthesia. 1980;35:804–6.
11. Vijayan S. TURP syndrome. Trends Anaesth Crit Care. 2011;1:46–50.

12. Hahn RG, Sandfeldt L, Nyman CR. Double-blind randomized study of symptoms associated with absorption of glycine 1.5% or mannitol 3% during transurethral resection of the prostate. J Urol. 1998;160:397–401.
13. Inman RD, Hussain Z, Elves AWS, Hallworth MJ, Jones PW, Coppinger SWV. A comparison of 1.5% glycine and 2.7% sorbitol-0.5% mannitol irrigants during transurethral prostate resection. J Urol. 2001;166:2216–20.
14. Mizutani AR, Parker J, Katz J, Schmidt J. Visual disturbances, serum glycine levels and transurethral resection of the prostate. J Urol. 1990;144:697–9.
15. Hahn RG. Hallucination and visual disturbances during transurethral prostatic resection. Intensive Care Med. 1988;14:668–71.
16. Hahn R, Andersson T, Sikk M. Eye symptoms, visual evoked potentials and EEG during intravenous infusion of glycine. Acta Anaesthesiol Scand. 1995;39:214–9.
17. Johansson J, Lindahl M, Gyllencreutz E, Hahn RG. Symptomatic absorption of isotonic saline during transcervical endometrial resection. Acta Anaesthesiol Scand. 2017;61:121–4.
18. Hahn RG. Ethanol monitoring of irrigating fluid absorption (review). Eur J Anaesth. 1996;13:102–15.
19. Hahn RG. Smoking increases the risk of large-scale fluid absorption during transurethral prostatic resection. J Urol. 2001;166:162–5.
20. Istre O, Bjoennes J, Naess R, Hornbaek K, Forman A. Postoperative cerebral oedema after transcervical endometrial resection and uterine irrigation with 1.5% glycine. Lancet. 1994;344:1187–9.
21. Arieff AI, Guisado R. Effects on the central nervous system of hypernatremic and hyponatremic states. Kidney Int. 1976;10:104–16.
22. Ayus JC, Krothapalli RK, Arieff AI. Treatment of symptomatic hyponatraemia and its relation to brain damage. N Engl J Med. 1987;317:1190–5.
23. Hoekstra PT, Kahnoski R, McCamish MA, Bergen W, Heetderks DR. Transurethral prostatic resection syndrome—a new perspective: encephalopathy with associated hyperammonaemia. J Urol. 1983;130:704–7.
24. Hahn RG, Stalberg HP, Gustafsson SA. Intravenous infusion of irrigating fluids containing glycine or mannitol with and without ethanol. J Urol. 1989;142:1102–5.
25. Hahn R, Berlin T, Lewenhaupt A. Irrigating fluid absorption and blood loss during transurethral resection of the prostate studied by a regular interval monitoring (RIM) method. Scand J Urol Nephrol. 1988;22:23–30.
26. Hahn RG. Natriuresis and "dilutional" hyponatremia after infusion of glycine 1.5%. J Clin Anesth. 2001;13:167–74.
27. Hahn RG, Gebäck T. Fluid volume kinetics of dilutional hyponatremia; a shock syndrome revisited. Clinics. 2014;69:120–7.
28. Woodcock TE, Woodcock TM. Revised Starling equation and the glycocalyx model of transvascular fluid exchange: an improved paradigm for prescribing intravenous fluid therapy. Br J Anaesth. 2012;108:384–94.
29. Hahn RG, Olsson J, Sótonyi P, Rajs J. Rupture of the myocardial histoskeleton and its relation to sudden death after overhydration with glycine 1.5% in the mouse. APMIS. 2000;108:487–95.
30. Arieff AI, Ayus JC. Endometrial ablation complicated by fatal hyponatremic encephalopathy. JAMA. 1993;270:1230–2.
31. Baggish MS, Brill AIO, Rosenweig B, Barbot JE, Indman PD. Fatal acute glycine and sorbitol toxicity during operative hysteroscopy. J Gynecol Surg. 1993;9:137–43.
32. Byard RW, Harrison R, Wells R, Gilbert JD. Glycine toxicity and unexpected intra-operative death. J Forensic Sci. 2001;46:1244–6.
33. Ichai C, Cialis JF, Roussel LJ, et al. Intravascular absorption of glycine irrigating solution during shoulder arthroscopy: a case report and follow-up study. Anesthesiology. 1996;85:1481–5.
34. Radal M, Jonville Bera AP, Leisner C, Haillot O, Autret-Leca E. [Adverse effects of glycolic irrigation solutions]. Therapie. 1999;54:233–6.
35. Hahn RG, Ekengren J. Patterns of irrigating fluid absorption during transurethral resection of the prostate as indicated by ethanol. J Urol. 1993;149:502–6.

36. Hermanns T, Grossman NC, Wettstein MS, et al. Absorption of irrigating fluid occurs frequently during high power 532 nm laser vaporization of the prostate. J Urol. 2015;193:211–6.
37. Ran L, He W, Zhu Z, Zhou Q, Gou X. Comparison of fluid absorption between transurethral enucleation and transurethral resection for benign prostate hyperplasia. Urol Int. 2013;91:26–30.
38. Ayus JC, Wheeler JM, Arieff AI. Postoperative hyponatremic encephalopathy in menstruant women. Ann Intern Med. 1992;117:891–7.
39. Okeke AA, Lodge R, Hinchliffe A, Walker A, Dickerson D, Gillatt DA. Ethanol-glycine irrigating fluid for transurethral resection of the prostate in practice. BJU Int. 2000;86:43–6.
40. Hahn RG, Larsson H, Ribbe T. Continuous monitoring of fluid absorption in transurethral surgery. Anaesthesia. 1995;50:327–31.
41. Bernstein GT, Loughlin KR, Gittes RF. The physiologic basis of the TUR syndrome. J Surg Res. 1989;46:135–41.
42. Hahn RG, Nilsson A, Hjelmqvist H, Zhang W, Rundgren M. Renal function during intravenous infusion of irrigating fluids in the sheep. Acta Anaesthesiol Scand. 1996;40:671–8.
43. Crowley K, Clarkson K, Hannon V, McShane A, Kelly DG. Diuretics after transurethral prostatectomy: a double-blind controlled trial comparing frusemide and mannitol. Br J Anaesth. 1990;65:337–441.

Relationship Between Central Venous Pressure and Acute Kidney Injury in Critically Ill Patients

23

P. M. Honoré, C. Pierrakos, and H. D. Spapen

23.1 Introduction

Central venous pressure (CVP) is the blood pressure within the vena cava relative to atmospheric pressure. The CVP is determined by the interaction between cardiac function and venous return, which in turn are influenced by total blood volume, vascular tone, cardiac output, right ventricular compliance and intrathoracic, abdominal, and pericardial pressures [1]. When correctly measured, CVP reflects right atrial pressure and volume status of the right and, to a lesser extent, the left ventricle [2]. In critically ill patients, CVP is used to assess cardiac preload and volume status and to assist in the diagnosis of right- and left-sided heart failure.

Adequate fluid loading is the first-line therapy for managing hypotension and shock. Expanding intravascular volume will increase stroke volume and cardiac output. The endpoint of fluid therapy in shock is to improve and optimize tissue perfusion. Measuring CVP is still considered to be useful for guiding fluid resuscitation in critically ill patients, especially when followed over time and in combination with cardiac output recording [3]. However, many studies have reported that dynamic measurements (e.g., passive leg raising, pulse pressure [PPV] and stroke volume [SVV] variation) better predict the effect of volume substitution than static CVP measurements [4].

Fluid administration is also imperative for preventing acute kidney injury (AKI) associated with circulatory failure. Maintaining a correct mean arterial pressure (MAP) has long been regarded as the primary goal in preventing AKI, especially in vasopressor-dependent patients. However, MAP does not reflect changes in renal

P. M. Honoré (✉) · C. Pierrakos
Department of Intensive Care, Centre Hospitalier Universitaire Brugmann, Brussels, Belgium
e-mail: Patrick.Honore@CHU-Brugmann.be

H. D. Spapen
Ageing & Pathology Research Group, Vrije Universiteit Brussel,
Brussels, Belgium

J.-L. Vincent (ed.), *Annual Update in Intensive Care and Emergency Medicine 2019*, Annual Update in Intensive Care and Emergency Medicine,
https://doi.org/10.1007/978-3-030-06067-1_23

hemodynamics that determine renal perfusion. Low diastolic arterial pressure, decreased mean perfusion pressure, and high CVP were associated with AKI in septic and post-cardiac surgery patients whereas a MAP deficit was not [5, 6].

Aggressive fluid resuscitation does not necessarily protect the kidney but may augment the risk of AKI by elevating the CVP. de Jong et al. first proposed the terms "glomerular pre- and afterload" [7] after showing that an increase in afferent arteriolar resistance diminished the transmission of MAP into the glomerular capillaries thereby decreasing glomerular capillary pressure by preload reduction. Ostermann et al. recently demonstrated that a low mean perfusion pressure, calculated as the difference between MAP and CVP, was independently associated with progression to AKI stage III [8]. Hence, keeping CVP low will beneficially influence the renal perfusion pressure gradient. A detailed discussion on the pathophysiological rationale of 'congestive kidney failure' is beyond the scope of this review. It is important to realize that volume (CVP!) has priority over arterial blood pressure in the autonomic regulation of cardiovascular and renal interaction [9].

This chapter will highlight the relationship between CVP and AKI in different disease states.

23.2 Sepsis and Septic Shock

Sepsis is the most common cause of AKI in critically ill patients. AKI occurs in almost half of patients with septic shock. For a long time, sepsis-induced AKI was thought to be a disease of the renal macrocirculation resulting from a decrease in renal blood flow, cellular damage and acute tubular necrosis [10]. Treatment aiming to prevent or reverse septic AKI therefore primarily focused on improving circulation, perfusion and oxygen delivery. This was accentuated by the Surviving Sepsis Campaign guidelines, which recommended early fluid administration targeting a CVP of 8–12 mmHg (12–15 mmHg in mechanically ventilated patients) to restore tissue perfusion in septic shock [11]. Yet, septic AKI can occur in the absence of hypoperfusion [12].

Legrand et al. retrospectively observed a strong association between CVP values and the risk of developing new or persistent AKI in 137 septic patients [13]. This association remained significant after adjustment for fluid balance and positive end-expiratory pressure (PEEP) levels. In patients with septic shock and AKI, Wong et al. reported a substantial deficit in mean renal perfusion pressure. Patients with a greater pressure deficit had higher AKI severity. Only CVP was independently associated with AKI progression and worsening [3]. In 124 septic patients, a high CVP and renal resistive index and a low diastolic perfusion pressure at admission were independent risk factors for sepsis-induced AKI [14]. Elevated CVP is also associated with increased mortality in pediatric patients with septic shock. Mortality risk increased more than twofold in patients with CVP >12 mmHg compared to those with minimally elevated CVP [15].

These studies underscore a crucial role for venous congestion and diastolic perfusion in the development of septic AKI. Preserving kidney function during sepsis and septic shock highly depends on improvement of renal perfusion pressure. However, fluid overload propagates CVP elevation with lowering of diastolic perfusion pressure resulting in diastolic flow reduction. CVP-targeted fluid resuscitation in septic shock might thus seriously compromise renal function. This concept is supported by recent trials reporting an association between fluid overload and mortality in critically ill patients with AKI or septic shock [16, 17]. From a therapeutic viewpoint, it is apparent that aggressive fluid resuscitation and subsequent venous congestion should be avoided. Fluid responsiveness should be evaluated better. This could be accomplished by using dynamic markers instead of empirically defined static measurements for guiding volume loading [18]. In addition, care must be taken to mobilize and evacuate excess fluid after successful resuscitation. Different strategies can be used to achieve a negative fluid balance and/or to reduce renal damage due to ongoing venous congestion (furosemide plus albumin, continuous renal replacement therapy [CRRT], hypertonic saline, ...). Randomized controlled trials are definitely needed to better determine individualized fluid needs by comparing the various methods for assessing fluid responsiveness and to evaluate the effect of de-resuscitation therapy on kidney function.

23.3 Left Heart Failure

Renal impairment is common and acts as an independent predictor of mortality in patients with acute or chronic heart failure. The term ‘cardiorenal syndrome’ is often used to describe worsening renal function despite intensive heart failure therapy. The pathophysiology of cardiorenal syndrome is complex [19]. Acute cardiorenal syndrome is characterized by acute heart failure leading to AKI. Although non-hemodynamic pathways are involved (activation of sympathetic and renin angiotensin-aldosterone system, inflammation, oxidative stress, intravascular volume depletion secondary to overzealous use of diuretics), hemodynamic mechanisms play a preponderant role by inducing a decrease in renal arterial flow and a fall in glomerular filtration rate (GFR). Patients typically present with increased systemic and/or pulmonary congestion. Chronic cardiorenal syndrome is characterized by chronic abnormalities in cardiac function leading to AKI. Neuro-hormonal activation, renal hypoperfusion, inflammation, underlying atherosclerosis and oxidative stress play an important pathophysiological role in chronic cardiorenal syndrome. In addition, high CVPs directly affect renal vein pressure and renal perfusion pressure and increase interstitial pressure causing tubular collapse. Along with increased renal venous pressure, proportional declines in GFR and in absolute and fractional sodium excretion are observed [20]. In the most severe stages of chronic cardiorenal syndrome, GFR becomes flow-dependent.

Worsening renal function is frequently observed in patients with advanced decompensated heart failure receiving intensive medical therapy. The strongest hemodynamic determinant of worsening renal function is venous congestion identified by elevated CVP. Worsening renal function occurs less frequently in patients who display a CVP <8 mmHg. Baseline CVP values >16 or >24 mmHg were associated with, respectively, a 60% and 75% increase in the incidence of worsening renal function [21].

Uthoff et al. measured CVP non-invasively using compression sonography in a large patient cohort admitted for acute heart failure [22]. They found that a low systolic blood pressure and a high CVP at presentation and discharge were significantly associated with lower GFR. However, in patients with normal to high systolic blood pressure, CVP had no effect on GFR.

Taken together, these data suggest that venous congestion, rather than reduced cardiac output, may be the primary hemodynamic factor driving worsening renal function in patients with acute and chronic heart failure.

23.4 Cardiac Surgery

According to the chosen definition, the incidence of AKI in cardiac surgery patients ranges from 5% to 20% [23]. Even after adjustment for comorbidities and procedural complications, AKI contributes significantly to morbidity and mortality [24]. Therapies aimed at mitigating preoperative anemia, peroperative hemodilution, perioperative red blood cell transfusions and surgical re-exploration may offer protection against AKI in cardiac surgery patients [25]. Controversy exists about the relationship between cardiopulmonary bypass (CPB) and postsurgical renal dysfunction. Off-pump revascularization surgery is associated with more intraoperative hemodynamic instability due to ventricular compression during cardiac manipulation [26] but also with reduced hospital morbidity and AKI occurrence in patients with preoperative non-dialysis-dependent renal insufficiency [27]. A twofold increase in the risk of AKI was noted in the cardiac surgery population as a whole when postoperative CVP values reached the threshold of 14 mmHg. A higher incidence of AKI was observed in conditions hallmarked by venous hypertension (e.g., tricuspid disease). The effect of CVP on renal function was found to be modulated by ventricular function class, etiology and acuity of venous congestion [28]. In a multi-institutional cohort of high-risk patients undergoing coronary bypass surgery, CVP measured at 6 h after surgery was, independently of cardiac index and other important clinical variables, associated with postoperative mortality and AKI [29]. Thus, acute and postoperative increases in CVP should be actively treated to avoid AKI in cardiac surgery patients, particularly in patients with poor ventricular function.

23.5 Myocardial Infarction

An early study by Collins et al. showed that CVP was raised above the normal range in 84% of patients admitted with acute myocardial infarction. Almost all had clinical and radiographic evidence of left heart failure. Raised mean CVP was associated with dysrhythmias and, if greater than 15 mmHg, with a fatal outcome [30]. Moderate or severe CVP elevation was also observed in a large proportion of ST segment elevation myocardial infarction (STEMI) patients without physical signs of left heart failure [31]. Khoury et al. evaluated 1336 STEMI patients who underwent primary percutaneous coronary intervention. Patients were stratified according to left ventricular ejection fraction (LVEF) and CVP. Variables associated with AKI included a LVEF ≤45%, time to reperfusion, mechanical ventilation and chronic kidney disease. Notably, a CVP ≥8 mmHg was associated with AKI irrespective of LVEF. Patients with a LVEF ≤45% and a CVP ≥8 mmHg had a tenfold increase in the incidence of AKI compared to patients with LVEF >45% and normal CVP [32]. As a consequence, any fluid challenge during angiographic reperfusion (e.g., before administration of intravenous contrast) may be inappropriate as a CVP increase might augment the risk of AKI.

23.6 Right Heart Failure

Systemic venous congestion caused by hypervolemia and right heart failure is particularly detrimental for renal function. Treatment of right heart dysfunction should not be based on inadvertent fluid loading but strive to decrease right ventricular afterload by lowering pulmonary vascular resistance while increasing ventricular inotropy [28].

23.7 Acute Respiratory Distress Syndrome

Darmon et al. analyzed 8029 patients, of whom 1879 were diagnosed with ARDS. AKI occurred in 31.3% of patients and was more common in patients with than those without ARDS (44.3% vs. 27.4%; $p < 0.001$). AKI doubled mortality in patients with ARDS [33]. The relationships between MAP, CVP and renal perfusion pressure in ARDS are complex and poorly studied. Levitt et al. showed that CVP values >15 mmHg were associated with a higher incidence of AKI only when renal perfusion pressure was <60 mmHg. A MAP target >60 mmHg did not minimize the risk of AKI in patients with elevated CVP and low renal perfusion pressure [34]. Thus, CVP at values seen in ARDS affects the risk of AKI by lowering renal perfusion pressure rather than by venous congestion.

23.8 Conclusion

The pathophysiology of AKI is multifactorial. Within a context of comorbidity and type, severity, or acuteness of disease, AKI is determined by impaired renal perfusion, inflammation, endothelial dysfunction, cellular damage and neurohormonal activation.

In a broad spectrum of patients with and without reduced cardiac function, a significant association between increased CVP and impaired renal function has been recognized. Increasing evidence points to a close relationship between venous congestion, as estimated by CVP, and AKI. Elevated CVP is independently correlated with prolonged treatment and poor outcome in critical care settings [35, 36]. We have summarized the most important findings in Table 23.1.

While awaiting more robust data, it is essential to recognize patients at risk of developing AKI. Maintaining diastolic arterial pressure and selectively lowering

Table 23.1 Summary of some of the important studies looking at central venous pressure (CVP) and acute kidney injury (AKI) under various conditions

	First author, year [ref]	Design, number of patients	Results	Conclusions	Limitations
Sepsis, septic shock	Song, 2018 [14]	Prospective cohort study, n = 124	A high CVP and renal resistive index and a low diastolic perfusion pressure at admission were independent risk factors for sepsis-induced AKI	The combination of renal resistive index and CVP was more valuable than either of the two parameters alone	Limited design, number of patients
Left ventricular failure	Mullens, 2009 [21]	Prospective cohort study, n = 145	Baseline CVP values >16 or >24 mmHg were associated with, respectively, a 60% and 75% increase in the incidence of worsening renal function	Taken together, these data suggest that venous congestion, rather than reduced cardiac output, may be the primary hemodynamic factor driving worsening renal function in patients with acute and chronic heart failure	Limited design, number of patients
Cardiac surgery	Williams, 2014 [29]	Observational cohort study, n = 2390	CVP at 6 h after CABG surgery was highly predictive of operative mortality or renal failure, independent of cardiac index and other important clinical variables	Future studies will need to assess whether interventions guided by postoperative CVP can improve patient outcomes	Observational design

Table 23.1 (continued)

	First author, year [ref]	Design, number of patients	Results	Conclusions	Limitations
Myocardial infarction	Khoury, 2018 [32]	Retrospective study, n = 1336	A CVP ≥8 mmHg was associated with AKI irrespective of LVEF	Patients with a LVEF ≤45% and a CVP ≥8 mmHg had a tenfold increase in the incidence of AKI compared to patients with LVEF >45% and normal CVP	Retrospective design
Right ventricular failure	Gambardella, 2016 [28]	Observational, subgroup analysis	Systemic venous congestion caused by hypervolemia and right heart failure is particularly detrimental for renal function	Treatment of right heart dysfunction should not be based on inadvertent fluid loading but strive to decrease right ventricle afterload by lowering pulmonary vascular resistance while increasing ventricular inotropy	Observational design, subgroup analysis
Acute respiratory distress syndrome	Levitt, 2015 [34]	Observational, substudy of ARDSNet-FACTT	CVP values >15 mmHg were associated with a higher incidence of AKI only when renal perfusion pressure was <60 mmHg. A MAP target >60 mmHg did not minimize the risk of AKI in patients with elevated CVP and low renal perfusion pressure	Thus, CVP at values seen in ARDS affects the risk of AKI through lowering renal perfusion pressure rather than by venous congestion	Observational design, only published in abstract form, substudy

CABG coronary artery bypass graft, *LVEF* left ventricular ejection fraction, *MAP* mean arterial pressure

CVP may reduce symptoms and signs of renal congestion, ameliorate GFR and improve prognosis in septic, cardiac and surgical patients. This also implies closer and probably more dynamic monitoring of volume resuscitation.

References

1. Gelman S. Venous function and central venous pressure: a physiologic story. Anesthesiology. 2008;108:735–48.
2. Magder S. Right atrial pressure in the critically ill: how to measure, what is the value, what are the limitations? Chest. 2017;151:908–16.
3. De Backer D, Vincent JL. Should we measure the central venous pressure to guide fluid management? Ten answers to 10 questions. Crit Care. 2018;22:43.
4. Monnet X, Marik PE, Teboul JL. Prediction of fluid responsiveness: an update. Ann Intensive Care. 2016;6:111.
5. Saito S, Uchino S, Takinami M, Uezono S, Bellomo R. Postoperative blood pressure deficit and acute kidney injury progression in vasopressor-dependent cardiovascular surgery patients. Crit Care. 2016;20:74.
6. Wong BT, Chan MJ, Glassford NJ, et al. Mean arterial pressure and mean perfusion pressure deficit in septic acute kidney injury. J Crit Care. 2015;30:975–81.
7. de Jong PE, Anderson S, de Zeeuw D. Glomerular preload and afterload reduction as a tool to lower urinary protein leakage: will such treatments also help to improve renal function outcome? J Am Soc Nephrol. 1993;3:1333–41.
8. Ostermann M, Hall A, Crichton S. Low mean perfusion pressure is a risk factor for progression of acute kidney injury in critically ill patients—a retrospective analysis. BMC Nephrol. 2017;18:151.
9. Charkoudian N, Martin EA, Dinenno FA, Eisenach JH, Dietz NM, Joyner MJ. Influence of increased central venous pressure on baroreflex control of sympathetic activity in humans. Am J Physiol Heart Circ Physiol. 2004;287:1658–62.
10. Zarbock A, Gomez H, Kellum JA. Sepsis-induced acute kidney injury revisited: pathophysiology, prevention and future therapies. Curr Opin Crit Care. 2014;20:588–95.
11. Dellinger RP, Levy MM, Rhodes A, et al. Surviving Sepsis Campaign Guidelines Committee including the Pediatric Subgroup. Surviving sepsis campaign: international guidelines for management of severe sepsis and septic shock: 2012. Crit Care Med. 2013;41:580–637.
12. Gomez H, Ince C, De Backer D, et al. A unified theory of sepsis-induced acute kidney injury: inflammation, microcirculatory dysfunction, bioenergetics, and the tubular cell adaptation to injury. Shock. 2014;41:3–11.
13. Legrand M, Dupuis C, Simon C, et al. Association between systemic hemodynamics and septic acute kidney injury in critically ill patients: a retrospective observational study. Crit Care. 2013;17:R278.
14. Song J, Wu W, He Y, Lin S, Zhu D, Zhong M. Value of the combination of renal resistance index and central venous pressure in the early prediction of sepsis-induced acute kidney injury. J Crit Care. 2018;45:204–8.
15. Choi SJ, Ha EJ, Jhang WK, Park SJ. Elevated central venous pressure is associated with increased mortality in pediatric septic shock patients. BMC Pediatr. 2018;18:58.
16. Payen D, de Pont AC, Sakr Y, Spies C, Reinhart K, Vincent JL. Sepsis Occurrence in Acutely Ill Patients (SOAP) Investigators: a positive fluid balance is associated with a worse outcome in patients with acute renal failure. Crit Care. 2008;12:R74.
17. Boyd JH, Forbes J, Nakada T, Walley KR, Russell JA. Fluid resuscitation in septic shock: a positive fluid balance and elevated central venous pressure are associated with increased mortality. Crit Care Med. 2011;39:259–65.

18. Honore PM, Spapen HD. Passive leg raising test with minimally invasive monitoring: the way forward for guiding septic shock resuscitation? J Intensive Care. 2017;5:36.
19. Di Lullo L, Bellasi A, Barbera V, et al. Pathophysiology of the cardio-renal syndromes types 1–5: an uptodate. Indian Heart J. 2017;69:255–65.
20. Firth JF, Raine AE, Ledingham JG. Raised venous pressure: a direct cause of renal sodium retention in edema. Lancet. 1988;1:1033–5.
21. Mullens W, Abrahams Z, Francis GS, et al. Importance of venous congestion for worsening of renal function in advanced decompensated heart failure. J Am Coll Cardiol. 2009;53:589–96.
22. Uthoff H, Breidthardt T, Klima T, et al. Central venous pressure and impaired renal function in patients with acute heart failure. Eur J Heart Fail. 2011;13:432–9.
23. Mangano CM, Diamondstone LS, Ramsay JG, et al. Renal dysfunction after myocardial revascularization: risk factors, adverse outcomes, and hospital resource utilization. The Multicenter Study of Perioperative Ischemia Research Group. Ann Intern Med. 1998;128:194–203.
24. Chertow GM, Levy EM, Hammermeister KE, et al. Independent association between acute renal failure and mortality following cardiac surgery. Am J Med. 1998;104:343–8.
25. Karkouti K, Wijeysundera DN, Yau TM, et al. Acute kidney injury after cardiac surgery: focus on modifiable risk factors. Circulation. 2009;119:495–502.
26. Beauford RB, Saunders CR, Niemeier LA, et al. Is off-pump revascularization better for patients with non-dialysis-dependent renal insufficiency? Heart Surg Forum. 2004;7:E141–6.
27. Ascione R, Nason G, Al-Ruzzeh S, et al. Coronary revascularization with or without cardiopulmonary bypass in patients with preoperative nondialysis-dependent renal insufficiency. Ann Thorac Surg. 2001;72:2020–5.
28. Gambardella I, Gaudino M, Ronco C, Lau C, Ivascu N, Girardi LN. Congestive kidney failure in cardiac surgery: the relationship between central venous pressure and acute kidney injury. Interact Cardiovasc Thorac Surg. 2016;23:800–5.
29. Williams JB, Peterson ED, Wojdyla D, et al. Central venous pressure after coronary artery bypass surgery: does it predict postoperative mortality or renal failure? J Crit Care. 2014;29:1006–10.
30. Collins JV, Clark TJ, Evans TR, Riaz MA. Central venous pressure in acute myocardial infarction. Lancet. 1971;1:373–5.
31. Bergstra A, Svilaas T, van Veldhuisen DJ, van den Heuvel AF, van der Horst IC, Zijlstra F. Haemodynamic patterns in ST-elevation myocardial infarction: incidence and correlates of elevated filling pressures. Neth Heart J. 2007;15:95–9.
32. Khoury S, Steinvil A, Gal-Oz A, et al. Association between central venous pressure as assessed by echocardiography, left ventricular function and acute cardio-renal syndrome in patients with ST segment elevation myocardial infarction. Clin Res Cardiol. 2018 May 9. https://doi.org/10.1007/s00392-018-1266-7. [Epub ahead of print].
33. Darmon M, Clec'h C, Adrie C, et al. Acute respiratory distress syndrome and risk of AKI among critically ill patients. Clin J Am Soc Nephrol. 2014;9:1347–53.
34. Levitt JE, Lin PY, Liu K, Goldstein BA, Truvit JP. Increased central venous pressure reduces renal perfusion pressure and increases risk of acute kidney injury in patients with acute respiratory distress syndrome. Am J Respir Crit Care Med. 2015;191:A3993 (Abst).
35. Li DK, Wang XT, Liu DW. Association between elevated central venous pressure and outcomes in critically ill patients. Ann Intensive Care. 2017;7:83.
36. Chen X, Wang X, Honore PM, Spapen HD, Liu D. Renal failure in critically ill patients, beware of applying (central venous) pressure on the kidney. Ann Intensive Care. 2018;8:91.

Fluid Management in Acute Kidney Injury

24

M. Ostermann, A. More, and S. Jog

24.1 Introduction

Acute kidney injury (AKI) is very common during critical illness affecting >50% of patients and associated with increased morbidity and mortality and high health care costs [1]. The traditional strategy for managing patients at risk or with established AKI often involves high volume fluid administration due to fear of untreated hypovolemia [2]. Whilst timely fluid administration may be beneficial if AKI is indeed precipitated by intravascular volume depletion, there is increasing evidence that excessive fluid resuscitation beyond correction of hypovolemia leads to adverse outcomes, including worsening of renal function [3–6]. Furthermore, there is clear evidence that certain types of fluids are nephrotoxic [3, 6–9].

In this chapter, we discuss different aspects of fluid management for the prevention and treatment of AKI, challenge some of the traditional beliefs and highlight existing uncertainties.

M. Ostermann (✉)
Department of Critical Care, King's College London, Guy's & St Thomas' Hospital, London, UK
e-mail: Marlies.Ostermann@gstt.nhs.uk

A. More
Division of Critical Care, Christian Medical College Hospital, Vellore, India

S. Jog
Department of Critical Care, Deenanath Mangeshkar Hospital and Research Center, Pune, India

J.-L. Vincent (ed.), *Annual Update in Intensive Care and Emergency Medicine 2019*, Annual Update in Intensive Care and Emergency Medicine,
https://doi.org/10.1007/978-3-030-06067-1_24

24.2 Aims of Fluid Resuscitation

The physiological rationale for fluid administration in AKI is to correct intravascular volume depletion and to increase cardiac output and perfusion pressure in the hope that this will improve renal blood flow and glomerular function. However, in established AKI, renal blood flow and glomerular filtration correlate poorly [5]. In fact, fluids aimed at increasing renal blood flow may not affect glomerular filtration rate, especially if cardiac output is increased. In AKI, the only indication for fluid administration is intravascular hypovolemia. Oliguria should trigger an assessment of volume status but not be viewed as an absolute indication for fluid administration.

24.3 Types of Fluid

Broadly, fluids are differentiated as crystalloids and colloids (Tables 24.1 and 24.2). Independent of the impact of fluid overload, there is clear evidence that renal function is affected by the type of fluid and that certain fluids increase the risk of AKI [3, 6–9].

24.3.1 Colloids

Colloids are crystalloid solutions containing oncotic macromolecules that largely remain in the intravascular space (Table 24.2). The physiological basis for using them is that they preserve intravascular oncotic pressure and expand the intravascular volume more effectively for a longer duration compared to crystalloids. However, recent data indicate that their fluid sparing effect is only modest in the range of 1.0:1.1–1.0:1.4 [6]. Furthermore, some types of colloids have been found to be nephrotoxic, in particular hydroxyethyl starches (HES). Several large randomized controlled trials (RCTs) and systematic reviews showed increased rates of AKI and use of renal replacement therapy (RRT) with HES in critically ill patients [7–9].

There are only limited data on the benefits and risks of gelatin-based colloids in AKI. Observational data suggest that the administration of gelatin contributes to the development of osmotic nephrosis-induced AKI in critically ill patients [10]. A systematic review including three trials of a total of 212 patients randomized to gelatin versus crystalloid/albumin concluded that the risk ratio for AKI was 1.35 (0.58–3.14) [11]. Although it remains unclear whether gelatin-based colloids can cause AKI or not, given the potential risks and the absence of clear benefits, gelatin-based fluids should be avoided in AKI.

Albumin is a natural colloid. When used for resuscitation, either as a 4%, 5% or 20% solution, albumin has not been shown to have a consistent survival benefit compared to crystalloids [12–14]. A recent network meta-analysis found no difference in the use of RRT with albumin versus crystalloid solutions in patients with sepsis [15]. Whilst albumin is considered safe in patients at risk of or with

Table 24.1 Composition of commonly used crystalloids compared with plasma

Parameter	Plasma	NaCl 0.9%	NaCl 0.18%/ glucose 4%	NaCl 0.45%/ glucose 4%	Glucose 5%	Hartmann's solution	Ringer's lactate	Ringer's acetate	Plasma-Lyte	Sterofundin	Isolyte S	$NaHCO_3$ 1.26%	$NaHCO_3$ 1.4%	$NaHCO_3$ 8.4%
Na^+ (mmol/L)	135–145	154	31	77	–	131	130	130	140	145	141	150	167	1000
K^+ (mmol/L)	3.5–4.5	–	–	–	–	5	4	5	5	4	5	–	–	–
Cl^- (mmol/L)	95–105	154	31	77	–	111	109	112	98	127	98	–	–	–
HCO_3^- (mmol/L)	24–32	–	–	–	–	29 (as lactate)	28 (as lactate)	27 (as acetate)	(as acetate + gluconate)	(as acetate + malate)	(as acetate + gluconate)	150	167	1000
Lactate (mmol/L)	1	–	–	–	–	29	28	–	–	–	–	–	–	–
Acetate (mmol/L)	–	–	–	–	–	–	–	27	27	24	27	–	–	–
Gluconate (mmol/L)	–	–	–	–	–	–	–	–	23	–	23	–	–	–
Ca^{2+} (mmol/L)	2.2–2.6	–	–	–	–	2	1.5	1	–	2.5	–	–	–	–
Mg^{2+} (mmol/L)	0.8–1.2	–	–	–	–	–	–	1	1.5	1	3	–	–	–
Phosphate (mmol/L)	0.8–1.2	–	–	–	–	–	–	–	–	–	1	–	–	–
Glucose (mmol/L)	3.5–6.0	–	236	278	252	–	–	–	–	–	–	–	–	–
pH	7.35–7.45	5.5	3.5–5.5	3.5–6.5	3.5–5.5	5.0–7.0	6.0–7.5	6–8	4.0–6.5	5.1–5.9	6.3–7.3	7.0–8.5	7.0–8.5	7.0–8.5
Osmolarity (mosmol/L)	275–295	308	284	406	278	278	273	277	295	309	295	301	333	2000

Ca calcium, *Cl* chloride, *K* potassium, *Mg* magnesium, *Na* sodium

Table 24.2 Composition of commonly used colloids in comparison with plasma

Parameter	Plasma	Albumin 5%	Albumin 20%	Haemaccel	Gelofusine	Geloplasma	Dextran 40	Dextran 70 in NaCl	Tetraspan 6% HES130/0.42	Hetastarch 6% HES130/0.4	Hetastarch 6% HES670/0.75
Colloid source	–	Human donor	Human donor	Bovine gelatin	Bovine gelatin	Bovine gelatin	Sucrose	Sucrose	Potato starch	Maize starch	Maize starch
Na^+ (mmol/L)	135–145	148	130	145	154	150	154	154	140	154	143
K^+ (mmol/L)	3.5–4.5	–	–	5.1	–	5	–	–	4	–	3
Cl^- (mmol/L)	95–105	128	77	120	120	100	154	154	118	154	124
HCO_3^- (mmol/L)	24–32	–	–	–	–	30 (as lactate)	–	–	–	–	28 (as lactate)
Lactate (mmol/L)	1	–	–	–	–	30	–	–	–	–	28
Ca^{2+} (mmol/L)	2.2–2.6	–	–	6.25	–	–	–	–	2.5	–	2.5
Mg^{2+} (mmol/L)	0.8–1.2	–	–	–	–	1.5	–	–	1	–	0.45
Glucose (mmol/L)	3.5–6.0	–	–	–	–	–	–	–	–	–	5
Acetate (mmol/L)	–	–	–	–	–	–	–	–	24	–	–
Malate (mmol/L)	–	–	–	–	–	–	–	–	5	–	–
Octanoate (mmol/L)	–	8	16	–	–	–	–	–	–	–	–
pH	7.35–7.45	6.4–7.4	6.7–7.3	7.4	7.4	7.4	3.0–7.0	4.5–7.0	5.6–6.4	4.0–5.5	5.9
MW (kDa)	–	69	69	30	30	30	40	63–77	130	130	670
Osmolarity (mosmol/L)	275–295	309	130	274–300	274	273	308–310	310	297	286–308	307
Effective half-life	–	15 h	15 h	5 h	2.5 h	2.5 h	12–24 h	12–24 h	12 h	6–12 h	24–48 h

Ca calcium, *Cl* chloride, *HES* hydroxyethyl starch, *K* potassium, *Mg* magnesium, *MW* molecular weight

established AKI, a beneficial role has not been established [6, 12]. Possible exceptions are patients with hepatorenal syndrome where the combination of albumin with a vasopressor analogue has been shown to be renoprotective, and patients with serum albumin less than 40 g/L before undergoing off-pump coronary artery surgery, in whom the preoperative administration of 20% albumin reduced the risk of postoperative AKI [16].

In conclusion, there is no role for colloids for routine resuscitation in patients at risk of AKI. Current recommendations are to use crystalloids instead of colloids for fluid resuscitation in critically ill patients, including those at risk of or with established AKI [17, 18]. Colloids may be considered in limited quantities for early resuscitation in patients with profound and refractory shock who are fluid responsive and not responding to crystalloids, but HES should be avoided.

24.3.2 Crystalloids

0.9% saline solution is still the most commonly used crystalloid in critically ill patients. However, rapid administration of moderate to large volumes of 0.9% saline can cause hyperchloremia and metabolic acidosis. Animal research and studies in healthy volunteers suggest that this may lead to renal vasoconstriction and reduction in glomerular filtration [19–21].

The electrolyte composition of balanced solutions, such as Ringer's lactate, Hartmann's solution and Plasma-Lyte, is similar to human plasma and there is no association with hyperchloremic acidosis (Table 24.1) Although balanced fluids contain potassium in small quantities, this only poses a risk in patients with AKI and severe hyperkalemia.

Clinical trials comparing different types of crystalloid fluids in critically ill patients at risk of AKI have revealed conflicting results [22–26]. In the Saline versus Plasma-Lyte 148 for ICU fluid Therapy (SPLIT) trial, 2278 ICU patients were randomized to Plasma-Lyte 148 or 0.9% saline [25]. There was no significant difference in the proportion of patients with moderate to severe AKI. In contrast, the SALT-ED investigators performed a cluster-randomized multiple-cross over trial in 5 ICUs at a single center and randomized 15,802 patients to 0.9% saline versus balanced solution [26]. They showed a significant reduction in the risk of major adverse kidney events (need for RRT, death and/or final serum creatinine ≥200% of baseline) within 30 days in the group of patients treated with balanced solutions (14.3% versus 15.4%; $p = 0.04$).

It has been hypothesized that the risk of saline-induced AKI may be dose dependent and only be seen in patients receiving large volumes of 0.9% saline. However, a recent study in ICU patients receiving large volume fluid resuscitation (>60 mL/kg fluids per 24 h) showed no association between chloride load and risk of AKI after adjusting for severity of illness [27].

Based on the current evidence, it is reasonable to preferably use balanced solutions for fluid resuscitation in patients at risk of AKI who do not have hypochloremia [3]. 0.9% saline is the preferred solution for patients with hypovolemia and hypochloremia, for example after prolonged vomiting. When used, chloride concentrations should be monitored. To date, there are no published clinical trials specifically comparing different crystalloid fluids in patients with established AKI.

24.4 Volume of Fluid

Large observational studies have shown an association between excessive fluid administration and development of AKI [28–30]. The potential mechanisms include intra-renal compartment syndrome and venous congestion as a result of the kidneys being encapsulated organs [3, 5]. Fluid administration may also impair the renal oxygen supply-demand relationship as a result of an increase in glomerular filtration rate (GFR) and sodium reabsorption [31]. For these reasons, fluids should only be administered until intravascular hypovolemia has been corrected. It is desirable to administer the minimum amount of intravenous fluid required to maintain perfusion and systemic oxygen delivery. If fluids are considered necessary, they should be administered in frequent small aliquots and under periodic reassessment of fluid responsiveness and hemodynamic status so that fluid overload is avoided.

24.4.1 Assessment of Volume Status

Fluid responsiveness is often viewed as a surrogate marker of intravascular hypovolemia, and lack of fluid responsiveness is considered as equivalent to euvolemia. However, it needs to be remembered that being fluid responsive is physiologic.

Classically, the assessment of fluid responsiveness involves giving a fluid challenge to a patient with decreased organ perfusion and checking whether this increases cardiac output and improves organ perfusion. It is typically done by ascertaining the response of stroke volume or pulse pressure to an increase in preload. If a significant increase in stroke volume or pulse pressure is seen, it is viewed as an indication that cardiac function lies on the steeper part of the Frank-Starling curve, and the patient is considered to be fluid responsive. To date, pulse pressure variation (PPV) is the marker of preload responsiveness that has accumulated most evidence [32].

Various invasive and non-invasive techniques have been developed to assess fluid responsiveness, including administration of internal fluid challenges using the passive leg raise (PLR) test [32]. Other methods of assessing volume status include the evaluation of static parameters like central venous pressure (CVP) and pulmonary artery occlusion pressure (PAOP), but they are generally considered to be of limited use for this purpose [33, 34].

Ultrasonography of the inferior vena cava (IVC) may demonstrate that the IVC is collapsed or has features of extreme variation with respiration, which are considered signs of intravascular hypovolemia. When applying this technique, it is important that right ventricular (RV) pathology, cardiac tamponade and intra-abdominal hypertension are ruled out beforehand. Importantly, a full IVC does not necessarily mean that the patient is no longer fluid responsive [35, 36].

In spontaneously breathing patients with intra-arterial blood pressure monitoring in place, the PLR test is the easiest and most reliable dynamic test to predict fluid responsiveness [37, 38]. It basically involves giving an internal fluid challenge by diverting the blood in the venous pool of the splanchnic bed and lower limbs to the central circulation and looking for a PPV >10%. This preload challenge of around 300 mL of blood can be repeated as often as necessary. The technique can also be used as a safety parameter during fluid administration to prevent fluid overload. An end-expiratory occlusion (EEO) test is another tool to assess preload responsiveness in patients receiving mechanical ventilation and who are spontaneously breathing. A significant increase in cardiac output of >5% measured by pulse contour analysis after 15 s of EEO can predict fluid responsiveness with good sensitivity and specificity [39, 40]. To use PPV as an indicator of fluid responsiveness in patients receiving full mechanical ventilation, a regular heart rhythm and controlled mechanical ventilation with large tidal volumes >8 mL/kg are required [41].

In spontaneously breathing patients not on mechanical ventilation, the assessment of fluid responsiveness includes the non-invasive assessment of stroke volume changes pre- and post-PLR test or bedside echocardiography. Newer assessment tools like the evaluation of changes in carotid blood flow and corrected carotid flow time pre- and post-PLR test show promise but are yet to be validated [42].

In general, the threshold to define fluid responsiveness depends on the change in cardiac preload induced by the test (e.g., 15% for fluid challenge, 10% for the PLR test, 5% for the EEO test). In any case, it is important to remember that fluid responsiveness is a normal physiologic condition and does not necessarily equate to being fluid deplete and 'needing fluids'. Fluids are only indicated if the patient also has signs of hypoperfusion (Fig. 24.1).

24.5 Duration of Fluid Therapy

The overall aim of fluid resuscitation is to correct hypovolemia and optimize preload in order to maintain renal perfusion. In patients with AKI, fluid resuscitation beyond correction of hypovolemia does not increase the chances of renal recovery and may in fact hinder recovery of renal function and reduce overall outcomes [30]. Fluid administration should be stopped when signs of circulatory failure have resolved, early signs of fluid overload appear and/or dynamic tests indicate that the patient is no longer fluid responsive.

The Conservative Versus Liberal Approach to Fluid Therapy of Septic Shock in Intensive Care (CLASSIC) trial showed that active fluid restriction is feasible and safe in patients with septic shock and may even improve outcomes [43]. In nine ICUs in Denmark and Finland, 151 patients with septic shock who were clinically euvolemic were randomized to restrictive fluid therapy or standard care. Although there were some baseline differences between groups, AKI was more likely to worsen in patients receiving standard care. Further studies are necessary to validate these findings.

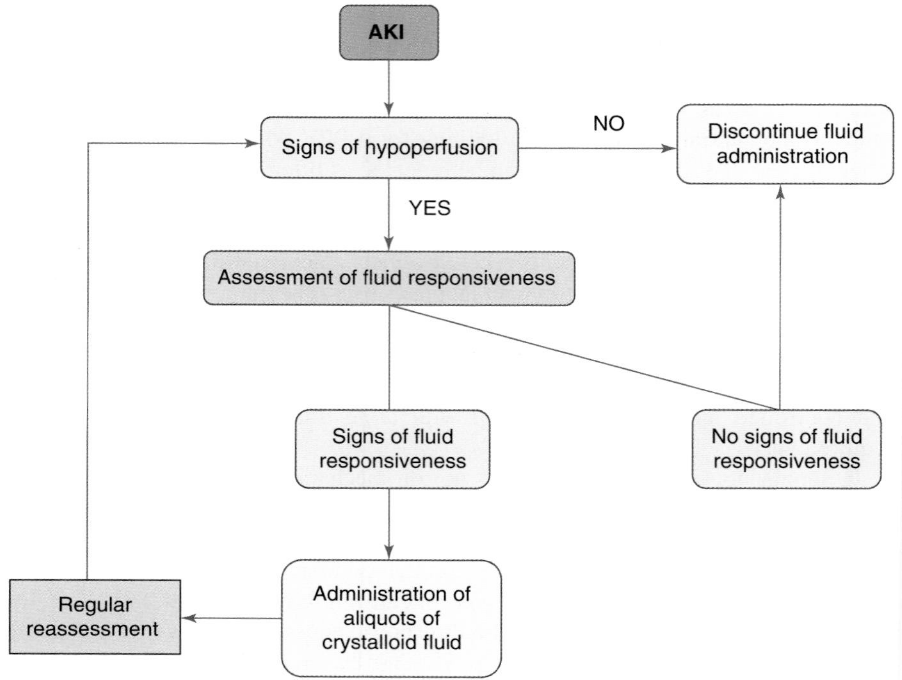

Fig. 24.1 Algorithm to guide fluid therapy in acute kidney injury (AKI)

In conclusion, patients at risk of or with established AKI should only be administered fluids until intravascular volume depletion has been corrected, ideally only in small aliquots under regular assessment of their hemodynamic status. If they remain hemodynamically unstable after hypovolemia has been corrected, support with vasopressors or inotropes should be considered.

24.6 Fluid Management in Specific Types of AKI

24.6.1 AKI in Liver Disease

Patients with liver disease are at high risk of AKI, mainly due to splanchnic vasodilation and relative intravascular hypovolemia [44, 45]. Volume expansion in combination with vasoconstrictors is an important component of resuscitation. Several studies have confirmed that the combination of vasopressin analogues and albumin has a beneficial effect on renal function [46, 47].

24.6.2 Obstructive AKI

Resolution of obstruction and correction of intravascular hypovolemia are the mainstay of treatment in obstructive AKI. Patients who develop post-obstruction polyuria may need large volume fluid resuscitation to keep up with diuresis. Balanced crystalloid solutions are the preferred fluids but occasionally additional electrolyte supplementation is necessary.

24.6.3 AKI in Congestive Cardiac Failure

Patients with cardiac disease are at high risk of AKI for multiple reasons, including impaired cardiac output, renal congestion due to RV dysfunction and potential drug nephrotoxicity. In this situation, fluid therapy is only indicated in case of true intravascular fluid depletion. Support with inotropes and vasopressors are more commonly needed, often in combination with diuretics and fluid removal.

24.6.4 AKI Treated with Renal Replacement Therapy

During RRT, fluid management should be guided by the fluid and hemodynamic status of the patient. Most patients on RRT need fluid removal and therefore fluid intake should be minimized. If fluid administration is necessary, the same principles as outlined earlier apply.

Determining the exact volume and speed of fluid removal during RRT is challenging, in particular if patients are hemodynamically unstable. In patients who develop hypotension, the rate of fluid removal should be decreased to allow vascular refilling. To facilitate timely and effective fluid removal without cardiovascular collapse, the patient's fluid and hemodynamic status and overall trajectory need to be assessed regularly so that the fluid removal rate can be adjusted accordingly. Continuous RRT provides more flexibility in this regard.

24.7 Conclusion

In patients with AKI, the only indication for fluid administration is correction or prevention of intravascular hypovolemia (Table 24.3). The optimal type of fluid remains unknown but starches should be avoided. There is no evidence that fluid administration beyond correction of intravascular hypovolemia is beneficial. Fluid responsiveness should not automatically be viewed as fluid depletion and should only trigger fluid administration if there are clinical signs of hypoperfusion. If fluids are considered to be necessary, boluses of small aliquots should be considered instead of rapid high volume fluid administration. In patients receiving RRT, the same principles apply.

Table 24.3 Dos and Don'ts of fluid management in acute kidney injury (AKI)

Factor	Do	Don't
Indication	Intravascular hypovolemia	Oliguria without hypovolemia
Type of fluid	Crystalloids	Starches
Volume	Boluses of small aliquots	High volumes
Duration	Until hypovolemia corrected	Until AKI resolved

References

1. Hoste EA, Bagshaw SM, Bellomo R, et al. Epidemiology of acute kidney injury in critically ill patients: the multinational AKI-EPI study. Intensive Care Med. 2015;41:1411–23.
2. Rhodes A, Evans LE, Alhazzani W, et al. Surviving sepsis campaign: international guidelines for management of sepsis and septic shock: 2016. Crit Care Med. 2017;45:486–552.
3. Finfer S, Myburgh J, Bellomo R. Intravenous fluid therapy in critically ill adults. Nat Rev Nephrol. 2018;14:541–57.
4. Martensson J, Bellomo R. Does fluid management affect the occurrence of acute kidney injury? Curr Opin Anesthesiol. 2017;30:84–91.
5. Prowle JR, Echeverri JE, Ligabo EV, Ronco C, Bellomo R. Fluid balance and acute kidney injury. Nat Rev Nephrol. 2010;6:107–15.
6. Perner A, Prowle J, Joannidis M, Young P, Hjortrup PB, Pettilä V. Fluid management in acute kidney injury. Intensive Care Med. 2017;43:807–15.
7. Mutter TC, Ruth CA, Dart AB. Hydroxyethyl starch (HES) versus other fluid therapies: effects on kidney function. Cochrane Database Syst Rev. 2013;7:CD007594.
8. Myburgh JA, Finfer S, Bellomo R, et al. Hydroxyethylstarch or saline for fluid resuscitation in intensive care. N Engl J Med. 2012;367:1901–11.
9. Perner A, Haase N, Guttomsen AB, et al. Hydroxyethyl starch 130/0.42 versus Ringer's acetate in severe sepsis. N Engl J Med. 2012;367:124–34.
10. Bayer O, Reinhart K, Kohl M, et al. Effects of fluid resuscitation with synthetic colloids or crystalloids alone on shock reversal, fluid balance, and patient outcomes in patients with severe sepsis: a prospective sequential analysis. Crit Care Med. 2012;40:2543–51.
11. Moeller C, Fleischmann C, Thomas-Rueddel D, et al. How safe is gelatin? A systematic review and meta-analysis of gelatin-containing plasma expanders vs crystalloids and albumin. J Crit Care. 2016;35:75–83.
12. Finfer S, Bellomo R, Boyce N, et al. A comparison of albumin and saline for fluid resuscitation in the intensive care unit. N Engl J Med. 2004;350:2247–56.
13. Myburgh J, Cooper DJ, Finfer S, et al. Saline or albumin for fluid resuscitation in patients with traumatic brain injury. N Engl J Med. 2007;357:874–84.
14. Caironi P, Tognoni G, Masson S, et al. Albumin replacement in patients with severe sepsis or septic shock. N Engl J Med. 2014;370:1412–21.
15. Rochwerg B, Alhazzani W, Gibson A, et al. Fluid type and the use of renal replacement therapy in sepsis: a systematic review and network meta-analysis. Intensive Care Med. 2015;41:1561–71.
16. Lee EH, Kim WJ, Kim JY, et al. Effect of exogenous albumin on the incidence of postoperative acute kidney injury in patients undergoing off-pump coronary artery bypass surgery with a preoperative albumin level of less than 4.0g/dL. Anesthesiology. 2016;124:1001–11.
17. KDIGO AKI Work Group. KDIGO clinical practice guideline for acute kidney injury. Kidney Int Suppl. 2012;2:1–138.
18. Joannidis M, Druml W, Forni LG, et al. Prevention of acute kidney injury and protection of renal function in the intensive care unit: update 2017: expert opinion of the Working Group on Prevention, AKI section, European Society of Intensive Care Medicine. Intensive Care Med. 2017;43:730–49.
19. Wilcox CS. Regulation of renal blood flow by plasma chloride. J Clin Invest. 1983;71:726–35.
20. Bullivant EM, Wilcox CS, Welch WJ. Intrarenal vasoconstriction during hyperchloremia: role of thromboxane. Am J Phys. 1989;256:F152–7.
21. Chowdhury AH, Cox EF, Francis ST, Lobo DN. A randomized, controlled, double-blind crossover study on the effects of 2-L infusions of 0.9% saline and plasma-lyte® 148 on renal blood flow velocity and renal cortical tissue perfusion in healthy volunteers. Ann Surg. 2012;256:18–24.
22. McCluskey SA, Karkouti K, Wijeysundera D, Minkovich L, Tait G, Beattie WS. Hyperchloremia after noncardiac surgery is independently associated with increased morbidity and mortality: a propensity-matched cohort study. Anesth Analg. 2013;117:412–21.

23. Raghunathan K, Shaw A, Nathanson B, et al. Association between the choice of IV crystalloid and inhospital mortality among critically ill adults with sepsis. Crit Care Med. 2014;42:1585–91.
24. Yunos NM, Bellomo R, Hegarty C, Story D, Ho L, Bailey M. Association between a chloride-liberal vs chloride-restrictive intravenous fluid administration strategy and kidney injury in critically ill adults. JAMA. 2012;308:1566–72.
25. Young P, Bailey M, Beasley R, et al. Effect of a buffered crystalloid solution vs saline on acute kidney injury among patients in the intensive care unit: the SPLIT randomized clinical trial. JAMA. 2015;314:1701–10.
26. Semler MW, Self WH, Wanderer JP, et al. Balanced crystalloids versus saline in critically ill adults. N Engl J Med. 2018;378:829–39.
27. Sen A, Keener CM, Sileanu FE, et al. Chloride content of fluids used for large-volume resuscitation is associated with reduced survival. Crit Care Med. 2016;45:e146–53.
28. Payen D, de Pont AC, Sakr Y, Spies C, Reinhart K, Vincent JL, Sepsis Occurrence in Acutely Ill Patients (SOAP) Investigators. A positive fluid balance is associated with a worse outcome in patients with acute renal failure. Crit Care. 2008;12:R74.
29. Garzotto F, Ostermann M, Martin-Langenwerf D, et al. The Dose Response Multicentre Investigation on Fluid Assessment (DoReMIFA) in critically ill patients. Crit Care. 2016;20:196.
30. Raimundo M, Crichton S, Martin JR, et al. Increased fluid administration after early acute kidney injury is associated with less renal recovery. Shock. 2015;44:431–7.
31. Skytte Larsson J, Bragadottir G, Krumbholz V, et al. Effects of acute plasma volume expansion on renal perfusion, filtration, and oxygenation after cardiac surgery: a randomized study on crytstalloid vs colloid. Br J Anaesth. 2015;115:736–42.
32. Monnet X, Marik PE, Teboul JL. Prediction of fluid responsiveness: an update. Ann Intensive Care. 2016;6:111.
33. Marik PE, Cavallazzi R. Does the central venous pressure predict fluid responsiveness? an updated meta-analysis and a plea for some common sense. Crit Care Med. 2013;41:1774–81.
34. Osman D, Ridel C, Ray P, et al. Cardiac filling pressures are not appropriate to predict hemodynamic response to volume challenge. Crit Care Med. 2007;35:64–8.
35. Zhang Z, Xu X, Ye S, Xu L. Ultrasonographic measurement of the respiratory variation in the inferior vena cava diameter is predictive of fluid responsiveness in critically ill patients: systematic review and meta-analysis. Ultrasound Med Biol. 2014;40:845–53.
36. Airapetian N, Maizel J, Alyamani O, et al. Does inferior vena cava respiratory variability predict fluid responsiveness in spontaneously breathing patients? Crit Care. 2015;19:400.
37. Cherpanath TG, Hirsch A, Geerts BF, et al. Predicting fluid responsiveness by passive leg raising: a systematic review and meta-analysis of 23 clinical trials. Crit Care Med. 2016;44: 981–91.
38. Monnet X, Marik P, Teboul JL. Passive leg raising for predicting fluid responsiveness: a systematic review and meta-analysis. Intensive Care Med. 2016;42:1935–47.
39. Silva S, Jozwiak M, Teboul JL, Persichini R, Richard C, Monnet X. End-expiratory occlusion test predicts preload responsiveness independently of positive end-expiratory pressure during acute respiratory distress syndrome. Crit Care Med. 2013;41:1692–701.
40. Yang X, Du B. Does pulse pressure variation predict fluid responsiveness in critically ill patients? A systematic review and meta-analysis. Crit Care. 2014;18:650.
41. Marik PE, Cavallazzi R, Vasu T, Hirani A. Dynamic changes in arterial waveform derived variables and fluid responsiveness in mechanically ventilated patients: a systematic review of the literature. Crit Care Med. 2009;37:2642–7.
42. Ma IWY, Caplin JD, Azad A, et al. Correlation of carotid blood flow and corrected carotid flow time with invasive cardiac output measurements. Crit Ultrasound J. 2017;9:10.
43. Hjortrup PB, Haase N, Bundgaard H, et al. Restricting volumes of resuscitation fluid in adults with septic shock after initial management: the CLASSIC randomised, parallel-group, multicentre feasibility trial. Intensive Care Med. 2016;42:1695–705.

44. Wong F. Recent advances in our understanding of hepatorenal syndrome. Nat Rev Gastroenterol Hepatol. 2012;9:382–91.
45. Bucsics T, Krones E. Renal dysfunction in cirrhosis: acute kidney injury and the hepatorenal syndrome. Gastroenterol Rep. 2017;5:127–37.
46. Israelsen M, Krag A, Allegretti AS, et al. Terlipressin versus other vasoactive drugs for hepatorenal syndrome. Cochrane Database Syst Rev. 2017;9:CD011532.
47. Singh V, Ghosh S, Singh B, et al. Noradrenaline vs. terlipressin in the treatment of hepatorenal syndrome: a randomized study. J Hepatol. 2012;56:1293.

Part IX

Altered Renal Function

25 Diagnostic Implications of Creatinine and Urea Metabolism in Critical Illness

R. W. Haines and J. R. Prowle

25.1 Introduction

The serum concentrations of urea and creatinine form the basis of our understanding of renal function and are requested and interpreted by critical care clinicians on a near daily basis for patients admitted to intensive care units (ICUs) worldwide. Changes in creatinine constitute the diagnostic criteria for acute kidney injury (AKI) while urea is commonly used as a marker of dehydration and as a potential trigger for initiation of renal replacement therapy (RRT). However, the interpretation of these routinely measured biomarkers of renal function has been brought under scrutiny as the complex impact of critical illness on the metabolism of urea and creatinine affects their interpretation. A more careful understanding of the changes in creatinine and urea metabolism during acute illness and in survivors of critical care is necessary to better inform decisions on diagnosis, treatment strategies and research of new interventions for AKI.

R. W. Haines
Adult Critical Care Unit, The Royal London Hospital, Barts Health NHS Trust, London, UK

William Harvey Research Institute, Queen Mary University of London, London, UK

J. R. Prowle (✉)
Adult Critical Care Unit, The Royal London Hospital, Barts Health NHS Trust, London, UK

William Harvey Research Institute, Queen Mary University of London, London, UK

Department of Renal Medicine and Transplantation, The Royal London Hospital, Barts Health NHS Trust, London, UK
e-mail: j.prowle@qmul.ac.uk

J.-L. Vincent (ed.), *Annual Update in Intensive Care and Emergency Medicine 2019*, Annual Update in Intensive Care and Emergency Medicine,
https://doi.org/10.1007/978-3-030-06067-1_25

25.2 Creatinine and Urea Metabolism in Health

The measurement of creatinine in human urine and blood, developed in the late 1900s [1], led to studies establishing the link between protein metabolism and creatinine appearance. Creatinine (from the Greek *kreas* meaning flesh), is formed from the daily, near constant, irreversible, non-enzymatic conversion of creatine or hydrolysis of phosphocreatine in muscle [2]. For example, a 70 kg man of average build contains roughly 120 g of creatine, of which 2 g/day is converted to soluble creatinine and excreted by the kidneys and is replaced by dietary replacement or *de novo* biosynthesis. Creatine and phosphocreatine, via the creatine kinase reaction, replenish adenosine triphosphate (ATP) in tissues with high energy demands such as skeletal muscle and play a key role in the development and function of brain tissue, as demonstrated by the impact of creatine deficiency syndromes on neurological development. The primary site of creatine production is the liver, but this process depends on metabolic pathways in the kidney and consequently the transport of intermediaries through blood; however the exact nature of these processes and contribution of different organ tissues to creatine synthesis remains unclear. A widely thought dominant pathway of creatine biosynthesis involves initial formation of the precursor guanidinoacetate in the kidney and subsequent uptake by the liver as a substrate for creatinine synthesis (Fig. 25.1). Another source of guanidinoacetate is the urea cycle in the liver itself via the conversion of arginine to glycine [3].

As a small, 113 Da molecule, creatinine is freely filtered in the glomerulus and appears unaltered in the urine together with a small amount of active tubular secretion (<10%). As renal clearance is high, non-renal excretion or degradation of creatinine in health is negligible, but in advanced renal failure when creatinine concentration is higher, bacterial activity has been shown to convert creatinine to creatine and other degradation products and limited gastrointestinal excretion may occur. As plasma creatinine is excreted predominantly by glomerular ultrafiltration, when glomerular filtration rate (GFR) decreases, creatinine accumulates. To fully interpret the meaning of alterations in plasma creatinine concentration, an understanding of kinetics of creatinine generation and excretion is required. First, as >90% of creatinine excretion is by glomerular ultrafiltration, net creatinine excretion approximates to the GFR (rate of plasma filtration) multiplied by the concentration of creatinine in the plasma. Second, at steady state (defined by constant plasma creatinine concentration over time) the rate of excretion must equal the rate of creatinine generation thus:

$$\text{GFR} \times [\text{Cr}]_{\text{P}} = \text{G}$$

where GFR is in L/min, $[\text{Cr}]_{\text{P}}$ is the plasma concentration of creatinine in μmol/L and G is the creatinine generation rate in μmol/min. Thus, at steady state, GFR is proportional to the reciprocal of the plasma creatinine. Assuming a creatinine change occurs and levels stabilize at a new steady state, a doubling of plasma creatinine will then imply an approximate halving of GFR, as long as the creatinine generation rate also remains constant. This relationship forms the basis of the use of

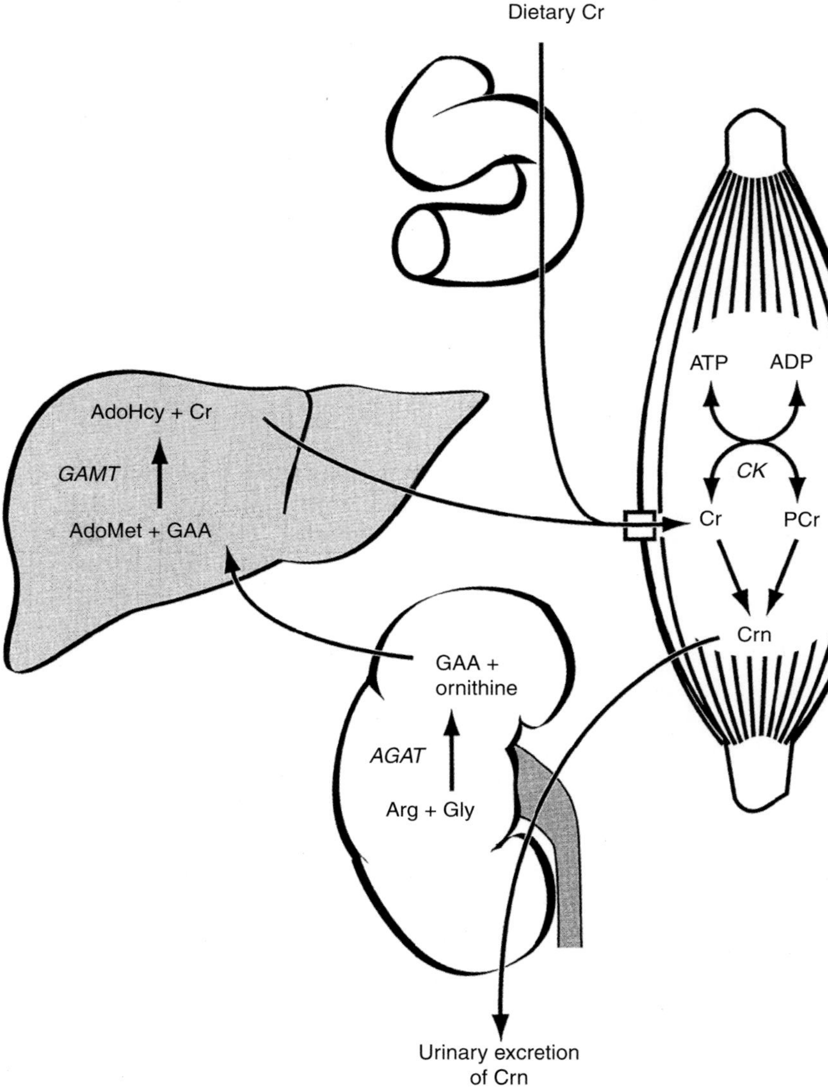

Dietary Cr
ATP ADP
AdoHcy + Cr
GAMT
AdoMet + GAA
CK
Cr PCr
Crn
GAA + ornithine
AGAT
Arg + Gly
Urinary excretion of Crn

Fig. 25.1 Creatinine generation and the source of creatine biosynthesis. Creatinine (Crn) is formed from the non-enzymatic breakdown of creatine (Cr) in the muscle and diffuses into the blood to be excreted by the kidney. Cr generation, thought to start in the kidney, involves the transfer of an amidino group of arginine (Arg) to glycine (Gly) catalyzed by L-arginine:glycine amidinotransferase (AGAT) to form guanidinoacetic acid (GAA) and ornithine. The liver then methylates GAA via the action of S-adenosyl-L-methionine (AdoMet): N-guanidinoacetate methyltransferase (GAMT) to Cr. Skeletal muscle and other tissues have specific Cr uptake transporters. Once in skeletal muscle, Cr is involved in the reversible creatine kinase (CK) reaction with adenosine triphosphate to yield adenosine diphosphate (ADP) and phosphocreatine (PCr). *AdoHcy* S-adenosyl-L-homocysteine. From [2] with permission

1.5–2- and 3-fold rises in creatinine above a baseline value to define severity of AKI in consensus definitions. It is crucial to stress, however, that this direct relationship between fold-increase in creatinine and fold-decrease in GFR only holds true when creatinine concentration has regained steady state and if creatinine generation is constant. Thus, despite its relatively predictable excretion, the incompletely understood complexities of creatinine and creatine metabolism that underlie creatinine generation and their variation in disease states implies that our interpretation of serum creatinine as a biomarker of renal function may be imperfect in a variety of disease states.

The urea (or ornithine) cycle was discovered through the work of Hans Krebs and Kurt Henseleit in 1932 [4]. It has the primary role of removing toxic ammonia produced from the deamination of amino acids. Once created, highly soluble and non-toxic urea is excreted via the kidney in urine and a smaller percentage hydrolyzed by bacterial ureases in the gut [5]. The urea cycle is therefore essential in controlling the excess ammonia produced from the body's handling of proteins. The degradation of proteins and subsequent alterations of amino acids is a key process in human physiology to allow formation of new amino acids, and other important metabolic substrates such as creatine [6]. Urea is further used by the kidney as the principal solute contributing to the renal medullary osmotic gradient while ureagenesis itself contributes to acid base balance via removal of bicarbonate ions and ammonium [7]. The metabolic machinery thought necessary for ureagenesis is confined to the liver.

25.3 Ureagenesis in Critical Illness

The rate of urea generation is directly related to the concentration of urea precursors: amino acids. Any increase in free amino acids either from protein degradation or exogenous amino acid delivery will therefore result in an increase in ureagenesis. Muscle proteolysis and protein breakdown is an early, near universal process occurring in critically ill patients [8, 9], and the resulting increase in energy intensive ureagenesis contributes to an overall catabolic state. Glucagon, cortisol and catecholamines along with relative insulin resistance have been proposed as the key determinants of protein catabolism and reduced amino acid uptake [6]. Increased ureagenesis in sepsis is well described in animal models [10, 11] as a by-product of the increased utilization of mobilized amino acids used as energy substrates in the liver and has been observed in critically ill patients with sepsis and trauma [12].

As the mechanisms of acute skeletal muscle wasting in critically ill patients are being further elucidated, increasing ureagenesis has been reviewed as a marker of effectiveness of interventional strategies that aim to improve incorporation of exogenous amino acids and potentially reduce the profound loss of skeletal muscle [13]. However, the use of ureagenesis is limited by the high incidence of AKI in critically ill patients, with the subsequent alteration in urea excretion by the kidney complicating the interpretation of serum urea measurements [14]. Despite these complexities, ureagenesis has been investigated in critically ill patients during acute and chronic phases of critical illness. Studies have explored the significance of serum urea changes in investigations of the phenotype of persistent critical illness, attributed to patients who survive the initial injury or acute illness and enter a state of unchecked catabolism with persistent inflammation a likely contributory factor [15]. Retrospective studies suggest that urea is an important marker of this deleterious metabolic phase [16] and associated with worse outcomes in pancreatitis [17], decompensated heart failure [18] and the elderly admitted to critical care units [19]. Although retrospective in design, there are growing data to support the role of ureagenesis and worse outcome in critically ill patients [20], especially in the growing group of patients who survive but require longer periods of critical care support.

25.4 Creatinine Generation in Critical Illness

Creatine and phosphocreatine biosynthesis in critical illness will determine the amount of creatinine released into the blood via continuous non-enzymatic breakdown. Additionally, loss of lean body mass will result in reduced creatinine generation as skeletal muscle is the primary reservoir of creatine. Clinicians continue to interpret changes in serum creatinine in the scenario of static creatinine generation, for example when applying the Kidney Disease: Improving Global Outcomes (KDIGO) creatinine criteria to diagnose AKI. Creatinine generation has been established from studies assessing urinary excretion of creatinine from healthy humans which shows a decrease with age and in females [21]. However, research has suggested that creatinine generation is not constant. Work by Pickering et al. [22] highlighted the potential impact of cardiac arrest on misclassification of AKI that could not be fully explained by the dilutional effect of initial fluid resuscitation on serum creatinine. They hypothesized that metabolic changes to creatine generation may account for such changes, with other investigators suggesting that unstable creatinine kinetics impact on the interpretation of creatinine in critically ill patients [23]. These concepts have been supported in several animal studies, including a mice cecal ligation and puncture sepsis model [24]. To eliminate the impact of AKI and explore non-renal factors contributing to creatinine generation, mice that had undergone bilateral nephrectomy were studied. Mice with sepsis had the slowest increase in creatinine (versus ischemia/reperfusion models). Mechanisms underlying creatinine production were further explored from mice data and supported by other studies and included an association with raised liver injury biomarkers in septic mice potentially resulting in reduced liver creatine production [25]; reduced microcirculatory perfusion reducing creatinine release from muscle [26]; and the neurohormonal impact of sepsis reducing energy production [27].

Reduced creatinine generation was demonstrated in a group of anuric, critically ill patients on continuous venovenous hemodialysis [28], in patients with acute renal failure [29] and in critically unwell adults [30]. Contradictory findings of a raised urinary creatinine excretion, suggestive of increased creatinine generation, have been described in cases of severe traumatic injury [31] and in pediatric cases of traumatic brain injury [32]. The increased urinary creatinine described in these cases is thought to herald the beginning of hypercatabolism with an initial rise then reduction in creatinine generation due to muscle loss. However this theory relies on a pool of creatinine to be readily released in acute illness for which clear evidence does not exist, and instead, the increased urinary excretion of creatinine could be explained by glomerular hyperfiltration, a recognized phenomenon in early stages of critical illness, especially trauma [33].

25.5 Creatine and Phosphocreatine in Critical Illness

Defining the metabolic phenotype of critical illness and understanding the impact of the bioenergetic changes is essential to developing interventions to combat the damaging sequelae of critical illness, such as skeletal muscle wasting. Phosphocreatine conversion to creatine and the release of ATP in tissues with high metabolic activity is a key biochemical process in the human body [2]. In exercising adults, there is evidence supporting creatine supplementation where it improves muscle strength and power [34] by increasing the pool of available creatine. Disturbances of phosphocreatine have been described in muscle biopsies from patients with sepsis and after trauma and in animal models and are often accompanied by reduced levels in other vital organs including the kidney and muscle [9]. In recent work by Puthucheary et al., there was a strong relationship between decreased availability of ATP, phosphocreatine and creatine with skeletal muscle wasting in a heterogeneous cohort of critically ill patients [35]. The decrease in creatine and phosphocreatine suggest that concordant reductions in creatinine generation are not solely due to loss of muscle mass and that strategies to help maintain the pool of high energy phosphates in conditions such as sepsis are a potential interventional target for future research.

25.6 Urea:Creatinine Ratio in Critical Illness

Historically, the urea:creatinine ratio was commonly used as a biochemical test to distinguish between ‘pre-renal failure’ and ‘acute tubular necrosis’ to then guide the subsequent fluid resuscitation strategy. The reasoning relied entirely on a focus on renal physiology as the explanation for changes in the urea:creatinine ratio, without any appreciation of the effect of relative changes in production of these metabolites. Improved understanding of the pathophysiology of AKI in critically ill patients, especially patients with sepsis where reduced renal blood flow has not been shown to be a universal phenomenon [36], cast doubt on the use of the urea:creatinine ratio to dichotomize subtypes of AKI that may not in reality exist as clear phenotypes. Work by Uchino et al. confirmed the weakness of this approach demonstrating in fact there was significantly higher risk of death in AKI patients with a raised urea:creatinine ratio, something that would have been traditionally regarded as more treatment-responsive ‘pre-renal failure’ [37]. In fact, the urea:creatinine ratio has been proposed as a marker of protein catabolism by incorporating the increase in ureagenesis and fall in creatinine due to loss of muscle mass and creatine generation, an interpretation based on differential production rather than differential excretion. In this framework, a raised urea:creatinine ratio has been used in neurohormonal studies of critical care-associated catabolism [13], however with the caveat that alteration in renal function could be a potential confounder of this use.

25.7 Limitations of Creatinine in AKI Diagnosis

Thus, while relative changes in plasma creatinine define AKI in consensus criteria, there are significant limitations to interpretation of creatinine values in critical illness. Use of plasma creatinine as a direct indication of relative change in GFR is dependent on having achieved a new steady-state concentration. After a change in GFR, time to reach steady state is dependent on both the magnitude of change in GFR and the underlying creatinine generation rate. In acute severe AKI, many days could be required for a new steady-state to be achieved and, until then, plasma creatinine will underestimate severity of renal dysfunction delaying full appreciation of the severity of AKI. Furthermore, changes in creatinine generation significantly impact plasma creatinine concentration. Reduction in muscle mass, dietary intake of creatine and hepatic creatine synthesis may all contribute to an acute fall in generation rate. Thus, incidence and severity of creatinine-assessed AKI may be underestimated in the critically ill and, similarly, renal recovery after AKI may be significantly overestimated [38]. Furthermore, as reduction in generation is related to length and severity of illness, the confounding effect of these changes on AKI diagnosis is likely to be greater in more severe illness (Fig. 25.2).

25.8 Towards a Better Interpretation of Serum Creatinine

The limitations on the use of serum creatinine for the diagnosis of AKI and chronic kidney disease during and after critical illness have been well illustrated [22, 39]. Loss of muscle mass experienced both during and after critical illness confounds the interpretation of serum creatinine and results in an overestimation of GFR. However, serum creatinine is an attractive marker of muscle mass with a direct correlation with total skeletal muscle, yet its diagnostic role in acute skeletal muscle wasting in critical illness remains complicated by the high prevalence of AKI in this population [40]. Previous studies have highlighted the loss of creatinine in critically ill populations despite AKI diagnosis and the association of a low serum creatinine with poorer outcomes [39, 41]. Cystatin C, which is produced from all nucleated cells and is less likely to be confounded by acute and chronic effects of ill-health on diet and muscle mass, may have the potential to improve the interpretation of creatinine and in some instances supersede its use as a renal functional biomarker in critically ill adults. In a population of critical care survivors, Ravn et al. demonstrated a 24 mL/min/1.73 m^2 median difference in estimated GFR (eGFR) based on cystatin C versus creatinine at ICU discharge [42]. Furthermore, cystatin C showed improved

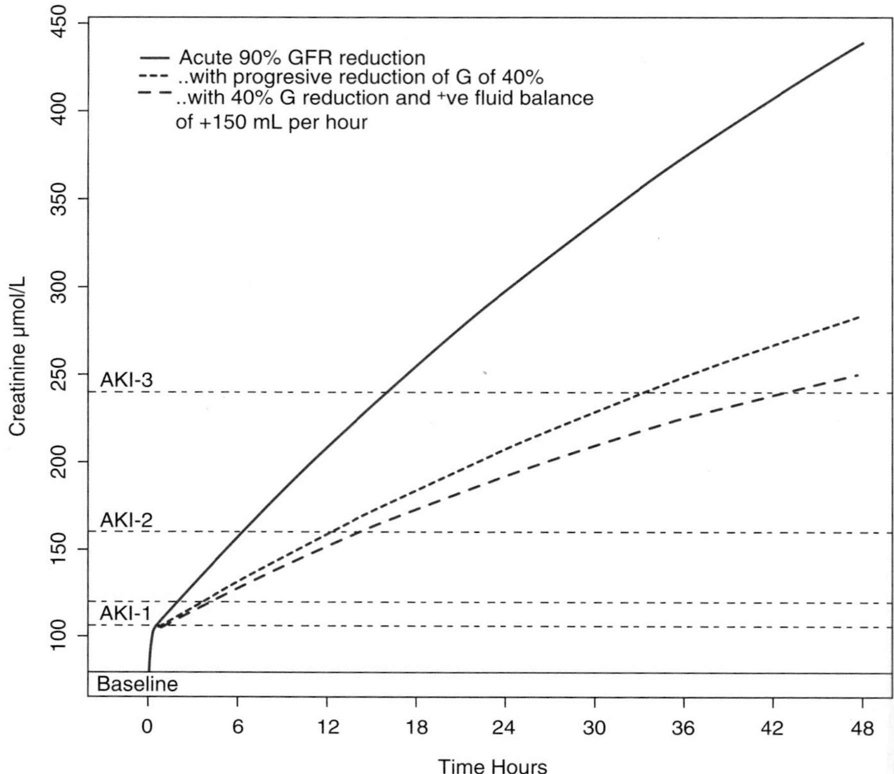

Fig. 25.2 Kinetic modeling of changes in plasma creatinine concentration after an acute 90% reduction in glomerular filtration rate (GFR) after major surgery in a 65-year old male with a baseline creatinine of 80 µmol/L. With such severe reduction in GFR, acute kidney injury (AKI)-1 criteria are rapidly achieved on a 26.5 µmol/L increase; however, full severity of AKI would take over 15 h to be apparent. However, when one factors in a creatinine generation rate (G) decreasing to 60% of baseline over 48 h and then the effect of a continuous positive fluid balance of 150 mL/h over the same period, creatinine increase is significantly retarded, delaying AKI-2 diagnosis by over 6 h and AKI-3 diagnosis by up to one-day despite likely greater illness-severity. From [45] with permission

association with age and comorbidity-adjusted short-term and 1-year mortality and may therefore by a superior method to monitor eGFR post-critical illness.

Recent work by Kashani et al. incorporated cystatin C and creatinine to create a novel index (serum creatinine-to-serum cystatin C ratio × 100) [43] and showed good correlation with skeletal muscle mass derived from computed tomography (CT) analysis. Similar work in a community population used a cystatin C and serum creatinine derived equation to estimate body mass and showed a strong correlation with total body muscle mass derived from dual-energy X-ray absorptiometry [44]. This work requires confirmation in prospective cohorts and remains limited by the measurement of body mass at single timepoints but does highlight that when combined with an accurate marker of renal function, plasma creatinine could be a potential biomarker of muscle wasting.

25.9 Conclusion

Changes in urea and creatinine metabolism provide insights into the impact of critical illness on organ function, body composition and the metabolic phenotype of patients. However, the effect of critical illness on changes to generation and clearance pose challenges to how best to interpret such changes in clinical context. Interesting associations of ureagenesis with catabolism, creatinine with body composition and urea:creatinine ratio with mortality accompanied by the incorporation of newer biomarkers such as cystatin C should form the basis of future research to explore their clinical utility as candidate markers of muscle mass, renal function and predictors of worse outcomes.

References

1. Behre J, Benedict S. Studies in creatine and creatinine metabolism. J Biol Chem. 1922;52:11–33.
2. Wyss M, Kaddurah-Daouk R. Creatine and creatinine metabolism. Physiol Rev. 2000;80:1107–213.
3. Brosnan JT, Brosnan ME. Creatine metabolism and the urea cycle. Mol Genet Metab. 2010;100(Suppl 1):S49–52.
4. Holmes FL. Hans Krebs and the discovery of the ornithine cycle. Fed Proc. 1980;39: 216–25.
5. Anonymous. Urea metabolism in man. Lancet. 1971;2:1407–8.
6. Meijer AJ, Lamers WH, Chamuleau RA. Nitrogen metabolism and ornithine cycle function. Physiol Rev. 1990;70:701–48.
7. Withers PC. Urea: diverse functions of a 'waste' product. Clin Exp Pharmacol Physiol. 1998;25:722–7.
8. Puthucheary ZA, Rawal J, McPhail M, et al. Acute skeletal muscle wasting in critical illness. JAMA. 2013;310:1591–600.
9. Friedrich O, Reid MB, Van den Berghe G, et al. The sick and the weak: neuropathies/myopathies in the critically ill. Physiol Rev. 2015;95:1025–109.
10. Beisel WR, Wannemacher RW. Gluconeogenesis, ureagenesis, and ketogenesis during sepsis. JPEN J Parenter Enteral Nutr. 1980;4:277–85.
11. Ohtake Y, Clemens MG. Interrelationship between hepatic ureagenesis and gluconeogenesis in early sepsis. Am J Phys. 1991;260:E453–8.
12. Hasselgren PO, Pedersen P, Sax HC, Warner BW, Fischer JE. Current concepts of protein turnover and amino acid transport in liver and skeletal muscle during sepsis. Arch Surg. 1988;123:992–9.
13. Van den Berghe G. On the neuroendocrinopathy of critical illness. Perspectives for feeding and novel treatments. Am J Respir Crit Care Med. 2016;194:1337–48.
14. Gunst J, Vanhorebeek I, Casaer MP, et al. Impact of early parenteral nutrition on metabolism and kidney injury. J Am Soc Nephrol. 2013;24:995–1005.
15. Griffith DM, Lewis S, Rossi AG, et al. Systemic inflammation after critical illness: relationship with physical recovery and exploration of potential mechanisms. Thorax. 2016;71:820–9.
16. Arihan O, Wernly B, Lichtenauer M, et al. Blood Urea Nitrogen (BUN) is independently associated with mortality in critically ill patients admitted to ICU. PLoS One. 2018;13:e0191697.

17. Faisst M, Wellner UF, Utzolino S, Hopt UT, Keck T. Elevated blood urea nitrogen is an independent risk factor of prolonged intensive care unit stay due to acute necrotizing pancreatitis. J Crit Care. 2010;25:105–11.
18. Kajimoto K, Minami Y, Sato N, et al. Serum sodium concentration, blood urea nitrogen, and outcomes in patients hospitalized for acute decompensated heart failure. Int J Cardiol. 2016;222:195–201.
19. Pan SW, Kao HK, Yu WK, et al. Synergistic impact of low serum albumin on intensive care unit admission and high blood urea nitrogen during intensive care unit stay on post-intensive care unit mortality in critically ill elderly patients requiring mechanical ventilation. Geriatr Gerontol Int. 2013;13:107–15.
20. Beier K, Eppanapally S, Bazick HS, et al. Elevation of blood urea nitrogen is predictive of long-term mortality in critically ill patients independent of "normal" creatinine. Crit Care Med. 2011;39:305–13.
21. Bjornsson TD. Use of serum creatinine concentrations to determine renal function. Clin Pharmacokinet. 1979;4:200–22.
22. Pickering JW, Ralib AM, Endre ZH. Combining creatinine and volume kinetics identifies missed cases of acute kidney injury following cardiac arrest. Crit Care. 2013;17:R7.
23. Wells M, Lipman J. Measurements of glomerular filtration in the intensive care unit are only a rough guide to renal function. S Afr J Surg. 1997;35:20–3.
24. Thiele RH, Isbell JM, Rosner MH. AKI associated with cardiac surgery. Clin J Am Soc Nephrol. 2015;10:500–14.
25. Cocchetto DM, Tschanz C, Bjornsson TD. Decreased rate of creatinine production in patients with hepatic disease: implications for estimation of creatinine clearance. Ther Drug Monit. 1983;5:161–8.
26. Piper RD, Pitt-Hyde M, Li F, Sibbald WJ, Potter RF. Microcirculatory changes in rat skeletal muscle in sepsis. Am J Respir Crit Care Med. 1996;154:931–7.
27. Singer M, De Santis V, Vitale D, Jeffcoate W. Multiorgan failure is an adaptive, endocrine-mediated, metabolic response to overwhelming systemic inflammation. Lancet. 2004;364:545–8.
28. Wilson FP, Sheehan JM, Mariani LH, Berns JS. Creatinine generation is reduced in patients requiring continuous venovenous hemodialysis and independently predicts mortality. Nephrol Dial Transplant. 2012;27:4088–94.
29. Clark WR, Mueller BA, Kraus MA, Macias WL. Quantification of creatinine kinetic parameters in patients with acute renal failure. Kidney Int. 1998;54:554–60.
30. Pesola GR, Akhavan I, Carlon GC. Urinary creatinine excretion in the ICU: low excretion does not mean inadequate collection. Am J Crit Care. 1993;2:462–6.
31. Schiller WR, Long CL, Blakemore WS. Creatinine and nitrogen excretion in seriously ill and injured patients. Surg Gynecol Obstet. 1979;149:561–6.
32. Carlotti AP, Bohn D, Matsuno AK, Pasti DM, Gowrishankar M, Halperin ML. Indicators of lean body mass catabolism: emphasis on the creatinine excretion rate. QJM. 2008;101:197–205.
33. Saour M, Klouche K, Deras P, Damou A, Capdevila X, Charbit J. Assessment of modification of diet in renal disease equation to predict reference serum creatinine value in severe trauma patients: lessons from an observational study of 775 cases. Ann Surg. 2016;263:814–20.
34. Weitzel LR, Sandoval PA, Mayles WJ, Wischmeyer PE. Performance-enhancing sports supplements: role in critical care. Crit Care Med. 2009;37:S400–9.
35. Puthucheary ZA, Astin R, Mcphail MJW, et al. Metabolic phenotype of skeletal muscle in early critical illness. Thorax. 2018;73:926–35.
36. Prowle JR, Ishikawa K, May CN, Bellomo R. Renal blood flow during acute renal failure in man. Blood Purif. 2009;28:216–25.
37. Uchino S, Bellomo R, Goldsmith D. The meaning of the blood urea nitrogen/creatinine ratio in acute kidney injury. Clin Kidney J. 2012;5:187–91.

38. Schetz M, Gunst J, Van den Berghe G. The impact of using estimated GFR versus creatinine clearance on the evaluation of recovery from acute kidney injury in the ICU. Intensive Care Med. 2014;40:1709–17.
39. Prowle JR, Kolic I, Purdell-Lewis J, Taylor R, Pearse RM, Kirwan CJ. Serum creatinine changes associated with critical illness and detection of persistent renal dysfunction after AKI. Clin J Am Soc Nephrol. 2014;9:1015–23.
40. Wang ZM, Gallagher D, Nelson ME, Matthews DE, Heymsfield SB. Total-body skeletal muscle mass: evaluation of 24-h urinary creatinine excretion by computerized axial tomography. Am J Clin Nutr. 1996;63:863–9.
41. Thongprayoon C, Cheungpasitporn W, Kashani K. Serum creatinine level, a surrogate of muscle mass, predicts mortality in critically ill patients. J Thorac Dis. 2016;8:E305–11.
42. Ravn B, Prowle JR, Mårtensson J, Martling CR, Bell M. Superiority of serum cystatin c over creatinine in prediction of long-term prognosis at discharge from ICU. Crit Care Med. 2017;45:e932–40.
43. Kashani KB, Frazee EN, Kukrálová L, et al. Evaluating muscle mass by using markers of kidney function: development of the sarcopenia index. Crit Care Med. 2017;45:e23–9.
44. Kim SW, Jung HW, Kim CH, Kim KI, Chin HJ, Lee H. A new equation to estimate muscle mass from creatinine and cystatin c. PLoS One. 2016;11:e0148495.
45. Prowle J, Forni L. Functional biomarkers. In: Ronco C, Bellomo R, Kellum J, Ricci Z, editors. Critical Care Nephrology. Philadelphia: Elsevier; 2019. p. 141–145.e141.

New Insights into the Renal Microcirculation in Sepsis-Induced Acute Kidney Injury

26

A. Harrois, N. Libert, and J. Duranteau

26.1 Introduction

Acute kidney injury (AKI) is a frequent complication during septic shock with the incidence of AKI ranging from 55% to 73% [1–3]. Sepsis-induced AKI is independently associated with mortality [4] and survivors have a greater risk of developing chronic and end-stage kidney disease [5]. Thus, understanding the pathophysiology of sepsis-induced AKI is essential for appropriate treatment. Renal microvascular alterations appear to play a role in the occurrence of septic AKI [6, 7], but the relative contribution of renal microvascular alterations in the pathophysiology of sepsis-induced AKI in septic patients remains to be determined. Indeed, without the possibility of assessment of the renal microcirculation, renal perfusion status remains poorly studied in patients with septic shock. Thus, in clinical practice during the resuscitation of septic shock, physicians hope that optimization of the macrocirculation (i.e., mean arterial pressure [MAP] and systemic oxygen delivery) will be beneficial to the renal microcirculation but are totally blind to the actual behavior of the renal microcirculation. To gain new insights into the pathogenesis of AKI in septic patients and in intensive care unit (ICU) patients, we need new techniques to evaluate kidney microcirculation. In this chapter, we focus on recent results that have clarified the contribution of renal microvascular alterations in sepsis-induced AKI in septic patients. We expect that these findings will improve the understanding and the clinical management (prevention and treatment) of sepsis-induced AKI.

A. Harrois · J. Duranteau (✉)
Département d'Anesthésie-Réanimation, Hôpitaux universitaires Paris-Sud, Hôpital de Bicêtre, Le Kremlin-Bicêtre, France
e-mail: jacques.duranteau@aphp.fr

N. Libert
Service d'Anesthésie-Réanimation, Hôpital d'instruction des armées Percy, Clamart, France

J.-L. Vincent (ed.), *Annual Update in Intensive Care and Emergency Medicine 2019*, Annual Update in Intensive Care and Emergency Medicine,
https://doi.org/10.1007/978-3-030-06067-1_26

26.2 Potential Mechanisms of Renal Microcirculatory Dysfunction in Sepsis-Induced AKI

Growing evidence suggests that the pathophysiology of septic AKI is multifactorial and that several mechanisms may be involved and may differ between patients [8]. These mechanisms include inflammation, oxidative stress, apoptosis of tubular cells, mitochondrial dysfunction and microvascular dysfunction. A recent review [9] proposed that sepsis-induced AKI is an early clinical and biochemical manifestation of an adaptive response of the tubular cells to an injurious, inflammatory danger signal (damage or pathogen-associated molecular patterns [DAMPs and PAMPs]) that may be magnified by microvascular dysfunction and that, in response, mitochondria within tubular cells orchestrate a complete metabolic downregulation and reprioritization which favors individual cell survival processes at the expense of 'kidney function' (i.e., tubular absorption and secretion of solutes).

The microcirculatory dysfunction leads to heterogeneity of tissue perfusion with low or no flow areas resulting in tissue hypoxia, while other areas have normal or high flow. This microcirculatory dysfunction has been reported independently of the total renal blood flow and an increase in total renal blood flow does not exclude the possibility of microcirculatory dysfunction [10]. In a porcine model of severe sepsis, reduced renal cortex microcirculatory flow occurred well before any changes in renal blood flow were observed [11]. These alterations can persist even after fluid resuscitation despite restoration of systemic hemodynamics [11].

The renal medulla appears to be particularly at risk of tissue hypoxia in sepsis-induced AKI because the medulla does not have a blood supply of its own and receives about 20% of the cortical blood flow from juxtamedullary efferent arterioles. In that respect, intrarenal blood flow redistribution with preserved cortical perfusion but decreased medullary perfusion has been described [10].

Several mechanisms have been proposed to explain the sepsis-induced microcirculatory alterations. Pressure in the glomeruli is tightly controlled through the vascular tone of afferent and efferent arterioles, which are regulated by the myogenic response, the tubuloglomerular feedback, and the balance between vasopressor factors (renal sympathetic nerve, renin-angiotensin-aldosterone system and endothelin) and vasodilatory factors (nitric oxide [NO], adenosine triphosphate [ATP] and prostaglandin). Sepsis may affect renal autoregulation with a decrease in glomerular filtration rate (GFR) through dominant efferent arteriole dilatation (compared to afferent arteriole) and subsequent decrease in glomerular filtration pressure ('intra-glomerular hypotension'). In sepsis-induced AKI, imbalance between vasopressor factors and vasodilator factors affect the flow, the capillary density and the capillary heterogeneity of the kidney microcirculation. For example, Langenberg et al. [12] reported in a sheep model of sepsis that cortical, but not medullary, expression of all NO synthase (NOS) isoforms was increased during sepsis-induced AKI. This selective increase in NOS expression in the cortex may induce intrarenal shunting, whereby blood is shunted away from the medulla during sepsis potentially leading to medullary ischemia. Inflammation increases leukocyte trafficking with an increase in the expression of adhesion molecules and leukocyte-endothelial interactions, resulting in capillary plugging. Sepsis also induces shedding of the glycocalyx with a breakdown of the oncotic pressure gradient, and inflammatory mediators induce disruption of the endothelial barrier with capillary leak, which results in tissue edema with a risk of tissue hypoxia. Indeed, tissue edema can impair tissue oxygenation by increasing the distance required for the diffusion of oxygen to cells and by decreasing microvascular perfusion due to an increase in interstitial pressure.

26.3 New Evidence That Renal Microvascular Alterations Play a Central Role in Sepsis-Induced AKI

The availability of new techniques capable of visualizing the kidney microcirculation is crucial to understand the contribution of renal microvascular alterations in sepsis-induced AKI. In addition, in daily practice we need techniques at the bedside to guide the resuscitation of the renal microcirculation and prevent any occult renal hypoperfusion despite optimization of macrovascular hemodynamic parameters. Several tools have been proposed to investigate renal microcirculatory perfusion at the bedside. Renal Doppler ultrasound measures the variations in intrarenal resistance and has been proposed to assess modification in renal perfusion (renal resistive index [RRI]) after fluid loading [13, 14] or vasopressor administration [15]. However, renal Doppler ultrasound does not directly quantify renal microcirculatory perfusion.

Contrast-enhanced ultrasonography (CEUS) is a recent non-invasive imaging modality enabling visualization and quantification of organ perfusion and microcirculation at the bedside. Renal CEUS has been proposed to quantify kidney microcirculation in patients in various conditions, including renal transplantation [16, 17] or vasopressor administration [18, 19].

CEUS uses microbubble contrast agents, which are composed of microbubbles of an injectable gas in a supporting shell (phospholipids or proteins). Their size (1–6 μm), similar to red blood cells (RBCs), enables the microbubbles to cross the capillary bed of the pulmonary circulation and to flow up to the capillary level of other organs, enabling assessment of their microcirculation (Figs. 26.1 and 26.2). At the same time, their size is large enough to ensure they do not cross the endothelium, making them truly intravascular agents. Ultrasound waves induce a non-linear oscillation of microbubbles and the backscattered signal consequently contains a range of frequencies in addition to that of the incident ultrasound field with a high echogenicity difference between the gas in the microbubbles and the soft tissue. The microbubbles can be injected as a bolus injection or as a constant infusion. When a constant infusion is administered, a 'destruction-replenishment' mode is applied in which higher power ultrasound pulses are used to destroy the bubbles followed by low-power ultrasound pulses to observe replenishment in the tissue. Signal-processing techniques have been developed to separate echoes generated by microbubbles from those generated by tissue. However, the existence of significant variations among animals or patients might be due to individual

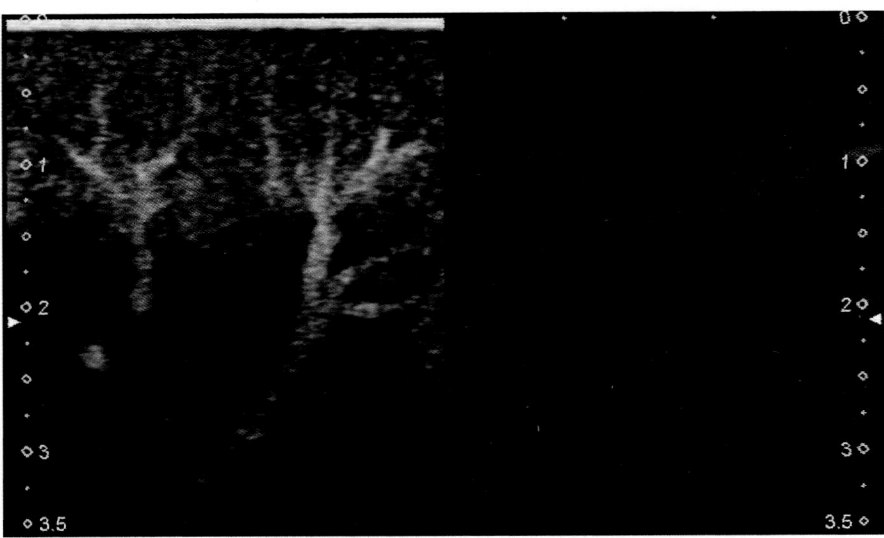

Fig. 26.1 Illustration of images of renal contrast-enhanced ultrasonography (CEUS) in pigs. The left part of the image shows contrast-image mode imaging and the right part the standard (B-mode) image

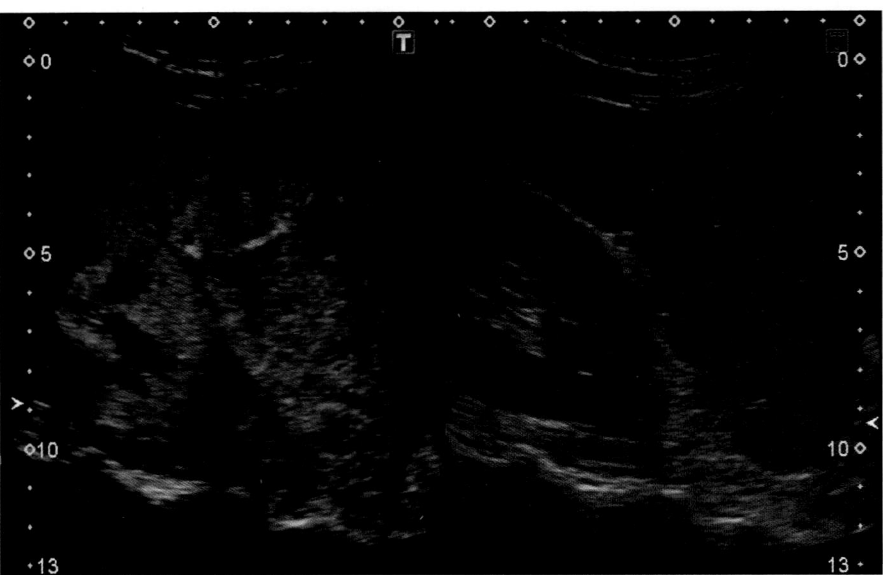

Fig. 26.2 Illustration of images of renal contrast-enhanced ultrasonography (CEUS) in septic shock patients. The left part of the image shows contrast-image mode imaging and the right part the standard (B-mode) image

differences and heterogeneities in the renal microcirculation but could also be related to ultrasound settings. It is of crucial importance that this issue is addressed, since this will identify the best CEUS variables for implementation in routine clinical practice.

Lima et al. [20], in a lipopolysaccharide (LPS)-induced shock model, validated the use of CEUS to identify renal microvascular alterations associated with shock against a recognized methodology for measuring the renal microcirculation: laser speckle imaging [21]. Reduced intrarenal blood flow could be estimated by measuring the microbubble transit times between the interlobar arteries and capillary vessels in the renal cortex. Such microcirculatory alterations were not normalized by fluid resuscitation despite normalization of MAP, central venous pressure (CVP) and cardiac output, probably because of an inflammatory-induced obstruction of the endothelial microcirculation and increased microvascular permeability with accumulation of fluids in the renal tissue (microvascular congestion) and tissue edema.

Schneider et al. [22] were the first authors to test the feasibility of CEUS in the assessment of the renal cortical microcirculation in ICU patients. The authors performed renal CEUS with destruction-replenishment sequences in 12 patients before elective cardiac surgery, on ICU admission and the day following the admission. The first result of this study was that the CEUS technique was safe in ICU patients without deleterious hemodynamic effects (absence of changes in systolic pulmonary pressure after contrast-agent administration). The second result was that when compared with baseline, no overall difference in CEUS-derived parameters (perfusion index, corresponding to the ratio of relative blood volume to mean transit time) was observed on ICU admission. However, 24 h after the operation, there was an overall 50% decrease in the perfusion index, suggestive of decreased renal cortical perfusion. These differences persisted after correction for hemoglobin, vasopressor use and MAP. Four patients developed AKI in the postoperative period. These results complete previous results from Redfors et al. [23] who reported that renal blood flow, measured by the thermodilution technique and the measurement of para-immuno hippurate clearance, was decreased in postcardiac surgery patients (−40%) who developed postoperative AKI despite similar cardiac index and MAP in patients with and without AKI.

Recently, Harrois et al. [24] evaluated cortical renal microcirculation in 20 patients with septic shock within the first 24 h, between 24 and 48 h and after 72 h of care. The first finding of this study was the highly variable renal cortical microcirculation in patients with septic shock despite similar restoration of systemic hemodynamic parameters. Indeed, the renal cortical microperfusion was decreased, normal or even increased during septic shock after restoration of systemic hemodynamic parameters. Thus, this study confirms that given the complex and heterogeneous renal microvascular alterations, it is impossible to predict renal microvascular perfusion based on the restoration of macrohemodynamic data. This requires that we develop bedside techniques capable of visualizing the

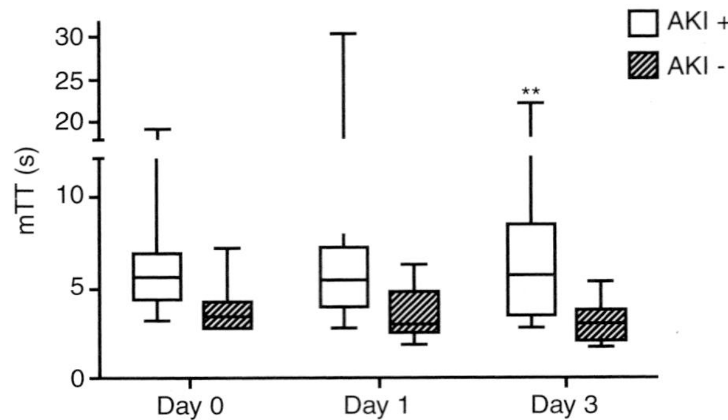

Fig. 26.3 Evolution of mean transit time (mTT) during the first 3 days in the ICU in septic shock patients with acute kidney injury (AKI) KDIGO 2 or 3 (AKI+) or in septic shock patients without AKI or with AKI KDIGO 1 (AKI−). $^{**}p = 0.005$ for group effect (with AKI or without AKI) with ANOVA on ranks. Box plots are median, interquartile (1;3) and maximum values. From [24] with permission

renal microcirculation. The second finding of the study by Harrois et al. [24] was that perfusion of the renal cortex microcirculation was significantly reduced in patients with septic shock developing severe AKI (KDIGO stages 2 or 3) compared to those who did not develop AKI (Fig. 26.3) and compared to a control group of ICU patients without septic shock. For the first time, an association between cortical renal perfusion and the occurrence of severe AKI in patients with septic shock was reported: the greater the alteration in mean transit time measured with CEUS, the higher the risk of severe AKI. This result highlights the central role of renal microvascular alterations in sepsis-induced AKI. In addition, the mean transit time at day 0 had the highest predictive value for severe AKI (area under the curve [AUC] = 0.82 [0.60–1.04]) compared to renal resistive index and cardiac index (Fig. 26.4).

CEUS can also be useful to test the microvascular effects of fluid resuscitation and vasopressor therapy in septic patients. For example, Schneider et al. [19] used CEUS to estimate the effect of an increase in MAP induced by norepinephrine infusion on renal microvascular cortical perfusion in critically ill patients (83% septic shock patients). Overall, there was no difference in perfusion indices measured with CEUS between measurements obtained at baseline with a MAP level of 60–65 mmHg and those obtained after a norepinephrine-induced increase in MAP to reach a MAP of 80–85 mmHg. However, at the individual level, large variations were observed with increase or decrease in kidney microcirculatory perfusion. A tailored MAP target aimed at restoring renal microcirculation based on CEUS parameters presents an interesting perspective.

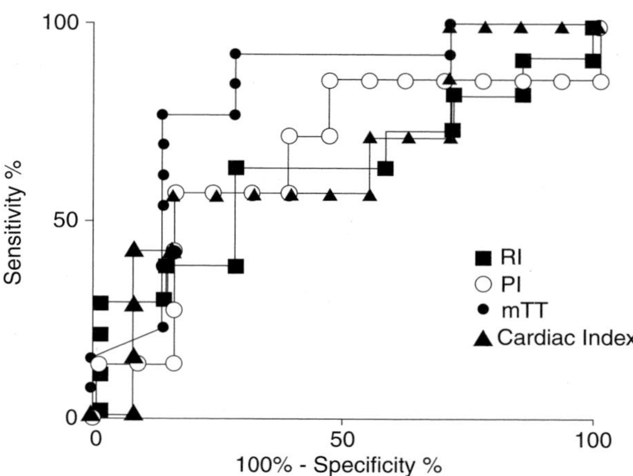

Fig. 26.4 Receiver operating characteristics (ROC) curves for prediction of severe AKI (KDIGO 2 or 3) during the first 72 h with microhemodynamic data (mean transit time [mTT], perfusion index [PI], resistive index [RI]) and macrohemodynamic data (cardiac index). From [24] with permission

26.4 Conclusion

The relative contribution of renal microvascular alterations in the pathophysiology of sepsis-induced AKI remains to be determined for appropriate treatment. The availability of new techniques capable of visualizing the renal microcirculation is crucial. In addition, in daily practice, we need techniques at the bedside to guide the resuscitation of the renal microcirculation and to prevent any occult renal hypoperfusion despite optimization of macrovascular hemodynamic parameters. CEUS is a recent non-invasive imaging modality enabling visualization and quantification of the renal microcirculation at the bedside. Recent results have demonstrated that given the complex and heterogeneous renal microvascular alterations, it is impossible to predict renal microvascular perfusion based on the restoration of macrohemodynamic parameters. In addition, perfusion of the renal cortex microcirculation is significantly reduced in patients with septic shock who develop severe AKI, proving that renal microvascular alterations play a central role in sepsis-induced AKI. The use of renal CEUS to guide renal perfusion resuscitation needs further investigation with larger groups of critically ill patients.

References

1. Sood M, Mandelzweig K, Rigatto C, et al. Non-pulmonary infections but not specific pathogens are associated with increased risk of AKI in septic shock. Intensive Care Med. 2014;40:1080–8.
2. Venot M, Weis L, Clec'h C, et al. Acute kidney injury in severe sepsis and septic shock in patients with and without diabetes mellitus: a multicenter study. PLoS One. 2015;10:e0127411.

3. Kellum JA, Chawla LS, Keener C, et al. The effects of alternative resuscitation strategies on acute kidney injury in patients with septic shock. Am J Respir Crit Care Med. 2016;193:281–7.
4. Nisula S, Kaukonen KM, Vaara ST, et al. Incidence, risk factors and 90-day mortality of patients with acute kidney injury in Finnish intensive care units: the FINNAKI study. Intensive Care Med. 2013;39:420–8.
5. Odutayo A, Wong CX, Farkouh M, et al. AKI and long-term risk for cardiovascular events and mortality. J Am Soc Nephrol. 2017;28:377–87.
6. Post EH, Kellum JA, Bellomo R, Vincent JL. Renal perfusion in sepsis: from macro- to microcirculation. Kidney Int. 2017;91:45–60.
7. Pettila V, Bellomo R. Understanding acute kidney injury in sepsis. Intensive Care Med. 2014;40:1018–20.
8. Langenberg C, Wan L, Egi M, May CN, Bellomo R. Renal blood flow and function during recovery from experimental septic acute kidney injury. Intensive Care Med. 2007;33:1614–8.
9. Gomez H, Ince C, De Backer D, et al. A unified theory of sepsis-induced acute kidney injury: inflammation, microcirculatory dysfunction, bioenergetics, and the tubular cell adaptation to injury. Shock. 2014;41:3–11.
10. Calzavacca P, Evans RG, Bailey M, Bellomo R, May CN. Cortical and medullary tissue perfusion and oxygenation in experimental septic acute kidney injury. Crit Care Med. 2015;43:e431–9.
11. Chvojka J, Sykora R, Krouzecky A, et al. Renal haemodynamic, microcirculatory, metabolic and histopathological responses to peritonitis-induced septic shock in pigs. Crit Care. 2008;12:R164.
12. Langenberg C, Gobe G, Hood S, May CN, Bellomo R. Renal histopathology during experimental septic acute kidney injury and recovery. Crit Care Med. 2014;42:e58–67.
13. Moussa MD, Scolletta S, Fagnoul D, et al. Effects of fluid administration on renal perfusion in critically ill patients. Crit Care. 2015;19:250.
14. Schnell D, Deruddre S, Harrois A, et al. Renal resistive index better predicts the occurrence of acute kidney injury than cystatin C. Shock. 2012;38:592–7.
15. Deruddre S, Cheisson G, Mazoit JX, Vicaut E, Benhamou D, Duranteau J. Renal arterial resistance in septic shock: effects of increasing mean arterial pressure with norepinephrine on the renal resistive index assessed with Doppler ultrasonography. Intensive Care Med. 2007;33:1557–62.
16. Mueller-Peltzer K, Negrao de Figueiredo G, Fischereder M, Habicht A, Rubenthaler J, Clevert DA. Vascular rejection in renal transplant: diagnostic value of contrast-enhanced ultrasound (CEUS) compared to biopsy. Clin Hemorheol Microcirc. 2018;69:77–82.
17. Schwenger V, Korosoglou G, Hinkel UP, et al. Real-time contrast-enhanced sonography of renal transplant recipients predicts chronic allograft nephropathy. Am J Transplant. 2006;6:609–15.
18. Schneider AG, Schelleman A, Goodwin MD, Bailey M, Eastwood GM, Bellomo R. Contrast-enhanced ultrasound evaluation of the renal microcirculation response to terlipressin in hepato-renal syndrome: a preliminary report. Ren Fail. 2015;37:175–9.
19. Schneider AG, Goodwin MD, Schelleman A, Bailey M, Johnson L, Bellomo R. Contrast-enhanced ultrasonography to evaluate changes in renal cortical microcirculation induced by noradrenaline: a pilot study. Crit Care. 2014;18:653.
20. Lima A, van Rooij T, Ergin B, et al. Dynamic contrast-enhanced ultrasound identifies microcirculatory alterations in sepsis-induced acute kidney injury. Crit Care Med. 2018;46:1284–92.
21. Basak K, Manjunatha M, Dutta PK. Review of laser speckle-based analysis in medical imaging. Med Biol Eng Comput. 2012;50:547–58.
22. Schneider AG, Goodwin MD, Schelleman A, Bailey M, Johnson L, Bellomo R. Contrast-enhanced ultrasound to evaluate changes in renal cortical perfusion around cardiac surgery: a pilot study. Crit Care. 2013;17:R138.
23. Redfors B, Bragadottir G, Sellgren J, Sward K, Ricksten SE. Effects of norepinephrine on renal perfusion, filtration and oxygenation in vasodilatory shock and acute kidney injury. Intensive Care Med. 2011;37:60–7.
24. Harrois A, Grillot N, Figueiredo S, Duranteau J. Acute kidney injury is associated with a decrease in cortical renal perfusion during septic shock. Crit Care. 2018;22:161.

Atypical Sepsis-Associated Acute Kidney Injury

27

J. A. Kellum, K. F. Kernan, and J. A. Carcillo

27.1 Introduction: AKI is a Major Public Health Problem and Sepsis-associated AKI is the Most Common Form

The overall incidence of acute kidney injury (AKI) in the USA is estimated to be about 7/1000 population [1]. Older adults and children are disproportionately affected in a bimodal distribution mirroring the incidence of sepsis [2], the leading cause of AKI [3–6]. Even mild forms of AKI are associated with increased risk of hospital mortality [6, 7], and AKI may result in chronic kidney disease and life-long morbidity, shortened survival and increased costs [8]. Moreover, severity of AKI varies by etiology and sepsis-associated AKI tends to be most severe. For example, KDIGO stage 3 occurs in <5% of patients undergoing cardiac surgery, but in >20% of patients with septic shock [9]. Once acquired, the consequences of AKI are also unequally distributed. Approximately one third of patients exhibit no reversal of renal dysfunction within the first few days of AKI. Roughly 25% will never recover, and experience a fivefold increase in mortality over the ensuing year [10]. Even among patients with sepsis-associated AKI, outcomes are heterogeneous and different mechanisms may be involved [11]—indeed, no fewer than six have been

J. A. Kellum (✉)
Center for Critical Care Nephrology, University of Pittsburgh, Pittsburgh, PA, USA

Department of Critical Care Medicine, University of Pittsburgh, Pittsburgh, PA, USA
e-mail: kellumja@upmc.edu

K. F. Kernan
Department of Critical Care Medicine, University of Pittsburgh, Pittsburgh, PA, USA

Children's Hospital of Pittsburgh of UPMC, Pittsburgh, PA, USA

J. A. Carcillo
Center for Critical Care Nephrology, University of Pittsburgh, Pittsburgh, PA, USA

Department of Critical Care Medicine, University of Pittsburgh, Pittsburgh, PA, USA

Children's Hospital of Pittsburgh of UPMC, Pittsburgh, PA, USA

J.-L. Vincent (ed.), *Annual Update in Intensive Care and Emergency Medicine 2019*, Annual Update in Intensive Care and Emergency Medicine,
https://doi.org/10.1007/978-3-030-06067-1_27

proposed [12]. Renal endothelial pathology is prevalent in experimental models of sepsis [12, 13]. Endothelial injury can reduce microcirculatory flow leading to perfusion abnormalities and interstitial infiltration of inflammatory cells [13]. However, the reasons some patients exhibit these pathologic features while others do not are obscure.

27.2 Little is Known About the Underlying Mechanisms of Sepsis-Associated AKI in Humans

Relatively little is known about the underlying mechanisms of AKI in humans and much has been written about the limitations of experimental models [14, 15]. Despite the fact that sepsis is the leading cause of AKI, especially in the critically ill, sepsis-associated AKI is understudied and poorly understood [12]. Pathology from humans with sepsis-associated AKI is limited and there is controversy as to the nature of the histopathology. Takasu and colleagues performed an elegant study comparing 14 kidneys from patients with sepsis to 9 from controls [16]. Rapid bedside postmortem exams were conducted with light and electron microscopy and immunohistochemical staining for markers of cellular injury including kidney injury molecule-1 (KIM-1). Patchy, acute tubular injury was present in 78% of septic kidneys, occurring in 10.3% and 32.3% of corticomedullary-junction tubules by conventional light microscopy and KIM-1 immunostains, respectively. Electron microscopy revealed increased tubular injury in sepsis, including hydropic mitochondria and increased autophagosomes, whereas glomeruli appeared normal [16]. By contrast, Augusto and colleagues performed kidney biopsies on 68 non-transplant patients with AKI (35% with sepsis) and found that 8 patients (12%) had evidence of thrombotic microangiopathy [17].

27.3 Atypical Hemolytic Uremic Syndrome is an Unusual Cause of AKI

Diseases of complement activation, including hemolytic uremic syndrome (HUS) and thrombotic thrombocytopenic purpura (TTP), cause microvascular thrombosis in the kidney and in other organs. The more common form of HUS is caused by strains of bacteria (mainly *Escherichia coli*) producing Shiga toxins (STEC-HUS) [18], whereas an atypical form (aHUS) is associated with genetic or acquired disorders leading to dysregulation of the complement system [19, 20]. Unlike typical HUS, aHUS occurs in the absence of Shiga toxin producing bacterial infection, when atypical infectious, drug or environmental triggers lead to a state of complement dysregulation, the clinical consequence of which is microangiopathy, thrombocytopenia and AKI. Cases can be familial or sporadic, and it is estimated that between 40–60% of cases harbor a rare variant that constitutes a genetic risk for disease [21]. More than 120 mutations affecting various complement components and regulators have been described to date (Table 27.1), accounting for 50–60% of cases—reviewed in Noris et al. [22]. Importantly, aHUS is thought to be an

Table 27.1 Main activators and regulators of the alternative complement pathway and their function with select examples of specific pathogenic variants described in atypical hemolytic uremic syndrome (aHUS)

Name (abbreviations)	Gene symbol	Variant	Amino acid change	MAF	Function
Complement Activators					
Complement component 3 (C3, C3a, C3b, AHUS5)	*C3*	c.784G>T c.1407G>C	p.Gly262Trp p.Glu469Asp	NF[a] 0.00394	The central zymogen of the complement cascade required for classical, alternative and lectin-mediated activation. Its cleavage products C3a and C3b act as direct chemoattractants, and amplification enzymes in the alternative pathway.
Complement factor B (BF, FB, AHUS4)	*CFB*	c.608G>A c.836A>G	p.Arg203Gln p.Asp279Gly	0.0000085 NF[a]	Circulating activating component of alternative pathway. Cleaved by factor D, its catalytic subunit Bb combines with C3b to form the C3bBb alternative pathway C3 convertase.
Complement Regulators					
Membrane cofactor protein (MCP, CD46, AHUS2)	*CD46*	c.1058C>T c.287-2A>G	p.Ala353Val	0.01532 0.00003	Binds C3b on cell surfaces and serves as a cofactor for CFI. Together CFI and CD46 inhibit complement by inactivating C3b deposits on cells.
Complement factor H (FH, CFH, AHUS1)	*CFH*	c.1139C>A c.3148A>T	p.Ser380Ter p.Asn1050Tyr	NF[a] 0.01512	Recognizes C3b and cell surfaces through the C-terminus, whereas the N-terminus mediates cofactor activity for CFI; CFH also directly accelerates the decay of C3-convertase C3b/Bb.
Complement factor I (CFI, FI, AHUS3)	*CFI*	c.1642G>C c.1421G>A	p.Glu548Gln p.Arg474Gln	0.00072 0.0000247	Plasma serine protease that cleaves C3b and C4b, inactivating complement, in the presence of soluble cofactors and/or membrane-bound complement regulators.

(continued)

Table 27.1 (continued)

Name (abbreviations)	Gene symbol	Variant	Amino acid change	MAF	Function
Complement factor H-related proteins (CFHRs)	*CFHR1* *CFHR5*	c.130C>T c.832G>A	p.Gln44Ter p.Gly278Ser	0.00014 0.00729	Secreted proteins of the complement factor H protein family.
Thrombomodulin	*THBD*	c.1456G>T c.127G>A c.1504G>C	p.Asp486Tyr p.Ala43Thr p.Gly502Arg	0.00764 0.00343 0.00227	Anticoagulant; involved in the generation of thrombin-activatable fibrinolysis inhibitor, a plasma carboxypeptidase B that cleaves C3a and C5a; binds to C3b, accelerating its inactivation by CFI in the presence of CFH

MAF minor allele frequency from ExAC. In most cases MAF is <1%

[a]Not found (NF) in ExAC, a population based human sequence database of 60,706 individuals, yielding a MAF of presumably <0.00001. Additional genes of interest include *CFB, CFHR3, CFHR4, PLG* and *DGKE*

extremely rare disease affecting fewer than 1 in a million adults and 3.5 per million children [23]. As a result, the disease is rarely considered, especially in patients with alternative explanations for AKI, thrombocytopenia and multiorgan failure—such as sepsis. We have discovered that more than 20% of patients in our center with sepsis and AKI develop severe thrombocytopenia (<50,000/μl) during their hospital course and yet only about 1% are diagnosed with a TMA disease (e.g., HUS, TTP). Strikingly, we have also identified genetic variation in some adults with septic shock, known to be consistent with aHUS [24] (see below).

27.4 Drug-Associated Thrombocytopenia

Of course, there are many causes of thrombocytopenia in the critically ill, especially in patients with sepsis. Multiple medications can induce thrombocytopenia. However, medications have also been linked to aHUS. In a case-series of for individuals with ticlopidine-associated TMA, complement factor H (CFH) sequencing was performed and three different rare variants were identified: c.2808G>T p.Glu936Asp, c.2850G>T p.Gln950His (ExAC MAF 0.00358), and c.3148A>T p.Asn1050Tyr [25]. The c.3148A>T p.Asn1050Tyr and c.2850G>T p.Gln950His variants have also been associated with aHUS [26–28]. While these disorders are distinct, the occurrence of a shared genetic risk allele emphasizes the pleotropic effects of complement mutations on kidney injury, further supporting a potential role in the pathogenesis of sepsis-associated AKI. In fact, the CFH c.2808G>T p.Glu936Asp variant (ExAC MAF 0.196) and the locus surrounding it plays a key role in determining host sensitivity to invasive meningococcal disease, again providing evidence for the loci's impact in infection [29]. This is likely related to the complement cascade's evolutionary role in the innate immune response. As complement activation is advantageous in pathogen clearance, the p.Glu936Asp variant lowers host-susceptibility to meningococcal infection [29], while concomitantly predisposing to inappropriate triggers in the setting of drug exposure [25] or inability to effectively downregulate the complement cascade once activated in aHUS [27] and potentially sepsis-associated AKI following infection.

27.5 Is It Really Possible that aHUS Is More Prevalent than Currently Thought or that Complement Activation Plays a Role in Some Cases of Sepsis-Associated AKI?

We appreciate that the idea that we are currently missing a critical diagnosis in a small but important number of patients might be seen as an outrageous assertion by some. However, consider the following. First, the ProCESS trial randomized 1351 patients with septic shock to 1 of 3 fluid resuscitation strategies [30]. Over 50% developed AKI [9]. We selected six patients with the highest ferritin levels as a screen for inflammation and performed whole exome sequencing with confirmation by Sanger sequencing [24]. Genetic variants linked to aHUS were seen in 50%, with one patient carrying two mutations (*CD46* c.1058C>T p. Ala353Val and *CFHR5* c.832G>A p.Gly278Ser). All patients were heterozygotes and were asymptomatic prior to developing sepsis (two were >60 years of age and the third was 32 years old). All three patients with aHUS variants had thrombocytopenia and renal dysfunction, but were not diagnosed with HUS or TTP; all three died. Second, more than 20% of patients in our center with sepsis and AKI develop severe thrombocytopenia (<50,000/μl) during their hospital course and yet only about 1% are diagnosed with a TMA disease (e.g., HUS, TTP). Finally, we found that diagnostic workups for these diseases occurred in relatively few patients, the majority of which were positive suggesting that the conditions are not being considered frequently enough. Even if our genetic screen found every patient with aHUS in the ProCESS cohort, the event rate would still be nearly 0.5% of patients with sepsis and AKI. For the US population this would translate to 9 per million adults per year—nearly 10 times the current estimate. Given that the condition is treatable and frequently progresses to death or end-stage renal disease without therapy, a substantial impact on outcome is possible.

27.6 New Treatments for Sepsis-Associated AKI Are Urgently Needed and Treatments Targeting Complement Activation are Currently Available with Several New Drugs in Development

Over the last 30 years, attempts to improve outcomes for patients with AKI have targeted hemodynamics [31–33], diuretics (including natriuretic peptides) [34, 35] and oxidative stress [36]. All have been failures [37]. One explanation for the failure to advance therapies is the flawed conceptual model that considers AKI a uniform disease. In reality, AKI is a loose collection of syndromes each with its own specific pathobiology [11, 38]. Our hypothesis is that even within a specific etiologic-subtype of AKI (i.e., sepsis), alternative molecular mechanisms exist. We hope that in isolating individuals with the TMA phenotype with a genetic variant associated with complement dysregulation, specific targeted therapy will be possible. For aHUS, paroxysmal nocturnal hemoglobinuria as well as other disorders characterized by hyperactive complement including age-related macular degeneration, myocardial infarction, ischemia reperfusion injury and autoimmune disorders [39, 40], complement activation is a viable drug target and several therapies are in the development pipeline [22]. Plasma exchange and eculizumab can both be used at present, but several other agents are being tested. Unlike eculizumab, some of these agents are small molecules, with the potentiality of oral bioavailability, lower costs and decreased immunogenicity [41]. Some of the compounds under development have more upstream targets than does eculizumab, acting at the level of C3. These compounds could theoretically be more effective by providing more complete complement blockade, while compounds targeting C5 and its activation products could be safer at the expense of reduced effectiveness due to unchecked upstream complement activation. In any case, no fewer than 15 compounds are in development [22] providing a rich pipeline for potential agents.

27.7 Other Advantages of Genetic Testing

Identification of the specific genetic defect carries crucial prognostic information in aHUS. CFH mutations are associated with the worst prognosis, with 70–80% of patients progressing to end-stage renal disease or dying, and a high prevalence of post-transplantation recurrences. At the other end of the spectrum are patients with membrane cofactor protein mutations, who rarely develop end-stage renal disease and, if they do so, have excellent transplant outcomes [19]. In addition, other diseases may be discovered in patients with sepsis, AKI and thrombocytopenia. In around 5% of cases of TTP, the enzyme deficiency is congenital owing to homozygous or compound heterozygous mutations in ADAMTS13 [42]. Rarely, this form of TTP first manifests in adulthood [43]. Other syndromes and mechanisms may be operating in these patients as well. For example, we recently reported on the role of Tie2 disruption as a sentinel event in septic disseminated intravascular dissemination (DIC) [44]. In endotoxemic mice, reduced Tie2 signaling preceded signs of overt DIC. Conversely, Tie2 activation normalized prothrombotic responses by inhibiting endothelial tissue factor and phosphatidylserine exposure. Mutations in *TEK* genes have been described, serving as an alternative target for investigation.

27.8 Conclusion

Despite its common occurrence in critically ill patients, little is understood about the mechanisms underlying sepsis-associated AKI and no specific treatments are available. aHUS is an acknowledged exception where mechanisms are known with targeted therapy available. However, aHUS is believed to be very rare. Recent findings challenge this assumption and we ask whether aHUS may explain more cases of sepsis-associated AKI than previously thought (perhaps as high as 5–10%). If confirmed, the treatment for sepsis-associated AKI and subsequent outcomes would be radically changed for this subgroup. Perhaps it would even change the treatment paradigm for sepsis-associated AKI in general by removing these patients from other treatment protocols and introducing genetic testing as a common management tool for patients with sepsis-associated AKI. Only the future will tell.

References

1. Al-Jaghbeer M, DeAlmeida D, Bilderback A, Ambrosino R, Kellum JA. Clinical decision support for in-hospital AKI. J Am Soc Nephrol. 2018;29:654–60.
2. Angus DC, Linde-Zwirble WT, Lidicker J, Clermont G, Carcillo J, Pinsky MR. Epidemiology of severe sepsis in the United States: analysis of incidence, outcome, and associated costs of care. Crit Care Med. 2001;29:1303–10.
3. Hoste EA, Bagshaw SM, Bellomo R, et al. Epidemiology of acute kidney injury in critically ill patients: the multinational AKI-EPI study. Intensive Care Med. 2015;41:1411–23.
4. Bagshaw SM, George C, Dinu I, Bellomo R. A multi-centre evaluation of the RIFLE criteria for early acute kidney injury in critically ill patients. Nephrol Dial Transplant. 2007;23:1203–10.
5. Uchino S, Kellum JA, Bellomo R, et al. Acute renal failure in critically ill patients: a multinational, multicenter study. JAMA. 2005;294:813.
6. Murugan R, Karajala-Subramanyam V, Lee M, et al. Acute kidney injury in non-severe pneumonia is associated with an increased immune response and lower survival. Kidney Int. 2010;77:527–35.
7. Sileanu FE, Murugan R, Lucko N, et al. AKI in Low-risk versus high-risk patients in intensive care. Clin J Am Soc Nephrol. 2015;10:187–96.
8. Chawla LS, Eggers PW, Star RA, Kimmel PL. Acute kidney injury and chronic kidney disease as interconnected syndromes. N Engl J Med. 2014;371:58–66.
9. Kellum JA, Chawla LS, Keener C, et al. The effects of alternative resuscitation strategies on acute kidney injury in patients with septic shock. Am J Respir Crit Care Med. 2016;193:281–7.
10. Kellum JA, Sileanu FE, Bihorac A, Hoste EA, Chawla LS. Recovery after acute kidney injury. Am J Respir Crit Care Med. 2017;195:784–91.
11. Kellum JA, Prowle JR. Paradigms of acute kidney injury in the intensive care setting. Nat Rev Nephrol. 2018;14:217–30.
12. Gomez H, Ince C, De Backer D, et al. A unified theory of sepsis-induced acute kidney injury: inflammation, microcirculatory dysfunction, bioenergetics, and the tubular cell adaptation to injury. Shock. 2014;41:3–11.
13. Post EH, Kellum JA, Bellomo R, Vincent JL. Renal perfusion in sepsis: from macro- to microcirculation. Kidney Int. 2017;91:45–60.
14. Agarwal A, Dong Z, Harris R, et al. Cellular and molecular mechanisms of AKI. J Am Soc Nephrol. 2016;27(5):1288–99.
15. Rabb H, Griffin MD, McKay DB, et al. Inflammation in AKI: current understanding, key questions, and knowledge gaps. J Am Soc Nephrol. 2016;27(2):371–9.
16. Takasu O, Gaut JP, Watanabe E, et al. Mechanisms of cardiac and renal dysfunction in patients dying of sepsis. Am J Respir Crit Care Med. 2013;187:509–17.
17. Augusto JF, Lassalle V, Fillatre P, et al. Safety and diagnostic yield of renal biopsy in the intensive care unit. Intensive Care Med. 2012;38:1826–33.
18. Tarr PI, Gordon CA, Chandler WL. Shiga-toxin-producing Escherichia coli and haemolytic uraemic syndrome. Lancet. 2005;365:1073–86.
19. Noris M, Remuzzi G. Atypical hemolytic-uremic syndrome. N Engl J Med. 2009;361:1676–87.
20. Kavanagh D, Goodship T. Genetics and complement in atypical HUS. Pediatr Nephrol. 2010;25:2431–42.

21. Osborne AJ, Breno M, Borsa NG, et al. Statistical validation of rare complement variants provides insights into the molecular basis of atypical hemolytic uremic syndrome and C3 glomerulopathy. J Immunol. 2018;200:2464–78.
22. Noris M, Mescia F, Remuzzi G. STEC-HUS, atypical HUS and TTP are all diseases of complement activation. Nat Rev Nephrol. 2012;8:622–33.
23. Zimmerhackl LB, Besbas N, Jungraithmayr T, et al. Epidemiology, clinical presentation, and pathophysiology of atypical and recurrent hemolytic uremic syndrome. Semin Thromb Hemost. 2006;32:113–20.
24. Kernan KF, Ghaloul-Gonzalez L, Shakoory B, Kellum JA, Angus DC, Carcillo JA. Adults with septic shock and extreme hyperferritinemia exhibit pathogenic immune variation. Genes Immun. 2018; Jul 6. https://doi.org/10.1038/s41435-018-0030-3. [Epub ahead of print].
25. Chapin J, Eyler S, Smith R, Tsai HM, Laurence J. Complement factor H mutations are present in ADAMTS13-deficient, ticlopidine-associated thrombotic microangiopathies. Blood. 2013;121:4012–3.
26. Besbas N, Gulhan B, Soylemezoglu O, et al. Turkish pediatric atypical hemolytic uremic syndrome registry: initial analysis of 146 patients. BMC Nephrol. 2017;18:6.
27. Caprioli J, Castelletti F, Bucchioni S, et al. Complement factor H mutations and gene polymorphisms in haemolytic uraemic syndrome: the C-257T, the A2089G and the G2881T polymorphisms are strongly associated with the disease. Hum Mol Genet. 2003;12:3385–95.
28. Le Quintrec M, Lionet A, Kamar N, et al. Complement mutation-associated de novo thrombotic microangiopathy following kidney transplantation. Am J Transplant. 2008;8:1694–701.
29. Davila S, Wright VJ, Khor CC, et al. Genome-wide association study identifies variants in the CFH region associated with host susceptibility to meningococcal disease. Nat Genet. 2010;42:772–6.
30. Yealy DM, Kellum JA, Huang DT, et al. A randomized trial of protocol-based care for early septic shock. N Engl J Med. 2014;370:1683–93.
31. Kellum JA, M Decker J. Use of dopamine in acute renal failure: a meta-analysis. Crit Care Med. 2001;29:1526–31.
32. Bove T, Zangrillo A, Guarracino F, et al. Effect of fenoldopam on use of renal replacement therapy among patients with acute kidney injury after cardiac surgery: a randomized clinical trial. JAMA. 2014;312:2244–53.
33. Murugan R, Kellum JA. Natriuretic peptides, acute kidney injury, and clinical evidence. Crit Care Med. 2008;36:996–8.
34. Ho KM, Power BM. Benefits and risks of furosemide in acute kidney injury. Anaesthesia. 2010;65:283–93.
35. Allgren RL, Marbury TC, Rahman SN, et al. Anaritide in acute tubular necrosis. N Engl J Med. 1997;336:828–34.
36. Ho KM, Morgan DJR. Meta-analysis of N-acetylcysteine to prevent acute renal failure after major surgery. Am J Kidney Dis. 2009;53:33–40.
37. Winkelmayer WC, Finkel KW. Prevention of acute kidney injury using vasoactive or antiplatelet treatment. JAMA. 2014;312:2221.
38. Kellum JA. Why are patients still getting and dying from acute kidney injury? Curr Opin Crit Care. 2016;22:513–9.
39. Ricklin D, Lambris JD. Complement-targeted therapeutics. Nat Biotechnol. 2007;25:1265–75.
40. Thurman JM, Le Quintrec M. Targeting the complement cascade: novel treatments coming down the pike. Kidney Int. 2016;90:746–52.
41. Woodruff TM, Nandakumar KS, Tedesco F. Inhibiting the C5-C5a receptor axis. Mol Immunol. 2011;48:1631–42.
42. Levy GG, Nichols WC, Lian EC, et al. Mutations in a member of the ADAMTS gene family cause thrombotic thrombocytopenic purpura. Nature. 2001;413:488–94.
43. Donadelli R, Banterla F, Galbusera M, et al. In-vitro and in-vivo consequences of mutations in the von Willebrand factor cleaving protease ADAMTS13 in thrombotic thrombocytopenic purpura. Thromb Haemost. 2006;96:454–64.
44. Higgins SJ, De Ceunynck K, Kellum JA, et al. Tie2 protects the vasculature against thrombus formation in systemic inflammation. J Clin Invest. 2018;128:1471–84.

Latest Developments in Perioperative Acute Kidney Injury

28

M. Meersch and A. Zarbock

28.1 Introduction

Acute kidney injury (AKI) is defined as an abrupt loss of kidney function occurring within hours to days. The scope of AKI ranges from subclinical to severe, dialysis-requiring AKI and from a reversible to an irreversible syndrome. This elucidates why finding the optimal management strategy for patients at high risk of developing of AKI is so challenging.

Sepsis, extended surgical procedures and nephrotoxic agents are the most common causes of AKI. Hence, it is not surprising that AKI is a frequent complication in the intensive care unit (ICU). Since the development of the various consensus criteria, awareness of this serious, life restricting complication has increased. The current Kidney Disease: Improving Global Outcomes (KDIGO) diagnostic criteria are based on urine output and/or serum creatinine (Box 28.1). These criteria reflect the fact that even mild changes in renal function are associated with adverse outcomes. However, both these markers have important limitations that need to be considered in clinical routine including the inability of providing an early diagnosis. However, early identification of high-risk patients is indispensable to effectively initiate preemptive strategies. New biomarkers can detect patients at high risk for the development of AKI suffering from kidney stress prior to changes in renal function. There are further clinical situations that might alter the risk for AKI in the perioperative period.

M. Meersch · A. Zarbock (✉)
Department of Anesthesiology, Intensive Care and Pain Medicine, University of Münster, Münster, Germany
e-mail: zarbock@uni-muenster.de

J.-L. Vincent (ed.), *Annual Update in Intensive Care and Emergency Medicine 2019*, Annual Update in Intensive Care and Emergency Medicine,
https://doi.org/10.1007/978-3-030-06067-1_28

Box 28.1 The Kidney Disease: Improving Global Outcomes (KDIGO) Staging Criteria For Acute Kidney Injury (AKI)

1. **AKI is defined as**
   - Increase in serum creatinine ≥0.3 mg/dL (26.5 μmol/L) within 48 h, OR
   - Increase in serum creatinine by ≥1.5-fold above baseline, known or presumed to have occurred within the last 7 days, OR
   - Urine volume <0.5 mL/kg/h for 6 h
2. **AKI severity is staged by the worst of either serum creatinine or oliguria**

Stage	Serum creatinine	Urine output
1	≥1.5 to 1.9 times baseline OR >0.3 mg/dL (26.5 μmol/L) increase	<0.5 mL/kg/h for 6–12 h
2	≥2.0 to 2.9 times baseline	<0.5 mL/kg/h for ≥12 h
3	≥3.0 times baseline OR Increase in serum creatinine to ≥4.0 mg/dL (353.6 μmol/L) OR RRT OR In patients <18 year, decrease in eGFR to <35 mL/min/1.73 m^2	<0.3 mL/kg/h for ≥24 h OR Anuria for ≥12 h

eGFR estimated glomerular filtration rate; *RRT* renal replacement therapy

28.2 Oliguria and the Effects of Fluids

28.2.1 Oliguria

Oliguria, when present long enough, can be a response to acute tubular necrosis or acute kidney injury. However, there are a large number of other reasons for oliguria, ranging from a maladaptive response to end-stage liver disease to congestive heart failure or a response to hypovolemia. The reliability of intraoperative urine output as a surrogate marker is frequently debated since other factors such as hemodynamic variability, e.g., due to anesthetic agents as well as hormone levels might alter the risk for oliguria and are not necessarily a result of renal dysfunction.

Isolated oliguria-based AKI has been shown to be more commonly associated with less severe adverse outcomes compared to isolated serum creatinine-based AKI [1–3]. However, recently a single center retrospective trial demonstrated that intraoperative oliguria was associated with the development of AKI, especially in patients with oliguria lasting more than 120 min [4]. The results of a logistic regression analysis showed that the odds for AKI increased significantly with the duration of oliguria (odds ratio [OR] 12.4 for patients with ≥300 min oliguria; $p < 0.001$) [4]. In another trial analyzing 320 living donors for liver transplantation, it was demonstrated that oliguria-based AKI was associated with adverse outcomes [5]. The results showed significantly increased ICU and hospital days, and a lower chronic kidney disease-free survival rate at day 90 in patients with isolated oliguria-based AKI as compared to patients with serum creatinine-based AKI. These studies highlight that oliguria-based AKI must not be underestimated because there appears to be an association with adverse outcomes.

28.2.2 Fluid Therapy

The administration of intravenous crystalloids in the perioperative period plays a crucial role to maintain hydration and to increase intravascular volume. However, it has been shown that the type of fluid may have an impact on the occurrence of AKI. 'Physiological' saline (0.9% sodium chloride) is still frequently used although it is known that it contains unphysiologically high sodium concentrations. With increasing doses, the risk of hyperchloremic acidosis with subsequent renal dysfunction caused by renal vasoconstriction has been described [6]. In non-cardiac surgical patients, it was demonstrated that approximately 22% of patients suffered from hyperchloremia [7] and that severe hyperchloremia was associated with an increased incidence of AKI [7, 8]. Recently published trials showed that the use of saline solutions resulted in a higher occurrence of the composite outcome consisting of death, persistent renal dysfunction or renal replacement therapy (RRT) compared with balanced crystalloids [9]. On the other hand, data from a further large randomized controlled trial (RCT) including 2278 critically ill patients showed no significant reduction in the occurrence of AKI if buffered solutions were used compared to saline administration (9.6% vs. 9.2%, $p = 0.77$) [10]. To date, it remains unclear whether balanced solutions are superior to saline regarding the occurrence of AKI. In addition, the amount of fluid administered might play a pivotal role. Several studies in critically ill patients have shown that fluid overload is associated with the development of organ edema which may lead to AKI and worsening of preexisting AKI [11, 12]. Since hypovolemia as well as hypervolemia are associated with increased morbidity and mortality, it appears reasonable to consider the application of intraoperative diuretics in hypervolemic situations. However, the KDIGO guidelines recommend the use of diuretics only for managing severe fluid overload and not for the prevention of AKI [13]. There is an association between the use and the dose of diuretics and the development of AKI, especially in patients with preexisting renal dysfunction so that they cannot be recommended [14].

28.2.3 Fluid Balance

The effect of intraoperative fluid balance has been investigated in several clinical trials. The underlying assumption is that intraoperative volume expansion improves hemodynamics including renal perfusion with less occurrence of AKI. Recently, the effect of two intraoperative fluid strategies (liberal 8–10 mL/kg/h vs. restrictive 2–4 mL/kg/h) on urine output has been investigated in patients undergoing

Box 28.2 Risk Factors for Acute Kidney Injury

Preoperative factors	Perioperative factors	Other factors
• Female • Congestive heart failure • Mechanical assist devices • Chronic kidney disease • IDDM • COPD • Age >70 years	• Hemodynamic instability • Cardiopulmonary bypass • Infection • Sepsis • MODS • Extended surgical procedures • Hypervolemia	• Antibiotics (amphotericin, aminoglycosides, vancomycin • Nephrotoxic agents (e.g., radiocontrast media) • Transfusion • Hyperchloremic fluids

IDDM insulin dependent diabetes mellitus; *MODS* multiorgan dysfunction syndrome; *COPD* chronic obstructive pulmonary disease

laparoscopic procedures [15, 16]. No difference in intraoperative urine output and in the occurrence of AKI was detected. However, these results were based on patients undergoing laparoscopic procedures in which an altered distribution of intravenous fluids might be the underlying cause for the results. In other clinical settings, e.g., abdominal surgery, a recently performed large RCT demonstrated that a restrictive fluid therapy providing a net zero fluid balance was associated with lower intraoperative urine output and with an increased occurrence of serum creatinine-based AKI in patients at high risk for perioperative complications [17]. Moreover, the risk of needing RRT was significantly higher in the restrictive group as compared to the liberal group (hazard ratio [HR] 3.27, 95% CI 1.01–2.85, $p = 0.048$).

In conclusion, isolated oliguria-based AKI is as important as serum creatinine-based AKI and should be critically appraised. There is evidence that buffered solutions are superior to saline solutions. However, the amount of crystalloids administered plays a pivotal role and the fluid management strategy needs to be individualized according to the patient's underlying condition (Box 28.2).

28.3 Preemptive Strategies

Realizing that it is too late to initiate preemptive strategies when changes in the two functional biomarkers, serum creatinine and urine output, become apparent, led to a new understanding of AKI.

Several studies have demonstrated that new renal biomarkers can detect 'subclinical AKI', kidney damage without or prior to a loss of renal function [18]. These biomarkers are able to detect AKI much earlier. However, the performance of the biomarkers has varied depending on the patient population. In a well-defined setting of AKI, i.e., in patients undergoing cardiac surgery, the performance of these

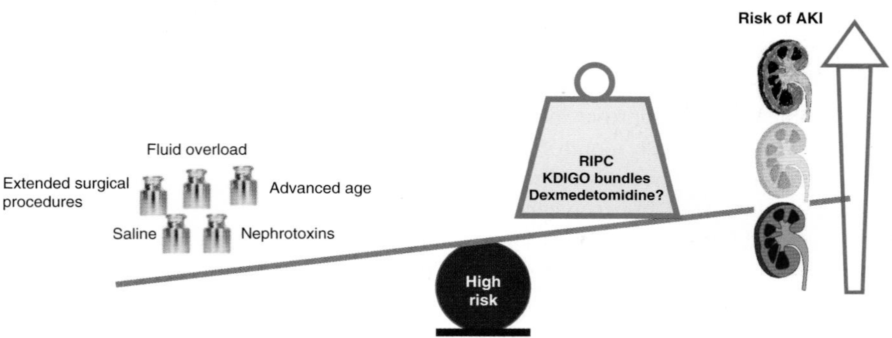

Fig. 28.1 Risk factors for acute kidney injury (AKI) and preemptive strategies. *RIPC* remote ischemic preconditioning; *KDIGO* Kidney Disease: Improving Global Outcomes

markers was very good [19], whereas in a heterogeneous patient population with a variable onset of AKI, biomarker performance was reduced [20]. Consequently, the "renal angina" concept was introduced, which combines clinical conditions, comorbidities and biomarkers. This significantly improved the negative predictive value of these markers [21].

There are some preventive measures that can protect the kidneys from an acute loss of kidney function (Fig. 28.1).

28.3.1 Remote Ischemic Preconditioning

Remote ischemic preconditioning is a simple and safe intervention with organ protective properties. It consists of transient episodes of sublethal ischemia and reperfusion injury to a remote tissue or organ before the subsequent injury occurs. Typically, remote ischemic preconditioning is performed by inflating a blood pressure cuff on the upper arm to 200 mmHg (or 50 mmHg higher than the systolic blood pressure) for several minutes to produce ischemia followed by a cuff deflation to mimic reperfusion. These cycles are repeated several times. The underlying protective mechanisms are unclear but the release of damage associated molecular patterns and the induction of cell cycle arrest with the release of cell cycle arrest markers seem to play a pivotal role.

Several trials have shown the renoprotective effects of remote ischemic preconditioning after surgery [22, 23] whereas other studies showed no effects [24, 25]. Different trial designs, different endpoints and the heterogeneity of the patient cohorts make it hard to compare the results. However, when deciding whether to implement remote ischemic preconditioning, it is important to note that some substances have a preconditioning-blocking effect (e.g., propofol) and therefore protective effects are mitigated [26–28]. Remote ischemic preconditioning remains a simple, economical and uneventful procedure and should consequently be considered as a preemptive strategy in high-risk patients.

28.3.2 KDIGO Bundles

According to the KDIGO guidelines, in patients at high risk for the development of AKI a bundle of supportive measures should be implemented. These supportive measures include close monitoring of serum creatinine and urine output, discontinuation and avoidance of nephrotoxic agents, use of alternatives to radio contrast agents, avoidance of hyperglycemia, maintenance of volume status and perfusion pressure, and functional hemodynamic monitoring [13]. A recently performed RCT analyzed whether this bundle truly affects the occurrence of AKI in patients undergoing cardiac surgery [29]. High-risk patients were defined as patients with elevated levels of biomarkers that have previously been shown to predict the occurrence of AKI [30]. The high-risk group showed an AKI incidence of 71.7% whereas in the low-risk group the incidence was only 21% indicating that this biomarker-based approach selected patients at high risk. Patients with high biomarker levels were randomly allocated to receive either strict implementation of the KDIGO bundle, including a predefined hemodynamic algorithm, or standard care. Patients in the intervention group had a significantly lower incidence of AKI compared to controls (absolute risk reduction 16.6%, 95% CI 5.5%–27.9%, $p = 0.004$). Additionally, a further trial on high-risk patients undergoing major abdominal surgery showed that optimizing fluid status using a predefined bundle reduced the incidence of moderate and severe AKI and reduced ICU and hospital lengths of stay [31].

Although most clinicians believe that some of the supportive measures recommended by the KDIGO guidelines are already implemented in every patient (e.g., avoidance of hyperglycemia, avoidance of nephrotoxic agents), the literature tells a different story. For example, hyperglycemia is a common complication after cardiac surgery. An occurrence rate of up to 74% in non-diabetic patients has been reported [32] reflecting that standard treatment may not be as good as expected. Moreover, some of the measures recommended, such as the implementation of functional hemodynamic monitoring which often implies invasive monitoring, cannot be recommended for every patient due to the associated risks.

In conclusion, in high-risk patients undergoing major surgery, close monitoring of metabolic and renal status and optimization of hemodynamics via functional hemodynamic monitoring to ensure perfusion pressure should be enforced.

28.3.3 Pharmacologic Options

Several pharmacologic options have been analyzed to protect the kidneys from injury. Statins, which are mainly used to reduce cholesterol levels to prevent cardiovascular disease, have been assumed to reduce the occurrence of AKI due to their pleiotropic effects. However, the most recent data in statin naïve cardiac surgery patients showed no benefit for patients receiving high-dose statin treatment with atorvastatin compared to patients receiving placebo [33]. The same was true for patients under pretreatment with statins where no reduction in the occurrence of AKI could be detected in patients receiving additional statin administration compared to placebo [33]. Additionally, in the ICU setting, especially in patients with community-acquired pneumonia, no effect of statins on the incidence of AKI could be detected resulting in the conclusion that there is no evidence for the preemptive use of statins.

Dexmedetomidine, a highly selective alpha-2 agonist that is commonly used in the ICU setting, has been shown to provide cytoprotection after renal ischemia and to ameliorate hypoxemia-induced apoptosis in proximal tubular epithelial cells in animal studies [34, 35]. In the clinical setting, several trials have focused on cardiac surgical patients. A recently performed meta-analysis analyzing the effects of dexmedetomidine on the prevention of cardiac surgery-associated AKI showed that overall dexmedetomidine was associated with a significantly reduced incidence of AKI compared to controls (relative risk 0.44, 95% CI 0.26–0.76, p = 0.003) [36]. However, currently there are only three RCTs with a relatively small patient cohort available. Therefore, due to the low evidence, a general recommendation for the use of dexmedetomidine for preventing AKI cannot be proposed.

28.4 Conclusion

AKI is an independent risk factor for worse outcomes. Warning signals, such as elevated biomarker levels or oliguria, should be recognized. Reducing the use of nephrotoxins and avoidance of hyperglycemia is recommended for every patient. In high-risk patients, the implementation of supportive measures as recommended by the KDIGO guidelines reduces the occurrence of AKI and should be considered. A multimodal approach including a strategy of risk assessment and risk identification seems to be a reasonable procedure.

References

1. Jin K, Murugan R, Sileanu FE, et al. Intensive monitoring of urine output is associated with increased detection of acute kidney injury and improved outcomes. Chest. 2017;152:972–9.
2. Kellum JA, Sileanu FE, Murugan R, Lucko N, Shaw AD, Clermont G. Classifying AKI by urine output versus serum creatinine level. J Am Soc Nephrol. 2015;26:2231–8.
3. Gameiro J, Neves JB, Rodrigues N, et al. Acute kidney injury, long-term renal function and mortality in patients undergoing major abdominal surgery: a cohort analysis. Clin Kidney J. 2016;9:192–200.
4. Shiba A, Uchino S, Fujii T, Takinami M, Uezono S. Association between intraoperative oliguria and acute kidney injury after major noncardiac surgery. Anesth Analg. 2018;127:1229–35.
5. Mizota T, Minamisawa S, Imanaka Y, Fukuda K. Oliguria without serum creatinine increase after living donor liver transplantation is associated with adverse post-operative outcomes. Acta Anaesthesiol Scand. 2016;60:874–81.
6. Bullivant EM, Wilcox CS, Welch WJ. Intrarenal vasoconstriction during hyperchloremia: role of thromboxane. Am J Physiol. 1989;256:F152–7.
7. McCluskey SA, Karkouti K, Wijeysundera D, Minkovich L, Tait G, Beattie WS. Hyperchloremia after noncardiac surgery is independently associated with increased morbidity and mortality: a propensity-matched cohort study. Anesth Analg. 2013;117:412–21.

8. Marttinen M, Wilkman E, Petaja L, Suojaranta-Ylinen R, Pettila V, Vaara ST. Association of plasma chloride values with acute kidney injury in the critically ill - a prospective observational study. Acta Anaesthesiol Scand. 2016;60:790–9.
9. Semler MW, Self WH, Wang L, et al. Balanced crystalloids versus saline in the intensive care unit: study protocol for a cluster-randomized, multiple-crossover trial. Trials. 2017;18:129.
10. Young P, Bailey M, Beasley R, et al. Effect of a buffered crystalloid solution vs saline on acute kidney injury among patients in the intensive care unit: The SPLIT randomized clinical trial. JAMA. 2015;314:1701–10.
11. Teixeira C, Garzotto F, Piccinni P, et al. Fluid balance and urine volume are independent predictors of mortality in acute kidney injury. Crit Care. 2013;17:R14.
12. Payen D, de Pont AC, Sakr Y, et al. A positive fluid balance is associated with a worse outcome in patients with acute renal failure. Crit Care. 2008;12:R74.
13. KDIGO. KDIGO clinical practice guideline for acute kidney injury. Kidney Int Suppl. 2012;2:1–138.
14. Wu X, Zhang W, Ren H, Chen X, Xie J, Chen N. Diuretics associated acute kidney injury: clinical and pathological analysis. Ren Fail. 2014;36:1051–5.
15. Matot I, Paskaleva R, Eid L, et al. Effect of the volume of fluids administered on intraoperative oliguria in laparoscopic bariatric surgery: a randomized controlled trial. Arch Surg. 2012;147:228–34.
16. Matot I, Dery E, Bulgov Y, Cohen B, Paz J, Nesher N. Fluid management during video-assisted thoracoscopic surgery for lung resection: a randomized, controlled trial of effects on urinary output and postoperative renal function. J Thorac Cardiovasc Surg. 2013;146:461–6.
17. Myles PS, Bellomo R, Corcoran T, et al. Restrictive versus liberal fluid therapy for major abdominal surgery. N Engl J Med. 2018;378:2263–74.
18. Ronco C, Kellum JA, Haase M. Subclinical AKI is still AKI. Crit Care. 2012;16:313.
19. Meersch M, Schmidt C, Van Aken H, et al. Urinary TIMP-2 and IGFBP7 as early biomarkers of acute kidney injury and renal recovery following cardiac surgery. PLoS One. 2014;9:e93460.
20. Golden D, Corbett J, Forni LG. Peri-operative renal dysfunction: prevention and management. Anaesthesia. 2016;71(Suppl 1):51–7.
21. Goldstein SL, Chawla LS. Renal angina. Clin J Am Soc Nephrol. 2010;5:943–9.
22. Zimmerman RF, Ezeanuna PU, Kane JC, et al. Ischemic preconditioning at a remote site prevents acute kidney injury in patients following cardiac surgery. Kidney Int. 2011;80:861–7.
23. Zarbock A, Schmidt C, Van Aken H, et al. Effect of remote ischemic preconditioning on kidney injury among high-risk patients undergoing cardiac surgery: a randomized clinical trial. JAMA. 2015;313:2133–41.
24. Meybohm P, Bein B, Brosteanu O, et al. A multicenter trial of remote ischemic preconditioning for heart surgery. N Engl J Med. 2015;373:1397–407.
25. Hausenloy DJ, Candilio L, Evans R, et al. Remote ischemic preconditioning and outcomes of cardiac surgery. N Engl J Med. 2015;373:1408–17.
26. Behmenburg F, van Caster P, Bunte S, et al. Impact of anesthetic regimen on remote ischemic preconditioning in the rat heart in vivo. Anesth Analg. 2018;126:1377–80.
27. Kottenberg E, Thielmann M, Bergmann L, et al. Protection by remote ischemic preconditioning during coronary artery bypass graft surgery with isoflurane but not propofol - a clinical trial. Acta Anaesthesiol Scand. 2012;56:30–8.
28. Ney J, Hoffmann K, Meybohm P, et al. Remote ischemic preconditioning does not affect the release of humoral factors in propofol-anesthetized cardiac surgery patients: a secondary analysis of the RIPHeart study. Int J Mol Sci. 2018;19:1094.
29. Meersch M, Schmidt C, Hoffmeier A, et al. Prevention of cardiac surgery-associated AKI by implementing the KDIGO guidelines in high risk patients identified by biomarkers: the PrevAKI randomized controlled trial. Intensive Care Med. 2017;3:1551–61.
30. Kashani K, Al-Khafaji A, Ardiles T, et al. Discovery and validation of cell cycle arrest biomarkers in human acute kidney injury. Crit Care. 2013;17:R25.
31. Gocze I, Koch M, Renner P, et al. Urinary biomarkers TIMP-2 and IGFBP7 early predict acute kidney injury after major surgery. PLoS One. 2015;10:e0120863.

32. Garg R, Grover A, McGurk S, Rawn JD. Predictors of hyperglycemia after cardiac surgery in nondiabetic patients. J Thorac Cardiovasc Surg. 2013;145:1083–7.
33. Billings FT, Hendricks PA, Schildcrout JS, et al. High-dose perioperative atorvastatin and acute kidney injury following cardiac surgery: a randomized clinical trial. JAMA. 2016;315:877–88.
34. Gu J, Sun P, Zhao H, et al. Dexmedetomidine provides renoprotection against ischemia-reperfusion injury in mice. Crit Care. 2011;15:R153.
35. Luo C, Yuan D, Yao W, et al. Dexmedetomidine protects against apoptosis induced by hypoxia/reoxygenation through the inhibition of gap junctions in NRK-52E cells. Life Sci. 2015;122:72–7.
36. Shi R, Tie HT. Dexmedetomidine as a promising prevention strategy for cardiac surgery-associated acute kidney injury: a meta-analysis. Crit Care. 2017;21:198.

29 Renal Replacement Therapy During Septic Renal Dysfunction

S. Romagnoli, Z. Ricci, and C. Ronco

29.1 Introduction

Sepsis-induced acute kidney injury (AKI) represents the leading cause of AKI in the intensive care unit (ICU). This syndrome is characterized by an acute deterioration of renal function and glomerular filtration in the context of sepsis and multiple organ damage. Sepsis-induced AKI is diagnosed in almost 50% of critically ill septic patients and 15–20% of them require renal replacement therapy (RRT) [1]. Moreover the syndrome is associated with short and long-term adverse outcomes including mortality and the development of chronic kidney disease [2]. Hemodynamic support and avoidance of toxic drugs (contrast media, non-steroidal anti-inflammatory drugs, antibiotics) still remain the most efficient strategies aimed at preventing or treating sepsis-induced AKI together with the administration of diuretics to balance fluid administration and the application of RRT in oligoanuric patients and/or those with severe acid base and electrolyte derangements [3]. Fifty to 60% of patients with sepsis-induced AKI receiving RRT in the ICU do not survive the hospital admission as also remarked in the Beginning and Ending Supportive Therapy for the Kidney (BEST Kidney) study in which patients with sepsis-induced AKI receiving continuous RRT (CRRT) had a longer hospital length of stay and

S. Romagnoli
Department of Anesthesiology and Intensive Care, Azienda Ospedaliero-Universitaria Careggi, Florence, Italy

Z. Ricci
Department of Cardiology and Cardiac Surgery, Pediatric Cardiac Intensive Care Unit, Bambino Gesù Children's Hospital, IRCCS, Rome, Italy

C. Ronco (✉)
Department of Nephrology, Dialysis and Transplantation, San Bortolo Hospital, Vicenza, Italy

International Renal Research Institute of Vicenza (IRRIV), Vicenza, Italy
e-mail: cronco@goldnet.it

J.-L. Vincent (ed.), *Annual Update in Intensive Care and Emergency Medicine 2019*, Annual Update in Intensive Care and Emergency Medicine, https://doi.org/10.1007/978-3-030-06067-1_29

higher mortality (70%) compared with those who received RRT outside the septic syndrome (52%) [4].

Renal support or replacement with continuous or intermittent modalities is usually applied to patients with more severe stages of AKI: KDIGO (Kidney Disease Improving Global Outcome) or AKIN (Acute Kidney Injury Network) AKI stage 3 [5]. In a sub-analysis of the Intensive Care Over Nations (ICON) audit, a multicenter worldwide study, including 4727 adult critically ill patients with AKI, RRT was performed in 4.0%, 5.7%, 6.8%, and 58.6% of patients without AKI and with AKI stage I, stage II, and stage III, respectively, with hemofiltration as the most frequent modality of RRT in sepsis-induced AKI vs non sepsis-induced AKI patients [5, 6]. Mortality rate was higher in patients receiving RRT (40%) compared to those without RRT (22%) with no difference between hemofiltration vs. hemodialysis. Until recently, our knowledge about RRT administration in sepsis-induced AKI has been derived largely from uncontrolled observational reports. More recently, large-scale controlled clinical studies have been conducted. Although most of these studies have been undertaken in heterogeneous groups of ICU patients with severe AKI, most of the patients had sepsis-induced AKI. Here we summarize current knowledge on RRT for patients with sepsis-induced AKI as a supportive measure in advanced stages of AKI. In addition, the application of RRT as blood purification therapy for sepsis (clearance of inflammatory mediators) will be addressed with a critical review of published studies.

29.2 Sepsis-Induced AKI: Pathophysiology and Rationale for Blood Purification

The 'endotype' sepsis-induced AKI is different from other forms of AKI in terms of pathogenesis, patient characteristics and clinical outcomes [7]. The hemodynamic derangements occurring during sepsis and septic shock have been considered as the main cause of AKI. Nevertheless, although our understanding of the pathogenesis of sepsis-induced AKI is still incomplete, it is now evident that hypoperfusion and ischemia do not completely explain the pathogenesis of sepsis-induced AKI because it can develop even in the presence of normal or even increased renal blood flow [8]. The mechanisms of sepsis-associated kidney damage come from blood flow redistribution and toxic and/or immunologic causes. Different to the pure hemodynamic mechanism, the pathophysiological theory of 'tubular injury' due to inflammatory mediators suggests that toxins in the bloodstream may be able to alter the renal microcirculation, induce apoptosis and functional alterations of tubular cells and concomitantly modulate the immune response in septic patients, representing the inciting mechanism for tubular stress and kidney damage [9]. Toxins causing tubular injury are grouped as pathogen-associated molecular patterns (e.g., lipopolysaccharide [LPS], porins, mannose-containing glycoproteins, lipoteichoic acid, flagellin, double strain RNA and quorum sensing molecules), damage-associated molecular patterns, endogenous molecules released by injured or necrotic cells (RNA, single/double strain DNA, ATP, histones and high-mobility group box 1

[HMBG1]), inflammatory cytokines and chemokines (interleukin [IL]-6, IL-8, IL-18, tumor necrosis factor [TNF]) and complement fragments [9]. These medium-sized molecules (molecular weight 8–60 kDa), are water soluble and do not bind to the plasma proteins [10]. They may reach the kidney by direct glomerular filtration and modulate the biological activities of epithelial tubular cells and, by acting on endothelial cells located in the peritubular capillaries, induce microvascular derangement. These toxins lead to alterations of tubular function at the basolateral compartment and biologic alterations, loss of cell polarity, apoptosis, enhanced senescence, and differentiation of tubular epithelial cells to fibroblasts [11]. The physical characteristics of such toxins make them theoretical targets for extracorporeal removal by RRT either with standard high flux membranes, with a nominal cut-off of 10–30 kDa or, more efficiently, with special membranes specifically manufactured for this purpose (see below) [10]. If the 'humoral pathogenesis' of sepsis-induced AKI is confirmed, RRT may be started as a specific treatment to protect and improve renal function, rather than to replace it in the phase of oligo-anuria.

29.3 Optimal Timing to Commence RRT in Sepsis

There is no clear consensus on the optimal timing for RRT in sepsis-induced AKI. Classic indications for starting RRT in patients with AKI (severe metabolic acidosis, hyperkalemia, uremia, oliguria/anuria and pulmonary edema unresponsive to diuretic therapy) are now universally accepted by nephrologists and intensive care physicians [3]. However, reasons for RRT in critically ill patients are frequently different from those indicated. Positive fluid balance, electrolyte disorders and metabolic acidosis are commonly observed in ICU patients with sepsis even with lower stages of AKI. In light of the inflammatory theory of sepsis-induced AKI, these insults, associated with an increase in serum concentration of inflammatory cytokines, may potentially cause additional damage to the kidney and lessen the chance of renal recovery [12]. Positive fluid balance and weight gain have been associated with multiple organ dysfunction and reduced survival in critically ill and surgical patients. Moreover, starting RRT early in patients with sepsis-induced AKI could limit fluid overload, organ injury, and, theoretically, contribute to managing the abnormal host response to infection [13]. By contrast, starting RRT too early, when renal function is clinically still acceptable or before a clear understanding of the possibility of rapid recovery, may expose patients to unnecessary risks: extracorporeal blood contact, anticoagulation, immobilization, unwanted loss of antibiotics or other drugs and electrolytes. Data from the literature have shown that early RRT may be associated with improved survival in patients with sepsis-induced AKI [14]. From the BEST Kidney study, a later RRT start in terms of both time and disease state (higher serum creatinine) was associated with worse outcomes in terms of renal recovery [15]. In a single-center retrospective study of 147 septic AKI patients, the group was divided according to serum urea into those who received RRT when serum urea was <36 mmol/L (early) and those who received RRT when the urea was >36 mmol/L (late) [16]. The mortality rate was significantly lower in the group with early RRT (52% vs. 68%, $p < 0.05$), but the dose and adequacy of RRT were not considered, and there may have been a selection bias because more than twice as many patients who started RRT late had cancer. A recent further retrospective analysis of the RENAL study, assessing RRT timing, investigated a subgroup of 439 patients (53% with sepsis). No significant relationships between RRT timing and mortality, duration of mechanical ventilation, ICU length of stay, or renal recovery were found. Importantly, patients without urgent indications for RRT and those with higher serum creatinine levels tended to have higher survival rates when RRT was started later [17]. Although some of these studies showed a benefit of earlier start of RRT in critically ill patients with AKI (before the onset of complications and of fluid overload), heterogeneity in patient populations, limited numbers of enrolled patients, design issues related to historical uncontrolled studies with marked publication bias, differences in definition of timing and renal failure, and variations in prescriptions and modalities suggest caution in drawing conclusions about 'when to start'.

Two randomized controlled trials (RCTs), published in 2016, investigated 'timing' as a critical variable affecting outcome of critically ill patients with AKI. Zarbock et al. [18] conducted a single center RCT that compared early (within 8 h of reaching KDIGO stage 2 AKI; n = 112) to delayed (within 12 h of stage 3 AKI or no initiation; n = 119) initiation of RRT and explored the 90-day all-cause mortality in the 231 critically ill patients enrolled. The authors showed that patients in the early group had significantly lower 90-day mortality compared with the delayed group (an absolute risk reduction of 15.4% [95% CI, −28.1% to −2.6%]; $p = 0.03$). Moreover, the early group showed shorter duration of RRT, shorter hospital length of stay, and higher rate of renal recovery by day 90. The second RCT, by Gaudry et al., including 80% septic patients, found no difference in survival between early and delayed RRT [19]. The study involved 620 patients with KDIGO stage 3 AKI requiring mechanical ventilation, vasopressors, or both but without life-threatening complications requiring immediate RRT. In the early group, patients had RRT initiated immediately after randomization whereas in the delayed strategy group, RRT was started if one of the following criteria was reached: severe hyperkalemia, metabolic acidosis, pulmonary edema, blood urea nitrogen level higher than 112 mg/dL, or oliguria for more than 72 h after randomization. No difference in survival rate at day 60 was found: 48.5% in the early-strategy group and 49.7% in the delayed-strategy group ($p = 0.79$). Interestingly, about half of the patients in the delayed group did not require RRT (recovery of spontaneous urine output) but had similar outcomes compared to those patients who did receive it and, different from the study by Zarbock et al., more than 50% of the patients received intermittent hemodialysis (IHD) as the first method of therapy and only 30% of them received CRRT as the sole method (with no intermittent dialysis at any time).

When evaluating these recent RCTs, significant differences in study design, populations, and choice of RRT modality should be taken into consideration before reaching any conclusion about RRT timing. Beyond isolated variables, such as the number of hours needed to start the RRT or a specific metabolic parameter or AKI stage, a more personalized good-sense approach should guide our clinical decisions [20]. It appears not to be particularly dangerous, in terms of survival probability and in highly specialized centers, to proactively start early treatment. However, this decision should be counterbalanced by the actual need of the treated patient (is a severe state of fluid overload present? Is the patient severely catabolic? Does the patient need to receive nephrotoxic drugs and/or parenteral nutrition? Does he/she require high transfusion volumes?); by his/her clinical condition (i.e., presence or not of sepsis-induced AKI, coagulation disorders, hemodynamic instability, ease of achieving vascular access); and finally, by the 50% possibility of a timely spontaneous urine flow recovery. New trials exploring optimal timing are ongoing and will probably clarify this controversial issue. The first of these is the The Standard versus Accelerated Initiation of Renal Replacement Therapy in Acute Kidney Injury (STARRT-AKI, ClinicalTrials.gov Identifier NCT02568722) trials. STARRT-AKI is an international multicenter study (130 sites involved so far) enrolling patients with severe AKI randomized to receive RRT (any mode) within 12 h or at the discretion of the clinician and it is currently at about 70% of target recruitment (2866 patients). The second study, the Initiation of Dialysis Early versus Delayed in the Intensive Care Unit (IDEAL-ICU, NCT01682590), is a French study, including patients with severe AKI (Risk, Injury, Failure, Loss of kidney function, and End-stage kidney disease [RIFLE] F stage) in early septic shock within 48 h of need for catecholamine infusion. RRT is allowed at any doses over 25 mL/kg/h (or IHD at least every 2 days for 4–6 h). This study has finished recruitment and publication of its final results is expected soon.

In conclusion, the optimal timing for RRT in sepsis-induced AKI is an unsolved and evolving issue. In addition to the absolute urgent/emergent indications for RRT, careful stratification based on organ dysfunction, main acute disease, chronic comorbidities, medications, nutritional needs and fluid status could better indicate the right time in the right patient with the right method. Moreover, the attempt to standardize the timing of RRT without evaluating each patient from a 'holistic' viewpoint may expose the patient to risks of both delayed and early strategies: in one case being too late and in the other being useless. Great attention, furthermore, should be payed to patients who would recover renal function with conservative treatment alone because these probably have a good chance of a good outcome. Finally, serum urea and creatinine are non-sensitive and non-specific biomarkers of renal function as they have variable rates of production, are influenced by hemodilution during critical illness, and do not accurately track kidney function and/or the need for RRT support. In this view, more sensitive and specific biomarkers may help to better stratify the indications for RRT although their exact relevance in sepsis-induced AKI remains unclear.

29.4 Standard and Special Filters: Variable Intensity, High Cut-off Membranes and Hemadsorption

The optimal intensity (product of [clearance (Cl) × time]) of RRT in critically ill patients with AKI is an open issue. Application of the convection modality of solute transport during RRT in patients with sepsis-induced AKI could be of advantage because inflammatory mediators, considered a contributing cause of organ injury and immune-dysregulation, can be cleared with the hemofilters. RCTs have investigated this application by testing intensive/higher-volume hemofiltration or hemodiafiltration versus less-intensive doses in septic patients. A key study by Ronco et al. performed in 425 patients, first showed that a survival benefit was associated with effluent rates of 35–45 mL/kg/h compared to 20 mL/kg/h (mortality 43% vs. 59%, $p < 0.01$) [21]. Subsequent controlled studies that addressed the dose of RRT applied to patients with severe AKI, the RENAL and the VA/NIH Acute Renal Failure Trial Network (ATN) studies, failed to replicate this result [22, 23]. Subsequent meta-analyses have concluded that higher doses of RRT (CRRT effluent >30 mL/kg/h, or 6 sessions of IHD per week), provide no survival or renal function recovery advantage over standard doses of RRT (CRRT effluent <30 mL/kg/h or 2–4 IHD sessions per week) [24]. These findings apply equally to patients with and without sepsis. Currently, KDIGO guidelines recommend a "standard" intensity of 20–25 mL/kg/h when continuous RRT is prescribed. However, a crucial point shown by the Dose Response Multicenter Investigation on Fluid Assessment (DoReMIFA) study [25] is that the actual delivered dose of RRT may by much lower than the prescribed one. Thus, prescribing a 30–35 mL/kg/h dose may be more appropriate when commencing CRRT, especially in sepsis-induced AKI in order to compensate for downtime.

In view of the opportunity to clear inflammatory mediators from the bloodstream with high flux hemofilters (membranes with ultrafiltration coefficient [K_{UF}] >25 mL/h/mmHg/m^2) [26], many studies have investigated the potential benefit of CRRT prescribed at high doses in septic patients. Although not unequivocally defined in the medical literature, high-volume hemofiltration (HVHF) is identified as continuous treatment with a convective target dose (prescribed) >35 mL/kg/h [27] whereas continuous treatments >45 mL/kg/h are classified as very high-volume hemofiltration (VHVHF) [27]. A total of five RCTs on RRT performed with standard high flux membranes, have been performed in septic patients with AKI. In 2009, Payen et al., in a prospective, randomized, open, multicenter study, investigated the effects of early (within 24 h after randomization) application of hemofiltration (continuous venovenous hemofiltration [CVVH]), in addition to standard management of sepsis, on organ dysfunction and plasma cytokine levels in patients with severe sepsis or septic shock [28]. The CVVH technique was performed with a heparin-coated polysulfone membrane of 1.2 m^2 surface with a cut-off coefficient of 30 kDa; blood flow was 150 mL/min and the ultrafiltration rate 2 L/h for all patients. Net ultrafiltration was set according to clinical needs. A total of 80 patients were enrolled within 24 h of development of the first sepsis-related organ failure and after the application of exclusion criteria 76 patients were randomized: 37 in the CVVH group and 39 in standard treatment. CVVH lasted at least 96 h and the hemofilter was replaced at 12, 24 and 48 h in order to preserve its efficiency. The study failed to demonstrate a benefit of early CVVH application and the number and severity of organ failures were significantly higher in the CVVH group. Moreover, no modifications in plasma cytokine levels were detected. Three years later, Zhang et al. published the results of a randomized trial in 280 patients with severe sepsis or septic shock and AKI treated with CVVH in a pre/post dilution ratio of 2/1 when at least one of the following criteria was met: oliguria (urine output <100 mL/6 h and unresponsive to fluid resuscitation), hyperkalemia >6.5 mmol/L, pH <7.2, serum creatinine >250 μmol/L or presence of severe organ edema (e.g., pulmonary edema). CRRT was performed with polysulfone filters at a blood flow rate of 250 mL/min. The patients were randomized to two different effluent doses for the first three days: 50 mL/kg/h (HVHF group) or 85 mL/kg/h (extra high-volume hemofiltration [EHVHF]) [29]. Depending on clinical needs, anticoagulation was avoided or performed with unfractionated heparin or low molecular weight heparin. A transmembrane pressure >250 mmHg was used as trigger for filter replacement. No difference in mortality or secondary outcomes was found at 28, 60, and 90 days even in a subgroup of patients with septic shock. In 2013, the prospective, randomized, open, multicenter clinical "hIgh VOlume in Intensive caRE" (IVOIRE) trial was published by Joannes-Boyau and collaborators. The study tested whether HVHF at 70 mL/kg/h was more efficient in reducing 28-day mortality in patients with septic shock and AKI compared to standard volume hemofiltration at 35 mL/kg/h (SVHF) for 96 h [30]. Hemofiltration was delivered in the CVVH mode with blood flow rate modified in order to maintain a filtration fraction <25% (average 200–320 mL/min). The hemofilter was changed every 48 h and anticoagulation was obtained with unfractioned heparin. A total of 137 patients were randomized to HVHF (66 patients) or SVHF (71 patients). Although the HVHF group had higher clearance yielding lower serum creatinine and urea, mortality at 28 days was not significantly different between treatment groups (HVHF 37.9% vs. SVHF 40.8%). Similarly, there were no statistically significant differences in any of the secondary endpoints between treatment groups, including 60- and 90-day mortality, duration of mechanical ventilation, duration of RRT, renal recovery, or ICU and hospital lengths of stay. It is of concern that hypophosphatemia and antibiotic clearance were markedly higher with HVHF. In 2015, Quenot and collaborators treated 29 patients with septic shock with VHVHF using a dose of 120 mL/kg/h for 48 h in a multicenter, prospective, randomized, open-label trial. The study did not demonstrate any beneficial effect of VHVHF in primary (catecholamine free days) or secondary (mechanical ventilation-free days, RRT-free days, or mortality at 7, 28 or 90 days) vs. usual care. In 2016, the HICORES trial, a prospective RCT, was conducted to investigate the effect of high CRRT intensity on inflammatory cytokine removal in addition to its influence on clinical outcomes [31]. Differently from the previous studies, RRT was performed by combining convection and diffusion mechanisms for solute transport as continuous venovenous hemodiafiltration (CVVHDF) with the following operating characteristics: blood flow rate 150 mL/min; effluent volume 40 mL/kg/h (conventional-dose group) or 80 mL/kg/h (high-dose group); replacement and dialysate volumes were set using the 1:1 balanced-predilution method; anticoagulation (no anticoagulation, heparin, or nafamostat mesilate) and volume control were managed by a nephrologist. The study showed no differences in 28-day or 90-day mortality in the standard dose group vs. the high dose group, no differences in lengths of ICU stay or total hospital stay among survivors, no differences in recovery of kidney function at 28 or 90 days after randomization. Cytokine measurements showed no differences in IL-6, IL-8, IL-1β or IL-10 levels at the dialyzer inlet or outlet but different levels were found between dialyzer inlet and outlet in the high dose group compared to the standard one. In addition, no difference in serum cytokine levels measured at baseline or 24 h after CVVHDF initiation was found between standard and high dose groups but serum IL-6 and IL-8 levels after 24 h of CVVHDF were significantly decreased compared to baseline in the high-dose group.

In 2017, a Cochrane meta-analysis on HVHF for sepsis was published [32]. The analysis included RCTs and quasi-randomized trials comparing HVHF or high-volume hemodiafiltration versus standard or usual dialysis therapy, as well as RCTs and quasi-randomized trials comparing HVHF or high-volume hemodiafiltration versus no similar dialysis therapy. All the studies involved adults treated in critical care units for sepsis-induced AKI. The analysis included four studies and a total of 201 patients. Investigators reported no adverse effects of HVHF (low-quality evidence) but, based on the limited number of studies and participants, no definitive answers could be reached and the authors concluded that new large RCTs are necessary to investigate HVHF in patients with sepsis. Possible reasons for a lack of benefit with HVHF are increased clearance of antimicrobials leading to inadvertent and potentially harmful sub-therapeutic levels, increase in electrolyte disturbances (e.g., hypokalemia, hypophosphatemia), depletion of micronutrients, and inability to effectively provide adequate mediators clearance at the cellular level rather than in the circulation. Therapeutic drug monitoring is crucial for patient receiving RRT for septic AKI because antibiotics are the mainstay of sepsis treatment and substantial changes in pharmacokinetic parameters occur in these patients, including increased volume of distribution, hypoalbuminemia, the presence of other extracorporeal circuits (e.g., extracorporeal membrane oxygenation [ECMO]), unnecessarily high RRT dose prescriptions and changes in renal and non-renal clearance. It recently became clearer that in critically ill patients, these aspects may exceed the reduced antibiotic clearance secondary to renal dysfunction. In general, careful dose adjustments should be provided. In addition, excessive fear of antibiotic toxicity (especially nephrotoxicity), and limited drug dosing resources may contribute to detrimental suboptimal antibiotic therapy whose clinical relevance may have been overlooked.

During recent years, developments in membranes and biomaterials have paralleled the evolution of all the CRRT machine components with the development of filters specifically dedicated to septic patients with the aim of potentiating the role of RRT as an adjuvant therapy. High cut-off (HCO) membranes, also known as 'super high flux filters', have been used for many years in patients with chronic kidney disease and more recently they have been proposed for septic patients needing clearance of inflammatory mediators. Clinically, the expression 'HCO membrane' describes membranes with a cut-off value that approximates the molecular weight of albumin, before exposure to blood or plasma [26]. Moreover, a recent classification method characterized HCO membranes with precision based on their molecular weight retention onset (MWRO) and molecular weight cut-off (MWCO) [33]. According to a study by Boschetti-de-Fierro et al., HCO filters have a MWRO and a MWCO of 15–20 kDa and 170–320 kDa, respectively; these values are respectively double and fivefold those of standard filters. Pore radius is increased to 8–12 nm, which is about double that of standard high flux filters for CRRT, and pore size distribution is expanded [33]. Currently available membranes achieve effective removal of substances in the range of 20–60 kDa; larger molecules are retained, although pores size ranges nominally reach larger values due to secondary layer formation and membrane fouling [34].

Excluding case reports, studies on animals, and *in vitro/ex vivo* studies, only 10 small clinical studies with variable but promising results on HCO treatment application have been published so far and recently summarized in a review article (Table 29.1) [34]. Very recently, Atan et al. performed a phase II double-blind randomized study comparing standard CVVH with HCO CVVH in critically ill patients with AKI requiring vasopressor support [10]. The primary endpoint was norepinephrine requirements expressed as hours of norepinephrine-free time within the first week of treatment. The investigators randomized patients in a 1:1 ratio to receive either standard or HCO CVVH within 12 h of a decision to commence hemofiltration. Patients requiring hemofiltration and norepinephrine for hemodynamic support were randomized. The criteria for initiating hemofiltration included either oliguria (<100 mL/6 h) unresponsive to fluid resuscitation, hyperkalemia (>6.5 mmol/L), pH <7.2, serum urea >25 mmol/L, serum creatinine >300 μmol/L, or clinically significant organ edema in the setting of acute renal failure (e.g., pulmonary edema). Patients were recruited if the clinician anticipated that the patient would require hemofiltration for at least 72 h. Patients underwent standard CVVH with custom manufactured polyethersulfone standard hemofilters with a nominal cut-off point of 30 kDa or CVVH with polyethersulfone HCO filters with a nominal cut-off point of 100 kDa (P2SH filters, 1.12 m^2; Gambro, Hechingen, Germany) depending on the allocation group. Blindness was respected for patients and all the investigators (healthcare personnel and researchers) since the two filters were indistinguishable. Operating characteristics of RRT were: blood flow at 200 mL/min, ultrafiltration rate at 25 mL/kg/h with bicarbonate-buffered replacement fluids. Anticoagulation was chosen at the discretion of the treating clinician. Secondary outcomes were the assessment of change in the levels of IL-1, IL-6 and IL-10, the percentage change in serum albumin levels, the total amount of albumin administered to each patient over the first 7 days, the filter life, the maximum rate of vasopressor infusion per day, and the duration of hemofiltration. Seventy-six patients were randomized, with 38 patients assigned to each group. Septic shock was the reason for vasopressor administration in 20 (55.6%) and 21 (55.3%) of the HCO and standard CVVH groups, respectively. A total of 226 filters were used for the HCO group with a median filter life of 9 h (4–17 h) versus 269 filters for the standard group with a median filter life of 10 h (5.5–19.8 h) ($p = 0.21$). Due to contraindications, no anticoagulation was used for 119 (52.7%) HCO filters and 118 (43.9%) standard filters. Unfractionated heparin was applied for 46.6% of the HCO filters and 28.3% of the standard filters. Regional citrate was applied for 3.8% of HCO filters and 7.5 of the standard filters. Median cumulative norepinephrine-free time over 7 days was 32 h (0–110.8 h) for HCO and 56 h (0–109.3 h) for standard CVVH after randomization ($p = 0.520$) and the maximum norepinephrine rates of infusion

Table 29.1 High cut-off (HCO) membrane: Human studies

First author, year [ref]	Study design and patients	RRT filters, modalities and prescription	Endpoint	Main findings
Morgera et al., 2003 [43]	RCT 28 septic patients with acute renal failure (14:14:3)	• High-flux polyamide hemofilter (P2SH, surface area 0.6 m^2)—1 L/h post-dilution • HCO-CVVH (12 h) alternated to C-HF (12 h) vs. C-HF for 60 h (vs. short HCO and C-HF in 3 healthy volunteers)—1 L/h, post-dilution	PBMC function restoration by HCO	No difference
Morgera et al., 2003 [44]	Observational 16 patients with septic shock and MOF	• High-flux polyamide hemofilter (P2SH, surface area 0.6 m^2)—1 L/h, post-dilution • HCO-CVVH (12 h) alternated to C-HF (12 h) for 5 days—1 L/h, post-dilution	IL-6 Cl: 12–17 mL/min TNF-α Cl: negligible	Non-significant improvement in SOFA score
Morgera et al., 2003 [45]	RCT 28 septic patients with acute renal failure (14:14:2)	• High-flux polyamide hemofilter (P2SH, surface area 0.6 m^2)—1 L/h, post-dilution • HCO-CVVH (12 h) alternated to C-HF (12 h) vs. C-HF for 60 h (vs. short HCO and C-HF in 2 healthy volunteers)—1 L/h, post-dilution	The PML phagocytosis rate measured at the end of the third HCO session was significantly decreased compared with baseline values	No difference
Morgera et al., 2004 [46]	24 patients with MOD due to septic shock (6:6:6:6)	• High-flux polyamide hemofilter (P2SH, surface area 1.1 m^2) • Group 1: CVVH 1 L/h; Group 2: CVVH 2.5 L/h; Group 3: CVVHD 1 L/h; Group 4: CVVHD 2.5 L/h 1 or 2.5 L/h post dilution hemofiltration vs. 1 or 2.5 hemodialysis for 72 h	IL-1ra Cl: 18–26 mL/min IL-6 Cl: 16–20 mL/min	No differences between groups in different severity scores
Morgera et al., 2006 [47]	RCT 30 patients with sepsis-induced acute renal failure (20:10) −2 HCO patients subsequently excluded	• High-flux polyamide hemofilter (P2SH, surface area 1.1 m^2)—2.5 L/h, post-dilution • HCO-CVVH vs. C-HF for 48 h—2.5 L/h, post-dilution	IL-1ra Cl: 39 mL/min IL-6 Cl: 36–40 mL/min	Slight reduction of SAPS score in the HCO group; significant reduction of adjusted norepinephrine dose

Haase et al., 2007 [48]	Double-blind, crossover, RCT. 10 septic patients with acute renal failure	• Polyflux filters (polyarylethersulfone) surface area of 1.1 m^2; custom-made—Blood flow at 200 mL/min and dialysate flow at 300 mL/min • 4 h of HCO-IHD and 4 h of standard HF-IHD in random order with 4 h wash-out (no treatment)—Blood flow at 200 mL/min and dialysate flow at 300 mL/min	IL-6 Cl: 9.6–14.1 mL/min; reduction in plasma levels of IL-6, IL-8 and IL-10	Non-significant greater reduction in norepinephrine dose in HCO group
Kade et al., 2016 [49]	Retrospective 28 patients with septic shock	• Polyarylethersulfone (PAES) membrane (Septex) • HCO-CVVHDF Blood flow 150 mL/min, dialysis flow 1200 mL/h. Predilution fluid 250 mL/h	IL-6 Cl: 59–75 mL/min	No difference
Chelazzi et al., 2016 [50]	Retrospective 24 septic patients with MDR Gram-negative infection (16:8)	• Polyarylethersulfone (PAES) membrane (Septex) • HCO-CVVHD vs. CVVHDF HCO: 35 mL/kg/h vs. CVVHDF 45 mL/kg/h	None	HCO group shorter ICU-LOS, days Lower ventilation days/ICU-LOS, vasopressor days/ICU-LOS, ICU mortality
Atan et al., 2016 [35]	Double blind RCT 14 patients with AKI and underlying shock requiring vasopressor infusion (6:8). A nested cohort of patients within a larger double-blind, randomized, parallel group, controlled trial.	• Polyethersulfone filters, surface area of 1.1 m^2—Blood flow 250 mL/min, 25 mL/kg/h pre-dilution • HCO-CVVH vs. CVVH—Blood flow 250 mL/min, 25 mL/kg/h pre-dilution	IL-6 Cl: 36 mL/min IL-8 Cl: 26 mL/min IL-10 Cl: 9.66 mL/min	No difference
Villa et al., 2017 [51]	Prospective, multicenter 38 patients with septic shock and AKI.	• Polyarylethersulfone (PAES) membrane (Septex) • HCO-CVVHD 35 mL/kg/h for 72 h (any KDIGO stage >0)	Decrease in IL-6, IL 10 and TNF-α especially in survivors	Survivors quick SOFA decrease. KDIGO stage and lactates associated with mortality

(continued)

Table 29.1 (continued)

First author, year [ref]	Study design and patients	RRT filters, modalities and prescription	Endpoint	Main findings
Atan et al., 2018 [10]	Single-center double-blind RCT >50% of each group with septic shock	• CVVH with custom manufactured polyethersulfone standard hemofilters—25 mL/kg/h • Polyethersulfone HCO filters (CVVH-HCO) (P2SH filters, 1.12 m²; Gambro, Hechingen, Germany)—25 mL/kg/h	Hours of norepinephrine-free time within the first week of treatment. Change in the levels of IL-1, IL-6, and IL-10, the percentage change in serum albumin levels, the total amount of albumin administered to each patient over the first 7 days, the filter life, the maximum rate of vasopressor infusion per day, and duration of hemofiltration.	No difference in primary and secondary outcome. Overall combined cytokine levels had fallen to 62.2% of baseline at 72 h for CVVH-HCO ($p < 0.0001$) and to 75.9% of baseline with standard CVVH ($p = 0.008$); there were no between group differences.

RCT randomized controlled trial; *RRT* renal replacement therapy; *CVVH* continuous venovenous hemofiltration; *CVVHD* continuous venovenous hemodialysis: *CVVHDF* continuous venovenous hemodiafiltration; *PBMC* peripheral blood mononuclear cells; *IL* interleukin; *TNF* tumor necrosis factor; *IHD* intermittent hemodialysis; *MOF* multiple organ failure; *MOD* multiple organ dysfunction; *PML* polymorphonuclear leukocyte; *Cl* clearance; *MDR* multidrug resistant: *LOS* length of stay; *SOFA* sequential organ failure assessment

per day (μg/min) were similar for both groups ($p = 0.75$). Changes in serum albumin levels within the first 7 days were not significantly different between the two groups ($p = 0.192$) with a median dose of intravenous albumin given over the first 7 days of 90 g (20–212 g) for HCO and 80 g (15–132 g) for standard CVVH ($p = 0.252$). There was no difference in time to permanent cessation of norepinephrine ($p = 0.358$) and time to permanent cessation of hemofiltration ($p = 0.563$) within the full 14-day treatment period. Interestingly, at 20 days about 70% patients in the standard vs. 50% in the HCO CVVH survived ($p = 0.052$). Changes in cytokine levels gave the following results [35]: by 72 h of treatment, IL-6 had decreased during both treatments ($p = 0.009$ and $p = 0.005$ respectively); IL-10 had decreased with standard CVVH ($p = 0.03$) but not with HCO CVVH ($p = 0.135$). There were no changes in levels of the other cytokines over time. There were no significant between-group differences in plasma levels for each cytokine over the 72 h treatment period. For all cytokines combined, however, the median sieving coefficient was higher for HCO CVVH (0.31 vs. 0.16; $p = 0.042$) as was the mass removal rate by ultrafiltration ($p = 0.027$). Although overall combined cytokine levels had fallen to 62.2% of baseline at 72 h for HCO CVVH ($p < 0.0001$) and to 75.9% of baseline with standard CVVH ($p = 0.008$) there were no significant between-group differences. This study unfortunately is a further confirmation that either our understanding of sepsis-induced AKI and sepsis pathogenesis in general is inadequate or the means so far utilized in order to control it are not efficient.

The technique known as coupled plasma filtration adsorption (CPFA) seems to be in the same category. During CPFA, plasma, separated from blood by a plasma-filter, is run through a synthetic resin cartridge (with adsorption capacity for inflammatory mediators) and then returned to the blood circuit where a hemofilter removes excess fluid and allows renal replacement [36]. CPFA is a sorbent technology based on RRT for removal of endotoxin, bacterial products and both pro- and anti-inflammatory endogenous substances in septic patients with AKI. A multicenter, randomized trial, the COMPACT (COMbining Plasma-filtration and Adsorption Clinical Trial) study, compared CPFA with standard care in the treatment of critically ill patients with septic shock [37]. No statistically significant differences were found in hospital mortality or in secondary endpoints (occurrence of new organ failure) or ICU-free days during the first 30 days. Because it was suggested that technical difficulties occurring during the treatments (early clotting) may have biased the results, a new trial, the COMPACT-2 study, including only patients achieving the prescribed CPFA treatment was planned (ClinicalTrials.gov Identifier: NCT01639664). The trial was prematurely terminated because of higher early mortality rates (within 72 h of randomization) in septic shock patients treated with CPFA compared to patients receiving standard therapy. After this *ad interim* analysis, the company delivered an urgent field safety notice reporting the results [38].

In recent years, other new membranes have been conceived with the specific aim of providing renal support combined with the attempt to treat sepsis-induced AKI. These membranes combine the enhanced clearance of middle to high molecular weight solutes of super high flux membranes with a particularly elevated adsorptive capacity. Adsorption implies the retention of some negatively charged molecules (inflammatory mediators, cytokines and proteins) within the membrane fibers after interaction with variable polarity ionic charges. The AN69 surface-treated (AN69ST) hemofilter is a derivative of the AN69, originally developed in 1969 as the world's first synthetic polymeric membrane, prepared by surface treatment of polyethyleneimine. The AN69ST membrane has excellent anti-thrombogenicity and its surface can be coated with heparin by priming with saline-containing heparin, further increasing its anti-thrombogenicity. AN69/AN69ST membranes have a hydrogel structure and are therefore highly hydrophilic. Research on the cytokine-adsorbing capacity of the AN69ST membrane is still limited. Yumoto et al. compared four different membrane hemofilters (AN69ST, polymethylmethacrylate [PMMA], HCO polyarylethersulfone [PAES] and polysulfone) for their capacity to remove HMBG1 proteins *in vitro*. The AN69ST had the highest efficiency for HMBG1 removal, followed by the PMMA membrane. The PAES and polysulfone membranes removed little HMGB-1 [39].

The oXiris® is a recently manufactured hemofilter using an AN69 membrane with polyethyleneimine surface coating and immobilized heparin. Compared with the AN69ST membrane, the oXiris® has three times more polyethyleneimine surface coating (in the second layer) and 10 times more pre-immobilized heparin (in the third layer). Therefore, oXiris® has excellent anti-thrombogenicity and is capable of adsorbing endotoxin to cationic polyethyleneimine in the second layer [40]. The deeper layer of the membrane remains negatively charged and thereby retains its ability to adsorb cytokines. The oXiris® membrane may therefore be able to adsorb both cytokines and endotoxin. Clinical application in large studies is still lacking. Whether cytokine/endotoxin-adsorbing hemofilters will be recognized as an effective adjunctive treatment of sepsis, septic shock and sepsis-induced AKI in the near future is unknown and dedicated RCTs are warranted.

29.5 Additional Aspects Related to RRT in Sepsis-induced AKI: Anticoagulation Strategies and Fluid Balance

Anticoagulation is required during CRRT to maintain circuit patency. Heparin has historically been the standard choice for anticoagulation but its use implies balancing the risk of bleeding complications with those of circuit clotting due to sub-therapeutic doses. Worldwide, unfractioned heparin is still widely used because of its low cost and relative ease of use (especially considering the availability of an antidote, protamine). In sepsis-induced AKI, the low levels of antithrombin and the putative inflammatory effects of heparin may lead to premature clotting of the circuit and intravenous administration of antithrombin is recommended to maintain levels higher than 60–70% [3]. Regional citrate anticoagulation (RCA) is recommended by KDIGO guidelines as a first approach to anticoagulation for CRRT [3] because it provides excellent anticoagulation within the circuit without increasing the risk of bleeding. Given these recommendations, and the development of safe, dedicated protocols, RCA is increasingly adopted in many centers, including smaller and non-academic hospitals with less experience of CRRT. Several studies have demonstrated the advantage of RCA compared to heparin in reducing bleeding and increasing circuit lifespan without clotting episodes [41]. Moreover, citrate may exert anti-inflammatory effects by reducing formation of platelet-leukocyte complexes and polymorphonuclear cell degranulation together with the induction of decreased levels of markers of oxidative stress and IL-1β [11]. Finally, RCA may be used in patients with heparin-induced thrombocytopenia. Careful application of RCA is required in patients with significant hemodynamic instability and/or systemic hypoperfusion due to the risk of citrate accumulation and reduced metabolism.

Retrospective and prospective studies have clearly shown that patients with AKI have higher mortality if they have a positive fluid balance. The DoReMIFA study [25] included a total of 991 patients (23.35% with sepsis on admission) and showed that hospital mortality increased by 1.075 (95% confidence interval 1.055–1.095) with every 1% increase in maximum fluid overload (peak value of fluid overload observed during the entire ICU stay). The observed phenomenon was a continuum and independent of thresholds. Moreover, the study showed that the speed of fluid accumulation was independently associated with ICU mortality. The evident relationship between fluid accumulation and mortality clearly suggests that net ultrafiltration (net fluid removal with the CRRT machine) and total fluid administration should be carefully monitored to avoid or limit a positive fluid balance whenever clinically possible. As confirmation of this, a *post hoc* analysis of the RENAL trial, initially conceived for the evaluation of different RRT intensities, clearly showed that the rapid (by the first 2–3 days of treatment) achievement of a negative fluid balance in critically ill patients with severe AKI was independently associated with improved survival [42].

29.6 Conclusion

Sepsis is a burdening epidemic condition syndrome associated with multiple organ failure, morbidity and mortality. Many patients with sepsis eventually develop AKI and most of them require RRT. Although the application of new RRT biotechnologies has opened new potential therapeutic strategies, these modified modalities and materials have yet to show cost-effectiveness and benefit in terms of mortality. Clinicians need to integrate the understanding of sepsis pathophysiology with the current evidenced-based strategies for multimodal treatments. Before prescribing any form of extracorporeal renal support, all efforts to prevent renal function deterioration must be attempted. Once RRT is indicated to prevent further renal and distal organ injury, the decision to start early should include the careful evaluation of hemodynamic status and the actual impossibility to further delay the treatment. Although convection is more efficient than diffusion in clearing middle molecules, there is insufficient evidence to recommend one technique over another in sepsis-induced AKI. Applications at doses over those suggested by the guidelines and use of special dedicated membranes for inflammatory mediator clearance have not produced any clinical benefit and remain in the research domain. Total fluid balance should always be carefully monitored since fluid overload is clearly associated with worse outcomes.

References

1. Prowle JR. Sepsis-associated AKI. Clin J Am Soc Nephrol. 2018;13:339–42.
2. Coca S, Yusuf B, Shlipak M. Long-term risk of mortality and other adverse outcomes after acute kidney injury: a systematic review and meta-analysis. Am J Kidney Dis. 2009;53:961–73.
3. Kidney Disease Improving Global Outcomes. Kidney Disease Improving Global Outcomes (KDIGO) clinical practice guideline for acute kidney injury. Kidney Int Suppl. 2012;2:1–138.
4. Uchino S, Bellomo R, Morimatsu H, et al. Continuous renal replacement therapy: a worldwide practice survey: the beginning and ending supportive therapy for the kidney (B.E.S.T. Kidney) investigators. Intensive Care Med. 2007;33:1563–70.
5. Peters E, Antonelli M, Wittebole X, et al. A worldwide multicentre evaluation of the influence of deterioration or improvement of acute kidney injury on clinical outcome in critically ill patients with and without sepsis at ICU admission: results from the intensive care over nations audit. Crit Care. 2018;22:188.
6. Vincent JL, Marshall JC, Ñamendys-Silva SA, et al. Assessment of the worldwide burden of critical illness: the intensive care over nations (ICON) audit. Lancet Respir Med. 2014;2:380–6.
7. Gomez H, Ince C, De Backer D, et al. A unified theory of sepsis-induced acute kidney injury: inflammation, microcirculatory dysfunction, bioenergetics, and the tubular cell adaptation to injury. Shock. 2014;41:3–11.
8. Post EH, Kellum JA, Bellomo R, Vincent JL. Renal perfusion in sepsis: from macro- to microcirculation. Kidney Int. 2017;91:45–60.
9. Dellepiane S, Marengo M, Cantaluppi V. Detrimental cross-talk between sepsis and acute kidney injury: new pathogenic mechanisms, early biomarkers and targeted therapies. Crit Care. 2016;20:61.
10. Atan R, Peck L, Care GC, et al. A double-blind randomized controlled trial of high cutoff versus standard hemofiltration in critically ill patients with acute kidney injury. Crit Care Med. 2018;46:e988–94.
11. Marengo M, Dellepiane S, Cantaluppi V. Extracorporeal treatments in patients with acute kidney injury and sepsis. Contrib Nephrol. 2017;190:1–18.
12. Heung M, Wolfgram DF, Kommareddi M, et al. Fluid overload at initiation of renal replacement therapy is associated with lack of renal recovery in patients with acute kidney injury. Nephrol Dial Transplant. 2012;27:956–61.
13. Singer M, Deutschman CS, Seymour CW, et al. The third international consensus definitions for sepsis and septic shock (sepsis-3). JAMA. 2016;315:801–10.
14. Karvellas C, Farhat M, Sajjad I, et al. A comparison of early versus late initiation of renal replacement therapy in critically ill patients with acute kidney injury: a systematic review and meta-analysis. Crit Care. 2011;15:R72.
15. Bagshaw SM, Uchino S, Bellomo R, et al. Timing of renal replacement therapy and clinical outcomes in critically ill patients with severe acute kidney injury. J Crit Care. 2009;24:129–40.
16. Carl DE, Grossman C, Behnke M, et al. Effect of timing of dialysis on mortality in critically ill, septic patients with acute renal failure. Hemodial Int. 2010;14:11–7.
17. Jun M, Bellomo R, Cass A, et al. Timing of renal replacement therapy and patient outcomes in the randomized evaluation of normal versus augmented level of replacement therapy study. Crit Care Med. 2014;42:1756–65.
18. Zarbock A, Kellum J, Schmidt C, et al. Effect of early vs delayed initiation of renal replacement. JAMA. 2016;315:2190–9.
19. Gaudry S, Hajage D, Schortgen F, et al. Initiation strategies for renal-replacement therapy in the intensive care unit. N Engl J Med. 2016;375:122–33.
20. Romagnoli S, Clark WR, Ricci Z, Ronco C. Renal replacement therapy for AKI: when? how much? when to stop? Best Pract Res Clin Anaesthesiol. 2017;31:371–85.
21. Ronco C, Bellomo R, Homel P, et al. Effects of different doses in continuous veno-venous haemofiltration on outcomes of acute renal failure: a prospective randomised trial. Lancet. 2000;356:26–30.

22. RENAL Replacement Therapy Study Investigators, Bellomo R, Cass A, et al. Intensity of continuous renal-replacement therapy in critically ill patients. N Engl J Med. 2009;361:1627–39.
23. The VA/NIH Acute Renal Failure Trial Network. Intensity of renal support in critically ill patients with acute kidney injury. N Engl J Med. 2008;359:7–20.
24. Van Wert R, Friedrich JO, Scales DC, et al. High-dose renal replacement therapy for acute kidney injury: systematic review and meta-analysis. Crit Care Med. 2010;38:1360–9.
25. Garzotto F, Ostermann M, Teng J, et al. The dose response multicentre investigation on fluid assessment (DoReMIFA) in critically ill patients. Crit Care. 2016;20:196.
26. Neri M, Cerdà J, Garzotto F, et al. Nomenclature for renal replacement therapy in acute kidney injury: basic principles. Crit Care. 2016;20:318.
27. Villa G, Neri M, Bellomo R, et al. Nomenclature for renal replacement therapy and blood purification techniques in critically ill patients: practical applications. Crit Care. 2016;20:283.
28. Payen D, Mateo J, Cavaillon JM, et al. Impact of continuous venovenous hemofiltration on organ failure during the early phase of severe sepsis: a randomized controlled trial. Crit Care Med. 2009;37:803–10.
29. Zhang P, Yang Y, Lv R, et al. Effect of the intensity of continuous renal replacement therapy in patients with sepsis and acute kidney injury: a single-center randomized clinical trial. Nephrol Dial Transplant. 2012;27:967–73.
30. Joannes-Boyau O, Honoré PM, Perez P, et al. High-volume versus standard-volume haemofiltration for septic shock patients with acute kidney injury (IVOIRE study): a multicentre randomized controlled trial. Intensive Care Med. 2013;39:1535–46.
31. Park JT, Kee YK, Oh HJ, et al. High-dose versus conventional-dose continuous venovenous hemodiafiltration and patient and kidney survival and cytokine removal in sepsis-associated acute kidney injury: a randomized controlled trial. Am J Kidney Dis. 2016;68:599–608.
32. Borthwick EM, Hill CJ, Rabindranath KS, Maxwell AP, McAuley DF, Blackwood B. High-volume haemofiltration for sepsis in adults. Cochrane Database Syst Rev. 2017;2017:CD008075.
33. Boschetti-de-Fierro A, Voigt M, Storr M, Krause B. Extended characterization of a new class of membranes for blood purification: the high cut-off membranes. Int J Artif Organs. 2013;36:455–63.
34. Ricci Z, Romagnoli S, Ronco C. High cut-off membranes in acute kidney injury and continuous renal replacement therapy. Int J Artif Organs. 2017;40:657–64.
35. Atan R, Peck L, Visvanathan K, et al. High cut-off hemofiltration versus standard hemofiltration: effect on plasma cytokines. Int J Artif Organs. 2016;39:479–86.
36. Ricci Z, Romagnoli S, Ronco C, La Manna G. From continuous renal replacement therapies to multiple organ support therapy. Contrib Nephrol. 2018;194:155–69.
37. Livigni S, Bertolini G, Rossi C, et al. Efficacy of coupled plasma filtration adsorption (CPFA) in patients with septic shock: a multicenter randomised controlled clinical trial. BMJ Open. 2014;4:e003536.
38. Teo D (2018) Urgent: field safety notice: CPFA coupled plasma filtration adsorption™ in patients with septic shock. Available at: http://www.hsa.gov.sg/content/dam/HSA/HPRG/Medical_Devices/Updates_and_Safety_reporting/Field_Safety_Corrective_Action/FSN/2018/April%202018/HSA%206004101-046-18-04_46%20FSN_Redacted.pdf. Accessed 10 Nov 2018.
39. Yumoto M, Nishida O, Moriyama K, et al. In vitro evaluation of high mobility group box 1 protein removal with various membranes for continuous hemofiltration. Ther Apher Dial. 2011;15:385–93.
40. Rimmelé T, Assadi A, Cattenoz M, et al. High-volume haemofiltration with a new haemofiltration membrane having enhanced adsorption properties in septic pigs. Nephrol Dial Transplant. 2009;24:421–7.
41. Liu C, Mao Z, Kang H, et al. Regional citrate versus heparin anticoagulation for continuous renal replacement therapy in critically ill patients: a meta-analysis with trial sequential analysis of randomized controlled trials. Crit Care. 2016;20:1–13.

42. RENAL Replacement Therapy Study Investigators, Bellomo R, Cass A, et al. An observational study fluid balance and patient outcomes in the randomized evaluation of normal vs. augmented level of replacement therapy trial. Crit Care Med. 2012;40:1753–60.
43. Morgera S, Haase M, Rocktäschel J, et al. High permeability haemofiltration improves peripheral blood mononuclear cell proliferation in septic patients with acute renal failure. Nephrol Dial Transplant. 2003;18:2570–6.
44. Morgera S, Rocktäschel J, Haase M, et al. Intermittent high permeability hemofiltration in septic patients with acute renal failure. Intensive Care Med. 2003;29:1989–95.
45. Morgera S, Haase M, Rocktäschel J, et al. Intermittent high-permeability hemofiltration modulates inflammatory response in septic patients with multiorgan failure. Nephron Clin Pract. 2003;94:c75–80.
46. Morgera S, Slowinski T, Melzer C, et al. Renal replacement therapy with high-cutoff hemofilters: impact of convection and diffusion on cytokine clearances and protein status. Am J Kidney Dis. 2004;43:444–53.
47. Morgera S, Haase M, Kuss T, et al. Pilot study on the effects of high cutoff hemofiltration on the need for norepinephrine in septic patients with acute renal failure. Crit Care Med. 2006;34:2099–104.
48. Haase M, Bellomo R, Baldwin I, et al. Hemodialysis membrane with a high-molecular-weight cutoff and cytokine levels in sepsis complicated by acute renal failure: a phase 1 randomized trial. Am J Kidney Dis. 2007;50:296–304.
49. Kade G, Lubas A, Rzeszotarska A, et al. Effectiveness of high cut-off hemofilters in the removal of selected cytokines in patients during septic shock accompanied by acute kidney injury-preliminary study. Med Sci Monit. 2016;22:4338–44.
50. Chelazzi C, Villa G, D'Alfonso MG, et al. Hemodialysis with high cut-off hemodialyzers in patients with multi-drug resistant gram-negative sepsis and acute kidney injury: a retrospective, case-control study. Blood Purif. 2016;42:186–93.
51. Villa G, Chelazzi C, Morettini E, et al. Organ dysfunction during continuous venovenous high cut-off hemodialysis in patients with septic acute kidney injury: a prospective observational study. PLoS One. 2017;12:e0172039.

30 Acid-Base Disorders and Regional Citrate Anticoagulation with Continuous Renal Replacement Therapy

C. Ichai, H. Quintard, and L. Velly

30.1 Introduction

Citrate delivery with continuous renal replacement therapy (CRRT) enables provision of real regional anticoagulation. Several meta-analyses have strongly confirmed that regional citrate anticoagulation (RCA) is more efficient (longer circuit lifespan) and safer (lower bleeding risk) than heparin [1–3]. Besides these beneficial effects, three recent high-quality randomized controlled trials (RCTs) have demonstrated that metabolic complications are now uncommon, transient and easily preventable when RCA is implemented using a formalized strategy [4–6]. Therefore, RCA is now recommended as the first choice for anticoagulation during CRRT [7, 8].

In this chapter, we summarize current knowledge on the interaction between CRRT and citrate metabolism and its consequences in terms of acid-base adverse effects. The final paragraph provides some practical management approaches aimed at preventing and treating these effects appropriately at the bedside.

C. Ichai (✉)
Polyvalent Intensive Care Unit, Hôpital Pasteur 2, University Hospital of Nice, University Côte D'Azur, Nice, France
e-mail: ichai@unice.fr

H. Quintard
Polyvalent Intensive Care Unit, Hôpital Pasteur 2, University Hospital of Nice, University Côte D'Azur, Nice, France

UMR 7275 CNRS, Valbonne, France

L. Velly
Department of Anesthesiology and Critical Care Medicine, Institut de Neuroscience de la Timone (INT), University Hospital La Timone, Aix Marseille University, Marseille, France

J.-L. Vincent (ed.), *Annual Update in Intensive Care and Emergency Medicine 2019*, Annual Update in Intensive Care and Emergency Medicine,
https://doi.org/10.1007/978-3-030-06067-1_30

30.2 Citrate in CRRT: General Considerations

Understanding the pharmacokinetics of citrate is essential to comprehend the development of acid-base disorders related to RCA during CRRT. Most commercialized citrate solutions exclusively contain trisodium citrate to provide a prolonged effect. Under physiological conditions, trisodium citrate is converted into citric acid within 30 min. This latter enters the tricarboxylic acid cycle and is finally metabolized into CO_2, H_2O and ATP through the mitochondrial oxidative phosphorylation pathway [9–11]. This reaction is mainly performed by the liver and to a lesser extent by skeletal muscle and the renal cortex. Citrate metabolism is characterized by a short systemic half-life of 5 min. This saturable reaction can be impaired and reduced in case of liver failure and in all conditions associated with an altered Kreb's cycle or mitochondrial oxidation caused by hypoxia or toxics. The major role of the liver in citrate metabolism has been confirmed by Kramer et al. [10]. These authors reported a substantial altered citrate metabolism, which was characterized by a 50% reduction in total body clearance in patients with compared to those without cirrhosis.

Trisodium citrate acts by chelating calcium, which is a major element of the coagulation cascade. Briefly, 2 trisodium molecules react with 3 molecules of calcium to produce a citrate-calcium (Cit-Ca^{++}) complex while releasing 6 molecules of sodium (Fig. 30.1). With usual doses of RRT, approximately 60% of these complexes are removed through the filter regardless of the convective or diffuse modality. However, because of its close relationship with the effluent rate (ultrafiltration/dialysate), this amount can vary. The remaining Ca^{++} released from the non-removed

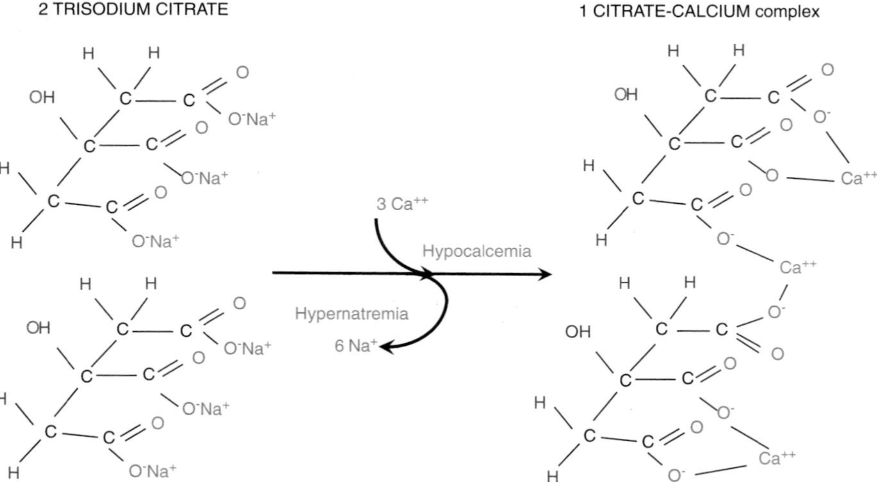

Fig. 30.1 Trisodium citrate and calcium chelation. Two molecules of trisodium citrate are converted into one complex of citrate-calcium leading to a simultaneous systemic ionized hypocalcemia (fixation of 3 molecules of ionized calcium) and hypernatremia (release of 6 molecules of sodium)

Cit-Ca^{++} induces a partial systemic ionized calcium (iCa^{++}) return in the total calcium blood pool. Therefore, blood calcium supplementation is needed to compensate for losses through the filter [9, 11, 12].

30.3 Acid-base Disorders and RCA

The Stewart approach is now accepted as the more comprehensive concept to precisely identify and quantify complex acid-base disorders [13–16]. Briefly, the Stewart concept assumes that the pH depends on three independent variables: $PaCO_2$, strong ion difference (SID) and weak anions (albuminate, phosphate) [17]. Any modification of one of these parameters causes pH variations. Accordingly, hypercapnia causes respiratory acidosis (and conversely). Metabolic abnormalities are the consequences of changes in SID or weak acids. In these situations, the absolute rule of electroneutrality, i.e., the equilibrium between positive (cations) and negative (anions) charges, lead to acidosis or alkalosis. As a consequence, any reduction in SID is responsible for a metabolic acidosis by decreasing bicarbonate concentration. An increase in any strong anion (hyperlactatemia, hyperketonemia) or decrease in strong cation (hyponatremia) induces a reduction in SID and, in turn, a metabolic acidosis (and conversely). Finally, changes in weak acid concentration represent the second cause of metabolic acid-base disturbances. Physiological weak acids are albuminate$^-$ and phosphate$^-$ while citrate$^-$ is an exogenous weak metabolizable anion. Elevation in weak acids is responsible for metabolic acidosis (hyperphosphatemia or hyperalbuminemia). In the absence of acid base disorders, the normal value of $PaCO_2$ is 40 mmHg, of SID is 39 meq/L (Fig. 30.2). Trisodium citrate can cause complex and various acid base disorders, depending on citrate load and a patient's capacity to metabolize it.

During RCA, metabolic acidosis may be the consequence of two different mechanisms which must be identified to deliver the appropriate treatment. First, metabolic acidosis caused by citrate accumulation occurs when citrate metabolism is impaired leading to hypercitratemia. As previously mentioned, the increase in the negatively charged citrate$^-$ leads to a decrease in bicarbonate concentration (the main plasma buffer) to maintain electroneutrality and creates metabolic acidosis. In this situation, the SID is normal and the cause of the problem is hypercitratemia (Figs. 30.3a and 30.4a). However, other anions, especially strong metabolizable anions (lactate) can participate partly to the development of metabolic acidosis. The presence of such anions is identified by a reduction in the SID and an increase in the strong ion gap (difference between the apparent and the effective SID), which indicates the presence of excessive strong metabolizable anion (Figs. 30.3b and 30.4b). Hyperlactatemia is frequently associated with hypercitratemia [18]. Finally, metabolic alkalosis related to hypoalbuminemia can counteract or minimize the acidifying effect of hypercitratemia or hyperlactatemia, and lead to an incorrect interpretation in case of normal pH.

Because the level of citratemia is not routinely available in clinical practice, citrate accumulation must be suspected and recognized from indirect warning

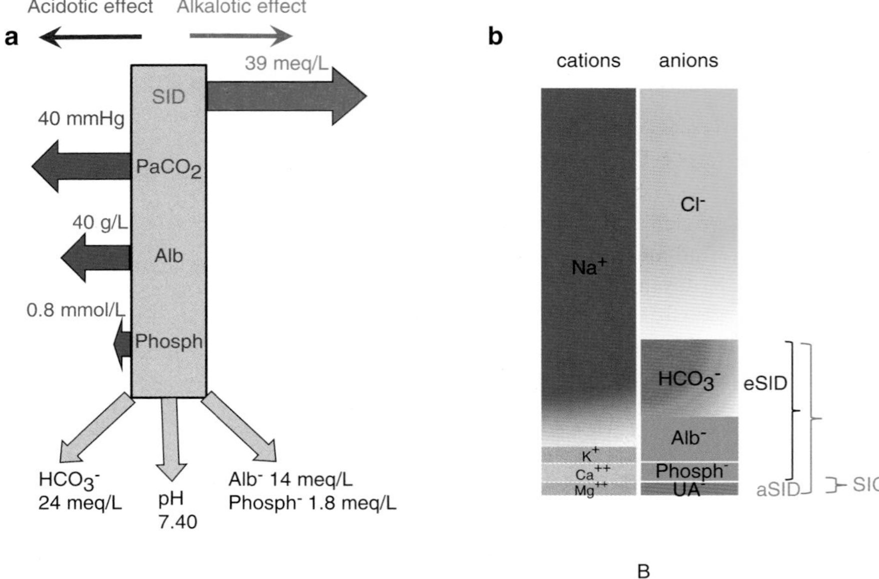

Fig. 30.2 Schematic representation of the acid base equilibrium in physiological conditions according to the Stewart concept. (**a**) The three independent variables of the pH value: $PaCO_2$, strong ion difference (SID) and weak acids (albuminate [Alb^-] and phosphate [$phosph^-$]). Hypercapnia causes respiratory acidosis (and conversely). Regardless of the specific cause, any reduction in SID or elevation in weak acid, is responsible for metabolic acidosis (and conversely). Normocapnia (40 mmHg) associated with a normal albumin (40 g/L), phosphate (0.8 mmol/L) and SID (39 meq/L) leads to an acid-base equilibrium within normal range. (**b**) Schematic representation of plasma electroneutrality with the major cations (positive charges) and anions (negative charges). The effective SID (eSID) is calculated using the following formula: eSID = (HCO_3^- + albuminate$^-$ + phosphate$^-$) = 39 meq/L; the apparent SID (aSID) = ($Na^+ + K^+ + Ca^{++} + Mg^{++}$) − ($Cl^-$) = 45 meq/L. The strong ion gap (SIG), which is the difference between the aSID and the eSID, indicates the presence of unmeasured strong anions (UA; normal value = 5–8 meq/L)

signs. The most popular of these is the increased total to ionized calcium ratio (Ca_{tot}/iCa^{++}) above 2.5: Ca_{tot} increases due to the accumulation of Cit-Ca^{++} complexes while iCa^{++} remains low and protein-bound calcium unchanged (Fig. 30.5) [19]. The Ca_{tot}/iCa^{++} ratio is closely correlated with citrate plasma level and a cut-off >2.5 mmol/L appears accurate to predict citrate accumulation [18–20]. Persistent ionized hypocalcemia, despite a progressive increase in calcium supplementation, seems to be the most sensitive and earliest sign of citrate accumulation. A trend towards abnormal values is probably a good and early marker of citrate accumulation rather than an absolute cut-off. Finally, hyperlactatemia is an interesting surrogate marker of altered citrate metabolism due to an impaired Krebs' cycle [18, 21, 22].

Second, metabolic acidosis caused by insufficient trisodium citrate delivery occurs when the amount of citrate is low (low blood flow) with respect to the amount of Cit-Ca^{++} removed (high ultrafiltration or dialysate flow). With such a setup, the

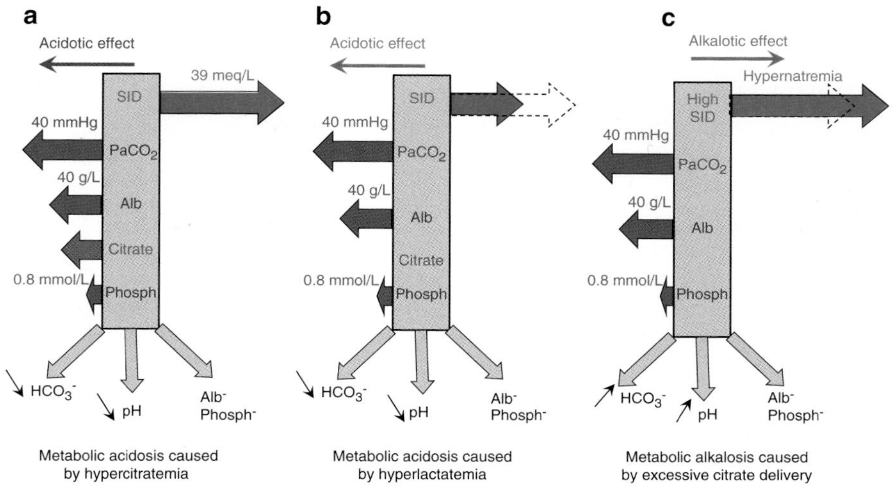

Fig. 30.3 Regional citrate anticoagulation-related metabolic acid base disorders according to the Stewart concept. (**a**) Because citrate is a weak metabolizable anion, hypercitratemia (citrate accumulation) causes metabolic acidosis (low pH and bicarbonate values) providing there is no change in other weak acids, $PaCO_2$ or strong ion difference (SID). (**b**) Because lactate is a strong metabolizable anion, hyperlactatemia causes metabolic acidosis by decreasing the SID (high pH and bicarbonate values) providing there is no change in weak acids or $PaCO_2$. (**c**) Because sodium is a strong non-metabolizable cation, hypernatremia, which results from excessive citrate delivery and metabolism, causes metabolic alkalosis by increasing the SID (low pH and bicarbonate level) providing there are no changes in weak acids or $PaCO_2$. *Alb* albumin; *Alb*$^-$ albuminate; *Phosph* phosphorus; *Phosph*$^-$ phosphate

low citrate delivery associated with high citrate removal does not enable a sufficient alkalinizing effect of citrate metabolism. Contrary to what happens with citrate accumulation, metabolic acidosis is associated with normal citrate metabolism.

Metabolic alkalosis caused by trisodium citrate overload occurs when the amount of trisodium citrate delivery is excessive or its filter clearance is insufficient while the Cit-Ca^{++} complexes are normally metabolized. According to the Stewart concept, when citrate is metabolized, the non-metabolizable cation, sodium, is simultaneously released and persists in the plasma. To maintain electroneutrality, bicarbonate increases and in turn, the SID too, leading to metabolic alkalosis (Figs. 30.3c and 30.4c) [13, 17]. However, because citrate produces H_2O and CO_2, the final alkalinizing effect of trisodium citrate depend on the patient's capacity to excrete CO_2. If there is altered CO_2 elimination, the metabolic alkalosis can be replaced by respiratory acidosis (hypercapnia).

In summary, RCA can be responsible for complex acid-base disorders. Citrate, which is a weak acid, is the cause of metabolic acidosis essentially due to an impairment in its metabolism, with citrate accumulation. The non-metabolizable cation, sodium, which is released when trisodium citrate is metabolized, is responsible for the development of metabolic alkalosis. This latter disorder indicates citrate overload.

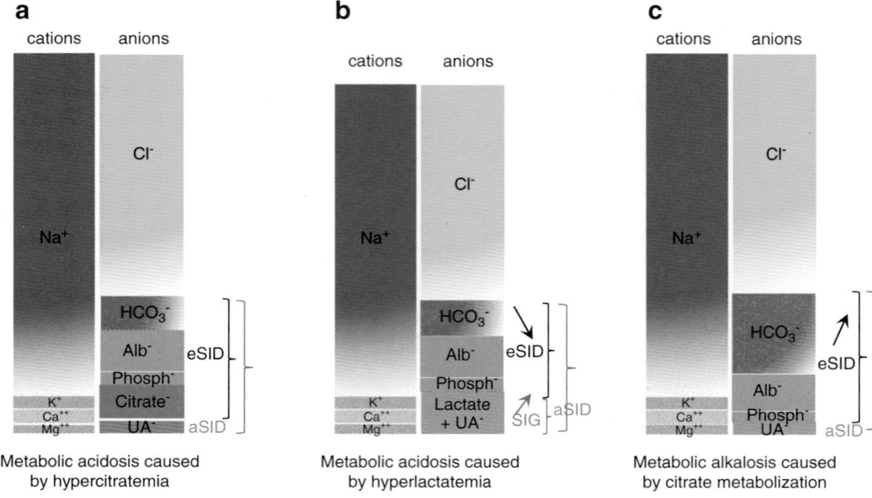

Fig. 30.4 Plasma electroneutrality during regional citrate anticoagulation (RCA)-related acid-base disorders. The effective strong ion difference (eSID) is calculated using the following formula: eSID = (HCO_3^- + albuminate$^-$ + phosphate$^-$); the apparent SID (aSID) = (Na^+ + K^+ + Ca^{++} + Mg^{++}) – (Cl^-). Strong ion gap (SIG) = aSID − eSID. (**a**) Metabolic acidosis caused by hypercitratemia (citrate accumulation). To maintain plasma electroneutrality, the accumulation of the weak anion, citrate$^-$, leads to a decrease in bicarbonate (the major plasma buffer) and pH. Neither eSID nor aSID change as there is no change in strong cations or anions. (**b**) Metabolic acidosis caused by hyperlactatemia. To maintain plasma electroneutrality, the accumulation of the strong anion, lactate$^-$, leads to a decrease in bicarbonate (the major plasma buffer) and pH. Consequently the eSID decreases while the SIG increases indicating the presence of abnormal strong anions, in this case, lactate$^-$. (**c**) Metabolic alkalosis caused by trisodium citrate metabolism. Metabolism of excessive trisodium delivery leads to the release of citrate, which disappears during metabolism, and sodium, which is non-metabolizable and remains in the plasma. To maintain plasma electroneutrality, hypernatremia induces an increase in the eSID by increasing the bicarbonate negative charges. As a result, plasma pH elevates. *Phosph*$^-$ phosphate; *Alb*$^-$ albuminate; *UA*$^-$ unmeasured strong anions (lactate, ketone bodies)

30.4 Practical Management of Acid-base Disorders Related to RCA

The reported incidence of RCA-related acid-base disorders varies in the literature [21, 23–29]. Multiple reasons likely contribute to this large variability, including the technique, the types of patients, the absence of appropriate setup and monitoring and above all the absence of formalized protocols, expertise and training of the team for this modality of anticoagulation [12, 30, 31]. The incidence of the syndrome of citrate accumulation with metabolic acidosis is now rare (approximately 5% of patients). A higher incidence was reported in patients with acute liver failure reaching up to 12% [5, 19, 23, 25, 27]. More recently, studies performed in patients with liver failure failed to demonstrate a greater risk of citrate accumulation provided a

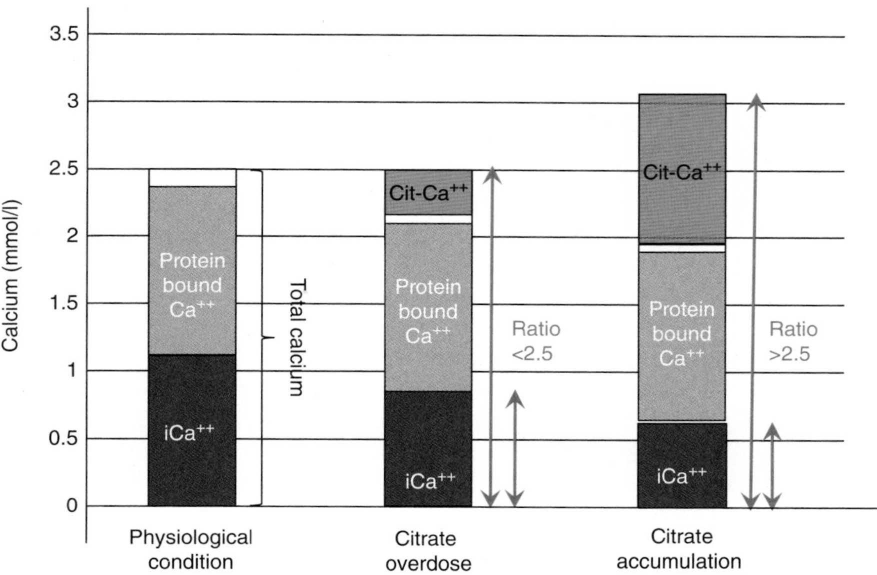

Fig. 30.5 Distribution of total plasma calcium in physiological conditions and during regional citrate anticoagulation with continuous renal replacement therapy. In physiological conditions, 50% of total plasma calcium (2.2–2.6 mmol/L) is distributed in an ionized form (iCa^{++} 1.1–1.3 mmol/L), 10% in complexed form (0.05 mmol/L) and 40% in protein-bound form (0.95–1.2 mmol/L). In citrate overdose, the presence of citrate-Ca^{++} complex (Cit-Ca^{++}) is associated with ionized hypocalcemia and usually with total hypocalcemia. The ratio of total calcium to iCa^{++} (Ca_{tot}/iCa^{++}) is <2.5 because protein Ca^{++} does not change. In citrate accumulation, the presence of high levels of Cit-Ca^{++} with ionized hypocalcemia leads to an elevation of Ca_{tot}/iCa^{++} to >2.5 as protein Ca^{++} does not change

formal protocol was used with close monitoring by an expert trained team [21, 28]. However, it is difficult to really predict this risk as usual laboratory tests (bilirubinemia, transaminase levels) poorly reflect liver dysfunction. Hyperlactatemia >3.4 mmol/L (and lactate kinetics) and a low prothrombin time (≤25%) seem to be the most accurate indicators of citrate accumulation in patients with severe liver dysfunction [21]. In these situations, patients also present with hyperlactatemic metabolic acidosis before starting citrate delivery due to severe hemodynamic instability. Although rare, citrate accumulation develops within the first 24 h and resolves rapidly with the appropriate treatment.

Metabolic alkalosis is the most common metabolic disorder caused by RCA during CRRT. Its incidence can reach up to 50% of patients [23, 28, 29]. Usually, metabolic alkalosis remains moderate without severe clinical consequences. It develops later than metabolic acidosis, within 48–72 h. Schultheiß et al. [21] found that metabolic acidosis was already present at baseline in 65% of patients with liver failure receiving RCA; normalization of bicarbonate was obtained after 24 h in 60% of cases but, after 72 h, metabolic alkalosis developed in 53% of patients.

30.4.1 Prevention of Acid-base Disorders Related to RCA

Three large RCTs have reported no differences in metabolic derangements, especially for acid-base adverse effects between RCA and heparin anticoagulation during CRRT. Regardless of the precise modality, these disorders were uncommon, transient and resolved early in experienced centers [4–6]. Two major recent meta-analyses confirmed that the incidence of metabolic alkalosis was comparable between RCA and heparin [1, 3], while another reported an increased risk [2]. Indeed, it is not the acid-base disorders by themselves, but rather the resulting ionized hypocalcemia, which is more frequently observed with RCA, that may cause severe clinical complications. Nevertheless, these data must be interpreted with caution as patients at risk were not included.

The prevention of RCA-related complications is based on the implementation of a proper technique including the choice of the most appropriate modality (dedicated machines and fluids), and education and training of the healthcare professionals involved in this management [30–32]. It is necessary to create an in-home formal protocol that includes as a minimum the optimal setup of the devices, patient and machine monitoring (especially the alarms) and regular evaluation of the quality of the management. In these conditions, RCA can be performed with all continuous diffuse and convective modalities with comparable efficiency and safety [9, 12, 31]. RCA requires a device equipped with a blood flow coupled to citrate delivery to maintain a stable citrate concentration. However, such a control loop forces reduced blood flows compared with heparin, to prevent excessive citrate delivery. Citrate solution is delivered in the arterial line. A citratemia target between 3 and 4 mmol/L provides effective anticoagulation with a minimal risk of bleeding. This objective is obtained by measuring the postfilter iCa^{++} with a value of 0.25–0.35 mmol/L. Such close monitoring is essential to prevent unplanned blocks of the circuit caused by clotting and risks of bleeding [33, 34]. However, the accuracy of this measurement is poor with large over- and underestimations according to the machine [35, 36]. Accordingly, it is strongly suggested that the targeted value of postfilter iCa^{++} should be adjusted and personalized using the bedside blood gas analyzer. Losses of Cit-Ca^{++} through the filter require calcium supplementation to be provided. Calcium infusion is performed after the filter on the 'venous' line as close as possible to the patient to avoid recalcification of the circuit. The target is to achieve physiological values of 1.1–1.3 mmol/L. Ionized hypocalcemia represents the most serious metabolic complication of RCA, affecting 12–18% of patients [37, 38]. Fortunately, the incidence of severe hypocalcemia associated with shock or profound hypotensive episodes remains low (2.5%). To prevent such a complication, it is recommended to favor devices with a feedback control between the citrate and the calcium supplementation pumps, to always normalize the patient's iCa^{++} before starting RCA and to monitor it closely during the therapy. Only specifically formulated dialysate and substitution solutions are available and must be calcium-free, with low concentrations of sodium and bicarbonate and high concentrations of chloride. This is essential to counteract the development of metabolic alkalosis and hypernatremia caused by the trisodium citrate solution. For similar reasons, it is preferable to favor calcium chloride rather than calcium gluconate. Exclusive convective modalities (continuous venovenous hemofiltration [CVVH]) are performed with low-concentration solutions (18 mmol/L of citrate) which lead to high predilution and may reduce the capacity of clearance. Therefore, ultrafiltration must be used exclusively in postdilution with a sufficient rate (20–25 mL/kg/h). Blood flow in CVVH must not exceed 150–160 mL/min. The disadvantage of this strategy is that the anticoagulation effect is coupled with the predilution volume, which partially determines the clearance. High trisodium citrate solution (140 mmoL/L) is required with the diffusive modality (continuous venovenous hemodialysis [CVVHD]) to reach the targeted concentration of citrate in the circuit while maintaining low blood flow to prevent citrate overdose. Blood flow must be less than with CVVH at between 80 and 120 mL/min and dialysate rate between 1500 and 2000 mL/h. Thanks to the dialysate solution, it is easily possible to modulate blood bicarbonate concentration and to compensate metabolic acid base disorders. Consequently, RCA with CVVHD cannot be performed in patients requiring high blood flows. As recommended with heparin, it is mandatory to correctly interpret the pressure alarms and to check and manage them appropriately.

RCA requires closer biological monitoring than when using heparin. Ionized hypocalcemia is the most serious complication that can worsen patient outcomes. To prevent it, it is crucial to measure baseline iCa^{++} and any initiation of RCA is strictly prohibited before normalizing this value. Approximately 15–30 min from the start of RCA, iCa^{++} must be checked, then hourly within the first 3 h and every 6 h in stable situations. Any new adjustment requires a new control measurement approximately 30 min later. The calculation of Ca_{tot}/iCa^{++} ratio is usually performed daily, but close monitoring (3 times per day) is necessary in conditions at risk of citrate accumulation. Baseline arterial blood gas and electrolyte (sodium, chloride, potassium, magnesium and phosphate) measurements are needed followed by repeated measurements every 6–8 h in stable situations. Hyperlactatemia and lack of normalization of lactate levels may be a good early indicator of citrate accumulation and must be checked regularly in patients at risk [18, 21]. An example of a protocol indicating how to approach biological monitoring in patients receiving RCA is summarized in Box 30.1.

In summary, all convective and diffusive modalities (CVVH, CVVHDF, CVVHD) are comparable in terms of efficiency and safety enabling control of citrate losses via the total effluent rate (ultrafiltration and/or dialysate rate). Despite substantial improvements in simplicity, ergonomy and automation of devices, the appropriate setting, close monitoring, and expertise of the healthcare team are needed to elaborate a formalized protocol and prevent RCA-related adverse effects, especially acid-base derangements.

Box 30.1: An Example of Patient and Filter Biological Monitoring During Regional Citrate Anticoagulation

The patient (arterial samples)	The circuit (postfilter samples)
Measure systemic iCa^{++} to adjust calcium supplementation	*Measure postfilter iCa^{++} to adjust citrate concentration*
• Baseline before starting • 15–30 min after initiation and 30 min after any adjustment • Every hour within the first 3 h • Every 6 h if iCa^{++} is stable	• 15 min after starting • The 1 h after initiation • 30–60 min after any adjustment • Every 6–8 h if postfilter iCa^{++} is stable and in the target range
Measure total systemic calcium to calculate the total calcium/iCa^{++} ratio	
• Daily if stable • Every 6–8 h in patients at risk of citrate accumulation (medical prescription)	
Arterial blood samples	
• Blood gas (pH, bicarbonates, $PaCO_2$), Na, Cl, K, magnesium, and phosphate daily	
Additional and more frequent measurements on medical prescription	

30.4.2 Treatment of Acid-base Disorders Related to RCA

30.4.2.1 Metabolic Acidosis Related to Citrate Accumulation

Citrate by itself is not toxic or dangerous except in cases of very high accumulation, which may result in vasodilation. The real clinical risk is the development of substantial hypotension or shock caused by the resulting persistent severe systemic ionized hypocalcemia. The two most frequent causes of citrate accumulation are a violation of protocol or use in patients at risk [11, 24]. However, liver failure, shock and some intoxications (metformin, cyclosporine, paracetamol) are not absolute contraindications for RCA during CRRT provided closer than usual monitoring is performed by an experienced team. In this condition, the risk of citrate accumulation is negligible, easily suspected and rapidly treated [11, 21, 28, 39]. The sole real treatment for citrate accumulation, especially with severe ionized hypocalcemia and metabolic acidosis, is to stop citrate delivery while increasing Cit-Ca^{++} complex clearance with a sufficient effluent rate (dialysate or ultrafiltration rate) and normalizing the systemic iCa^{++} value. The removal of citrate will lead to an 'endogenous' alkalization and a progressive restoration of a normal pH. If citrate accumulation and metabolic acidosis are slight and caused by an incorrect circuit setup, an adjustment consisting of a reduction in blood flow (to decrease citrate delivery) associated with an increase in the effluent rate (to elevate citrate losses) can be cautiously proposed aimed at a rapid normalization of metabolic disorders (Box 30.2).

Acute Kidney Injury and Delirium: Kidney–Brain Crosstalk

31

R. Y. Y. Wan and M. Ostermann

31.1 Introduction

Delirium is widely recognized as a form of fluctuating dysfunction of the brain and occurs in up to 70% of the critically ill [1]. It is associated with increased morbidity, longer hospital stay, cognitive decline with associated loss of quality of life, and death [1–4]. Recognition of delirium remains a challenge. Completion of delirium screening involves first using a validated sedation scale to assess eligibility for cognitive assessment, followed by a validated delirium screening tool. This may not be possible to complete if patients are in a coma, unable to understand the language or have established cognitive dysfunction (e.g., dementia, mental disorders) [5, 7]. Furthermore, delirium assessments will only reflect the cognitive state of the patient at the time of the assessment, making it difficult to capture this fluctuating cognitive disorder. As a result, the prevalence of delirium is likely to be underestimated. Furthermore, with no proven effective pharmacological therapy, delirium in the critically ill continues to pose a healthcare burden and a management conundrum for clinicians [8–10].

The mechanisms leading to critical care delirium remain poorly understood. The pathophysiology is likely multifactorial given the diversity of etiologic mechanisms associated with encephalopathy in the context of liver disease, sepsis, drug interactions, metabolic derangements and alcohol withdrawal [11]. Its acute onset presentation is likely to be the failure of the brain's resilience to withstand a response to

R. Y. Y. Wan
Department of Pharmacy, Guy's & St Thomas' NHS Foundation Trust, London, UK

M. Ostermann (✉)
Departments of Critical Care and Nephrology, King's College London, Guy's & St Thomas' NHS Foundation Trust, London, UK
e-mail: Marlies.Ostermann@gstt.nhs.uk

J.-L. Vincent (ed.), *Annual Update in Intensive Care and Emergency Medicine 2019*, Annual Update in Intensive Care and Emergency Medicine,
https://doi.org/10.1007/978-3-030-06067-1_31

noxious insults during critical illness, coupled with a series of punctuated declines and major medical insults which can lead to lasting cognitive dysfunction [12]. The impact on healthcare resources is substantial [4].

Despite the development of delirium prediction tools, the prevention and early identification of patients at risk remains a challenge [13, 14]. To date, only multicomponent non-pharmacologic approaches have proven to be effective in delirium prevention [9, 15, 16]. Delirium has a substantial impact on patients, their relatives, healthcare providers and resources [4], and remains one of the top three research areas in importance to patients, carers and health professionals as identified by the James Lind Alliance Priority Setting Partnerships for intensive care research.

31.2 Diagnosing Delirium in the Critically Ill

Delirium presents as three major subtypes: hyperactive (agitated), hypoactive (quiet) and mixed (features of both hyperactive and hypoactive), with hypoactive and mixed the most common presentations in critically ill patients over 65 years old [17]. There are several validated screening tools for delirium in adult patients, [5, 6, 18]. The two most well-known, widely used tools, endorsed by the Society of Critical Care Medicine (SCCM) Pain Agitation and Delirium (PAD) guideline, are the Confusion Assessment Method for the ICU (CAM-ICU) and the Intensive Care Delirium Screening Checklist (ICDSC) [19, 20]. The ICDSC has some advantages over CAM-ICU as it is scored cumulatively over an entire 24-h period of nursing observation whereas three of the four CAM-ICU features are based on performance at a single time point. The ICDSC gives a score that potentially identifies subsyndromal delirium in patients but, conversely, also increases the likelihood of false-positive assessments. The advantage of CAM-ICU includes being more extensively validated against American Psychiatric Association's Diagnostic and Statistical Manual of Mental Disorders (DSM) reference raters in 12 studies across both critically ill and non-critically ill patients than the ICDSC [21, 22]. Implementation of the ICDSC into clinical practice depends heavily on the training and experience of each member of the nursing staff [23] whereas the CAM-ICU tool is simpler and can be easily used by all healthcare professionals caring for the patient.

31.3 Risk Factors for Intensive Care Delirium

Over 100 risk factors have been investigated for potential association with intensive care delirium. However, studies are heterogeneous in design, methods used to detect delirium and patient populations [24]. Despite the heterogeneity, there are risk factors relevant to the critically ill patient that can be broadly categorized as predisposing vulnerability factors and hospital-related precipitating factors [25–28] (Box 31.1).

Box 31.1: Common Risk Factors for Delirium During Critical Illness

Predisposing vulnerability factors	Precipitating hospital-related factors
Age	Severity of illness
Dementia predisposing cognitive impairment	Benzodiazepines (especially lorazepam and midazolam)
Alcohol use disorder	Mechanical ventilation (and need for sedation)
Charlson Comorbidity Index	Metabolic disturbances
	Sepsis
	Sleep alterations

31.4 Acute Brain Dysfunction during Critical Illness

Acute brain dysfunction in critical illness includes both delirium and coma, and the leading concepts involve inflammatory and immune-related processes associated with critical illness, disturbances of the neuro-endocrine system and alterations in pharmacokinetics and pharmacodynamics of drugs leading to alterations in neurotransmitter synthesis, function and/or availability. In animal models of acute sepsis, activation of the immune system led to the rapid release of one or more of the following cytokines, interleukin (IL)-1β, Toll-like receptor (TLR)4, tumor necrosis factor (TNF)-α and IL-6 [29]. This was thought to be associated with post-septic behavioral impairment. Interestingly, it has also been shown in mice that cognitive dysfunction occurred after critical illness had peaked [30]. The acetylcholinergic neurotransmitter system appears to play an important role in the control of brain inflammation. These changes in neurotransmitters including deficiencies in acetylcholine and/or melatonin availability, excess in dopamine, norepinephrine, and/or glutamate release, and variable alterations in serotonin, histamine, and/or γ-aminobutyric acid are thought to drive acute brain dysfunction during critical illness and prolonged delirium with dementia on follow-up [31, 32].

31.5 Acute Brain Dysfunction in Renal Disease

Chronic kidney disease (CKD) has long been linked to cognitive decline, and at a faster exponential rate compared to age-related cognitive decline [33]. The exact pathophysiological mechanisms leading to cognitive decline are not fully understood, but it is thought that associated complications, such as cardiovascular disease, exposure to uremia-induced oxidative stress, and electrolyte and fluid disturbances, play a role [33]. Interestingly, cognitive decline seen in CKD has been shown to be reversible following renal transplantation with reported sustained cognitive improvement [34, 35].

Unsurprisingly, acute kidney injury (AKI) has also been reported to be associated with delirium during critical illness [25, 36]. The sharp decline in renal function seen in AKI, typically within 48 h, is common among the critically ill, affecting up to 60% of patients [37, 38]. It is plausible that similar pathophysiological mechanisms exist for the development of delirium as with those seen with CKD-associated cognitive decline.

AKI is a syndrome with multiple potential etiologies. By consensus, it is defined by the Kidney Disease Improving Global Outcomes (KDIGO) staging criteria based on changes in serum creatinine or urine output but this classification is not without controversy [39]. Serum creatinine and urine output are neither renal-specific nor early markers of renal dysfunction. Serum creatinine concentrations depend on liver function and muscle mass and may also be affected by acute illness (e.g., major trauma, sepsis) [40]. Elucidating baseline renal function can be challenging in clinical practice as historical serum creatinine results are not always available. As such, AKI may be over- or under-diagnosed [41, 42]. Moreover, serum creatinine has a non-linear relationship with glomerular filtration rate (GFR) and requires time to accumulate, which contributes to delays in detection of important changes in kidney function. Urine output can also be misleading when driven by drugs such as diuretics, or as a natural physiological response to hypovolemia or endogenous secretion of anti-diuretic hormone [39, 43].

31.5.1 Pathophysiology of Acute Brain Dysfunction in AKI

AKI is considered an inflammatory condition. It is known to be associated with neurological complications including confusion, seizures and coma [44]. The pathophysiological mechanisms during AKI include endothelial injury, leukocyte infiltration, release of cytokines and inflammatory mediators, induction of apoptosis, and local activation of the coagulation system. The promotion of leukocyte infiltration into the kidneys has been found in animal models to induce the production of cytokines and chemokines, including IL-1, IL-6, IL-10 and TNF, and subsequent release into the systemic circulation, extending effects to other organs including the brain [45, 46]. Furthermore, animal model studies utilizing this concept have identified increased brain vascular permeability, microvascular protein leakage, neuronal pyknosis and microgliosis in the hippocampus, and disruption of the blood-brain barrier in AKI [46]. It is this disruption to the blood-brain barrier that is thought to allow infiltration of metabolites and toxins into the brain and central nervous system that ultimately leads to brain dysfunction.

31.6 Kidney–Brain Interaction and Critical Illness

During critical illness, AKI leads to electrolyte imbalances, fluid shifts and amplification of inflammatory processes. This augmented inflammation is likely to be a result of multifaceted mechanisms categorized by: (1) release of cytokines and inflammatory mediators by the kidney; (2) decreased renal clearance of cytokines and chemokines prolonging their exposure on both the brain and kidney; (3) acute uremic state with imbalance of electrolyte and volume homeostasis; and (4) exposure of blood to the extracorporeal circuit during renal replacement therapy (RRT).

Many critically patients with AKI require sedatives and opioid analgesia, both of which are known risks factors associated with delirium. During AKI, drug dosing is very challenging as renal function often changes quickly and is difficult to assess and quantify [47]. Furthermore, there have only been a few small pharmacokinetic studies conducted on a limited number of antibiotics making them difficult to generalize to the wider critical care population [48]. In addition, as AKI augments the inflammatory response in critical illness, it remains unclear how drugs and their metabolites are affected and to what degree they cross the altered blood-brain barrier. In the case of antibiotics, both under-and over-dosing have been described in critically ill patients with sepsis and AKI [49].

From a follow-up study of AKI patients who required RRT, patients had an increased risk of dementia after critical illness independent of severe sepsis and prolonged delirium duration [50]. It remains unclear, even when RRT is administered as a therapy, whether the risk of delirium and long-term cognitive impairment is modifiable. During critical illness there appears to be growing evidence to suggest AKI and brain dysfunction are linked (Fig. 31.1). The delayed cognitive dysfunction seen in critical care survivors may be due to critical illness itself but emerging theories of kidney–brain crosstalk suggest that AKI could contribute to the risk of delirium and long-term cognitive impairment in the critically ill.

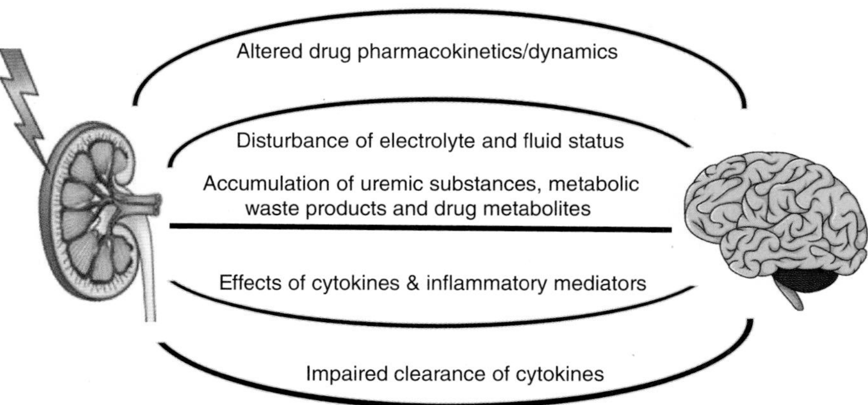

Fig. 31.1 Acute kidney injury-induced brain dysfunction. The reasons for brain dysfunction in patients with acute kidney injury are multifactorial and include the effects of accumulated waste products and fluid overload, the impact of altered drug metabolism and the effects of cytokines and inflammatory mediators

31.7 Conclusion

Delirium remains highly prevalent in the critically ill and difficult to diagnose in patient groups where there is uncertainty over baseline cognitive impairment, neurological injury, and often inability to partake in delirium screening assessments. Modifiable risk factors associated with critical care delirium are influenced by kidney–brain crosstalk interactions through amplification of inflammation, impaired clearance of chemokines and cytokines, alteration of drug clearance, electrolyte imbalances and fluid shifts. Interventions directed at preventing or reducing delirium and preserving renal function may mitigate brain injury associated with critical illness. Although the role of RRT on ameliorating brain injury appears hopeful, to date RRT's ability to modify delirium risk is unclear and requires further research. It is accepted that those who survive their critical illness are at increased risk of long-term cognitive impairment, though less is known regarding whether AKI *per se* contributes to this. It remains unknown whether it is the initial AKI insult that increases the risk of delirium and cognitive dysfunction and whether this is reversible. More research is urgently needed.

References

1. Pandharipande P, Jackson J, Ely EW. Delirium: acute cognitive dysfunction in the critically ill. Curr Opin Crit Care. 2005;11:360–8.
2. Ely EW, Shintani A, Truman B, et al. Delirium as a predictor of mortality in mechanically ventilated patients in the intensive care unit. JAMA. 2004;291:1753–62.
3. Pisani MA, Kong SY, Kasl SV, Murphy TE, Araujo KL, Van Ness PH. Days of delirium are associated with 1-year mortality in an older intensive care unit population. Am J Respir Crit Care Med. 2009;180:1092–7.
4. Svenningsen H, Tonnesen EK, Videbech P, Frydenberg M, Christensen D, Egerod I. Intensive care delirium - effect on memories and health-related quality of life - a follow-up study. J Clin Nurs. 2014;23:634–44.
5. Ely EW, Inouye SK, Bernard GR, et al. Delirium in mechanically ventilated patients: validity and reliability of the confusion assessment method for the intensive care unit (CAM-ICU). JAMA. 2001;286:2703–10.
6. Bergeron N, Dubois MJ, Dumont M, Dial S, Skrobik Y. Intensive care delirium screening checklist: evaluation of a new screening tool. Intensive Care Med. 2001;27:859–64.
7. Reade MC, Eastwood GM, Peck L, Bellomo R, Baldwin I. Routine use of the confusion assessment method for the intensive care unit (CAM-ICU) by bedside nurses may underdiagnose delirium. Crit Care Resusc. 2011;13:217–24.
8. Jubran A, Lawm G, Kelly J, et al. Depressive disorders during weaning from prolonged mechanical ventilation. Intensive Care Med. 2010;36:828–35.
9. Al-Qadheeb NS, Balk EM, Fraser GL, et al. Randomized ICU trials do not demonstrate an association between interventions that reduce delirium duration and short-term mortality: a systematic review and meta-analysis. Crit Care Med. 2014;42:1442–54.
10. Sharma A, Malhotra S, Grover S, Jindal SK. Incidence, prevalence, risk factor and outcome of delirium in intensive care unit: a study from India. Gen Hosp Psychiatry. 2012;34:639–46.
11. Williams ST. Pathophysiology of encephalopathy and delirium. J Clin Neurophysiol. 2013;30:435–7.

12. Abraham CM, Obremskey WT, Song Y, Jackson JC, Ely EW, Archer KR. Hospital delirium and psychological distress at 1 year and health-related quality of life after moderate-to-severe traumatic injury without intracranial hemorrhage. Arch Phys Med Rehabil. 2014;95:2382–9.
13. Wassenaar A, Schoonhoven L, Devlin JW, et al. Delirium prediction in the intensive care unit: comparison of two delirium prediction models. Crit Care. 2018;22:114.
14. van den Boogaard M, Pickkers P, Slooter AJ, et al. Development and validation of PRE-DELIRIC (PREdiction of DELIRium in ICu patients) delirium prediction model for intensive care patients: observational multicentre study. BMJ. 2012;344:e420.
15. Abraha I, Trotta F, Rimland JM, et al. Efficacy of non-pharmacological interventions to prevent and treat delirium in older patients: a systematic overview. The SENATOR project ONTOP Series. PLoS One. 2015;10:e0123090.
16. Schweickert WD, Pohlman MC, Pohlman AS, et al. Early physical and occupational therapy in mechanically ventilated, critically ill patients: a randomised controlled trial. Lancet. 2009;373:1874–82.
17. Peterson JF, Pun BT, Dittus RS, et al. Delirium and its motoric subtypes: a study of 614 critically ill patients. J Am Geriatr Soc. 2006;54:479–84.
18. Van Rompaey B, Schuurmans MJ, Shortridge-Baggett LM, Truijen S, Elseviers M, Bossaert L. A comparison of the CAM-ICU and the NEECHAM Confusion Scale in intensive care delirium assessment: an observational study in non-intubated patients. Crit Care. 2008;12:R16.
19. Barr J, Fraser GL, Puntillo K, et al. Clinical practice guidelines for the management of pain, agitation, and delirium in adult patients in the intensive care unit: executive summary. Am J Health Syst Pharm. 2013;70:53–8.
20. Arumugam S, El-Menyar A, Al-Hassani A, et al. Delirium in the intensive care unit. J Emerg Trauma Shock. 2017;10:37–46.
21. Neto AS, Nassar AP Jr, Cardoso SO, et al. Delirium screening in critically ill patients: a systematic review and meta-analysis. Crit Care Med. 2012;40:1946–51.
22. Gusmao-Flores D, Salluh JI, Chalhub RA, Quarantini LC. The confusion assessment method for the intensive care unit (CAM-ICU) and intensive care delirium screening checklist (ICDSC) for the diagnosis of delirium: a systematic review and meta-analysis of clinical studies. Crit Care. 2012;16:R115.
23. Devlin JW, Marquis F, Riker RR, et al. Combined didactic and scenario-based education improves the ability of intensive care unit staff to recognize delirium at the bedside. Crit Care. 2008;12:R19.
24. Pandharipande PP, Ely EW, Arora RC, et al. The intensive care delirium research agenda: a multinational, interprofessional perspective. Intensive Care Med. 2017;43:1329–39.
25. Pisani MA, Murphy TE, Van Ness PH, Araujo KL, Inouye SK. Characteristics associated with delirium in older patients in a medical intensive care unit. Arch Intern Med. 2007;167:1629–34.
26. Pandharipande P, Shintani A, Peterson J, et al. Lorazepam is an independent risk factor for transitioning to delirium in intensive care unit patients. Anesthesiology. 2006;104:21–6.
27. Serafim RB, Dutra MF, Saddy F, et al. Delirium in postoperative nonventilated intensive care patients: risk factors and outcomes. Ann Intensive Care. 2012;2:1–6.
28. Van Rompaey B, Elseviers MM, Schuurmans MJ, Shortridge-Baggett LM, Truijen S, Bossaert L. Risk factors for delirium in intensive care patients: a prospective cohort study. Crit Care. 2009;13:R77.
29. Volpe BT, Berlin RA, Frankfurt M. The brain at risk: the sepsis syndrome and lessons from preclinical experiments. Immunol Res. 2015;63:70–4.
30. Anderson ST, Commins S, Moynagh PN, Coogan AN. Lipopolysaccharide-induced sepsis induces long-lasting affective changes in the mouse. Brain Behav Immun. 2015;43:98–109.
31. Maldonado JR. Neuropathogenesis of delirium: review of current etiologic theories and common pathways. Am J Geriatr Psychiatry. 2013;21:1190–222.
32. van Gool WA, van de Beek D, Eikelenboom P. Systemic infection and delirium: when cytokines and acetylcholine collide. Lancet. 2010;375:773–5.

33. Lu R, Kiernan MC, Murray A, Rosner MH, Ronco C. Kidney–brain crosstalk in the acute and chronic setting. Nat Rev Nephrol. 2015;11:707–19.
34. Van Sandwijk MS, Ten Berge IJ, Majoie CB, et al. Cognitive changes in chronic kidney disease and after transplantation. Transplantation. 2016;100:734–42.
35. Griva K, Thompson D, Jayasena D, Davenport A, Harrison M, Newman SP. Cognitive functioning pre- to post-kidney transplantation – a prospective study. Nephrol Dial Transplant. 2006;21:3275–82.
36. Siew ED, Fissell WH, Tripp CM, et al. Acute kidney injury as a risk factor for delirium and coma during critical illness. Am J Respir Crit Care Med. 2016;195(12):1597–607.
37. Hoste EA, Bagshaw SM, Bellomo R, et al. Epidemiology of acute kidney injury in critically ill patients: the multinational AKI-EPI study. Intensive Care Med. 2015;41:1411–23.
38. Piccinni P, Cruz DN, Gramaticopolo S, et al. Prospective multicenter study on epidemiology of acute kidney injury in the ICU: a critical care nephrology Italian collaborative effort (NEFROINT). Minerva Anestesiol. 2011;77:1072–83.
39. Ostermann M. Diagnosis of acute kidney injury: Kidney Disease Improving Global Outcomes criteria and beyond. Curr Opin Crit Care. 2014;20:581–7.
40. Ostermann M, Joannidis M. Acute kidney injury in 2016: diagnosis and diagnostic workup. Crit Care. 2016;20:299.
41. de Mendonca A, Vincent JL, Suter PM, et al. Acute renal failure in the ICU: risk factors and outcome evaluated by the SOFA score. Intensive Care Med. 2000;26:915–21.
42. Okusa MD, Davenport A. Reading between the (guide)lines--the KDIGO practice guideline on acute kidney injury in the individual patient. Kidney Int. 2014;85:39–48.
43. Rewa O, Bagshaw SM. Acute kidney injury-epidemiology, outcomes and economics. Nat Rev Nephrol. 2014;10:193–207.
44. Grams ME, Rabb H. The distant organ effects of acute kidney injury. Kidney Int. 2012;81:942–8.
45. Akcay A, Nguyen Q, Edelstein CL. Mediators of inflammation in acute kidney injury. Mediat Inflamm. 2009;2009:137072.
46. Yap SC, Lee HT. Acute kidney injury and extrarenal organ dysfunction: new concepts and experimental evidence. Anesthesiology. 2012;116:1139–48.
47. Ostermann M, Chawla LS, Forni LG, et al. Drug management in acute kidney disease – report of the ADQI XVI meeting. Br J Clin Pharmacol. 2018;84:396–403.
48. Shaw AR, Chaijamorn W, Mueller BA. We underdose antibiotics in patients on CRRT. Semin Dial. 2016;29:278–80.
49. Eyler RF, Mueller BA. Antibiotic dosing in critically ill patients with acute kidney injury. Nat Rev Nephrol. 2011;7:226–35.
50. Guerra C, Linde-Zwirble WT, Wunsch H. Risk factors for dementia after critical illness in elderly Medicare beneficiaries. Crit Care. 2012;16:R233.

Part X

The Neurological Patient

32 Brain Ultrasound in the Non-neurocritical Care Setting

C. Robba, L. Ball, and P. Pelosi

32.1 Introduction

The clinical applications of ultrasound in intensive care and perioperative medicine have expanded enormously over the past decades. In particular, brain ultrasonography and transcranial Doppler (TCD) can help with early detection of neurological emergencies and provide real-time information on the cerebral hemodynamics of critically ill patients. Ultrasound enables assessment of brain structures and detection of anatomy, as well as calculation of basic and TCD-derived parameters. Among these, non-invasive assessment of intracranial pressure (ICP), cerebral perfusion pressure (CPP) and autoregulation mechanisms have gained particular interest and can have useful clinical applications also outside the specialized neurocritical care unit.

In this chapter, we will present and discuss clinical applications of brain ultrasound intended for use in the non-neurocritical care setting, with particular regard to specific clinical conditions commonly seen in the polyvalent intensive care unit (ICU), operating room and emergency department where these techniques can integrate other commonly used diagnostic techniques.

C. Robba
Anaesthesia and Intensive Care, San Martino Policlinico Hospital, IRCCS for Oncology, Genoa, Italy

L. Ball · P. Pelosi (✉)
Anaesthesia and Intensive Care, San Martino Policlinico Hospital, IRCCS for Oncology, Genoa, Italy

Department of Surgical Sciences and Integrated Diagnostics, University of Genoa, Genoa, Italy
e-mail: paolo.pelosi@unige.it

J.-L. Vincent (ed.), *Annual Update in Intensive Care and Emergency Medicine 2019*, Annual Update in Intensive Care and Emergency Medicine,
https://doi.org/10.1007/978-3-030-06067-1_32

32.2 Methods to Evaluate Cerebral Perfusion and Intracranial Pressure

Brain ultrasound can be used to infer information regarding the ICP, CPP and their interaction through autoregulation mechanisms. These ultrasound-based methods have been widely studied thanks to their non-invasiveness, low cost, repeatability, and availability at the bedside without the need for particular software or probes [1]. These techniques may also be applied in emergency settings outside the hospital for early detection of brain functional abnormalities.

TCD measures the blood flow velocity (FV) through the major intracranial vessels. Because of its easy availability and safety, the non-invasive evaluation of ICP using TCD has been widely explored [1]. The Gosling pulsatility index, calculated as $Pulsatility\ index = \frac{FV_{systolic} - FV_{diastolic}}{FV_{mean}}$, is often considered an estimate of distal cerebrovascular resistance to blood flow; however its relation with resistance and ICP is complex and its usefulness as a single indicator of cerebral perfusion impairment is very limited [2].

Hence, more complex formulas have been proposed to estimate CPP. Since arterial blood pressure, CPP and ICP are linked by the formula $CPP = arterial\ blood\ pressure - ICP$, computing CPP from Doppler-derived measures can provide an indirect estimate of ICP. Different formulas and mathematical approaches have been proposed for non-invasive ICP and CPP estimation [3]. Schmidt et al. [4] proposed the following formula for estimation of CPP (nCPP), and therefore ICP:

$$nCPP = arterial\ blood\ pressure \cdot \frac{FV_{diastolic}}{FV_{systolic}} + 14$$

The authors showed that the absolute difference between this estimate and the actual CPP was less than 10 mmHg in 89% of measurements and less than 13 mmHg in 92% of measurements in a cohort of brain-injured patients. In a validation study, Rasulo et al. found a high sensitivity of this method in a cohort of head trauma patients, suggesting that it could be a valuable tool to rule out intracranial hypertension [5].

Autoregulation is a physiologic mechanism aimed at maintaining an adequate perfusion in response to changes in CPP: in each patient there is a range of CPP values where this mechanism is preserved, outside of which perfusion may be impaired. Ultrasound techniques based on TCD can measure both static and dynamic autoregulation [1]. The measurement of static autoregulation requires blood pressure manipulation using vasopressors or carotid compression or reducing venous return by using a tilting test or thigh cuff release. However, static assessment of autoregulation is simplistic, as it does not take in account a number of factors including the between-patient differences in autoregulation mechanisms.

A recent approach used TCD for the investigation of dynamic cerebral autoregulation given its high temporal resolution, which enabled measurement of the timing of the changes in cerebral blood flow in response to the changes in CPP. The mean flow index has been proposed as an indicator of adequacy of autoregulation mechanisms. It is computed as the correlation coefficient between the mean cerebral flow velocity and CPP: a mean flow index value of zero or negative indicates preserved autoregulation, whereas a positive correlation indicates impaired autoregulation [1].

Another ultrasound-based method to screen for ICP increase is based on the measurement of the diameter of the optic nerve sheath diameter. The optic nerve sheath is continuous with the dura mater; as such, the space within the sheath is continuous with the cranial subarachnoid space. When ICP increases, the pressure in this anatomical space increases linearly, increasing the optic nerve sheath diameter [6]. Measurement of the optic nerve sheath diameter with ultrasound has gained interest over the last years, as it is a promising bedside tool for the non-invasive detection of increased ICP, with several studies suggesting that this technique provides good diagnostic accuracy [7, 8]. The cut-off value for normal optic nerve sheath diameter ranges from 5.2 to 5.9 mm, higher values suggesting the presence of intracranial hypertension. A recent meta-analysis [6], including 320 patients from seven studies assessing the accuracy of optic nerve sheath diameter measurement for detection of intracranial hypertension, found a pooled diagnostic odds ratio >65, a pooled likelihood ratio of 5.35 and an area under the receiver-operating characteristic curve (AUC) of 0.938. Although these concepts have been widely explored in the settings of neurocritical care, all authors agree that although these non-invasive tools have several advantages, their accuracy is not good enough compared with invasive devices and, therefore, they cannot substitute for invasive methods [7]. In fact, for both TCD and optic nerve sheath diameter measurement, their ability is not to measure ICP and CPP, but rather to perform a preliminary estimation, aimed at ruling out or corroborating the hypothesis of intracranial hypertension. Table 32.1 resumes the characteristics of some of the discussed parameters.

In this context, these methods may find a useful application in patients at risk of intracranial hypertension especially outside of the neurocritical care setting where invasive ICP is easily available and often indicated. These settings include the polyvalent ICU, the emergency department and the operating room, as illustrated in Fig. 32.1.

32.3 Brain Ultrasound in Liver Failure

Cerebral edema and intracranial hypertension are common during acute liver failure and severe encephalopathy, and are major causes of morbidity and mortality [9]. However, invasive ICP monitoring often has an unfavorable risk-benefit ratio, the major concern being coagulopathy and the risk of intracranial hemorrhage, the incidence of which is estimated at between 2.5% and 10% [10]. Therefore, optic nerve sheath diameter assessment and TCD-derived ICP estimation can play an important role in this group of patients.

Recently, Rajajee et al. [11] compared different non-invasive ICP methods with invasive ICP in a retrospective cohort of 41 patients with liver failure. According to their results, all the methods had a significant correlation with ICP, but the TCD-derived estimation formula had the best ability to predict intracranial hypertension, with an

Table 32.1 Some characteristics of some brain ultrasound parameters

Probe	Mode	Anatomic structures	Findings and parameters	Clinical applications
Cardiac	B-mode	• Mesencephalon • Basal cisterns • Intracerebral ventricles • Brain parenchyma	• Midline shift • Intracerebral haemorrhage • Cerebral ischemia • Hydrocephalus	• Rapid assessment of brain injury in the emergency room, operating room • Evaluation of patients at risk of intracerebral bleeding (coagulopathy, ECMO, liver failure etc.)
	B-mode Color Doppler	• Willis circle • Main brain vessels	• Pulsatility index • Non-invasive cerebral perfusion pressure • Non-invasive intracranial pressure estimation	• Assessment of brain perfusion homeostasis in patients with organ failure (*e.g.* in sepsis, respiratory failure, liver failure) • Effects on cerebral flow of extracorporeal life support • Assessment of cerebral function in pregnancy-related neurological complications
			• Critical closing pressure • Cerebral compliance • Autoregulation mechanisms	• Individualization of cerebral perfusion pressure targets
Linear	B-mode	• Eye • Optic nerve sheath	• Optic nerve sheath diameter	• Screening of intracranial hypertension in the emergency room • Semi-quantitative evaluation of intracranial pressure in patients in whom invasive monitoring is not available or contraindicated

ECMO extracorporeal membrane oxygenation

AUC of0.90. Few studies have described changes in optic nerve sheath diameter during liver failure. In a cohort of 20 liver transplant recipients with end-stage liver disease, optic nerve sheath diameter was measured at the pre-induction, pre-anhepatic, anhepatic, reperfusion and neohepatic phases [12]; optic nerve sheath diameter was increased especially during the reperfusion phase and directly correlated with arterial carbon dioxide concentration, suggesting that the carbon dioxide with consequent cerebral vasodilation can play a key role in increasing optic nerve sheath diameter and ICP during hepatic graft reperfusion. Zheng et al. used TCD to compute the autoregulation index and found that autoregulation was impaired in most patients undergoing liver transplantation and was strongly related to neurologic complications after surgery [13].

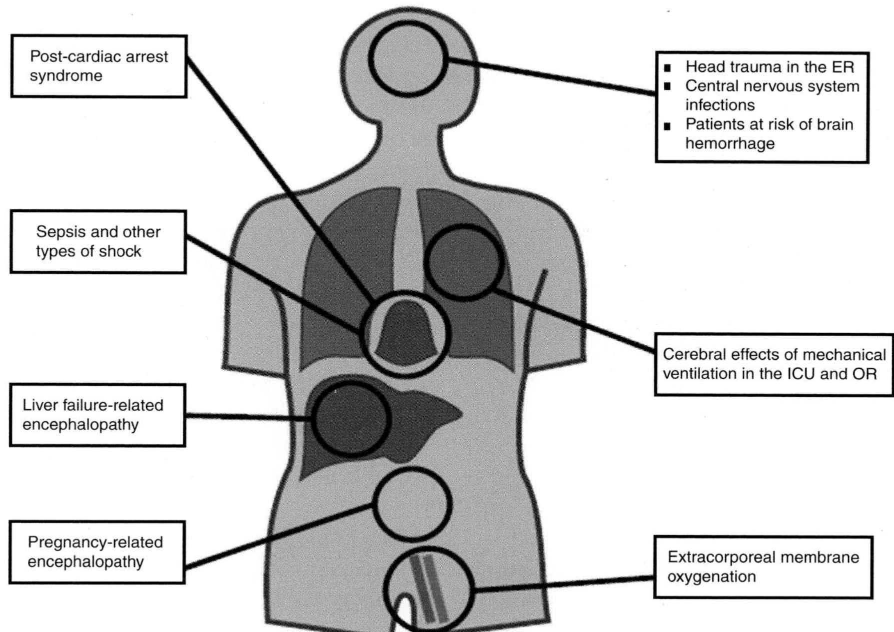

Fig. 32.1 Applications for brain ultrasound and transcranial Doppler in the non-critical care setting. *ER* emergency room, *OR* operating room, *ICU* intensive care unit

The role of the pulsatility index is less clear, as it seems to be a poor predictor of patient outcome according to several studies [14]. However, Abdo et al. [15] demonstrated that a large number of patients with acute liver failure had a low-flow sonographic pattern with increased cerebrovascular resistance and that a higher pulsatility index was correlated with neurological deterioration and mortality. These findings suggest that structural vascular damage and loss of vascular autoregulation are implicated in the pathophysiology of hepatic encephalopathy, but the role of the pulsatility index as a prognostic factor to assess the severity of disease needs further clarification.

The use of non-invasive TCD-based ICP estimation might be helpful to stratify the risk of intracranial hypertension in patients with severe liver failure admitted to the ICU or scheduled for surgery.

32.4 Brain Ultrasound in Sepsis and Septic Shock

In sepsis and septic shock, brain function is frequently affected even in the absence of infection of the central nervous system, in a condition referred to as septic encephalopathy.

Among the putative mechanisms of septic encephalopathy, cytokine-induced damage of the blood-brain barrier can result in brain edema, microvascular failure and loss of cerebral autoregulation. Also, a reduction in CPP related to systemic hypotension can lead to cerebral ischemia and edema.

Although TCD is only an indirect measure of cerebral blood flow, it could potentially provide indirect information about autoregulation, non-invasive CPP as well as cerebrovascular reactivity to carbon dioxide in patients with sepsis [16]. Cerebral blood flow changes can occur during sepsis and septic shock and some authors have demonstrated that the alterations in pulsatility index, as an indicator of peripheral vascular resistance, are associated with the severity of clinical symptoms and might have a correlation with the development of delirium [17].

Pfister et al. showed that cerebral autoregulation is often impaired in patients with septic shock, and that high levels of carbon dioxide may further compromise cerebral autoregulation in these patients [18]. Furthermore, low CPP is significantly correlated with elevated levels of protein S-100β, a biomarker of brain damage, thus suggesting that the combination of hypotension and damaged autoregulation can determine brain injury in septic patients [18].

Although robust evidence is still lacking in this field, brain ultrasound might be considered as a complement to conventional diagnostic tools to optimize the hemodynamic management of septic patients, targeting systemic pressure values that are not only sufficient to maintain peripheral organ perfusion, but also to minimize the impact on brain homeostasis.

32.5 Brain Ultrasound in Cardiac Arrest

Early prediction of severe hypoxic encephalopathy after cardiac arrest is of extreme interest to optimize post-resuscitation care. However, prediction of long-term neurologic outcome is challenging and very few parameters are available. Optic nerve sheath diameter measurement could have a role as a prognostic indicator of hypoxic encephalopathy. In a small group of patients resuscitated after cardiac arrest, the mean optic nerve sheath diameter of the group with a poor outcome was significantly larger than in patients with a good outcome (6.1 mm vs 5.0 mm), and a cut-off of 5.4 mm was an indicator of prognosis, with a sensitivity of 83% and specificity of 73% [19]. Similarly, in an observational study of comatose post-arrest patients, non-survivors showed significantly higher optic nerve sheath diameter values than survivors, with a threshold of 5.75 mm for predicting mortality with a specificity of 100% [20]. These results suggest that neurologic outcome after cardiac arrest is related to the presence of intracranial hypertension, and that optic nerve sheath diameter could have a role in its detection [21]. However, the results of these small-sample studies need larger validation.

Few studies are available describing the application of TCD after cardiac arrest, most of them describing cerebrovascular hemodynamics in comatose patients. Although some authors suggest that TCD can reflect an increase in cerebrovascular resistance secondary to arteriolar vasoconstriction distal to the point of insonation of the middle cerebral artery during ventricular tachycardia and fibrillation [22], results are not consistent, and the correlation between TCD findings and prognosis is still unclear.

Thus TCD and optic nerve sheath diameter might be considered as part of multimodal prognostication of post-cardiac arrest patients, including electroencephalography, pupillometry and neuroimaging [23].

32.6 Brain Ultrasound During Extracorporeal Membrane Oxygenation

Cerebrovascular complications are common in patients treated with extracorporeal membrane oxygenation (ECMO), because one of the major risks during ECMO is the development of ischemic stroke, caused by solid or gaseous microemboli due to thrombosis within the circuit or cannula, or hemorrhagic complications, due to systemic anticoagulation. According to a recent study, TCD is able to detect microembolic signals in real time during ECMO, demonstrating a prevalence of 26% in veno-venous ECMO patients and in more than 80% of veno-arterious ECMO patients [24]. However, in this study, no correlation was found between microemboli detection and clinical neurological impairment at 6 months follow-up. Pulsatility index can have very low values during veno-arterial ECMO and is directly correlated with changes in the ejection fraction, due to the non-pulsatile nature of the ECMO flow [25]. In this setting, changes in pulsatility index mostly depend on the severity of myocardial dysfunction and should not be mistakenly attributed to cerebral vasodilation or cerebral circulatory arrest. Moreover, increased pulsatility index in these patients can represent a phase of improvement in cardiac function and should not be confused with elevated ICP [25].

In neonatal ECMO candidates, brain ultrasound examination has been proposed as the screening technique of choice for assessing pre-existing neurological damage. Ultrasound can detect intracranial abnormalities, such as parenchymal hemorrhage infarcts, cerebellar hemorrhage, and diffuse edema as well as providing ancillary tests to support the diagnosis of irreversible brain injury and brain death during ECMO [26].

Due to the high incidence of neurologic complications during ECMO, further research is warranted to better clarify the role of brain ultrasound and TCD to improve the clinical management of these patients.

32.7 Brain Ultrasound in Patients with Acute Respiratory Failure

Respiratory and cerebral monitoring are complex aspects of critical care management [27]. Many ventilation strategies commonly used in patients with respiratory failure, in particular the use of positive pressure ventilation, are potentially associated with an increased risk of intracranial hypertension; furthermore, lung protective ventilation and consequent permissive hypercarbia, may aggravate a preexisting alteration of cerebral autoregulation [28]. Moreover, in chronically hypercapnic patients, mechanical ventilation can dramatically affect the blood levels of carbon dioxide, with potentially relevant effects on the cerebral perfusion.

Positive airway pressure and, in particular, the use of positive end-expiratory pressure (PEEP), can have dangerous effects on cerebral physiology by impeding cerebral venous return and decreasing arterial pressure and carries the risk of decreasing cerebral perfusion. However, several authors suggest that the reduction in CPP is possibly secondary to hypocapnic vasoconstriction and systemic blood pressure reduction rather than being directily related to PEEP application [29]. Similarly, prone positioning and recruitment maneuvers can potentially increase ICP, and their use in brain injured patients must be carefully balanced against the risks. Overall, ventilator strategies may affect ICP, and because invasive neuromonitoring is not indicated in these patients, brain ultrasound can be useful for the non-invasive assessment of ICP and CPP as well as for the calculation of complex parameters such as autoregulation.

In a cohort of non-brain injured patients undergoing spine surgery, non-invasive ICP was estimated with TCD and optic nerve sheath diameter during prone positioning and PEEP application [30]. The mean values of optic nerve sheath diameter and TCD-derived ICP significantly increased after changes from supine to prone position, whereas the effect of PEEP was negligible.

Non-invasive methods may be applicable in clinical practice to monitor cerebrovascular changes non-invasively during mechanical ventilation, to monitor the cerebral effects of ventilation.

32.8 Brain Ultrasound in Pregnancy-Related Pathology

Pregnancy is associated with changes in maternal physiology that predispose to several neurologic disorders. Pregnancy-related systemic changes are well known, especially the major hemodynamic changes that occur during pregnancy with increase in cardiac output and circulating plasma. However, the changes in central nervous system physiology are poorly understood and it is not clear whether these modifications can predispose pregnant patients to neurological complications [31].

Because of its non-invasiveness, brain ultrasound has been used to assess cerebrovascular changes during pregnancy. Some authors found that the pulsatility index has a peak in mid-pregnancy between 8 and 29 gestational weeks and that CPP drops to its lowest levels in mid-pregnancy and after delivery. Also, middle cerebral artery mean velocity decreases with advancing gestation and increases to non-pregnant values in the immediate puerperium [31]. According to some authors, dynamic cerebral autoregulation does not differ in pregnant and non-pregnant women [32].

Preeclampsia is associated with endothelial dysfunction and impaired autonomic function, which is hypothesized to cause cerebral hemodynamic abnormalities, including altered cerebrovascular response to breath holding; therefore, brain ultrasound has been proposed to predict the development of eclamptic encephalopathy. Recent studies showed that optic nerve sheath diameter is larger in preeclamptic versus healthy pregnant women at delivery with 20–43% of preeclamptic patients having optic nerve sheath diameter values compatible with ICP >20 mmHg [33]. Similarly, preeclampsia may severely affect the cerebral circulation leading to impairment of cerebral autoregulation. In a prospective cohort analysis, autoregulation determined by TCD was significantly reduced in preeclamptic women compared with normotensive women, without any correlation between the autoregulation index and blood pressure, thus suggesting cerebral complications might occur even without sudden or excessive changes in blood pressure [34].

Cerebrovascular complications in pregnant patients are associated not just with preeclampsia, but also with other hypertensive disorders of pregnancy, including isolated hemolysis, elevated liver enzymes, and low platelet count syndrome, chronic hypertension and gestational hypertension, which are believed to be associated with impaired cerebral autoregulation. In a recent study assessing autoregulation in patients with preeclampsia, gestational hypertension and chronic hypertension, the autoregulatory index was reduced in preeclampsia and chronic hypertension, but not in gestational hypertension when compared with control subjects [34]. These findings suggest that in patients with preeclampsia, hyperperfusion and vasogenic edema with loss of autoregulation are the most probable pathophysiological mechanisms responsible for neurological complications.

Brain ultrasound could be a complementary tool to assess pregnant women at increased risk for neurologic complications, such as in preeclampsia.

32.9 Brain Ultrasound in Central Nervous System Infections

In patients with central nervous system infections, the development of cerebral edema precipitates the neurologic conditions of the patient, but invasive monitoring of ICP is contraindicated. In these patients, the pulsatility index seems to be increased, especially in patients with poor neurologic state, which may be attributed to focally increased ICP, peripheral vasospasm of distal arterial branches or hyperemia. Serial TCD evaluations revealed that the decrease in pulsatility index coincided with symptom improvement [35]. A recent case report described the clinical application of non-invasive methods as targets for an ICP lowering protocol in a woman with meningoencephalitis [36]. In this case, the patient presented with meningitis and cerebral edema and was therefore at high risk for intracranial hypertension, but invasive ICP monitoring was contraindicated because the patient was receiving anticoagulation. Therefore, continuous TCD and regular assessments of optic nerve sheath diameter were used for non-invasive ICP monitoring with excellent results.

Although there is not enough evidence to apply non-invasive methods as targets for ICP management protocols in patients with central nervous system infections where invasive ICP monitoring is contraindicated but the patient is at risk of intracranial hypertension, brain ultrasound could be an acceptable substitute.

32.10 Brain Ultrasound in Stroke

Brain ultrasound can play several roles in patients with stroke: discriminate ischemic from hemorrhagic forms, unravel the mechanism of stroke, monitor temporal evolution of stroke and predict stroke outcome. In addition to the common application as screening for vasospasm, TCD can be used to detect hemorrhage itself, as an echo-dense parenchymal lesion in the acute phase, with progressive decrease in the echogenicity in the central region over time.

In patients with an adequate transtemporal acoustic window, accuracy in the detection of the size and site of an intracranial hematoma is high, potentially comparable to that of computed tomography (CT): supratentorial intracranial hemorrhages are easily detected when larger than 1 mL, with excellent correlation between ultrasound and CT measurements, with a sensitivity of 94%, specificity of 95%, positive predictive value of 91% and negative predictive value of 95% [37] in the differentiation between intracerebral hemorrhage and ischemic stroke [38]. Enlargement of the optic nerve sheath diameter can also be detected in the hyperacute phases of acute intracerebral hemorrhage within 6 h of the onset of symptoms, with optic nerve sheath diameter >0.66 mm suggesting hemorrhage volume >2.5 mL with 90% accuracy [39].

Because the hematoma volume is an important determinant of outcome and a predictor of clinical deterioration in patients with intracerebral hemorrhage, TCD can be applied to assess hemodynamic changes following hemorrhage. Although CPP, resistance area product, and cerebral blood flow are more sensitive parameters than the absolute velocity values to detect hemorrhage, the severity of the changes does not correlate with the volume of the hemorrhage in the acute stage.

The common applications of TCD used in neurocritical settings, might be extended to non-neurointensivists, especially to provide a first rapid assessment of patients at risk of developing acute cerebrovascular events, e.g., in the emergency room.

32.11 Brain Ultrasound in the Emergency Department

In the specific context of the emergency department, in addition to other applications, brain ultrasound has gained particular interest as part of the clinical assessment of the patient in the early phases of trauma in the emergency room. Ultrasound can be performed rapidly with adequate image quality in the majority of critically ill patients and frequently enables an early assessment of brain injury as well as the screening of patients at risk of developing secondary damage [40]. Brain ultrasound can detect early intracranial hypertension, intracerebral hemorrhage, hydrocephalus and midline shift, and could potentially be included in the focused assessment with sonography for trauma (FAST) protocol, for the rapid diagnosis and treatment decision making of patients with intracranial emergencies in point-of-care settings [41–44]. Bouzat et al. recently demonstrated that a pulsatility index of more than 1.25 and diastolic blood flow velocity <25 cm/s in the two middle cerebral arteries had 80% sensitivity and 79% specificity to predict neurologic worsening [45]. Similarly, optic nerve sheath diameter has been studied in the emergency setting. Tayal et al. conducted a small prospective study on adult emergency department patients with suspected intracranial injury who underwent sonographic measurement of optic nerve sheath diameter, finding high sensitivity but low specificity in detecting elevated ICP [40]. Similarly, Blaivas et al. [41] found a good agreement between enlarged optic nerve sheath diameter and CT findings compatible with increased ICP, such as the presence of a mass effect with a midline shift, a collapsed third ventricle, hydrocephalus, the effacement of sulci with evidence of significant edema, and abnormal mesencephalic cisterns.

Overall, results from studies on optic nerve sheath diameter as a reliable predictor for increased mean intracranial hypertension show that this method could be an easy, cheap, and non-invasive method that can be used to support the diagnosis and evaluation of patients with acute brain injury presenting in the emergency department. We conducted a meta-analysis of six studies that used optic nerve sheath diameter as a predictor for the presence of signs of intracranial hypertension on CT scan [40–44, 46]. In these studies, the optic nerve sheath diameter cut-off ranged from 4.5 to 6 mm. We synthetized studies with a diagnostic random-effects model using the DerSimonian-Laird method, finding a pooled sensitivity of 0.92 (95% confidence interval [CI] 0.82–0.97, $I^2 = 40\%$, $p = 0.14$) and specificity of 0.87 (95% CI 0.71–0.95, $I^2 = 87\%$, $p < 0.001$). The cumulative receiver-operating curve is illustrated in Fig. 32.2. Overall, the analysis suggests that the optic nerve sheath

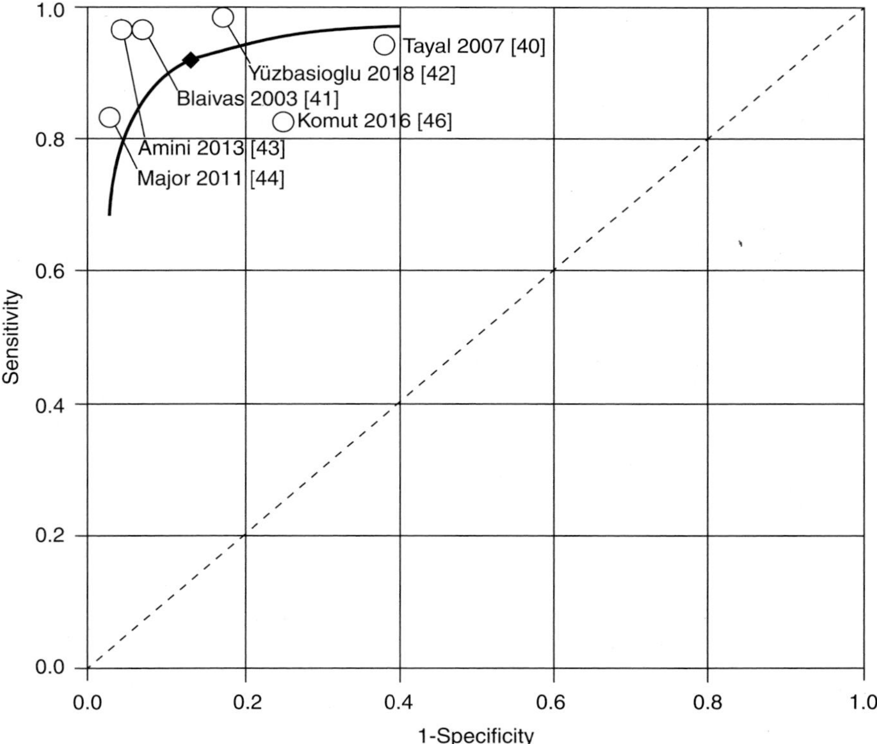

Fig. 32.2 Receiver-operating curve for the prediction of raised intracranial pressure using optic nerve sheath diameter in the emergency room. White circles: single study estimates, black diamond: pooled estimate. In all studies the reference was the presence of signs of intracranial hypertension on computed tomography scan

diameter could be a promising tool in the emergency room to screen for the presence of intracranial hypertension, but statistical heterogeneity is moderate-to-high and further validation studies are warranted.

32.12 Brain Ultrasound in the Operating Room

Intraoperative use of brain ultrasound has gained popularity over the years as an easily available and safe neuromonitoring tool in procedures at risk for neurological complications. Potentially, it could be used in the perioperative management of various groups of surgical patients, to monitor the occurrence of neurological complications during anesthesia including intracerebral bleeding, ischemia and stroke. Brain ultrasound has raised interest in specific perioperative settings. Cardiac surgery requires specific anesthetic management related to the need for extracorporeal circulation and hypothermia in most surgical procedures. In this context, neurological complications are common, and the mechanisms responsible for cerebral complications include micro-emboli, cerebral hypoperfusion and loss of autoregulation. Clinical studies measuring cerebral blood flow during deep hypothermia have demonstrated altered cerebrovascular autoregulation and association with poor outcome and neurological complications [47].

The use of TCD has also been widely used in vascular surgery and in particular during carotid endoarterectomy as a monitoring tool during carotid clamping, declamping, external carotid artery occlusion and risk of chronic embolization, or a site for extended thrombosis during wound closure. TCD can identify microembolic signals enabling prediction of the risk for development of new postoperative ischemic lesions, and could reduce the use of carotid shunting [47].

Another important application of brain ultrasound in the intraoperative setting is in patients undergoing laparoscopic surgery. This technique requires application of a pneumoperitoneum and often a concomitant steep head-down position, thus increasing the risk of decreased venous return, variation in mean arterial pressure and systemic vascular resistance, hypercapnia and therefore an increase in ICP. Because an increase of ICP >20 mmHg has been detected in around 10% of patients without neurological disease [48], a non-invasive ICP measurement method could be useful to identify patients at higher risk of postoperative neurologic impairment. Ultrasound-based, non-invasive ICP monitoring during pneumoperitoneum and Trendelenburg position has been studied by several authors demonstrating a significant increase in optic nerve sheath diameter and TCD-derived ICP [48]. Finally, non-invasive neuromonitoring could be useful even in orthopedic surgery, and in particular for shoulder surgery in the beach-chair position. This peculiar position can be associated with a reduction in cerebral oxygenation, venous return, cardiac output, CPP and blood pressure especially during general anesthesia which alters cardiovascular reflex responses [49].

Some authors have reported neurologic injury occurring in healthy patients in the beach chair position, including stroke, spinal cord ischemia, and transient visual loss and stroke. Pohl and Cullen [50] reported cases of catastrophic perioperative central nervous system infarction associated with shoulder surgery in the sitting position. There are few published reports on the use of TCD in the beach chair position for the assessment of cerebral hemodynamics, and most used the flow velocity as the main measure [50]. Cerebral hypoperfusion can be the main mechanism for a low cerebral blood flow velocity pattern with loss of optimal cerebral autoregulation. Moreover, estimated CPP <60 mmHg may indicate that patients were on the verge of the lower limit of autoregulation, a physiological state in which flow velocity decreases passively with decreasing CPP.

32.13 Conclusion

Brain ultrasound is a safe and quick bedside technique, which enables identification of several structures within the brain parenchyma and monitoring of various aspects of cerebrovascular pathophysiology. The non-invasiveness of this technique, together with its safety and low cost as a neuromonitoring system, determine its applicability in multiple settings, also in the non-neurocritical care setting, in cases where invasive monitoring is warranted but not available or contraindicated. Brain ultrasound assessment of cerebral perfusion assessment is still a poorly developed technique and is not routinely performed in critical care. Future studies should aim to further validate these techniques and explore the role of monitoring in different settings and the effect on patient outcome.

References

1. Robba C, Cardim D, Sekhon M, Budohoski K, Czosnyka M. Transcranial Doppler: a stethoscope for the brain-neurocritical care use. J Neurosci Res. 2018;96:720–30.
2. De Riva N, Budohoski KP, Smielewski P, et al. Transcranial doppler pulsatility index: what it is and what it isn't. Neurocrit Care. 2012;17:58–66.
3. Robba C, Donnelly J, Bertuetti R, et al. Doppler non-invasive monitoring of ICP in an animal model of acute intracranial hypertension. Neurocrit Care. 2015;23:419–26.
4. Schmidt EA, Czosnyka M, Gooskens I, Piechnik SK, Matta BF, Whitfield PC. Preliminary experience of the estimation of cerebral perfusion pressure using transcranial Doppler ultrasonography. J Neurol Neurosurg Psychiatry. 2001;70:198–204.
5. Rasulo FA, Bertuetti R, Robba C, et al. The accuracy of transcranial Doppler in excluding intracranial hypertension following acute brain injury: a multicenter prospective pilot study. Crit Care. 2017;21:44.
6. Robba C, Santori G, Czosnyka M, et al. Optic nerve sheath diameter measured sonographically as non-invasive estimator of intracranial pressure: a systematic review and meta-analysis. Intensive Care Med. 2018;44:1284–94.
7. Robba C, Cardim D, Tajsic T, et al. Ultrasound non-invasive measurement of intracranial pressure in neurointensive care: a prospective observational study. PLoS Med. 2017;14:e1002356.
8. Geeraerts T, Launey Y, Martin L, Pottecher J, Duranteau J, Benhamou D. Ultrasonography of the optic nerve sheath may be useful for detecting raised intracranial pressure after severe brain injury. Intensive Care Med. 2007;33:1704–11.
9. Thumburu KK, Taneja S, Vasishta RK, Dhiman RK. Neuropathology of acute liver failure. Neurochem Int. 2012;60:672–5.

10. Vaquero J, Fontana RJ, Larson AM, et al. Complications and use of intracranial pressure monitoring in patients with acute liver failure and severe encephalopathy. Liver Transpl. 2005;11:1581–9.
11. Rajajee V, Williamson CA, Fontana RJ, Courey AJ, Patil PG. Noninvasive intracranial pressure assessment in acute liver failure. Neurocrit Care. 2018;8:1–11.
12. Seo H, Kim YK, Shin WJ, Hwang GS. Ultrasonographic optic nerve sheath diameter is correlated with arterial carbon dioxide concentration during reperfusion in liver transplant recipients. Transplant Proc. 2013;45:2272–6.
13. Zheng Y, Villamayor AJ, Merritt W, et al. Continuous cerebral blood flow autoregulation monitoring in patients undergoing liver transplantation. Neurocrit Care. 2012;17:77–84.
14. Stewart J, Särkelä M, Koivusalo AM, et al. Frontal electroencephalogram variables are associated with the outcome and stage of hepatic encephalopathy in acute liver failure. Liver Transpl. 2014;20:1256–65.
15. Abdo A, Pérez-Bernal J, Hinojosa R, et al. Cerebral hemodynamics patterns by transcranial Doppler in patients with acute liver failure. Transplant Proc. 2015;47:2647–9.
16. Oddo M, Taccone FS. How to monitor the brain in septic patients? Minerva Anestesiol. 2015;81:776–88.
17. Pierrakos C, Antoine A, Velissaris D, et al. Transcranial doppler assessment of cerebral perfusion in critically ill septic patients: a pilot study. Ann Intensive Care. 2013;3:28.
18. Pfister D, Siegemund M, Dell-Kuster S, et al. Cerebral perfusion in sepsis-associated delirium. Crit Care. 2008;12:R63.
19. Ueda T, Ishida E, Kojima Y, Yoshikawa S, Yonemoto H. Sonographic optic nerve sheath diameter: a simple and rapid tool to assess the neurologic prognosis after cardiac arrest. J Neuroimaging. 2015;25:927–30.
20. Ertl M, Weber S, Hammel G, Schroeder C, Krogias C. Transorbital sonography for early prognostication of hypoxic-ischemic encephalopathy after cardiac arrest. J Neuroimaging. 2018;28:542–8.
21. Chelly J, Deye N, Guichard JP, et al. The optic nerve sheath diameter as a useful tool for early prediction of outcome after cardiac arrest: a prospective pilot study. Resuscitation. 2016;103:7–13.
22. Grubb BP, Durzinsky D, Brewster P, Gbur C, Collins B. Sudden cerebral vasoconstriction during induced polymorphic ventricular tachycardia and fibrillation: further observations of a paradoxic response. Pacing Clin Electrophysiol. 1997;20:667–72.
23. Heimburger D, Durand M, Gaide-Chevronnay L, et al. Quantitative pupillometry and transcranial Doppler measurements in patients treated with hypothermia after cardiac arrest. Resuscitation. 2016;103:88–93.
24. Marinoni M, Migliaccio ML, Trapani S, et al. Cerebral microemboli detected by transcranial doppler in patients treated with extracorporeal membrane oxygenation. Acta Anaesthesiol Scand. 2016;60:934–44.
25. Kavi T, Esch M, Rinsky B, Rosengart A, Lahiri S, Lyden PD. Transcranial Doppler changes in patients treated with extracorporeal membrane oxygenation. J Stroke Cerebrovasc Dis. 2016;25:2882–5.
26. Taylor GA, Fitz CR, Miller MK, Garin DB, Catena LM, Short BL. Intracranial abnormalities in infants treated with extracorporeal membrane oxygenation: imaging with US and CT. Radiology. 1987;165:675–8.
27. Ball L, Sutherasan Y, Pelosi P. Monitoring respiration: what the clinician needs to know. Best Pract Res Clin Anaesthesiol. 2013;27:209–23.
28. Meng L, Gelb AW. Regulation of cerebral autoregulation by carbon dioxide. Anesthesiology. 2015;122:196–205.
29. Shapiro HM, Marshall LF. Intracranial pressure responses to PEEP in head-injured patients. J Trauma. 1978;18:254–6.
30. Robba C, Bragazzi L, Bertuccio A, et al. Effects of prone position and positive end-expiratory pressure on noninvasive estimators of ICP: a pilot study. J Neurosurg Anesthesiol. 2017;29:243–50.

31. Lindqvist PG, Maršál K, Pirhonen JP. Maternal cerebral Doppler velocimetry before, during, and after a normal pregnancy: a longitudinal study. Acta Obstet Gynecol Scand. 2006;85:1299–303.
32. Janzarik WG, Ehlers E, Ehmann R, et al. Dynamic cerebral autoregulation in pregnancy and the risk of preeclampsia. Hypertension. 2014;63:161–6.
33. Dubost C, Le Gouez A, Jouffroy V, et al. Optic nerve sheath diameter used as ultrasonographic assessment of the incidence of raised intracranial pressure in preeclampsia: a pilot study. Anesthesiology. 2012;116:1066–71.
34. Van Veen TR, Panerai RB, Haeri S, Griffioen AC, Zeeman GG, Belfort MA. Cerebral autoregulation in normal pregnancy and preeclampsia. Obstet Gynecol. 2013;122:1064–9.
35. Kargiotis O, Safouris A, Magoufis G, Stamboulis E, Tsivgoulis G. Transcranial color-coded duplex in acute encephalitis: current status and future prospects. J Neuroimaging. 2016;26:377–82.
36. Sheehan JR, Liu X, Donnelly J, Cardim D, Czosnyka M, Robba C. Clinical application of non-invasive intracranial pressure measurements. Br J Anaesth. 2018;121:500–1.
37. Mäurer M, Shambal S, Berg D, et al. Differentiation between intracerebral hemorrhage and ischemic stroke by transcranial color-coded duplex-sonography. Stroke. 1998;29:2563–7.
38. Albert AF, Kirkman MA. Clinical and radiological predictors of malignant middle cerebral artery infarction development and outcomes. J Stroke Cerebrovasc Dis. 2017;26:2671–9.
39. Školoudík D, Herzig R, Fadrná T, et al. Distal enlargement of the optic nerve sheath in the hyperacute stage of intracerebral haemorrhage. Br J Ophthalmol. 2011;5:217–21.
40. Tayal VS, Neulander M, Norton HJ, Foster T, Saunders T, Blaivas M. Emergency department sonographic measurement of optic nerve sheath diameter to detect findings of increased intracranial pressure in adult head injury patients. Ann Emerg Med. 2007;49:508–14.
41. Blaivas M, Theodoro D, Sierzenski PR. Elevated intracranial pressure detected by bedside emergency ultrasonography of the optic nerve sheath. Acad Emerg Med. 2003;10:376–81.
42. Yüzbaşioğlu Y, Yüzbaşioğlu S, Coşkun S, et al. Bedside measurement of the optic nerve sheath diameter with ultrasound in cerebrovascular disorders. Turk J Med Sci. 2018;48:93–9.
43. Amini A, Kariman H, Arhami Dolatabadi A, et al. Use of the sonographic diameter of optic nerve sheath to estimate intracranial pressure. Am J Emerg Med. 2013;31:236–9.
44. Major R, Girling S, Boyle A. Ultrasound measurement of optic nerve sheath diameter in patients with a clinical suspicion of raised intracranial pressure. Emerg Med J. 2011;28:679–81.
45. Bouzat P, Almeras L, Manhes P, et al. Transcranial Doppler to predict neurologic outcome after mild to moderate traumatic brain injury. Anesthesiology. 2016;125:346–54.
46. Komut E, Kozacı N, Sönmez BM, et al. Bedside sonographic measurement of optic nerve sheath diameter as a predictor of intracranial pressure in ED. Am J Emerg Med. 2016;34:963–7.
47. Smith B, Vu E, Kibler K, et al. Does hypothermia impair cerebrovascular autoregulation in neonates during cardiopulmonary bypass? Paediatr Anaesth. 2017;27:905–10.
48. Robba C, Cardim D, Donnelly J, et al. Effects of pneumoperitoneum and Trendelenburg position on intracranial pressure assessed using different non-invasive methods. Br J Anaesth. 2016;117:783–91.
49. Buhre W, Weyland A, Buhre K, et al. Effects of the sitting position on the distribution of blood volume in patients undergoing neurosurgical procedures. Br J Anaesth. 2000;84:354–7.
50. Pohl A, Cullen DJ. Cerebral ischemia during shoulder surgery in the upright position: a case series. J Clin Anesth. 2005;17:463–9.

Brain Fog: Are Clearer Skies on the Horizon? A Review of Perioperative Neurocognitive Disorders

33

S. Saxena, A. Joosten, and M. Maze

33.1 Introduction

Postoperative cognitive decline is a complication in which a typically elderly surgical patient inadvertently substitutes one illness for another. The change in cognitive performance can be defined by postoperative deterioration in completing neuropsychological tests and requires preoperative testing and testing after the surgical intervention. Unlike postoperative delirium, an acute onset of cognitive impairment in which no preoperative testing is required to make the postoperative diagnosis, postoperative cognitive decline is defined by a significant deterioration from the patient's preoperative capabilities. As formal preoperative neurocognitive testing is not the current standard of clinical care, postoperative cognitive decline and its sequelae, are currently under-reported [1].

S. Saxena
Center for Cerebrovascular Research, Department of Anesthesia and Perioperative Care, Zuckerberg San Francisco General Hospital & Trauma Center, University of California, San Francisco, CA, USA

Department of Anesthesia, Erasme University Hospital, Université Libre de Bruxelles, Brussels, Belgium

A. Joosten
Department of Anesthesia, Erasme University Hospital, Université Libre de Bruxelles, Brussels, Belgium

Department of Anesthesia and Intensive Care, Hôpitaux Universitaires Paris-Sud, Université Paris-Sud, Université Paris-Saclay, Hôpital De Bicêtre, Assistance Publique Hôpitaux de Paris (APHP), Le Kremlin-Bicêtre, France

M. Maze (✉)
Center for Cerebrovascular Research, Department of Anesthesia and Perioperative Care, Zuckerberg San Francisco General Hospital & Trauma Center, University of California, San Francisco, CA, USA
e-mail: Mervyn.maze@ucsf.edu

J.-L. Vincent (ed.), *Annual Update in Intensive Care and Emergency Medicine 2019*, Annual Update in Intensive Care and Emergency Medicine,
https://doi.org/10.1007/978-3-030-06067-1_33

33.2 Epidemiology/Incidence of Postoperative Cognitive Decline

According to the Center for Disease Control, more than 40% of surgical procedures in the USA are performed on patients aged 65 or older, the cohort that is especially likely to develop either postoperative cognitive decline or postoperative delirium [2].

The incidence of postoperative delirium ranges from 13% to 42% and postoperative cognitive decline occurs in 9–46% of patients [3–5]. Both postoperative delirium and postoperative cognitive decline are associated with higher mortality, increased incidence of other postoperative complications, longer duration of hospital stay, greater utilization of social financial assistance and earlier retirement [6].

33.3 History of Postoperative Cognitive Decline

Postoperative cognitive decline was first described in 1887 by the prominent British psychiatrist, Sir George Savage, who documented cases of "insanity" after anesthesia/surgery. In one of the cases he mentions that the surgeon noticed upon emergence from anesthesia that his patient was restless, incoherent, repeating meaningless expressions and remained in this state for a few weeks after discharge. Savage concluded his paper by positing whether a previous attack of insanity could subsequently affect the postoperative prognosis and advising against performing operations "that are not essential for the prolonging or saving life" [7].

Professor Manny Papper mooted postoperative psychosis as an important complication of both spinal and general anesthesia in aged surgical patients in which family anecdotally stated words to the effect that "grandfather has not been the same after his surgery". Papper speculated that the cause may be related to cerebral anoxia [8].

Bedford published a report containing a retrospective series of patients who developed cognitive changes following surgery under general anesthesia in which he reported on a "transitory confusion state" following operations under general anesthesia. Bedford included 251 postoperative assessments and he reported that 18 patients suffered from some degree of "dementia" after surgery. Bedford, reiterated Savage's admonition that "operations on elderly patients should be confined to unequivocally necessary cases". Further, Bedford cautioned against the use of certain techniques such as hypotensive anesthesia, as well as the routine use of premedication, and the administration of powerful opiate analgesics, all in elderly surgical patients. Bedford also recommended careful attention to optimizing blood-pressure, hemoglobin concentration and oxygenation [9].

In 1998, the International Study on Postoperative Cognitive Dysfunction (ISPOCD) reported on a seminal multicenter study in which 1218 surgical patients aged 60 and above received general anesthesia. In this cohort, postoperative cognitive decline, identified by a set of postoperative criteria, was found to be present in 25.8% of patients one week after surgery and in 9.9% of patients (not necessarily the same patients) 3 months after surgery. Unlike the prior warnings of hypoxemia and hypotension, the ISPOCD did not attribute a causal relationship to these physiological derangements as had been suggested by others. Rather, the most important risk factors for "early" postoperative cognitive decline appeared to be increasing age, duration of anesthesia, low educational attainment, a second operation, postoperative infections and respiratory complications; only advanced age was associated with "late-onset" postoperative cognitive decline [10].

A decade later, Dr. Terri Monk and her colleagues examined the prevalence of postoperative cognitive decline in different age strata of 1064 non-cardiac surgical patients and noted that postoperative cognitive decline was present at discharge in 37% of young (18–39 years old), 30% of middle-aged (40–59 years old), and 41% of elderly (60 years or older) patients after non-cardiac surgery. At 3-months post-surgery, postoperative cognitive decline was present in 6% of young, 6% of middle-aged, and 13% of elderly patients. The independent risk factors for postoperative cognitive decline at 3 months after surgery were increasing age, low educational attainment, a history of previous cerebral vascular accident with no residual impairment, and postoperative cognitive decline at hospital discharge [11].

33.4 Nomenclature and Clinical Syndromes

Recently, a group of experts in postoperative cognitive disturbances devised a new terminology aligned to existing psychiatric diagnoses although only delirium is currently defined in the most recent Diagnostic and Statistical Manual (DSM) [12].

In their opinion, "perioperative neurocognitive disorder", is the over-arching term that covers all forms of this condition. Postoperative delirium is diagnosed by several criteria including clouding of consciousness with reduced awareness of the environment and difficulty in sustaining and/or shifting attention. In addition, postoperative delirium is characterized by changes in cognition that affect memory, language and orientation in time/space. Postoperative delirium is further classified by duration and level of activity, such as hyperactive, hypoactive or mixed delirium.

Perioperative neurocognitive disorder has been known to occur up to 12 months after intervention and can have a major impact on one's daily quality of life. The link between postoperative delirium and less immediate perioperative neurocognitive disorder is being investigated; both postoperative delirium and ICU delirium are associated with delayed neurocognitive recovery [13–15].

Although hotly contested, perioperative neurocognitive disorders may ultimately morph into chronic and progressive dementia [16].

33.5 Etiology

Initially, anesthesiologists had maintained a Pollyannish view of general anesthetics as agents that produced a profound alteration in the state of consciousness, which was transient with the patient returning to their pristine preoperative condition as soon as these short-acting drugs were eliminated. However, general anesthetics are capable of producing residual physiological changes after complete washout of the drug [17]. The pendulum then swung to a 'belief' that general anesthetics were in fact the culprit, a view that was supported by clinical studies that demonstrated long-lasting cognitive decline in aged rats exposed to volatile anesthetics [18]. Yet, there appeared to be no difference in the incidence of postoperative cognitive decline whether the surgical patient received a volatile or an intravenous general anesthetic [19, 20]; furthermore, there was no difference in the prevalence of postoperative cognitive decline whether the surgical patient was randomized to receive a general or a regional anesthetic technique [21]. Confoundingly, the patients in the regional anesthetic group may also have received sedative/hypnotic agents that may have 'contaminated' a comparison between regional and general anesthesia.

Beginning with the observation that neuroinflammation is a consequence of the aseptic trauma of peripheral surgery [22], a body of evidence has evolved around the possibility that the immune response to surgery, so vital for the healing of wounds, may be a possible culprit. It had long been appreciated that the syndrome of "sickness behavior," comprising a constellation of behavioral alterations, including cognitive decline, develops as a defense mechanism to preserve the organism in response to illness and/or trauma [23]. How the process of sickness behavior begins, and perhaps more importantly, how it resolves, has led to the conclusion that the innate immune response to trauma, may be pivotal to understanding why postoperative neurocognitive disorders develop (Fig. 33.1).

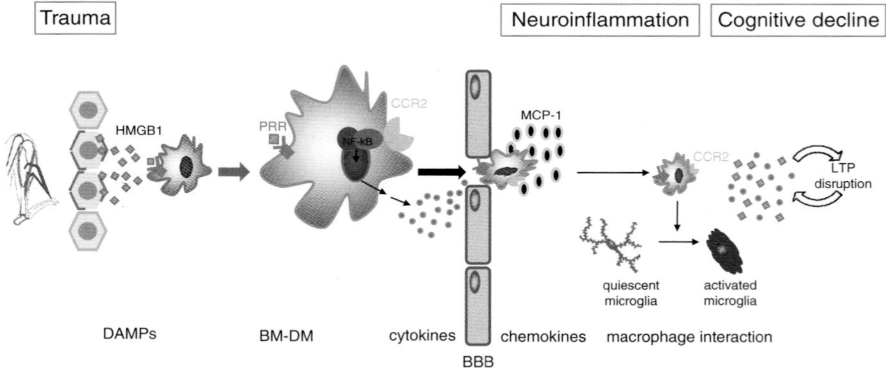

Fig. 33.1 From trauma to cognitive decline (from left to right). Following surgery/peripheral trauma (tibia fracture), high mobility group box protein 1 (HMGB1) is released. This damage-associated molecular pattern (DAMP) binds to pattern recognition receptors (PRR) on circulating bone marrow-derived monocytes (BM-DMs). Through an intracellular signaling pathway, the transcription factor nuclear factor-kappa B (NF-κB) passes into the nucleus, is activated and increases expression and release of pro-inflammatory cytokines. These in turn disrupt the blood-brain barrier (BBB). Within the brain parenchyma the chemokine monocyte chemoattractant protein (MCP)-1 (also referred to as CCL2) is upregulated and attracts the BM-DMs through binding to its receptor, CCR2. In turn, this activates the resident quiescent microglia. Together, the BM-DMs and activated microglia release HMGB1 and pro-inflammatory cytokines that disrupt long-term potentiation (LTP) thereby blocking synaptic plasticity changes that are required for the cognitive functions of learning and memory

High mobility group box 1 protein (HMGB1), a damage-associated molecular pattern (DAMP), is released from the cytosolic compartment of traumatized tissue and engages the innate immune system by binding to pattern recognition receptors on circulating immunocytes to induce translocation of the transcription factor nuclear factor-kappa B (NF-κB) into the nucleus where it enhances the transcription and translation of pro-inflammatory cytokines [24–26]. The released cytokines are capable of disrupting the blood-brain barrier facilitating the migration of circulating bone marrow-derived monocytes into the brain, attracted by an upregulation of the chemokine monocyte chemoattractant protein-1 (MCP-1) from microglia [27]. Within the central nervous system, the bone marrow-derived monocytes interact with microglia to release pro-inflammatory cytokines, such as interleukin (IL)-1β and IL-6 within the parenchyma; both of these cytokines can disrupt synaptic plasticity thereby preventing long-term potentiation, the neurobiologic correlate of learning and memory [28, 29].

A combination of humoral factors (derived from fatty acids) and neural mechanisms, principally vagal activation, resolve the peripheral and neuroinflammation and restore cognitive function to the pre-morbid state [30, 31].

Based upon these mechanisms, we hypothesize that the development of postoperative neurocognitive disorders is due to either the initiation of an exaggerated inflammatory response or the failure to appropriately resolve the inflammation. Risk factors known to influence the development of postoperative neurocognitive disorders have been shown to enhance the initiation, or thwart resolution, of inflammation in a predictable manner adding credence to the immunologic basis for this postoperative complication.

Whether there is a mechanistic link between anesthetics and Alzheimer's disease is under active investigation. Certain anesthetics increase aggregation and oligomerization of the amyloid-beta (Aβ) peptide and enhance accumulation and hyperphosphorylation of tau protein [32–34]. Nonetheless, studies have not shown that anesthesia exposure is associated with Alzheimer's disease [35–37]. Alternatively, neuroinflammation features prominently in both postoperative neurocognitive disorders (see above) and Alzheimer's disease; surgery enhanced microglial activation, amyloidopathy and tauopathy in a murine Alzheimer's disease model [38].

33.6 Interventions

There are currently no treatment options for postoperative neurocognitive disorders. Experts have therefore prioritized preventative strategies especially in patients that are at high risk (elderly, metabolic syndrome etc). Prehabilitation is defined as the "process of enhancing an individual's functional capacity to enable her/him to withstand a forthcoming stressor (such as major surgery)" [39]. Among the several prehabilitative measures that have been advocated, we favor the biologic plausibility of exercise. Aerobic exercise has immune-modulatory properties. Healthy young sedentary adult volunteers who were randomized to a 12-week high intensity training program had significantly less inflammatory response when stimulated with lipopolysaccharide [40]. Six weeks of preoperative exercise in a rat model of metabolic syndrome resulted in significantly less postoperative neuroinflammation and cognitive decline [41].

The risk-mitigation strategy of 'brain training' or 'cognitive training' has also been advocated. Chu-Man et al. noted that teaching neophytes to play mahjong over a period of 12 weeks resulted in higher overall scores indicating improved short-term memory, logical reasoning and attentiveness [42]. Three 1-h sessions of mnemonic training resulted in an overall lower incidence of postoperative cognitive decline 1 week after surgery (15.9% versus 36.1% in the control group; $p < 0.05$) [43]. An ongoing study is currently investigating whether engaging in preoperative "mental gymnastics" will prevent delirium. The mental gymnastics in this study consists of 1 h/day of electronic tablet-based cognitive exercise for 10 days prior to surgery (ClinicalTrials.gov Identifier: NCT02230605).

33.7 Conclusion

Described for the first time over a century ago, postoperative cognitive impairment remains a major and debilitating surgical complication. At present, there are no demonstrably efficacious pre-emptive actions or interventions for this condition. Although the inflammatory cascade described above is resolved in most patients through neural and humoral mechanisms, elderly patients and those with lower education levels are more prone to the non-resolution of this process leading to long-term postoperative neurocognitive disorder. Preoperative brain training and exercise demonstrate promising results. Future research should be aimed at defining patients at risk of perioperative neurocognitive disorders prior to surgery. With this information, physicians can optimize perioperative patient care in order to promote the resolution of neuroinflammation and so reduce the risk of development of postoperative neurocognitive disorders.

References

1. Berger M, Nadler JW, Browndyke J, et al. Postoperative cognitive dysfunction: minding the gaps in our knowledge of a common postoperative complication in the elderly. Anesthesiol Clin. 2015;33:517–50.
2. CDC/NCHS National Hospital Discharge Survey. Number and standard error of discharges from short-stay hospitals with and without procedures and percentage with procedures and standard error by selected characteristics: United States, 2010. 2010. Available at http://www.cdc.gov/nchs/data/nhds/4procedures/2010pro_numberpercentage.pdf. Accessed 11 Nov 11 2018.
3. Robinson TN, Raeburn CD, Tran ZV, Angles EM, Brenner LA, Moss M. Postoperative delirium in the elderly: risk factors and outcomes. Ann Surg. 2009;249:173–8.
4. Silverstein JH, Timberger M, Reich DL, Uysal S. Central nervous system dysfunction after noncardiac surgery and anesthesia in the elderly. Anesthesiology. 2007;106:622–8.
5. Ansaloni L, Catena F, Chattat R. Risk factors and incidence of postoperative delirium in elderly patients after elective and emergency surgery. Br J Surg. 2010;97:273–80.

6. Androsova G, Krause R, Winterer G, Schneider R. Biomarkers of postoperative delirium and cognitive dysfunction. Front Aging Neurosci. 2015;7:112.
7. Savage GH. Insanity following the use of anaesthetics in operations. BMJ. 1887;3:1199–200.
8. Papper M. Anesthesia in the aged. Bull N Y Acad Med. 1956;32:635–42.
9. Bedford PD. Adverse cerebral effects of anaesthesia on old people. Lancet. 1955;269:259–63.
10. Moller JT, Cluitmans P, Rasmussen LS, et al. Long-term postoperative cognitive dysfunction in the elderly ISPOCD1 study. ISPOCD investigators. International study of post-operative cognitive dysfunction. Lancet. 1998;351:857–61.
11. Monk TG, Weldon BC, Garvan CW, et al. Predictors of cognitive dysfunction after major noncardiac surgery. Anesthesiology. 2008;108:18–30.
12. American Psychiatric Association. Diagnostic and Statistical Manual of Mental Disorders. 5th ed. Washington: APA Press; 2013.
13. Hshieh TT, Saczynski J, Gou RY, et al. Trajectory of functional recovery after postoperative delirium in elective surgery. Ann Surg. 2017;265:647–53.
14. Brown CH 4th, Probert J, Healy R, et al. Cognitive decline after delirium in patients undergoing cardiac surgery. Anesthesiology. 2018;129:406–16.
15. Pandharipande PP, Girard TD, Jackson JC, et al. Long-term cognitive impairment after critical illness. N Engl J Med. 2013;369:1306–16.
16. Lundström M, Edlund A, Bucht G, Karlsson S, Gustafson Y. Dementia after delirium in patients with femoral neck fractures. J Am Geriatr Soc. 2003;51:1002–6.
17. Spiss CK, Smith CM, Tsujimoto G, Hoffman BB, Maze M. Prolonged hyporesponsiveness of vascular smooth muscle contraction after halothane anesthesia in rabbits. Anesth Analg. 1985;64:1–6.
18. Culley DJ, Baxter MG, Crosby CA, Yukhananov R, Crosby G. Impaired acquisition of spatial memory 2 weeks after isoflurane and isoflurane-nitrous oxide anesthesia in aged rats. Anesth Analg. 2004;99:1393–7.
19. Tang N, Ou C, Liu Y, Zuo Y, Bai Y. Effect of inhalational anaesthetic on postoperative cognitive dysfunction following radical rectal resection in elderly patients with mild cognitive impairment. J Int Med Res. 2014;42:1252–61.
20. Schoen J, Husemann L, Tiemeyer C, et al. Cognitive function after sevoflurane- vs propofol-based anaesthesia for on-pump cardiac surgery: a randomized controlled trial. Br J Anaesth. 2011;106:840–50.
21. Rasmussen LS, Johnson T, Kuipers HM, et al. Does anaesthesia cause postoperative cognitive dysfunction? A randomised study of regional versus general anaesthesia in 438 elderly patients. Acta Anaesthesiol Scand. 2003;47:260–6.
22. Wan Y, Xu J, Ma D, Zeng Y, Cibelli M, Maze M. Postoperative impairment of cognitive function in rats: a possible role for cytokine-mediated inflammation in the hippocampus. Anesthesiology. 2007;106:436–43.
23. Dantzer R. Cytokine-induced sickness behavior: where do we stand? Brain Behav Immun. 2001;15:7–24.
24. Vacas S, Degos V, Tracey KJ, Maze M. High-mobility group box 1 protein initiates postoperative cognitive decline by engaging bone marrow-derived macrophages. Anesthesiology. 2014;120:1160–7.
25. Vacas S, Maze M. Initiating mechanisms of surgery-induced memory decline: the role of HMGB1. J Clin Cell Immunol. 2016;7:481.
26. Levy RM, Mollen KP, Prince JM, et al. Systemic inflammation and remote organ injury following trauma require HMGB1. Am J Physiol Regul Integr Comp Physiol. 2007;293:R1538–44.
27. Bianconi V, Sahebkar A, Atkin SL, Pirro M. The regulation and importance of monocyte chemoattractant protein-1. Curr Opin Hematol. 2018;25:44–51.
28. Cibelli M, Fidalgo AR, Terrando N, et al. Role of interleukin-1beta in postoperative cognitive dysfunction. Ann Neurol. 2010;68:360–8.
29. Pickering M, O'Connor JJ. Pro-inflammatory cytokines and their effects in the dentate gyrus. Prog Brain Res. 2007;163:339–54.

30. Chandrasekharan JA, Sharma-Walia N. Lipoxins: nature's way to resolve inflammation. J Inflamm Res. 2015;8:181–92.
31. Capó X, Martorell M, Busquets-Cortés C. Resolvins as proresolving inflammatory mediators in cardiovascular disease. Eur J Med Chem. 2018;153:123–30.
32. Fodale V, Santamaria LB, Schifilliti D, Mandal PK. Anaesthetics and postoperative cognitive dysfunction: a pathological mechanism mimicking Alzheimer's disease. Anaesthesia. 2010;65:388–95.
33. Mardini F, Tang JX, Li JC, Arroliga MJ, Eckenhoff RG, Eckenhoff MF. Effects of propofol and surgery on neuropathology and cognition in the 3xTgAD Alzheimer transgenic mouse model. Br J Anaesth. 2017;119:472–80.
34. Li C, Liu S, Xing Y, Tao F. The role of hippocampal tau protein phosphorylation in isoflurane-induced cognitive dysfunction in transgenic APP695 mice. Anesth Analg. 2014;119:413–9.
35. Aiello Bowles EJ, Larson EB, Pong RP. Anesthesia exposure and risk of dementia and Alzheimer's disease: a prospective study. J Am Geriatr Soc. 2016;64:602–7.
36. Woodhouse A, Fernandez-Martos CM, Atkinson RAK, et al. Repeat propofol anesthesia does not exacerbate plaque deposition or synapse loss in APP/PS1 Alzheimer's disease mice. BMC Anesthesiol. 2018;18:47.
37. Sprung J, Roberts RO, Knopman DS, et al. Mild cognitive impairment and exposure to general anesthesia for surgeries and procedures: a population-based case-control study. Anesth Analg. 2017;124:1277–90.
38. Tang JX, Mardini F, Janik LS, et al. Modulation of murine Alzheimer pathogenesis and behavior by surgery. Ann Surg. 2013;257:439–48.
39. Topp R, Ditmyer M, King K, Doherty K, Hornyak J 3rd. The effect of bed rest and potential of prehabilitation on patients in the intensive care unit. AACN Clin Issues. 2002;13:263–76.
40. Sloan RP, Shapiro PA, Demeersman RE, et al. Aerobic exercise attenuates inducible TNF production in humans. J Appl Physiol (1985). 2007;103:1007–11.
41. Feng X, Uchida Y, Koch L, et al. Exercise prevents enhanced postoperative neuroinflammation and cognitive decline and rectifies the gut microbiome in a rat model of metabolic syndrome. Front Immunol. 2017;8:1768.
42. Chu-Man L, Chang MY, Chu MC. Effects of mahjong on the cognitive function of middle-aged and older people. Int J Geriatr Psychiatry. 2015;30:995–7.
43. Saleh AJ, Tang GX, Hadi SM, et al. Preoperative cognitive intervention reduces cognitive dysfunction in elderly patients after gastrointestinal surgery: a randomized controlled trial. Med Sci Monit. 2015;21:798–805.

Uncovering Consciousness in Unresponsive ICU Patients: Technical, Medical and Ethical Considerations

34

B. Rohaut, A. Eliseyev, and J. Claassen

34.1 Introduction

Over a decade ago, researchers published the first case of a patient who had been clinically unresponsive for years after traumatic brain injury (TBI) and demonstrated command following using motor imagery paradigms visualized by functional magnetic resonance imaging (fMRI) [1]. The term "cognitive motor dissociation" is gaining popularity to describe this scenario of an inability to behaviorally express preserved cognitive processes [2]. Alternative labels are covert or hidden consciousness and functional locked-in syndrome [3] (see Table 34.1). A flurry of subsequent studies using fMRI and functional electroencephalogram (fEEG) approaches explored the boundaries of human consciousness following brain injury. This growing body of knowledge is now being discussed in the lay press and is starting to affect clinical medicine, challenging the classical taxonomy of disorders of consciousness ([4] see Table 34.1). Until very recently, researchers have focused their attention on patients suffering from chronic disorders of consciousness and have generated estimates of cognitive motor dissociation of around 15% using convenience samples of these patients [5]. Detection of cognitive motor dissociation in the acute phase of brain injury may have prognostic significance as these patients are more likely to also recover behavioral command following and have better long-term functional outcomes.

Few data exist for the early phase after brain injury, such as in the intensive care unit (ICU) setting, when decisions regarding withdrawal of care are more frequently made and prognostic information is needed. Detection of cognitive motor dissociation in the acute setting will face unique challenges including logistics, safety and ethical considerations but also offer great opportunities to affect management. Even though the exploration of consciousness in the acutely brain injured

B. Rohaut · A. Eliseyev · J. Claassen (✉)
Neurocritical Care, Department of Neurology, Columbia University, New York, NY, USA
e-mail: jc1439@cumc.columbia.edu

J.-L. Vincent (ed.), *Annual Update in Intensive Care and Emergency Medicine 2019*, Annual Update in Intensive Care and Emergency Medicine,
https://doi.org/10.1007/978-3-030-06067-1_34

Table 34.1 Definitions of common states of consciousness

	Definition	Other terminologies similar or very close
Behaviorally defined states		
Coma [4]	State of unresponsiveness in which the patient lies with eyes closed and cannot be aroused to respond appropriately to stimuli even with vigorous stimulation (no eye opening or adapted motor response even to painful stimuli).	Coma-1a or 1b[a] (based on EEG compatibility [1a; e.g., slow unreactive predominant delta] or not [1b; e.g., reactive predominant alpha]). Some authors use a Glasgow coma scale cut-off (e.g., <8) but this is very misleading since this can include UWS or even MCS patients in whom the ascending reticular activating system (ARAS) is likely to be functional
Unresponsive wakefulness syndrome (UWS) [9]	State of unresponsiveness in which the patient shows spontaneous eye opening without any behavioral evidence of self or environmental awareness	Vegetative state (VS), coma vigil, apallic state, UWS/VS-2a or2b[a] (CMS excluded [2a] or not [2b] by functional MRI or EEG)
Minimally conscious state (MCS) [8]	State of severely impaired consciousness with minimal but definite behavioral evidence of self or environmental awareness Distinction between MCS "minus" and "plus" has been proposed [3] • MCS–minus: visual fixation/pursuit or adapted motor reaction to pain • MCS-plus: evidence of language processing (e.g., command following, verbalization...)	Cortically Mediated State[a] (CMS, in that case CMS-3b as based on behavior alone).
Locked-in syndrome (LIS) [4]	State in which the patient is actually conscious but de-efferented, resulting in paralysis of all four limbs and the lower cranial nerves	De-efferented state, Conscious state-4b[a]
Conscious state[b] [4]	State of full awareness of the self and one's relationship to the environment, evidenced by verbal or non-verbal (e.g., purposeful motor behavior) behavior	Exit-MCS (or EMCS) when the patient emerged from MCS, Conscious state-4b[a]
Brain functional imaging defined states (e.g., fMRI, fEEG, fNIRS, fPET, fMEG)		
Higher-order cortex motor dissociation (HMD) [26]	Comatose, UWS or MCS-minus (clinically defined) patients that show association cortex responses to language stimuli	CMS-3a[a]

Table 34.1 (continued)

	Definition	Other terminologies similar or very close
Cognitive motor dissociation (CMD) [2]	Comatose[c], UWS or MCS-minus clinically defined patients that show MRI or electrophysiologic evidence of command following	Functional locked-in syndrome, Conscious state-4a[a]
Communicating-CMD (Com-CMD)	CMD defined patients able to communicate using a brain computer interface (BCI)	Conscious state-4a[a]

fMRI functional magnetic resonance imaging, *fEEG* functional electroencephalography, *fNIRS* function near-infrared spectroscopy, *fPET* functional positron emission tomography, *fMEG* functional magnetoencephalography

[a]Terminology recently proposed by Naccache [50] ranging from 1 to 4 and, taking into account both behavioral ("b") and brain functional imaging ("a") evidence. Note that as a consequence, the Cortically Mediated State (CMS) and the Conscious state appear both in the behaviorally and the brain functional imaging sections of this table

[b]Note that as there is no consensus definition of consciousness yet, provided here is a pragmatic operational definition that would match the currently most commonly used definitions. It corresponds to the access consciousness, using the subjective report criterion

[c]The original description actually did not include the comatose state but was included here since the absence of eye opening cannot rule out the possibility of CMD

patient is in its infancy, emerging data demonstrating cognitive motor dissociation in patients who are clinically unresponsive raise a number of questions. These questions can be organized around three overarching themes: technical, medical and ethical aspects.

34.2 Technical Considerations

34.2.1 How Can We Probe Consciousness in Unresponsive Patients?

34.2.1.1 Clinical Exam

Intensivists are used to probing the consciousness of brain injured patients during rounds using standard neurological examination techniques. The general principle of the clinical approach for assessment of consciousness is to probe behavior that is non-reflexive and can be considered as intentional. The most common items assessed are reactivity to sound and touch and, if necessary, responsiveness to nociceptive stimuli: is the patient able to open his/her eyes, is he/she attentive or eventually tracking? Clinicians also use simple verbal commands such as "stick out your tongue" and "show me two fingers". These commands are often combined with a visual cue of the expected response also known as 'mimicking'. This is employed for patients to minimize the impact of acoustic (i.e., deafness) or speech perception problems (i.e., aphasia). This clinical assessment requires good neurological examination skills to minimize the risk of misinterpretation (e.g., motor responses as part of reflexive responses to pain are thought to be intentional). However, even when performed by experienced clinicians, non-standardized neurological examinations have a high error rate (estimated to be as high as 40% in the chronic setting [6]).

As a part of the neurological exam, many clinicians quantify impairment of consciousness using the Glasgow Coma Scale (GCS). Even though this scale was originally developed to triage acute neurosurgical interventions for TBI patients and to assist prognostication, it may have some utility when applied for this purpose. However, the GCS is a very crude assessment of consciousness, especially when applied to tracheally intubated patients. The Full Outline of Unresponsiveness (FOUR) score may offer an alternative and has been rigorously validated [7]. Since the FOUR does not require verbal responses, it is more applicable for tracheally intubated patients. Probing visual tracking, it also allows a better detection of patients in minimally conscious and locked-in states (Table 34.2). Currently, the most widely accepted clinical scale designed for assessment of consciousness is the Coma Recovery Scale-Revised (CRS-R) [8]. This comprehensive scale is the gold standard in the field of consciousness research. CRS-R scoring ranges from 0 to 23

Table 34.2 Approaches to assess consciousness

	Principle(s)	Pros/cons
Behavioral approaches		
Glasgow Coma Scale (GCS)	Probing non-reflexive and/or intentional behavior, spontaneous or in response to stimulations (auditory, tactile or nociceptive)	• Most widely used • Verbal response difficult to assess in intubated ICU patients • Not designed to quantify consciousness • No protocolized assessment of visual tracking • Mimicking not assessed (aphasic or deaf patients categorized as unconscious) • Sum score misleading
Full Outline of Unresponsiveness (FOUR)		• Designed for (intubated) ICU patients • Includes assessment of visual tracking and brainstem reflexes • Not designed to quantify consciousness • Sum score misleading
Coma Recovery Scale-Revised (CRS-R)		• Specifically designed to assess consciousness • Recommends the use of a mirror for visual tracking assessment • Captures non-verbal command following • Validated as research tool for consciousness assessment • Time consuming application

Table 34.2 (continued)

	Principle(s)	Pros/cons
Brain physiologic measures tested at rest • Pro: no patient participation required • Con: conscious thought not directly assessed: use of surrogate biomarkers compared to a database of (usually clinically) labeled patients, more assumptions needed in interpretation of physiologic responses		
FDG-PET	Cerebral metabolism	• Provides insights into spatial distribution of physiologic changes • Risks related to patient transport • Expensive
Multivariate EEG classification	Spontaneous electrical activity analyzed by spectral, complexity and/or connectivity measures	• Bedside procedure • Convenient for repeat assessments • Need a large dataset for training of classifier
Resting state MRI	Cerebral perfusion, Functional connectivity	• Controversial statistical processing required • Impact of large structural lesions • Risks and costs related to patient transport
TMS-EEG PCI	Dynamics and complexity of brain activity in response to magnetic brain stimulation	• Challenging but not impossible to perform at bedside (number of electrodes, neuro-navigation, TMS machine) • Expensive
Brain physiologic measures tested with active paradigms • Pro: conscious thought directly assessed, less assumptions needed in interpretation of physiologic responses • Con: need a functional sensory pathway and relatively preserved cognitive functions (e.g., language, memory, executive functions, etc.) in addition to consciousness to complete the active paradigm instructions; patient participation required		
Local-Global	Electrical correlates of conscious processing of sounds	• Bedside procedure • Convenient for repetitive assessments
Mental imagery fMRI paradigm	Blood flow changes in response to neuronal activation	• Allows analysis of the spatial activation pattern • Risks related to patient transport • Expensive
Motor imagery EEG paradigm	Electrical activity in response to neuronal activation	• Bedside procedure • Convenient for repetitive assessments

FDG-PET fluorodeoxyglucose position emission tomography, *PCI* perturbational complexity index, *TMS* transcranial magnetic stimulation, *EEG* electroencephalography, *(f)MRI* (functional) magnetic resonance imaging, *ICU* intensive care unit

according to the presence or the absence of behavioral responses on a set of hierarchically ordered items testing auditory, visual, motor, oromotor, communication and arousal function. State of consciousness is determined by specific key behaviors (and not the total score) probed during the CRS-R assessment. For example, visual pursuit, reproducible movements to command and/or complex motor behavior scores distinguish minimally conscious state from the unresponsive wakefulness syndrome [9], also called vegetative state (see Table 34.1). However, application of the CRS-R in the ICU can be challenging since assessments of patients may at times require up to 45 min of examination. Another issue is that patients can fluctuate so exams need to be repeated several times before drawing any conclusions. All behavioral scales may incorrectly classify aphasic patients as unconscious but the FOUR score and CRS-R include assessments using visual cues, which may detect signs of awareness in aphasic patients.

34.2.1.2 Assessing Biomarkers That Correlate with Level of Consciousness

The fundamental concept of this approach is based on using neurophysiologic correlates of brain activity as surrogates for levels of consciousness. Such markers include measures of brain metabolism, blood flow and electrical activity. These measures are assessed in a resting condition and correlated with current or future behavioral states. Comparisons are made of the obtained measures in patients appearing unconscious and healthy volunteers. Brain metabolism evaluated using 18F-fluorodeoxyglucose (FDG) position emission tomography (PET)-scans showed that hypometabolism in frontal and parietal cortices is seen in unresponsive wakefulness syndrome [10]. More generally, consciousness seems to vanish when brain metabolism drops below normal activity. Similar approaches have been developed using MRI arterial spin labelling sequences [11].

EEG can, amongst other approaches, be analyzed by decomposing it into spectral patterns, and quantifying complexity and connectivity. Spectral analysis is based on a Fourier transformation and provides information on the power distribution within the respective frequency bands (typically in the δ, θ, α, β and γ bands). Complexity of the EEG can be assessed by entropy measures (e.g., spectral entropy, K complexity, or permutation entropy). Functional connectivity between distant electrodes can be assessed using the spectral dimension (e.g., the debiased weighed phase lag index [wdPLI]) or information theoretical approaches (e.g., the weighed symbolic mutual information [wSMI]) [12, 13]. Similar methodologies assessing cortical functional connectivity have been developed using fMRI [14]. Candidate EEG features can then be used to train on an existing dataset of patients with known level of consciousness using a multivariate classifier to evaluate the EEG of a new patient [15].

Among these techniques, markers derived from resting state EEG seem to be the most promising in the ICU as imaging tests cannot be easily repeated and transport-related risks need to be considered for these sick patients. One study found a correlation between these EEG features (associating spectral, complexity and connectivity measures) and level of consciousness in ICU patients [16]. It is worth noting that the success of any multivariate classification approaches not only relies on the feature's selection and the quality of the EEG processing but also largely on the quality of the labels provided to the algorithm as a training set. So far, these labels are usually based on behavioral assessments with obvious limitations.

34.2.1.3 Detecting Correlates of Conscious Processing

Another approach to probe consciousness in unresponsive patients derives from neuroscientific and neuropsychological studies that have proposed physiological signatures of conscious processing in response to a given stimulus. One of these techniques focused on a late component of the evoked potential called P300 (it derives its name from the fact that it appears as a positive voltage around 300 ms following a stimulus). One of the most studied paradigms using this phenomenon in consciousness research is called the "Local-Global" paradigm [17]. Schematically this paradigm consists of delivering a subject sequences of sounds that embed two levels of auditory regularity, respectively at a local (within trial) and at a global (across trials) time scale. Whereas detection of local regularity can occur without awareness, detection of global regularity is highly correlated with access consciousness [17] (see [18] for a recent review).

A more recent approach that is at the boundaries between the two approaches described above (i.e., assessing biomarkers that correlate with the level of consciousness as well as detecting correlates of conscious processing itself) consists of measuring the complexity of brain responses to a direct stimulation of the brain using transcranial magnetic (TMS) pulses directly delivered to the parietal cortex. Using a specially designed EEG measure called perturbational complexity index, it is possible to estimate one's level of consciousness with great accuracy in different settings (i.e., sleep, anesthesia and following brain injury) [19, 20]. This measure summarizes the complexity of the response as well as the functional connectivity in its temporal dynamic dimension. This technique paved the way for alternative interpretations of late evoked brain responses (e.g., the N70) to sensory stimulations observed during the acquisition of somatosensory evoked potentials (SSEP). These brain responses have been associated with prognosis of comatose patients but clinical application has been primarily limited due to a much larger degree of variability when compared to early components of evoked potentials (i.e., the N20 of the SSEP) [21]. Revisiting the neuro-correlates of these late components that follow the classical N20 using new computational measures that quantify connectivity (e.g., wdPLI, wSMI), complexity measures (e.g., permutation entropy) or the perturbational complexity index may provide innovative approaches at the bedside in the ICU to quantify measures that not only correlate with the current state but with future recovery of consciousness.

34.2.1.4 Detecting Correlates of Command Following

Measuring physiologic changes to verbal commands allows the investigator to identify the state of cognitive motor dissociation. This approach has been the first to reliably demonstrate the existence of covert consciousness in patients that clinically meet the criteria of unresponsive wakefulness syndrome [1]. Using fMRI, it is possible to detect whether a patient is able to follow a simple verbal command (e.g., "imagine playing tennis" vs "imagine visiting your home") by comparing the elicited blood oxygen level dependent (BOLD) imaging signal changes in an unresponsive appearing patient to those seen in a group of healthy volunteers. The first large study suggested that 10% of patients with unresponsive wakefulness syndrome are able to reliably do this [22], a state later termed cognitive motor dissociation [2]. Subsequently, the feasibility of using fEEG paradigms to detect cognitive motor dissociation in unresponsive patients was demonstrated by several teams using a motor imagery EEG paradigm at the bedside [23–27]. Patients with cognitive motor dissociation should be distinguished from patients who are able to process language stimuli (using EEG or fMRI) but without evidence of conscious processing (coined high-order cortex motor dissociation [HMD] [26], see Table 34.1).

34.2.2 Pitfalls and Caveats of these Techniques in the ICU

34.2.2.1 Technical Aspects

Limitations of the clinical examination for assessing consciousness have been discussed extensively above. Imaging techniques allow spatial assessments of physical properties of interest (e.g., metabolism, blood flow) but for the purposes of studying ICU patients with impaired consciousness also have limitations in the real world. MRI and PET-scans both require transportation of the patient to the scanner, which potentially exposes patients to multiple risks (e.g., inferior monitoring, non-optimal environment in case of emergency, risk of accidental dislodging of tubes and catheters). To safely acquire MRI scans, sedation and paralytics may be required. Probing for correlates of consciousness under sedation is suboptimal. PET-scans are less problematic since the tracer can be administered just before the scan and the imaging can then be acquired under sedation. However, even for PET scans, transport will be necessary with all of the above outlined risks. Logistical challenges created include the additional personnel required to safely transport patients (e.g., nurse, physician, respiratory technician, MRI technician).

Among all the available techniques, EEG based approaches have enormous advantages in the ICU setting. EEG can be acquired at the bedside within the safe ICU environment. Associated costs for these tests will depend on local reimbursement and healthcare structures. Regardless, imaging tests like MRI or PET scans will likely be much more expensive in most health care systems when compared to EEG or evoked potentials. Additionally, EEG can be repeated many times per day, which is a huge advantage as consciousness is not a static phenomenon but may fluctuate throughout the day (see discussion about clinical limitations above). Assessments before and after interventions, for example, the administration of a medication, are more easily facilitated if repeat testing is easily available. Challenges unique to EEG assessments include electrical noise, which is very prevalent in the ICU environment, and artifacts created by involuntary movements such as myoclonus, respiratory artifact, and coughing. Seizures and other epileptiform patterns are additional major confounders to detect clear signatures of consciousness on the EEG. EEG leads may, in the hectic ICU environment, be removed to allow emergent head CT scans to be obtained to evaluate neurological changes, and placement of EEG leads may be limited by surgical wounds or bandages.

Mental imagery tasks are used both for fMRI and fEEG and are essentially very similar. These probe command following mostly to verbal commands and are fundamentally extensions of the neurological examination. Typically, patients are asked to perform (or to imagine) a motor movement that is thought to elicit a consistent BOLD or EEG signal change to be detected by fMRI or EEG, respectively. Major limitations are that patients need to be able to understand the command (challenging in patients that speak a different language, are deaf or aphasic), are interested in participating (challenging in patients with poor attention, abulia, delirium or in pain), and can keep the command in their working memory long enough to perform the task and to allow the classifier to detect the different brain activities (challenging in patients with advanced dementia). Importantly, both with fMRI and fEEG, patients can be identified that are conscious but for the reasons outlined above, consciousness cannot be ruled out for any of the patients that are classified as unconscious.

34.2.2.2 Confounding Factors

Among the major confounding factors for the assessment of consciousness in the ICU setting, the following take a central role: sedation and delirium. Determining the exact level of consciousness is usually not a major concern for the clinician treating deeply sedated patients (e.g., those receiving treatment of refractory status epilepticus or intracranial hypertension). Medications used in this context include those used for general anesthesia. On the other hand, in patients who receive lower doses of sedation, assessments of consciousness can be very challenging. However, pharmacodynamics and pharmacokinetics are altered in deeply sedated patients in the ICU receiving prolonged courses of sedatives. Inferring absence of consciousness from the absence of responsiveness may lead to the erroneous assumption of unconsciousness in sedated patients as recently demonstrated in a study revealing that conscious experiences may occur under propofol-induced unresponsiveness [28].

Another caveat is the high prevalence (30%) of delirium in the ICU [29]. Although it is relatively easy to diagnose the classical form of delirium and to demonstrate consciousness (even though in an altered form), the commonly coined 'hypoactive delirium' that can represent half of the delirium can be more difficult to identify [30]. Delirious patients usually have attention deficit that could hamper the focus required for the detection of signature of conscious processing of a stimulus (e.g., the Local-Global paradigm) or the sustained attempt to follow verbal commands.

34.2.3 What Are We Detecting Exactly?

Applying the above introduced techniques, three different kinds of signals as surrogates of covert consciousness can be detected in an unresponsive ICU patient: (1) a physiological biomarker that correlates with level of consciousness at the group level (e.g., FDG-PET scan measure of global brain metabolism or multivariate analysis of EEG features [perturbational complexity index]); (2) a correlate of conscious processing of a given stimulus at the individual level (e.g., the P3b using the Local-Global paradigm, perturbational complexity index); and (3) appropriate and sustainable brain activities in response to verbal commands at the individual level (e.g., using the motor imagery EEG paradigm). We propose that the last category represents at this point the most direct and convincing evidence of covert consciousness that has been termed cognitive motor dissociation. Indeed, physiologic biomarkers that correlate with consciousness have been developed on models trained on large datasets using clinical labels. Consequently, the confidence of how accurately a given patient is classified using these approaches mainly relies on the quality of the labels used in the training set. These labels are derived from clinical examinations which we know are imprecise. The relevance of neural correlates of conscious processing such as the P3b are still debated. In addition, evidence of conscious processing of simple stimuli does not imply the existence of conscious processing of more complex mental contents. Following commands revealed by fMRI or fEEG appears as the strongest evidence since it usually relies on statistics performed at the patient level (using for instance machine learning and permutation test).

34.3 Medical Considerations

34.3.1 Prognostication and Medical Decision Making

Prognostication in the acutely unconscious patient is one of the most challenging problems that intensivists face when taking care of brain injured patients. Determining goals of care is paramount in a setting where survival can mostly be provided but may not be desirable if the quality of survival is clearly against the patient's pre-stated wishes. Actual and predicted recovery of consciousness are major factors that physicians and families take into account when deciding about goals of care. Prognostication is frequently inaccurate but clinicians usually take into account the clinical examination, structural neuroimaging, biomarkers and electrophysiological testing. In addition, they need to consider the dynamic nature of the brain injury as well as potential confounding factors, such as sedation, metabolic derangement, and or mental disturbance (e.g., delirium). The premorbid condition and age of the patient play a role for most conditions. Disease specific prognosis markers can help predict long-term functional outcome (usually 6–12 months) [31] but uncertainty usually remains and clinicians should be aware of the risks of 'flawed reasoning' given the high degree of complexity that may occur as a result of cognitive biases [32].

Caution is warranted therefore against any studies that further add to the degree of complexity in assessing these patients. However, the existence of cognitive motor dissociation during the acute stage of brain injury, if confirmed, will likely dramatically change the assessment of prognostication of these patients. The recently published guidelines by the American Academy of Neurology for the management of patients suffering from chronic disorders of consciousness may serve as an indicator for what may occur for acutely brain injured patients. These guidelines underline the possibility of improvement for unresponsive patients months following acute brain injury and, accordingly, urge to replace the term 'permanent' vegetative state by 'chronic' vegetative state (or unresponsive wakefulness syndrome) [6]. The acknowledgement of this high degree of uncertainty at the subacute stage of acute brain injury, and usually with fewer data than in the chronic setting, should be remembered when elaborating a poor prognosis based on limited data a few days after acute brain injury.

34.3.2 Pain Management

Considering that 15–40% [5, 26, 27] of unresponsive patients might be actually conscious and able to experience pain without any way to express suffering, caregivers need to consider pain medications whenever a medical condition is bound to generate nociceptive inputs. Invasive procedures in unconscious appearing patients should be performed using the same analgo-sedative management approach as in an awake, communicative patients.

34.3.3 Recovery of Communication Abilities

A common challenge for patients in the ICU is their inability to consistently and effectively communicate their most fundamental physical needs [33]. Conscious patients in the ICU commonly suffer from unrecognized pain, discomfort, feelings of loss of control and insecurity, depersonalization, anxiety, sleep disturbances, fear and frustration [34]. The primary means of communication for these patients is the use of non-vocal techniques, such as lip reading and gestures; however these methods are often inadequate for effective communication [35]. In addition, the recent description of cognitive motor dissociation during the acute phase of brain injury increases the potential number of patients in a situation of inefficient communication [26].

Brain-computer interface (BCI) systems have recently generated interest as a method to facilitate contact with the ICU patients. BCIs translate the patient's cerebral electrical activity, typically recorded by EEG, into computer commands bypassing other body functions (Fig. 34.1). Although a variety of BCI systems have been proposed for rehabilitation purposes [36, 37], the number of BCIs, assisting with communication of the typical physical and emotional needs of the critically ill, remains significantly limited [38, 39].

The main restriction for practical application of BCI systems in the ICU is lack of reliability due to the considerable number of distractions, possible extinction of goal-directed thinking, deterioration of patient attention control, etc. Another specific challenge includes eyelid apraxia or other visual impairments that preclude the use of classical visual cues. In addition, owing to extended bedrest and skin breakdown, and pain medication, the tactile input channel is also sometimes impaired. Auditory cues allow only very limited information to be transferred, like simple questions or commands. Moreover, many training sessions could be required to teach patients to use BCI technology which will be challenging with distracted patients in pain and evolving medical conditions. Therefore, current BCIs in the ICU focus on quick and reliable signaling (e.g., 'yes'/'no' binary signals [38, 39] or

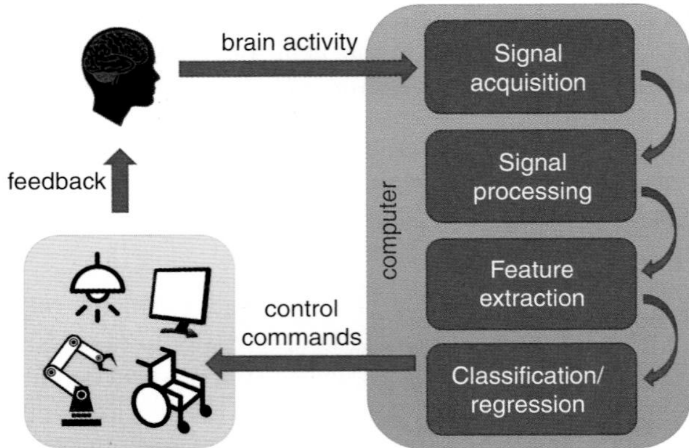

Fig. 34.1 Brain-computer interface systems. Brain-computer interface systems use state-of-the-art machine learning methods to decode brain activity. A brain-computer interface system is realized using several components: (1) brain signal activity acquisition: electroencephalogram (EEG), electrocorticography (ECoG), functional magnetic resonance imaging (fMRI), functional near-infrared spectroscopy (fNIRS), etc.; (2) signal processing: band-pass filtering, outlier removal, artifact correction, normalization, etc.; (3) feature extraction: gain task-relevant information from acquired data; (4) classification/regression: decode the intended action of the subject by applying machine learning methods; (5) control commands to external devices: screen, wheelchair, exoskeleton, etc.; (6) feedback: the subject receives feedback about how well he/she performed in a certain training task

steady-state visual evoked potential (SSVEP) based communication [38, 39]) rather than spelling of words or sentences.

Despite the limitations, BCI technology has the potential to significantly increase patient autonomy allowing more efficient pain management as well as better interaction with the external environment (e.g., bed position, call button, lights, television, etc.). Portable EEG-based BCI has been used in one study for the detection of consciousness [40]. It uses Pavlovian semantic conditioning to discriminate between cognitive 'yes' and 'no' responses. However, it demonstrated reliable level of performance only for offline classifiers in one out of three locked-in state patients.

To improve the reliability of BCI systems, utilization of hybrid BCIs, combining either sequential or simultaneous integration of different data sources, has been proposed [41]. In hybrid BCIs, EEG data could be complemented with other brain as well as non-brain modalities, such as functional near infrared spectroscopy (fNIRS), electrooculography (EOG), and electromyography (EMG), heart rate, hemodynamic response, etc. [42]. Due to their advanced reliability, hybrid BCIs could be especially efficient for ICU application.

Despite the drawbacks of current BCI systems, their main advantage is the potential for instant data processing. Moreover, computationally efficient methods proposed for robust treatment and adaptive modeling of complex data streams in real-time [43], allow implementation of BCIs into a personal computer or even tablet for easy installation in the ICU. Fast feedback of the real-time BCI systems simplifies the training process for patients and enables the medical staff to respond more rapidly to the time-sensitive needs of the patients.

The proportion of patients with cognitive motor dissociation who would be able to use a BCI to communicate (that could be called "communicating cognitive motor dissociation" [Table 34.1]) remains to be determined. According to the obstacles described above, we can hypothesize that only cognitive motor dissociation patients with preserved high cognition capacities (language, memory, executive function, etc.) will be able to use a BCI. However, it is worth noting that these devices would also benefit a larger disabled patient population, such as lock-in syndrome, hemiplegic or paraplegic patients.

34.4 Ethical Considerations

Currently, the majority of brain injured patients who die in the ICU do so as a direct consequence of withdrawal of life-sustaining therapies [44]. Lack of consciousness has a major impact on medical decision making, particularly withdrawal of life-sustaining therapies. Indeed, many prognostication tools (e.g., following cardiac arrest, intracranial hemorrhage, subarachnoid hemorrhage) attribute a huge weight on the level of consciousness (usually crudely assessed by the GCS). From that perspective, the use of the most accurate technique to detect consciousness and capture cognitive motor dissociation needs to be a major focus of our efforts. Consciousness is an irreducible component of personhood and a central tenet of the Belmont Report [45].

Decisions to withdraw life-sustaining therapies are frequently made within the first weeks following brain injury, frequently within hours or days of the injury. Increasingly, however, studies show that delayed recovery is more common than previously thought. Consciousness is not systematically quantified to improve prognostic tools. Concerns relative to these failures of our moral obligations to probe residual consciousness and to elaborate a prognosis as precise as possible have been raised to reduce our 'neglect' [46]. In that context, recent recommendations by an association of British critical care medical societies to (1) extend the observation time window; (2) use multiple exploration techniques; and (3) consider the involvement of a "neuroscience team" are a step in the right direction [31]. These recommendations should be put to test in cost-effectiveness studies and undergo open public debate. Caregivers are torn between on the one hand providing the highest level of care (which includes providing sufficient time to achieve a reliable prognosis) and on the other hand to guarantee equity by providing as many patients as possible access to the scarce resource of a highly specialized critical care unit (constraints of limited resources). The question of how much money a given society is willing to invest in order to maximize chances of recovery should be openly discussed considering the number of patients that could benefit from this service. Societal burden of potential long-term survival with disability also needs to be considered. To date these considerations are unfortunately handled locally by caregivers and are at the roots of a great variability in practice and differences in provided level of care.

34.4.1 Ethical Aspects Raised By Covert Consciousness in the ICU

The potential existence of covert consciousness in unresponsive patients in the ICU raises many concerns. For example, considering the pain management discussed above, one might want to preserve any suffering or pain and administer sedatives and pain killers whenever a doubt exists [45]. On the other hand, one might want to preserve covert consciousness in order to maximize the chances of detection to support prognostication and possibly provide a communication channel with these patients in the future. This dilemma has been known for years by clinicians assessing consciousness using fMRI of EEG on a regular basis.

34.5 Conclusion

Forty-five years ago, Jennet and Plum acknowledged that the absence of behavioral evidence of awareness could erroneously suggest the absence of consciousness ("it seems that there is wakefulness without awareness"), stating that there is no "reliable alternative available to the doctor at the bedside, which is where decisions have to be made" [47]. This visionary prediction is now reality. Given the available data it is clear that behavioral criteria alone are not sufficient to accurately define consciousness states and it is no wonder that recent discoveries on consciousness disorders have led to revisiting of the taxonomy of patients with disorders of consciousness [48–50]. For example, recent debate has emphasized the lack of homogeneity of the minimally conscious state (minimally conscious state minus/plus dichotomy [3]) category and even challenged assumptions of the nature of consciousness in minimally conscious state (proposing to replace this term by cortically mediated state, to avoid any inference from a patient's subjectivity) [50]. Increasing diagnostic precision is bound to increase prognostic accuracy and will hopefully lead to tailored therapeutic interventions. The intensivist needs to stay in tune with this rapidly evolving area that tackles some of the most complex neuroscientific concepts (i.e., consciousness, neuro-prognosis, neuro-repair), cutting edge technologies (advanced brain imagery and signal processing) and fundamental ethical questions (autonomy, equity, quality of life and life or death decisions).

References

1. Owen AM, Coleman MR, Boly M, et al. Detecting awareness in the vegetative state. Science. 2006;313:1402.
2. Schiff ND. Cognitive motor dissociation following severe brain injuries. JAMA Neurol. 2015;72:1413–5.
3. Bruno MA, Vanhaudenhuyse A, Thibaut A, et al. From unresponsive wakefulness to minimally conscious PLUS and functional locked-in syndromes: recent advances in our understanding of disorders of consciousness. J Neurol. 2011;258:1373–84.
4. Plum F, Posner JB. The Diagnosis of Stupor and Coma. 3rd ed. Philadelphia: Oxford University Press; 1980.

5. Kondziella D, Friberg CK, Frokjaer VG, et al. Preserved consciousness in vegetative and minimal conscious states: systematic review and meta-analysis. J Neurol Neurosurg Psychiatry. 2016;87:485–92.
6. Giacino JT, Katz DI, Schiff ND, et al. Practice guideline update recommendations summary: disorders of consciousness. Neurology. 2018;91:450–60.
7. Wijdicks EFM, Kramer AA, Rohs T, et al. Comparison of the full outline of unresponsiveness score and the Glasgow coma scale in predicting mortality in critically ill patients. Crit Care Med. 2015;43:439–44.
8. Giacino JT, Ashwal S, Childs N, et al. The minimally conscious state: definition and diagnostic criteria. Neurology. 2002;58:349–53.
9. Laureys S, Celesia GG, Cohadon F, et al. Unresponsive wakefulness syndrome: a new name for the vegetative state or apallic syndrome. BMC Med. 2010;8:68.
10. Stender J, Gosseries O, Bruno MA, et al. Diagnostic precision of PET imaging and functional MRI in disorders of consciousness: a clinical validation study. Lancet. 2014;384:514–22.
11. Liu AA, Voss HU, Dyke JP, et al. Arterial spin labeling and altered cerebral blood flow patterns in the minimally conscious state. Neurology. 2011;77:1518–23.
12. King JR, Sitt JD, Faugeras F, et al. Information sharing in the brain indexes consciousness in noncommunicative patients. Curr Biol. 2013;23:1914–9.
13. Chennu S, Annen J, Wannez S, et al. Brain networks predict metabolism, diagnosis and prognosis at the bedside in disorders of consciousness. Brain. 2017;140:2120–32.
14. Demertzi A, Antonopoulos G, Heine L, et al. Intrinsic functional connectivity differentiates minimally conscious from unresponsive patients. Brain. 2015;138(Pt 9):2619–3.
15. Sitt JD, King JR, El Karoui I, et al. Large scale screening of neural signatures of consciousness in patients in a vegetative or minimally conscious state. Brain. 2014;137:2258–70.
16. Claassen J, Velazquez A, Meyers E, et al. Bedside quantitative electroencephalography improves assessment of consciousness in comatose subarachnoid hemorrhage patients. Ann Neurol. 2016;80:541–53.
17. Bekinschtein TA, Dehaene S, Rohaut B, et al. Neural signature of the conscious processing of auditory regularities. Proc Natl Acad Sci U S A. 2009;106:1672–7.
18. Rohaut B, Naccache L. Disentangling conscious from unconscious cognitive processing with event-related EEG potentials. Rev Neurol (Paris). 2017;173:521–8.
19. Casali AG, Gosseries O, Rosanova M, et al. A theoretically based index of consciousness independent of sensory processing and behavior. Sci Transl Med. 2013;5:198ra105.
20. Casarotto S, Comanducci A, Rosanova M, et al. Stratification of unresponsive patients by an independently validated index of brain complexity. Ann Neurol. 2016;80:718–29.
21. Zandbergen EGJ, Koelman JHTM, Haan RJ, et al. SSEPs and prognosis in postanoxic coma only short or also long latency responses. Neurology. 2006;67:583–6.
22. Monti MM, Vanhaudenhuyse A, Coleman MR, et al. Willful modulation of brain activity in disorders of consciousness. N Engl J Med. 2010;362:579–89.
23. Cruse D, Chennu S, Chatelle C, et al. Bedside detection of awareness in the vegetative state: a cohort study. Lancet. 2011;378:2088–94.
24. Goldfine AM, Victor JD, Conte MM, et al. Determination of awareness in patients with severe brain injury using EEG power spectral analysis. Clin Neurophysiol. 2011;122:2157–68.
25. Cruse D, Chennu S, Chatelle C, et al. Relationship between etiology and covert cognition in the minimally conscious state. Neurology. 2012;78:816–22.
26. Edlow BL, Chatelle C, Spencer CA, et al. Early detection of consciousness in patients with acute severe traumatic brain injury. Brain. 2017;140:2399–414.
27. Curley WH, Forgacs PB, Voss HU, et al. Characterization of EEG signals revealing covert cognition in the injured brain. Brain. 2018;141:1404–21.
28. Radek L, Kallionpää RE, Karvonen M, et al. Dreaming and awareness during dexmedetomidine- and propofol-induced unresponsiveness. Br J Anaesth. 2018;121:260–9.
29. Salluh JI, Wang H, Schneider EB, et al. Outcome of delirium in critically ill patients: systematic review and meta-analysis. BMJ. 2015;350:h2538.
30. Hosker C, Ward D. Hypoactive delirium. BMJ. 2017;357:j2047.

31. Harvey D, Butler J, Groves J, et al. Management of perceived devastating brain injury after hospital admission: a consensus statement from stakeholder professional organizations. Br J Anaesth. 2018;120:138–45.
32. Rohaut B, Claassen J. Decision making in perceived devastating brain injury: a call to explore the impact of cognitive biases. Br J Anaesth. 2018;120:5–9.
33. Happ MB, Garrett K, Thomas DD, et al. Nurse-patient communication interactions in the intensive care unit. Am J Crit Care. 2011;20:e28–40.
34. Carroll SM. Nonvocal ventilated patients perceptions of being understood. West J Nurs Res. 2004;26:85–103.
35. Menzel LK. Factors related to the emotional responses of intubated patients to being unable to speak. Heart Lung. 1998;27:245–52.
36. Daly JJ, Huggins JE. Brain-computer interface: current and emerging rehabilitation applications. Arch Phys Med Rehabil. 2015;96:S1–7.
37. Chaudhary U, Birbaumer N, Curado MR. Brain-machine interface (BMI) in paralysis. Ann Phys Rehabil Med. 2015;58:9–13.
38. Dehzangi O, Farooq M. Portable brain-computer interface for the intensive care unit patient communication using subject-dependent SSVEP identification. Biomed Res Int. 2018;2018:9796238.
39. Chatelle C, Spencer CA, Cash SS, et al. Feasibility of an EEG-based brain-computer interface in the intensive care unit. Clin Neurophysiol. 2018;129:1519–25.
40. De Massari D, Ruf CA, Furdea A, et al. Brain communication in the locked-in state. Brain. 2013;136:1989–2000.
41. Pfurtscheller G, Allison BZ, Brunner C, et al. The hybrid BCI. Front Neurosci. 2010;4:30.
42. Hong KS, Khan MJ. Hybrid brain-computer interface techniques for improved classification accuracy and increased number of commands: a review. Front Neurorobot. 2017;11:35.
43. Eliseyev A, Auboiroux V, Costecalde T, et al. Recursive exponentially weighted n-way partial least squares regression with recursive-validation of hyper-parameters in brain-computer interface applications. Sci Rep. 2017;7:16281.
44. Turgeon AF, Lauzier F, Simard JF, et al. Mortality associated with withdrawal of life-sustaining therapy for patients with severe traumatic brain injury: a Canadian multicentre cohort study. CMAJ. 2011;183:1581–8.
45. Fins JJ, Bernat JL. Ethical, palliative, and policy considerations in disorders of consciousness. Neurology. 2018;91:471–5.
46. Fins JJ. Constructing an ethical stereotaxy for severe brain injury: balancing risks, benefits and access. Nat Rev Neurosci. 2003;4:323–7.
47. Jennett B, Plum F. Persistent vegetative state after brain damage. A syndrome in search of a name. Lancet. 1972;1:734–7.
48. Bayne T, Hohwy J, Owen AM. Reforming the taxonomy in disorders of consciousness. Ann Neurol. 2017;82:866–72.
49. Bernat JL. Nosologic considerations in disorders of consciousness. Ann Neurol. 2017;82:863–5.
50. Naccache L. Minimally conscious state or cortically mediated state? Brain. 2018;141:949–60.

Part XI

Infection and Antibiotics

From Influenza-Induced Acute Lung Injury to Multiorgan Failure

35

B. M. Tang, T. Cootes, and A. S. McLean

35.1 Introduction

Influenza viruses are among the most common causes of human respiratory infection, causing high morbidity and mortality. In the United States, influenza results in approximately 200,000 hospitalizations and 36,000 deaths during a seasonal epidemic [1]. During a pandemic, up to 50% of the population can be infected by influenza, increasing the number of deaths [2]. In 1918, the worst influenza pandemic recorded in history caused up to 50 million deaths worldwide, with elderly, infants, and people with underlying illness having the highest risk of fatality [3].

The modes of death in severe influenza patients are well recognized. They range from hypoxic respiratory failure to multiorgan failure. However, it remains unclear which host factors drive these processes. A better understanding of the host factors associated with severe disease is clinically important; it may help discover pathogenic pathways that determine disease progression and enable researchers to identify new therapeutic targets. Identifying new therapeutic targets is particularly important given that currently available antiviral therapy (e.g., neuraminidase inhibitors) has limited efficacy in reducing influenza-related fatality. Therefore,

B. M. Tang (✉)
Department of Intensive Care Medicine, Nepean Hospital, Kingswood, NSW, Australia

Centre for Immunology and Allergy Research, Westmead Institute for Medical Research, Westmead, NSW, Australia
e-mail: benjamin.tang@sydney.edu.au

T. Cootes
Department of Infectious Diseases and Immunology, Central Clinical School, University of Sydney, Darlington, NSW, Australia

A. S. McLean
Department of Intensive Care Medicine, Nepean Hospital, Kingswood, NSW, Australia

J.-L. Vincent (ed.), *Annual Update in Intensive Care and Emergency Medicine 2019*, Annual Update in Intensive Care and Emergency Medicine,
https://doi.org/10.1007/978-3-030-06067-1_35

delineating influenza-related host factors is a critical first step in improving patient outcome in influenza infection. Here, we examine the host factors underpinning both innate and adaptive immune response to influenza virus (Box 35.1).

Box 35.1: Innate and Adaptive Immune Responses in Influenza Infection

Innate immune response	Adaptive immune response
Alveolar macrophages—resident local immune cells in lung; early contact with influenza virus; initiate phagocytosis and antigen presentation of influenza virus to activate other immune cells.	**B cells**—produce influenza virus-specific antibodies in a CD4 T-cell-dependent manner; important in humoral response to influenza virus infection; important for vaccine development.
Neutrophils—first wave of recruited immune cells to lung; critical in antiviral response; also aid activation of CD8 T cells. However, can exacerbate tissue inflammation in infected lung.	**Cytotoxic CD8 T cells**—major driver of the cellular response; enable killing of influenza virus and elimination of virally infected host cells; critical for viral clearance and resolution of infection.
Monocytes—influx elicits potent inflammatory cascade; also aid the activation of CD8 T cells.	**Memory CD8 T cells**—initiate the recall response to secondary infection; thus, very important for vaccine development.
Natural killer cells—kill influenza-infected host cells; important not only for innate immune response but also for initiating adaptive immune response.	**CD4 T cells**—augment CD8 and B-cell response to influenza infection; also, have their own antiviral effects that are independent of CD8 and B-cell activity.
Dendritic cells—cross-present influenza virus antigens or peptides to CD4 and CD8 T cells; also potent producer of antiviral molecules such as interferons.	**Regulatory T cells (Treg)**—highly suppressive to CD4 and CD8 effector cells; usually required for initiating resolution of the immune response after infection.

35.2 Innate Immune Response

The innate response is critical for early protection against influenza virus and plays a key role in the induction and regulation of adaptive immune response. Innate immunity provides a vital bridge between first exposure of the naïve host and subsequent elaboration of specific antibody and T-cell responses, which is extremely important for clearing virus. Viral RNA is recognized through a variety of pattern recognition receptors (PRRs), including Toll-like receptor (TLR)3, TLR7, TLR8, retinoic acid-inducible gene I (RIG)-I and nucleotide-binding domain-like receptor protein (NLRP)3. Once viral RNA is recognized by PRRs, pro-inflammatory cytokines are secreted, such as type I interferons (IFNs), which induce an antiviral state in neighboring cells. Cytokine secretion leads to the recruitment of innate immune cells, which instruct the adaptive immune response for specific killing of influenza-infected cells [4].

Neutrophils are the first wave of recruited immune cells that respond to influenza virus infection; they provide critical protection by acting to limit viral replication [5, 6]. Some studies have suggested that neutrophils are mediators of immunopathology and mortality due to their excessive inflammatory response [7, 8]. However, there is also evidence supporting the protective role neutrophils perform in influenza virus infection [4]. In particular, neutrophil-depleted mice had reduced virus elimination from the infected site over time [9]. Additionally, neutrophils have also been shown to be vital in sustaining effective $CD8^+$ T-cell responses in the respiratory tract of influenza virus-infected mice, which is important for virus clearance [10].

Resident alveolar macrophages in lungs are involved in the first line of defense. In addition to phagocytosis of virions and virus-infected cells, alveolar macrophages contribute to recognition of the virus to present to the adaptive arm of the immune system [10]. Following recognition, alveolar macrophages produce an array of pro-inflammatory cytokines, including tumor necrosis factor (TNF)-α, interleukin (IL)-1, IL-6 and IFN-α/β, which further limit viral replication. In an animal study, mice depleted of alveolar macrophages had exacerbated disease severity, increased virus replication and a higher mortality when infected with influenza virus [11].

Monocytes are one of the predominant cell types upregulated during influenza virus infection and consequently circulate in high numbers. During inflammation, the bone marrow receives signals from pro-inflammatory cytokines and TLR ligands to increase monocyte production. Respiratory epithelial cells secrete monocyte chemoattractant protein (MCP)-1, which facilitates monocyte trafficking into the lungs [12]. Excessive numbers of monocytes drive immune pathology in severe influenza; however, by reducing recruitment of inflammatory monocytes to the lung, there is a decreased $CD8^+$ T-cell response leading to compromised viral clearance [13]. Recruited monocytes also respond to influenza virus infection by differentiating into monocyte-derived macrophages and monocyte-derived dendritic cells [14].

Natural killer (NK) cells are granular lymphocytes that contribute to the control of viral replication and production of cytokines that modulate the immune response to influenza virus [15]. The contribution of NK cells to the antiviral immune response has been extensively studied in mouse models of viral infections, demonstrating that NK cells not only contain viral replication by killing infected cells during earlier stages of infection, but also play a critical role during the development of adaptive immunity [16]. Defects in NK cell activity result in delayed viral clearance and increased morbidity and mortality [15].

Dendritic cells are a critical component in early detection of viral infection and transfer of viral antigens to draining lymph nodes, bridging innate and adaptive immunity. The major function of dendritic cells during the antiviral response is to process and present viral antigenic peptides to antigen-specific $CD8^+$ and $CD4^+$ T cells to establish an adaptive immune response [17]. Dendritic cells mainly obtain viral proteins via ingestion of virus-infected cells, as few viruses directly infect dendritic cells. Following ingestion, viral particles are mainly presented on MHC class I molecules through a process known as cross-presentation. Cross-presentation is important as it enables dendritic cells to activate $CD8^+$ T cells, which are required for viral clearance [18].

35.3 Adaptive Immune Response

The cellular and humoral arms of adaptive immunity are both activated in response to influenza virus infection. The humoral arm of the adaptive immune response involves B cells, which secrete antibodies to effectively prevent infection by neutralizing the virus [19]. B-cell responses to influenza infection are largely T-dependent, where maximal antiviral IgG responses rely on CD4$^+$ T cells and their interaction with B cells [20].

The cellular arm of the adaptive immune response involves T cells, which are critical for viral clearance. Following dendritic cell presentation of viral antigens in the draining lymph nodes, naïve virus-specific T cells undergo a process of activation, proliferation and differentiation to become effector T cells that can migrate to the site of infection and mediate antiviral immune responses [21]. Infection with influenza virus induces differentiation of effector CD4$^+$ and CD8$^+$ T cells, however the contribution of CD4$^+$ T cells to virus clearance is minor, compared to CD8$^+$ T cells. In influenza infection, the primary role of CD4$^+$ T cells involves supporting the activation and differentiation of B cells, leading to antibody production, and memory responses. Effector CD8$^+$ T cells are major players in viral clearance and are essential for elimination of infected cells [22]. CD8$^+$ effector T cells mediate viral clearance through three distinct mechanisms. First, CD8$^+$ T cells can induce lysis of infected cells through exocytosis of perforin and granzyme containing granules. Second, CD8$^+$ T cells can trigger TNF receptor (TNFR) family-dependent apoptosis in infected or stressed cells through either Fas ligand or TNF-related apoptosis-inducing ligand (TRAIL). Third, when encountered with virus-infected cells, CD8$^+$ T cells can produce pro-inflammatory mediators, such as IFN-γ, which is important for viral clearance [21].

35.4 Which Host Factor Is Most Directly Linked to Influenza Fatality?

The preceding sections demonstrate that a myriad of host factors is involved in mounting an immune response to influenza virus. A key question is, among these host factors identified, which host factor is primarily responsible for influencing disease progression? Several studies have addressed this question. A study by Brandes et al. evaluated all the common host factors implicated in influenza pathogenesis [7]. From this evaluation, the authors discovered that a neutrophil-driven response was the most dominant host factor in disease progression. Notably, the authors identified a neutrophil-driven inflammatory loop that could directly amplify tissue damage and exacerbate inflammation. Thus, the authors concluded that excessive neutrophil activation was the main host factor associated with poor outcome in influenza infection.

Another recent study provides further insight into the mechanism underpinning the neutrophil-driven response in severe influenza. In their study, Narasaraju et al. [8] examined neutrophil influx into the infected lung after influenza infection. Their findings confirmed that neutrophils were primarily responsible for causing immunopathology, lung inflammation and subsequently the development of acute respiratory distress syndrome (ARDS). Importantly, the authors further discovered that neutrophil extracellular trap (NET) formation correlated with tissue damage. By examining lung histopathology and NET activity, they found that NETs directly caused tissue damage to alveoli, epithelium and the vascular structure in the infected lung. Thus, this study provides strong etiological evidence that aberrant or excessive neutrophil response was the dominant causative factor in severe influenza.

An important caveat of the above studies is that they were mostly performed in animal models. Thus, it was uncertain whether the mechanistic findings obtained from these studies could be applied to infected humans. Two recent human studies have been performed to address this issue. A study by Dunning et al. examined the host response profile in 131 influenza infected humans (with either H1N1 or H3N2 influenza virus). The patient cohort include those with mild infection (n = 47), moderate infection (n = 34) and severe infection (n = 28) [23]. The findings of this study confirmed previous animal studies; they showed that neutrophil response was the primary host factor in determining the course of illness. Indeed, an excessive neutrophil response was consistently found in most patients with severe disease. Another study by Guan et al. investigated the host response profile of severe influenza infection, using a small case-series of patients with severe H7N9 infection [24]. This study also identified neutrophil response as the most critical factor in severe disease. Collectively, these human studies confirm findings from previous animal studies and pinpoint an aberrant neutrophil response as the main cause of disease progression in influenza infection.

35.5 How Does Influenza Virus Interact with Host Factors?

Influenza virus likely interacts with systemic host factors (e.g., circulating neutrophils) during the course of infection. Unravelling this interaction is key to understanding influenza pathogenesis and, in particular, to exploring the mechanism by which influenza infection evolves from lung inflammation to multiorgan failure. Most influenza infection begins in airway and the infection spreads locally to other parts of the lung. The mechanism by which the virus interacts with local immune cells is well studied and much of the molecular/cellular details have already been elucidated. By contrast, the mechanism by which influenza virus interacts with host factors outside the lung, such as circulating immune cells, remains relatively unknown. This is largely due to the established dogma that influenza virus does not circulate outside the lung and, by extension, influenza virus is not expected to interact with circulating immune cells (e.g., neutrophils). This 'lung-centric' paradigm has recently been challenged by new evidence. Several studies showed that influenza virus can indeed be carried by immune cells from lung to non-lung tissues [25–27]. These 'virus carrying' immune cells include professional antigen presenting cells such as monocytes, macrophage and dendritic cells [28–30]. These cells pick up influenza virus RNA during their encountering and processing of virus infected cells

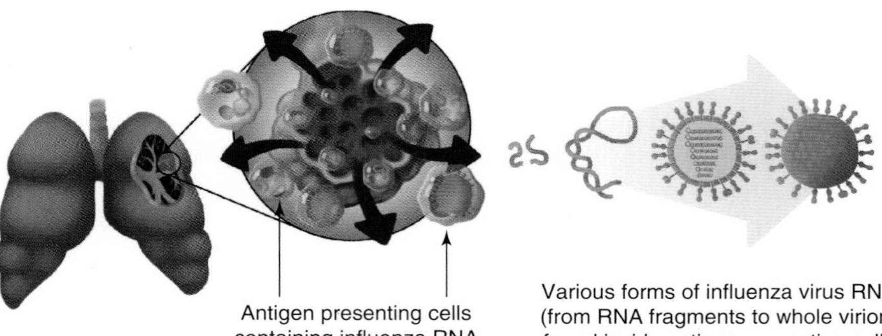

Fig. 35.1 Dissemination of influenza virus from infected lung tissue. Left side: antigen presenting cells carry influenza virus RNA; these 'carrier cells' disseminate influenza RNA from within infected airway/alveoli to outside the lung. Right side: the influenza RNA is carried inside antigen presenting cells in various forms, including (from left to right) (1) a short influenza RNA segment, (2) an intact full influenza RNA segment, (3) a non-replicating whole influenza virus, or (4) a whole influenza virus that is actively replicating and infecting other host cells

(e.g., epithelium) in the early phase of infection (Fig. 35.1). After processing of dead/infected cells, these cells carry influenza virus RNA within them, migrate towards local draining lymph nodes and subsequently into the systemic circulation.

The influenza virus RNA carried inside these 'carrier' immune cells consists mostly of fragments of the virus RNA (which cannot infect other cells) and a few replicating whole RNA virions (which can infect other cells). Collectively, these RNA molecules are known as the 'influenza virus transcriptome' (Fig. 35.1). Steuerman et al. recently successfully measured the influenza virus transcriptome in infected lung tissues (e.g., epithelium and endothelium) and circulating immune cells (e.g., monocytes, T cells, B cells and NK cells) [31]. Their findings provide strong support to the notion that the influenza virus transcriptome is transported by 'carrier' immune cells (e.g., macrophages or dendritic cells) within the systematic circulation, thereby enabling the dissemination of influenza virus transcriptome loads to distant organs [28, 32].

35.6 Influenza Virus Transcriptome Triggers a Systemic Inflammatory Response

The influenza virus transcriptome can be cross-presented by 'carrier' immune cells to circulating neutrophils (Fig. 35.2). Neutrophils are recruited to the infected tissue as part of the host response to influenza virus. These cells traffic from the systemic circulation towards the lung, as guided by released of chemoattractants from infected tissue. During this migration, neutrophils encounter 'carrier' immune cells in the systemic circulation, in transit towards the lung or after they have arrived within the infected

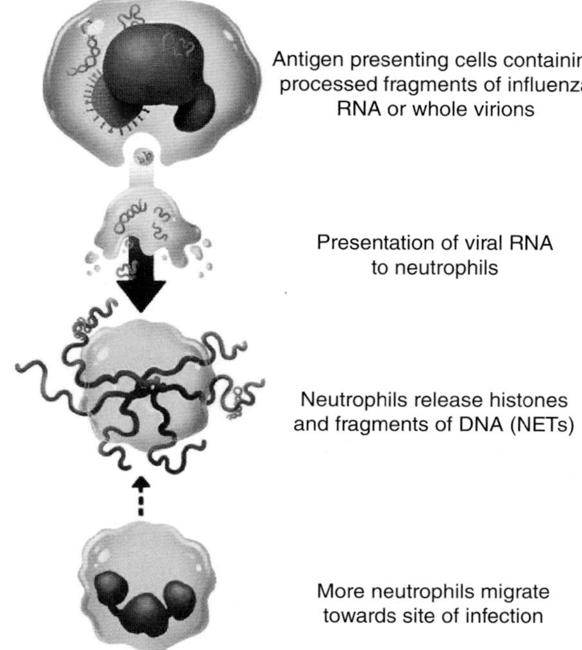

Fig. 35.2 Neutrophil extracellular traps (NETs) released by neutrophils upon encountering antigen presenting cells

lung. This encounter triggers a release of a massive amount of NETs (Fig. 35.2). NETs consist of a cellular 'debris' of nuclear contents (histones and DNA fibers) externalized by activated neutrophils in response to bacterial or viral infection.

Although NET formation is an evolutionarily conserved response to microbes, excessive NET release in the infected lung leads to endothelial damage, thrombosis, worsening inflammation. In a recent study, Narasaraju et al. showed that the excessive release of NET in infected lung exacerbated lung inflammation and directly caused the development of acute lung injury [8].

35.7 From Acute Lung Injury to Multiorgan Failure

It is clear, from the review above, that lung injury in influenza infection is partly a direct result of the cytopathic effects on host cells (e.g., epithelium or alveoli) by influenza virus and partly an indirect result of a dysregulated host response associated with NETs. Both direct and indirect processes may extend beyond the infected lung, since 'carrier' immune cells can transport influenza virus transcriptome to distant organs where a further encounter with recruited neutrophils may trigger local release of NETs into the affected organs. Indeed, in animal models, influenza virus transcriptome can be detected in major organs in the infected host (heart, spleen, kidney, brain, liver) [32]. Furthermore, a recent study showed that neutrophils can be infected by influenza virus [33]. Once infected, these neutrophils become 'carrier' immune cells themselves. They

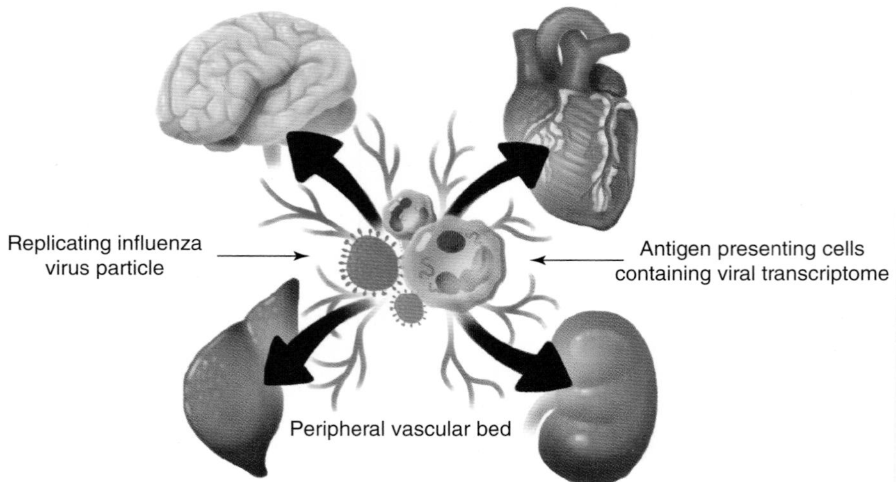

Fig. 35.3 A new multisystem view of influenza pathogenesis

then go on to spread neutrophil-induced inflammation (e.g., NETs, myeloperoxidase, reactive oxygen species) elsewhere or allow actively replicating virions to 'seed' the target organs. Collectively, both direct and indirect tissue injury mechanisms extend an initially lung-centered pathology to other major organs with the ensuing development of organ dysfunction (e.g., myocarditis, acute kidney injury). In light of this, the traditional 'lung-centric' view of influenza pathogenesis requires revision to incorporate a multisystem view of organ dysfunction influenza pathogenesis (Fig. 35.3).

35.8 Conclusion

Severe influenza infection remains an important clinical challenge to critical care physicians. The potentially high morbidity and mortality of this condition has remained unchanged over the last few decades, due mainly to a lack of effective new therapies to treat such patients. In recent years, we have gained a much better understanding of the disease mechanism. This improved understanding points to the pivotal roles played by immune dysregulation in causing severe disease. Agents that modulate the host response therefore hold particularly great promise in correcting the dysregulated immune response and may help reduce morbidity/mortality.

References

1. Thompson WW, Shay DK, Weintraub E, et al. Mortality associated with influenza and respiratory syncytial virus in the United States. JAMA. 2003;289:179–86.
2. Simonsen L. The global impact of influenza on morbidity and mortality. Vaccine. 1999;17(Suppl 1):S3–10.

3. Taubenberger JK, Morens DM. The pathology of influenza virus infections. Annu Rev Pathol Mech Dis. 2008;3:499–522.
4. Tripathi S, White MR, Hartshorn KL. The amazing innate immune response to influenza A virus infection. Innate Immun. 2015;21:73–98.
5. Camp JV, Jonsson CB. A role for neutrophils in viral respiratory disease. Front Immunol. 2017;8:11.
6. Iwasaki A, Pillai PS. Innate immunity to influenza virus infection. Nature. 2014;14:315–28.
7. Brandes M, Klauschen F, Kuchen S, Germain RN. A systems analysis identifies a feedforward inflammatory circuit leading to lethal influenza infection. Cell. 2013;154:197–212.
8. Narasaraju T, Yang E, Samy RP, et al. Excessive neutrophils and neutrophil extracellular traps contribute to acute lung injury of influenza pneumonitis. Am J Pathol. 2011;179:199–210.
9. Fujisawa H. Inhibitory role of neutrophils on influenza virus multiplication in the lungs of mice. Microbiol Immunol. 2001;45:679–88.
10. Tate MD, Brooks AG, Reading PC, Mintern JD. Neutrophils sustain effective CD8(+) T-cell responses in the respiratory tract following influenza infection. Immunol Cell Biol. 2012;90:197–205.
11. Kim HM, Lee YW, Lee KJ, et al. Alveolar macrophages are indispensable for controlling influenza viruses in lungs of pigs. J Virol. 2008;82:4265–74.
12. Herold S, von Wulffen W, Steinmueller M, et al. Alveolar epithelial cells direct monocyte transepithelial migration upon influenza virus infection: impact of chemokines and adhesion molecules. J Immunol. 2006;177:1817–24.
13. Cole SL, Ho LP. Contribution of innate immune cells to pathogenesis of severe influenza virus infection. Clin Sci. 2017;131:269–83.
14. Auffray C, Sieweke MH, Geissmann F. Blood monocytes: development, heterogeneity, and relationship with dendritic cells. Annu Rev Immunol. 2009;27:669–92.
15. Jost S, Altfeld M. Control of human viral infections by natural killer cells. Annu Rev Immunol. 2013;31:163–94.
16. Schultz-Cherry S. Role of NK cells in influenza infection. Curr Top Microbiol Immunol. 2015;386:109–20.
17. Grayson MH, Holtzman MJ. Emerging role of dendritic cells in respiratory viral infection. J Mol Med. 2007;85:1057–68.
18. Belz GT, Wilson NS, Kupresanin F, Mount AM, Smith CM. Shaping naive and memory CD8+ T cell responses in pathogen infections through antigen presentation. Adv Exp Med Biol. 2007;590:31–42.
19. Sealy R, Surman S, Hurwitz JL, Coleclough C. Antibody response to influenza infection of mice: different patterns for glycoprotein and nucleocapsid antigens. Immunology. 2003;108:431–9.
20. Sangster MY, Riberdy JM, Gonzalez M, Topham DJ, Baumgarth N, Doherty PC. An early CD4 +T cell–dependent immunoglobulin A response to influenza infection in the absence of key cognate T–B interactions. J Exp Med. 2003;198:1011–21.
21. Braciale TJ, Sun J, Kim TS. Regulating the adaptive immune response to respiratory virus infection. Nat Rev Immunol. 2012;12:295–305.
22. Sridhar S, Begom S, Bermingham A, et al. Cellular immune correlates of protection against symptomatic pandemic influenza. Nat Med. 2013;19:1305–12.
23. Dunning J, Blankley S, Hoang LT, et al. Progression of whole-blood transcriptional signatures from interferon-induced to neutrophil-associated patterns in severe influenza. Nat Immunol. 2018;19:625–35.
24. Guan W, Yang Z, Wu NC, et al. Clinical correlations of transcriptional profile in patients infected with avian influenza H7N9 virus. J Infect Dis. 2018;368:1888–11.
25. Korteweg C, Gu J. Pathology, molecular biology, and pathogenesis of avian influenza A (H5N1) infection in humans. Am J Pathol. 2008;172:1155–69.
26. Likos AM, Kelvin DJ, Cameron CM, et al. Influenza viremia and the potential for blood-borne transmission. Transfusion. 2007;47:1080–8.

27. Choi SM, Xie H, Campbell AP, et al. Influenza viral RNA detection in blood as a marker to predict disease severity in hematopoietic cell transplant recipients. J Infect Dis. 2012;206:1872–7.
28. Short KR, Brooks AG, Reading PC, Londrigan SL. The fate of influenza A virus after infection of human macrophages and dendritic cells. J Gen Virol. 2012;93:2315–25.
29. Hou W, Gibbs JS, Lu X, et al. Viral infection triggers rapid differentiation of human blood monocytes into dendritic cells. Blood. 2012;119:3128–31.
30. Hoeve MA, Nash AA, Jackson D, Randall RE, Dransfield I. Influenza virus A infection of human monocyte and macrophage subpopulations reveals increased susceptibility associated with cell differentiation. PLoS One. 2012;7:e29443.
31. Steuerman Y, Cohen M, Peshes-Yaloz N, et al. Dissection of influenza infection vivo by single-cell RNA sequencing. Cell Syst. 2018;7:1–13.
32. Fislova T, Gocnik M, Sladkova T, et al. Multiorgan distribution of human influenza A virus strains observed in a mouse model. Arch Virol. 2009;154:409–19.
33. Zhang Z, Huang T, Yu F, et al. Infectious progeny of 2009 A (H1N1) influenza virus replicated in and released from human neutrophils. Sci Rep. 2015;5:1–11.

Multidrug Resistant Gram-Negative Bacteria in Community-Acquired Pneumonia

36

C. Cillóniz, C. Dominedò, and A. Torres

36.1 Introduction: Why Is This Topic Important?

Community-acquired pneumonia (CAP) is associated with high morbidity and mortality worldwide [1]. Although several different bacteria and respiratory viruses can be responsible for CAP, *Streptococcus pneumoniae* (pneumococcus) remains the most common causative pathogen. A small proportion of CAP cases are caused by Gram-negative bacteria, especially *Pseudomonas aeruginosa*, *Klebsiella pneumoniae*, *Acinetobacter baumannii* and *Stenotrophomona maltophilia* [2, 3]. The main problem concerning the treatment of Gram-negative bacterial infections is their related antibiotic resistance, reported as multidrug resistant (MDR = resistant to at least one agent in three or more groups of antibiotics), extensively drug resistant (XDR = resistant to at least one agent in all but two or fewer groups of antibiotics) and pan-drug resistant (PDR = resistant to all groups of antibiotics) [4]. This makes the clinical management of pneumonia caused by such pathogens a challenge for physicians. Taking into account the clinical severity that may be associated with CAP caused by Gram-negative bacteria (respiratory failure, bacteremia, shock, acute respiratory distress syndrome [ARDS]) the magnitude of the global health problem is tremendous.

C. Cillóniz · A. Torres (✉)
Department of Pneumology, Hospital Clinic of Barcelona, Barcelona, Spain

August Pi i Sunyer Biomedical Research Institute (IDIBAPS), Barcelona, Spain

University of Barcelona, Barcelona, Spain

Biomedical Research Networking Centres in Respiratory Diseases (CIBERES), Barcelona, Spain
e-mail: atorres@clinic.cat

C. Dominedò
Department of Anesthesiology and Intensive Care Medicine, Fondazione Policlinico Universitario A. Gemelli, Università Cattolica del Sacro Cuore, Rome, Italy

J.-L. Vincent (ed.), *Annual Update in Intensive Care and Emergency Medicine 2019*, Annual Update in Intensive Care and Emergency Medicine,
https://doi.org/10.1007/978-3-030-06067-1_36

We are currently living through an antibiotic resistance crisis, mainly because antibiotics tend to lose their efficacy over time due to the emergence and dissemination of resistance among bacterial pathogens, principally caused by the overuse and inappropriate use of antibiotics, as well as the extensive use of antibiotics in agriculture and the food industry. The Global Point Prevalence Survey (Global-PPS), an international network set up to measure antimicrobial prescription and resistance in the hospital setting, recently published its findings [5]. Pneumonia was the most common illness to receive antibiotic therapy worldwide, accounting for 19% of patients treated. The most frequently prescribed antibiotics for community-acquired infections were penicillins with a β-lactamase inhibitor (29%); amoxicillin with a β-lactamase inhibitor accounted for 16% and piperacillin with a β-lactamase inhibitor accounted for 8%. Third-generation cephalosporins were the second most commonly prescribed antibiotics for community-acquired infections (mainly ceftriaxone, 16%), followed by fluoroquinolones (14%).

Antibiotic resistance is a natural phenomenon in bacteria that cannot be stopped; however various measures can be taken in order to reduce the rate of its development and devise more effective strategies to control its spread [6].

Because CAP caused by MDR Gram-negative bacteria is an important clinical concern, we review the main findings concerning the epidemiology, diagnosis and clinical impact of CAP.

36.2 CAP Caused by *Pseudomonas aeruginosa*

36.2.1 The Pathogen: Why Is It Difficult to Treat?

P. aeruginosa is an opportunistic Gram-negative, non-fermentative bacterium that inhabits the soil and surfaces in aqueous environments. Its high intrinsic antibiotic resistance, broad metabolic versatility and adaptability make it especially difficult to treat. Several studies have shown that the physical characteristics (phenotype) of *P. aeruginosa* isolates vary between those derived from chronic infections, such as cystic fibrosis, and those from acute infections, such as pneumonia [7]. Common chromosomal mutations in the mucA gene can convert a non-mucous phenotype into a mucous phenotype. The adaptation of *P. aeruginosa,* which includes complex physiological changes, confers a selective advantage since it can better survive in different habitats [8].

P. aeruginosa has intrinsic, adaptive and acquired mechanisms of resistance, the main ones including the presence of β-lactamases, alterations in membrane permeability due to the presence of ejection pumps, and mutations of transmembrane porins. Furthermore, the capacity to form biofilms (intricate, highly organized bacterial communities, embedded in a matrix composed of exopolysaccharides, DNA and proteins that is attached to a surface and hinders antimicrobial action) favors the persistence of *P. aeruginosa* and makes it more difficult to treat, due to the inherent protection that biofilms provide [8] (Table 36.1).

Table 36.1 Main resistance mechanisms in Gram-negative pathogens

Microorganism	Mechanism
Pseudomonas aeruginosa	Efflux pumps
	Mutant topoisomerases
	Modifying enzymes
	AmpC/porin reduction combinations
	Metallo-b-lactamases
	Outer membrane permeability
	Extended spectrum β-lactamases
Acinetobacter baumannii	β-lactamases
	Efflux pumps
	Membrane permeability
	Aminoglycoside-modifying enzymes
	Alteration of target sites
Klebsiella pneumoniae	Modifying enzyme
	Efflux pumps
	Mutant topoisomerases
	Extended spectrum β-lactamases
	Carbapenemases
Stenotrophomonas maltophilia	β-lactamases (L1 and L2)
	Multidrug efflux pumps
	Antibiotic-modifying enzymes
	Mutations of bacterial topoisomerase and gyrase genes
	Reduction in outer membrane permeability

A large number of intrinsic *P. aeruginosa* virulence factors are required to establish infection [7]. Moreover, the differential presence or expression of some of these virulence factors may determine major inter-strain variability in virulence and thus potentially have a major impact on disease severity and mortality [8].

In conclusion, the pathogenesis of *P. aeruginosa* CAP is very complex, in addition to the broad antimicrobial resistance that limits antibiotic therapy; the virulence of *P. aeruginosa* is certainly a major driver of pneumonia severity and outcome, as well as the different phenotypes described. The capacity to form biofilms provides the bacteria with a further possibility to escape the effects of antibiotics, turning it into a superbug.

36.2.2 Prevalence: What Is the Prevalence?

The reported prevalence of CAP caused by *P. aeruginosa* is controversial, largely due to data being limited to single-center studies and because of differences in the study populations [9] (Table 36.2). Recently, a multinational point-prevalence study analyzed data from 3193 CAP patients in 222 hospitals in 54 countries [10]. The study showed a low prevalence of CAP caused by *P. aeruginosa* (4.2%), which corresponded to only 11.3% of patients with culture-positive pneumonia. The prevalences of antibiotic-resistant and MDR *P. aeruginosa* were also low (2% and 1% respectively). Interestingly, the study reported the prevalence of *P. aeruginosa* in CAP in different continents: 3.8% in Europe, 4.3% in North America, 5.2% in Asia,

Table 36.2 Incidence and risk factors for *Pseudomonas aeruginosa* community-acquired pneumonia (CAP)

Study/year	Population/Country	Prevalence of *P. aeruginosa*	Risk factors for *P. aeruginosa* CAP
Aliberti et al. 2013 [2]	Prospective study of two cohorts (Barcelona and Edinburgh) n = 1591 CAP patients	Barcelona: 6.5% (32 cases) of these 12 cases (38%) were MDR *P. aeruginosa* Edinburgh: 1.6% (9 cases) of these 3 cases (30%) were MDR *P. aeruginosa*	Nursing home; hospitalization in the previous 90 days; history of chronic lung disease
Shindo et al. 2013 [51]	Prospective study of CAP and HCAP cases from Japan n = 1431	CAP 3.7% (33 cases) HCAP 8.7% (46 cases)	
Prina et al. 2015 [50]	Prospective study of CAP from Spain n = 1597	4.5% *P. aeruginosa*	Previous antibiotic use, chronic respiratory diseases, PO_2/FiO_2 ratio <200
Cillóniz et al. 2016 [11]	Prospective study of adult patients with CAP with definitive etiology n = 2023	4% *P. aeruginosa* 1.08% MDR *P. aeruginosa*	Male sex, chronic respiratory diseases, C-reactive protein <12.35 mg/dL, PSI IV to V Prior antibiotic treatment risk factor for MDR *P. aeruginosa*
Restrepo et al. 2018 [10]	Multicenter, point-prevalence study of CAP patients (22 hospitals in 54 countries) n = 3193	4.2% of all population 11.3% of cases with defined etiology 2% antibiotic-resistant *P. aeruginosa* 1% MDR *P. aeruginosa*	Prior pseudomonas infection/colonization, prior tracheostomy, bronchiectasis, IRVS, very severe COPD

HCAP healthcare-associated pneumonia; *IRVS* intensive respiratory or vasopressor support; *PSI* pneumonia severity index; *COPD*: chronic obstructive pulmonary disease

4.9% in South America, 5.5% in Africa and 3.1% in Oceania. The prevalence of antibiotic-resistant *P. aeruginosa* in CAP was 1.6% in Europe, 2.5% in North America, 2.2% in Asia, 3.0% in South America, and 3.9% in Africa; there were no reported cases of *P. aeruginosa* antibiotic resistance in Oceania. Finally, the prevalence of MDR *P. aeruginosa* in CAP was 0.9% in Europe, 1.2% in North America, 0.5% in Asia, 2% in South America, and 2.3% in Africa; there were no cases of MDR *P. aeruginosa* in Oceania.

Similarly, a Spanish study of clinical outcomes and risk factors for CAP caused by MDR and non-MDR *P. aeruginosa* reported a prevalence of MDR *P. aeruginosa* of 1.1% in a prospective cohort study of 2023 culture-positive CAP patients [11]. The authors also reported that *P. aeruginosa* was an individual risk factor associated with mortality in the study population.

A study by Ferrer et al. [12] of 664 severe CAP cases requiring mechanical ventilation showed that 336 patients had a final microbiological diagnosis; *P. aeruginosa* was reported in 7% (n = 25) of cases (4% in the non-invasive mechanical ventilation group and 5% in the invasive mechanical ventilation group).

36.2.3 *P. aeruginosa* Risk Factors

Antibiotic therapy for *P. aeruginosa* is totally different from the standard antimicrobial therapy used to treat common CAP pathogens. Current recommendations provided by international guidelines stratify therapy on the basis of *Pseudomonas* risk factors [1, 13].

Risk factors for *P. aeruginosa* include structural lung disease (bronchiectasis, chronic obstructive pulmonary disease [COPD]), nursing home residence, C-reactive protein (CRP) <12.35 mg/dL, prior use of oral steroids, antibiotic therapy within the previous 90 days, and malnutrition [1, 11]. Chronic *P. aeruginosa* colonization in patients with bronchiectasis and COPD can be an important preliminary step to pneumonia. Non-cystic fibrosis bronchiectasis and COPD account for 2–55% and for 20–46% of CAP cases, respectively. These two structural lung conditions facilitate chronic colonization by *P. aeruginosa*, mainly due to failure to eradicate the bacterium during acute infections. As mentioned earlier, *P. aeruginosa* can transform from a non-mucous phenotype to a mucous phenotype which can then adapt to the lung environment and grow as a biofilm.

Interestingly, a recent case-control study [14] identified risk factors for pneumonia due to *P. aeruginosa* susceptible to all routinely tested antipseudomonal β-lactams (APBL-S) and resistant to at least one antipseudomonal β-lactam (APBL-R). The authors identified bronchiectasis, interstitial lung disease, prior airway colonization with *P. aeruginosa* and recent exposure to an antipseudomonal β-lactam as risk factors for APBL-S P. *aeruginosa* in adults with acute bacterial pneumonia.

In the last few years, cases of *P. aeruginosa* infection in previously healthy individuals have been reported; in the majority, heavy exposure to aerosols of contaminated water has been identified [15].

P. aeruginosa can establish polymicrobial interactions, mainly with *Staphylococcus aureus* and *Candida albicans* that may affect disease management. The relationship between *S. aureus* and *P. aeruginosa* is competitive in nature. The association of *C. albicans* with *P. aeruginosa* or *S. aureus* enhances disease severity in several ways. *In vivo* studies in rats have shown that pre-colonization of lung tissue by *C. albicans* increases the rate of pneumonia caused by *P. aeruginosa.* This microbial interaction should be taken into account in patients with COPD or non-cystic fibrosis bronchiectasis who are frequently colonized with *P. aeruginosa* and *S. aureus* [16].

According to a recent study, prior antibiotic treatment is a risk factor for *P. aeruginosa*, especially for MDR *P. aeruginosa* [11]. It has been demonstrated that low levels of antibiotics contribute to strain diversification in *P. aeruginosa*; sub-inhibitory and sub-therapeutic antibiotic concentrations induce alterations that effect changes in gene expression, horizontal gene transfer and mutagenesis, which can promote and spread antibiotic resistance.

Given that *P. aeruginosa* CAP has been related to poor clinical outcomes, largely because of inappropriate empiric antibiotic treatment, it is recommended to use empiric anti-pseudomonal cover in all cases of highly suspected MDR *P. aeruginosa* CAP. Risk stratification should take into account the local ecology (prevalence of the pathogen in a specific area) and the patient's risk factors, especially in cases of severe CAP that are associated with higher mortality rates (20–50%) [1].

36.3 CAP Caused by *Acinetobacter baumanii*

36.3.1 The Pathogen: How Important Is *A. baumanii* In CAP?

A. baumannii is an aerobic Gram-negative coccobacillus. In 2017, the World Health Organization (WHO) included it in the list of "Priority Pathogens", a group of bacteria that poses the greatest threat to human health and for which new antibiotics are urgently needed [17].

In recent years, isolates of *A. baumannii* have been recovered from multiple extra-hospital sources, such as vegetables, water treatment plants, fish and shrimp farms, apart from its known natural habitat (soil and humid environments). This broad source of the bacteria may explain the occurrence of community-acquired infections [18].

A. baumannii has a natural resistance to desiccation due to morphological changes that justify its viability for months. Infections caused by *A. baumannii* may be very difficult to treat due to the ability of the bacterium to evade the host immunity and to form biofilm. Furthermore, *A. baumannii* has several resistance mechanisms, including β-lactamases, multidrug efflux pumps, aminoglycoside-modifying enzymes, permeability defects and modifications of target sites [19] (Table 36.1).

The majority of *A. baumannii* isolates from CAP have a lower antibiotic resistance than isolates from nosocomial infections. Despite this lower rate of antibiotic resistance, severe CAP is the most frequent clinical presentation of *A. baumannii* pneumonia. Caution should be taken when choosing the empirical antibiotic therapy. Although use of a ß-lactam plus a macrolide or a fluoroquinolone is the current international guideline recommendation for severe CAP [1], these drug combinations do not completely cover *A. baumannii*, mostly because of its frequent resistance to ceftriaxone [20].

Several studies have reported isolates of MDR *A. baumannii* in community-dwelling patients and in nursing-home patients. Recently, a prospective cohort study of 651 newly admitted patients in six nursing facilities in the USA reported that 95% of patients were admitted for post-acute care; 57% of patients were colonized with MDR pathogens at enrollment. Prolonged hospitalization (>14 days), functional disability, antibiotic use, or device use were the main risk factors for colonization at enrollment. The rate per 1000 patient-days of acquiring a new resistant Gram-negative bacillus was 13.6%. MDR colonization at discharge for resistant Gram-negative bacilli was 34% [21].

In a study from west China [22], investigating the antimicrobial susceptibility of 32 isolates of *A. baumannii* causing CAP, the authors reported that 30% of the isolates were resistant to the majority of the antibiotics; the resistant rates to imipenem and meropenem were 19% and 9%, respectively. An important finding of this study is that approximately 80% of the patients had had a previous hospital admission.

An MDR *A. baumannii* was recently isolated in a previously healthy patient with CAP from Hong Kong. The patient was treated with intravenous colistin and oral monocycline and recovered fully [23]. This case is not isolated and more and more reports of cases of CAP caused by MDR *A. baumannii* are being published.

In conclusion, although *A. baumannii* is not a frequent cause of CAP, the capacity to rapidly develop resistance mechanisms to antibiotics and the fulminant clinical presentation (with a mortality rate around 50%) make this pathogen an important health problem, especially in tropical and subtropical areas.

36.3.2 Prevalence: What Is the Prevalence?

During the last 10 years, *A. baumannii* has been described as a rare cause of CAP but with clinical relevance. The great majority of CAP cases caused by *A. baumannii* occurs in countries with tropical or sub-tropical climates. *A. baumannii* is an emerging pathogen in the regions of Asia-Pacific, with a higher prevalence in Hong Kong, Singapore, Taiwan, South Korea and Australia [24, 25].

CAP cases caused by *A. baumannii* are very rare in Europe and USA. A recent USA case report of severe CAP and review of the literature found that 19 cases of CAP caused by *A. baumannii* have been reported in the USA to date [26].

Unlike nosocomial pneumonia caused by *A. baumannii,* CAP cases caused by *A. baumannii* have a seasonal presentation, with the highest prevalence during the warm and humid months of the year [25].

36.3.3 *A. baumannii* Risk Factors

The clinical presentation of *A. baumannii* CAP is fulminant with acute onset of fever, dyspnea and rapid progression to respiratory failure and shock. *A. baumannii* CAP is associated with a mortality rate ranging from 40% to 60% especially in cases presenting with bacteremia and shock. The main risk factors related to this infection are alcoholism, diabetes mellitus and chronic lung disease [24].

It is known that alcohol abuse impacts on the innate and adaptive immune response. A study published in 2013 described the impact of alcohol on macrophage-like cell antimicrobial functions in *A. baumannii* infections [27]. The authors demonstrated that alcohol plays an important role in inhibiting nitric oxide (NO) production which is essential to eradicate bacteria exposed to macrophages after phagocytosis. Alteration of intra- and extra-cellular NO production promotes microbial survival, facilitating intracellular replication. Furthermore, macrophages exposed to alcohol have lower production of pro-inflammatory tumor necrosis factor (TNF)-α, interleukin (IL)-1β, and IL-12 and increased levels of IL-6. This imbalance in the production of cytokines affects the differentiation of naïve T cells into Th1 cells because of low IL-12 production, and the production of interferon (IFN)-γ from T and natural killer (NK) cells. Moreover, it is known that low levels of TNF-α and IL-1β are associated with septic shock and the risk of bacterial infections [27].

A related study recently published by Kamoshida et al. [28] described for the first time the ability of *A. baumannii* to inhibit the formation of neutrophil extracellular traps (NETs), thus suppressing neutrophil adhesion. It is well known that the main role of NETs is to prevent microbial dissemination and to eradicate pathogens. The ability of *A. baumannii* to escape the immune response may explain the fulminant clinical presentation of CAP caused by this pathogen.

An Australian study suggested that microaspiration of pharyngeal *A. baumannii* may be responsible for CAP in alcoholic patients [29]. In this study, 10% of community residents attending the Emergency Department in the wet-season (March–April) with non-respiratory diseases, no episode of previous hospitalization and a history of alcohol abuse (alcohol intake >6 standard drinks/day) had *A. baumannii* in their throat [29].

The susceptibility to pneumonia in patients with diabetes can be ascribed to several factors. Patients with diabetes have an increased risk of hyperglycemia (which reduces the mobilization of polymorphonuclear leukocytes, chemotaxis and phagocytic activity), increased risk of aspiration, impaired immunological defenses, and deterioration in lung function and chronic complications, such as neuropathy [30].

Patients with underlying chronic lung disease, such as COPD or bronchiectasis, also show reduced innate defense mechanisms. Generally, these patients are smokers, passive smokers or ex-smokers and the frequent use of inhaled corticosteroids make them more vulnerable to infections such as pneumonia [10, 11, 27].

In conclusion, because of its possible fulminating course, CAP caused by *A. baumannii* should be suspected in patients with specific risk factors and a severe presentation of pneumonia. Early recognition and prompt initiation of broad empirical antibiotic coverage are mandatory to limit the high mortality related to this infection.

36.4 CAP Caused by *Klebsiella pneumoniae*

36.4.1 The Pathogen: What Is So Special About *K. pneumoniae* in CAP?

K. pneumoniae is a Gram-negative capsulate bacterium responsible for severe pneumonia especially in immunocompromised patients. In the last two decades, there has been an increase in antibiotic resistance in *K. pneumoniae* isolates globally. The emergency of MDR and hypervirulent *K. pneumoniae* strains has been reported in immunocompromised patients and in healthy persons [31].

The main mechanisms of antibiotic resistance in *K. pneumoniae* are the expression of extended spectrum β-lactamases (ESBLs), which confers resistance against penicillins, cephalosprins and monobactams, and the expression of carbapenemases, which confers resistance against all β-lactams including carbapenems (Table 36.1).

Interestingly, hypervirulent *K. pneumoniae* strains produce a hypercapsule, also known as being hypermucoviscous. The capsule, a polysaccharide matrix that coats the cell, is necessary for *K. pneumoniae* virulence and is arguably the most thoroughly studied virulence factor of *K. pneumoniae* [31]. Although antimicrobial resistance in hypervirulent *K. pneumoniae* is generally lower than in non-hypervirulent *K. pneumoniae* strains, cases with more resistant strains of hypervirulent *K. pneumoniae* have recently been reported [32].

K. pneumoniae has the ability to avoid phagocytosis. A recent experimental study found that the capsule is dispensable for intracellular *Klebsiella* survival if bacteria are not opsonized. *K. pneumoniae* survives the killing by macrophages by manipulating phagosome maturation, which may contribute to *Klebsiella* pathogenesis [33].

In conclusion, CAP caused by MDR and hypervirulent *K. pneumoniae* represents a great challenge in terms of treatment and management, especially in Asian countries, where the majority of cases are reported.

36.4.2 Prevalence: What Is the Prevalence?

A recent 5-year study in a French ICU [34] described 59 infections caused by *K. pneumoniae*; 26 (44%) of them were community-onset infections. Interestingly, the authors reported 12 hypervirulent *K. pneumoniae* strains in the group of community-onset infections, 6 (50%) of which were isolated from patients with CAP. The authors observed that hypervirulent *K. pneumoniae* cases had higher rates of organ failure compared with non-hypervirulent cases. However, mortality rates were similar in the two groups.

In a study performed in Cambodia [35], 2315 patients with acute lower respiratory infections were enrolled, including 587 (25%) whose bacterial etiology could be assigned. *K. pneumoniae* was identified in 8% (n = 47) of the microbiologically-confirmed cases. ESBL-producing strains were found in 8 (17%) patients. The main risk factors related to *K. pneumoniae* infection were female sex and diabetes mellitus. The overall mortality rate due to *K. pneumoniae* infection was 38%.

Approximately 1–7% of cases of CAP are caused by *K. pneumoniae*, with 5–36% of these being MDR strains [2, 36]. Interestingly, in Asian countries (Taiwan, Cambodia, Shanghai) *K. pneumoniae* is described as a frequent pathogen causing bacteremia [37, 38]. Although reports of cases from Europe and USA are generally rare, an increasing incidence from these regions has been registered in recent years [34, 39].

36.4.3 *K. pneumoniae* Risk Factors

The recognized risk factors for K. pneumoniae CAP are female sex, diabetes mellitus and alcoholism. MDR *K. pneumoniae* can be recognized as a virulent pathogen causing severe CAP, frequently associated with septic shock, respiratory failure and bacteremia. Morbidity and mortality rates are high especially in Asian countries were the pathogen is reported in younger patients with no chronic conditions. This pattern may be explained by the virulence of the strains (especially hypervirulent *K. pneumoniae*) and the high rate of antibiotic consumption in these regions [35, 40].

36.5 CAP Caused by *Stenotrophomonas maltophilia*

36.5.1 The Pathogen: What Is So Special About *S. maltophilia* in CAP?

S. maltophilia is a motile, aerobic, non-fermentative Gram-negative bacillus with the ability to survive on any humid surface, form biofilm and colonize humid surfaces. It is an emerging opportunistic pathogen with multidrug resistance, which particularly affects immunocompromised patients (i.e., with malignances, post-organ transplantation) worldwide [41, 42].

S. maltophilia is intrinsically resistant to carbapenems and frequently carries genetic elements that provide resistance to other β-lactams, fluoroquinolones, aminoglycosides and tetracyclines. *S. maltophilia* has the ability to acquire genes involved in antibiotic resistance from other bacterial species. The most relevant mechanisms of antibiotic resistance include β-lactamase (L1 and L2) production, multidrug efflux pumps (which confer resistance to macrolides, quinolones, aminoglucosydes, polymyxins), antibiotic-modifying enzymes, mutations of bacterial topoisomerase and gyrase genes and reduction in outer membrane permeability [42] (Table 36.1).

Although *S. maltophilia* has been reported in patients with cystic fibrosis, it can affect healthy individuals through contaminated wounds or infected catheters [43, 44]. Transmission of *S. maltophilia* may occur through direct contact with contaminated source such as contaminated water or medical devices [42].

In conclusion, CAP caused by *S. maltophilia* is associated with high mortality rates. Hemorrhagic pneumonia is one of the most severe forms of *S. maltophilia* infection [45]. It is associated with poor outcome despite appropriate antibiotic therapy.

36.5.2 Prevalence: What Is the Prevalence?

There is limited information on the worldwide prevalence of community-acquired *S. maltophilia* pneumonia. The majority of data comes from case reports [46]. *S. maltophilia* has been reported as an important cause of CAP in patients with hematologic diseases, with a prevalence of bacteremia ranging between 2% and 7%. The mortality rate is approximately 35% (ranging between 30% and 40%) in this special population.

36.5.3 *S. maltophilia* Risk Factors

The majority of patients affected by this pathogen have previous chronic comorbidities, such as COPD, cystic fibrosis, malignancy (especially hematologic diseases), human immunodeficiency virus (HIV)-infection (acquired immunodeficiency syndrome [AIDS]) or other immunodeficiencies. Patients with prior antimicrobial therapy, prolonged hospitalization, indwelling catheters, mechanically ventilated and receiving corticosteroids have an increased risk of *S. maltophilia* CAP [42, 46].

36.6 Diagnosis: Is It Possible to Predict Gram-Negative MDR Pathogens in CAP?

The reference microbiological diagnostic tools for bacteria causing respiratory tract infections remain the Gram stain and semi-quantitative conventional cultures from direct respiratory samples. Bacterial identification is currently based on matrix-assisted latex laser desorption/ionization time-of-flight mass spectrometry (MALDI-TOF MS) and susceptibility testing. As a consequence of the time needed for microbiological diagnosis, many patients initially receive inappropriate antibiotic treatment, which may increase morbidity and mortality.

Molecular techniques based on multiplex PCR have also been developed in recent years in order to simultaneously identify and quantify multiple respiratory pathogens from different types of samples in a single procedure [47]. However, the main challenge for the rapid diagnosis of respiratory infections is the early detection of the antibiotic resistance profile of the various bacteria. The biggest obstacle in the use of molecular techniques for detecting resistance is the discrepancy between genotype and phenotype, the continuous discovery of new resistance mechanisms and, as a result, the potential presence of unknown mechanisms, which may lead to false negative results using molecular techniques [47].

Recognizing patients at risk of colonization with MDR Gram-negative bacteria, such as patients with bronchiectasis or COPD (frequently colonized by *P. aeruginosa*), is essential, since several studies have reported the association between previous colonization and risk of pneumonia [48, 49].

Currently, there is no specific score to predict MDR Gram-negative pathogens in CAP. However, several scoring systems have been proposed to identify patients with risk factors for developing CAP caused by MDR pathogens. The Aliberti score [2] takes into account different variables and gives a specific score to each of them: chronic renal failure (5 points), prior hospitalization (4 points), nursing home residence (3 points) and other variables (0.5 points each). CAP patients with an Aliberti score ≥3 points have a reported prevalence of MDR of 38%, whereas CAP patients with an Aliberti score of ≤0.5 have a reported prevalence of MDR of 8%. The PES (*P. aeruginosa*, Enterobacteriaceae ESBL-positive, methicillin-resistant *S. aureus* [MRSA]) score includes 1 point each for age 40–65 years and male sex; 2 points each for age >65 years, previous antibiotic use, chronic respiratory disorder, and impaired consciousness; 3 points for chronic renal failure; and minus 1 point if fever is present initially. The risk of MDR pathogens is higher with 5 points or more [50]. Unfortunately, studies validating the Aliberti and PES score do not include immunocompromised patients. The ability of these scores to identify risk factors for CAP by MDR pathogens in this population is still unclear.

An important study by Shindo et al. [51] investigated the main risk factors for MDR pathogens in 1413 patients with CAP. Six risk factors were identified: prior hospitalization, immunosuppression, previous antibiotic use, use of gastric acid-suppressive agents, tube feeding and non-ambulatory status. Unlike the Aliberti and PES studies, Shindo's study included immunocompromised patients. Interestingly, the authors analyzed risk factors for Gram-positive (MRSA) and Gram-negative pathogens separately. The authors observed that the risk of MDR Gram-negative pathogens did not increase in the presence of ≥3 risk factors; conversely, for Gram-positive (MRSA) pathogens, the risk increased in the presence of ≥2 risk factors, especially if one of the risk factors was specific for MRSA, such as previous colonization or previous hospitalization.

36.7 Therapy: How is it Possible to Treat These Pathogens?

Since antibiotic treatment for *P. aeruginosa* is completely different from standard therapy to cover the most common pathogens in CAP, current international guidelines for severe CAP stratify therapy recommendations on the basis of *P. aeruginosa* risk factors [1]. MDR *P. aeruginosa* should be covered only in cases that are strongly suspected because of concurrent risk factors. It is important to underline that prior antibiotic therapy has been reported as the only risk factor for MDR *P. aeruginosa* in CAP patients [11].

Empirical antibiotic treatment based on the evaluation of the patient's risk factors is also of pivotal importance in the management of *A. baumannii* CAP.

Because CAP caused by *A. baumannii* has a fulminant clinical presentation with a high mortality rate (approximately 50%), greater attention should be paid in elderly patients with multi-comorbidities, and patients with alcohol abuse, chronic lung disease and prior antibiotic therapy, especially in Asian countries where this pathogen is frequently reported. Early appropriate antimicrobial therapy is critical. Recommended empirical antibiotic therapy for *A. baumannii* CAP includes anti-pseudomonal penicillins, aminoglycoside, ciprofloxacin, and imipenem. Tigecycline, colistin, ceftazidime, doxycycline, minocycline, piperacillin/tazobactam, tobramycin, rifampin, fosfomycin and levofloxacin are active against variable percentages of strains. The treatment should include an association of two or more of these antibiotics according to the antibiogram of the isolated pathogen. Moreover some countries, notably Asia [52] and Australia [53], have implemented specific antibiotic recommendations in cases of severe CAP in order to cover pathogens such as *A. baumannii*.

In CAP caused by *K. pneumoniae*, depending on the clinical severity and the risk of infection by a strain with resistance mechanisms (production of ESBLs, cefaminases or carbapenemases), a 3rd generation cephalosporin (cefotaxime or ceftriaxone) or a fluoroquinolone (ciprofloxacin or levofloxacin) should be used. Another possibility, in case of infection by carbapenemase-producing or carbapenem-resistant strains (due to loss of porin and hyperproduction of Amp-C), is the use of associations of two or three of the following antibiotics: colistin, tigecycline, fosfomycin (if the strain is sensitive), an aminoglycoside (amikacin or gentamicin) and meropenem (if the minimum inhibitory concentration [MIC] = 16 mg/L), administered in high doses and by continuous perfusion. Hypervirulent strains (serotypes K1 and K2) are usually more sensitive to antibiotics, but production of *K. pneumoniae*-type carbapenemase has also been observed.

For the antibiotic treatment of *S. maltophilia* pneumonia, trimethoprim-sulfamethoxazole (TMP-SMX) is still considered the drug of choice despite increasing resistance. It is preferably used in association with another antibiotic depending on the severity of the pneumonia and the sensitivity of the pathogen. Other alternative antibiotics include β-lactams (i.e., ceftazidime), fluoroquinolones (i.e., levofloxacin, moxifloxacin), minocycline or tigecycline. *In vitro*, the following associations are often synergistic: cotrimoxazole with colistin, tigecycline, ceftazidime and rifampicin; colistin with tigecycline, ceftazidime and rifampin; ceftazidime with levofloxacin, moxifloxacin and aztreonam.

Figure 36.1 proposes an algorithm for the empiric antibiotic therapy of CAP in patients with risks factors for MDR pathogens.

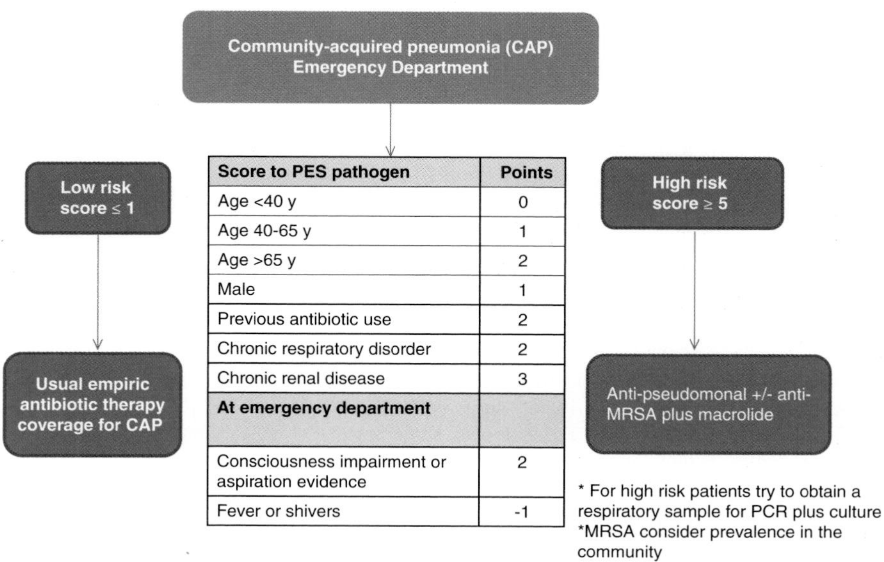

Fig. 36.1 Proposed algorithm for empiric antibiotic therapy in community-acquired pneumonia for patients with risk of multidrug resistant (MDR) pathogens using the PES (*Pseudomonas aeruginosa*, Enterobacteriaceae extended-spectrum β-lactamase-positive, methicillin-resistant *Staphylococcus aureus* [MRSA]) score from [50]. *PCR* polymerase chain reaction

36.8 Conclusion

Correct identification of CAP patients suspected of being infected with MDR Gram-negative pathogens is crucial. Specific risk factors, local ecology and resistance patterns should always be considered in order to determine the adequate empirical antibiotic therapy. Early hemodynamic and respiratory support is critical in these patients since the majority of cases of pneumonia may become fulminant systemic disease with both respiratory failure and multiple organ dysfunction.

The collaboration of a multidisciplinary team (critical care specialists, pneumologist, infectious disease specialists, microbiologists) improves management of the most severe cases. The role of the microbiology laboratory, in particular, is of pivotal importance to determine the antimicrobial susceptibility pattern of the pathogen causing CAP, so that appropriate antibiotic therapy can be initiated as soon as possible, avoiding excessive use of broad spectrum antimicrobials, which increase the selection of resistant pathogens.

Acknowledgement Dr Cillóniz is the recipient of a Postdoctoral Grant (Strategic plan for research and innovation in health-PERIS 2016-2020).

References

1. Mandell LA, Wunderink RG, Anzueto A, et al. Infectious Diseases Society of America/ American Thoracic Society consensus guidelines on the management of community-acquired pneumonia in adults. Clin Infect Dis. 2007;44(Suppl 2):S27–72.
2. Aliberti S, Cilloniz C, Chalmers JD, et al. Multidrug-resistant pathogens in hospitalised patients coming from the community with pneumonia: a European perspective. Thorax. 2013;68:997–9.
3. Cillóniz C, Ewig S, Polverino E, et al. Microbial aetiology of community-acquired pneumonia and its relation to severity. Thorax. 2011;66:340–6.
4. Magiorakos A-P, Srinivasan A, Carey RB, et al. Multidrug-resistant, extensively drug-resistant and pandrug-resistant bacteria: an international expert proposal for interim standard definitions for acquired resistance. Clin Microbiol Infect. 2012;18:268–81.
5. Versporten A, Zarb P, Caniaux I, et al. Antimicrobial consumption and resistance in adult hospital inpatients in 53 countries: results of an internet-based global point prevalence survey. Lancet Glob Health. 2018;6:e619–29.
6. European Antimicrobial Resistance Surveillance Network. Surveillance of antimicrobial resistance in Europe 2016. 2016. Available at: https://ecdc.europa.eu/sites/portal/files/documents/AMR-surveillance-Europe-2016.pdf. Accessed 19 Nov 2018.
7. Gellatly SL, Hancock REW. Pseudomonas aeruginosa: new insights into pathogenesis and host defenses. Pathog Dis. 2013;67:159–73.
8. Crousilles A, Maunders E, Bartlett S, et al. Which microbial factors really are important in Pseudomonas aeruginosa infections? Future Microbiol. 2015;10:1825–36.
9. von Baum H, Welte T, Marre R, et al. Community-acquired pneumonia through Enterobacteriaceae and Pseudomonas aeruginosa: diagnosis, incidence and predictors. Eur Respir J. 2010;35:598–605.
10. Restrepo MI, Babu BL, Reyes LF, et al. Burden and risk factors for pseudomonas aeruginosa community-acquired pneumonia: a multinational point prevalence study of hospitalised patients. Eur Respir J. 2018;52:1709910.

11. Cillóniz C, Gabarrús A, Ferrer M, et al. Community-acquired pneumonia due to multidrug and non-multidrug resistant Pseudomonas aeruginosa. Chest. 2016;150:415–25.
12. Ferrer M, Travierso C, Cilloniz C, et al. Severe community-acquired pneumonia: characteristics and prognostic factors in ventilated and non-ventilated patients. PLoS One. 2018;13:e0191721.
13. Lim WS, Baudouin SV, George RC, et al. BTS guidelines for the management of community acquired pneumonia in adults: update 2009. Thorax. 2009;64(Suppl 3):iii1–55.
14. Al-Jaghbeer MJ, Justo JA, Owens W, et al. Risk factors for pneumonia due to beta-lactam-susceptible and beta-lactam-resistant Pseudomonas aeruginosa: a case-case-control study. Infection. 2018. May 11, https://doi.org/10.1007/s15010-018-1147-z [Epub ahead of print]
15. John TJ, Lalla U, Taljaard JJ, et al. An outbreak of community-acquired pseudomonas aeruginosa pneumonia in a setting of high water stress. QJM. 2017;110:855–856.
16. Cillóniz C, Civljak R, Nicolini A, Torres A. Polymicrobial community-acquired pneumonia: an emerging entity. Respirology. 2016;21:65–75.
17. WHO. High levels of antibiotic resistance found worldwide, new data shows. 2018. Available at: WHO. http://www.who.int/mediacentre/news/releases/2018/antibiotic-resistance-found/en/. Accessed 25 Jun 2018.
18. Eveillard M, Kempf M, Belmonte O, et al. Reservoirs of Acinetobacter baumannii outside the hospital and potential involvement in emerging human community-acquired infections. Int J Infect Dis. 2013;17:e802–5.
19. Wong D, Nielsen TB, Bonomo RA, et al. Clinical and pathophysiological overview of acinetobacter infections: a century of challenges. Clin Microbiol Rev. 2017;30:409–47.
20. Dexter C, Murray GL, Paulsen IT, Peleg AY. Community-acquired Acinetobacter baumannii: clinical characteristics, epidemiology and pathogenesis. Expert Rev Anti-Infect Ther. 2015;13:567–73.
21. Mody L, Foxman B, Bradley S, et al. Longitudinal assessment of multidrug-resistant organisms in newly admitted nursing facility patients: implications for an evolving population. Clin Infect Dis. 2018;67:837–44.
22. Peng C, Zong Z, Fan H. Acinetobacter baumannii isolates associated with community-acquired pneumonia in West China. Clin Microbiol Infect. 2012;18:E491–3.
23. Son YW, Jung IY, Ahn MY, et al. A case of community-acquired pneumonia caused by multidrug-resistant Acinetobacter baumannii in Korea. Infect Chemother. 2017;49: 297–300.
24. Ong CWM, Lye DCB, Khoo KL, et al. Severe community-acquired Acinetobacter baumannii pneumonia: an emerging highly lethal infectious disease in the Asia-Pacific. Respirology. 2009;14:1200–5.
25. Kim YA, Kim JJ, Won DJ, Lee K. Seasonal and temperature-associated increase in community-onset Acinetobacter baumannii complex colonization or infection. Ann Lab Med. 2018;38:266–70.
26. Serota DP, Sexton ME, Kraft CS, Palacio F. Severe community-acquired pneumonia due to Acinetobacter baumannii in North America: case report and review of the literature. Open Forum Infect Dis. 2018;5:ofy044.
27. Eugenin EA. Community-acquired pneumonia infections by Acinetobacter baumannii: how does alcohol impact the antimicrobial functions of macrophages? Virulence. 2013;4:435–6.
28. Kamoshida G, Kikuchi-Ueda T, Nishida S, et al. Pathogenic bacterium Acinetobacter baumannii Inhibits the formation of neutrophil extracellular traps by suppressing neutrophil adhesion. Front Immunol. 2018;9:178.
29. Anstey NM, Currie BJ, Hassell M, Palmer D, Dwyer B, Seifert H. Community-acquired bacteremic Acinetobacter pneumonia in tropical Australia is caused by diverse strains of Acinetobacter baumannii, with carriage in the throat in at-risk groups. J Clin Microbiol. 2002;40:685–6.
30. Peleg AY, Weerarathna T, McCarthy JS, Davis TME. Common infections in diabetes: pathogenesis, management and relationship to glycaemic control. Diabetes Metab Res Rev. 2007;23:3–13.

31. Lee CR, Lee JH, Park KS, et al. Antimicrobial resistance of hypervirulent Klebsiella pneumoniae: epidemiology, hypervirulence-associated determinants, and resistance mechanisms. Front Cell Infect Microbiol. 2017;7:483.
32. Gu D, Dong N, Zheng Z, et al. A fatal outbreak of ST11 carbapenem-resistant hypervirulent Klebsiella pneumoniae in a Chinese hospital: a molecular epidemiological study. Lancet Infect Dis. 2018;18:37–46.
33. Cano V, March C, Insua JL, et al. Klebsiella pneumoniae survives within macrophages by avoiding delivery to lysosomes. Cell Microbiol. 2015;17:1537–60.
34. Rafat C, Messika J, Barnaud G, et al. Hypervirulent Klebsiella pneumoniae, a 5-year study in a French ICU. J Med Microbiol. 2018;67:1083–9.
35. Rammaert B, Goyet S, Beauté J, et al. Klebsiella pneumoniae related community-acquired acute lower respiratory infections in Cambodia: clinical characteristics and treatment. BMC Infect Dis. 2012;12:3.
36. Ishida T, Ito A, Washio Y, et al. Risk factors for drug-resistant pathogens in immunocompetent patients with pneumonia: evaluation of PES pathogens. J Infect Chemother. 2017;23:23–8.
37. Lin YT, Jeng YY, Chen TL, Fung C-P. Bacteremic community-acquired pneumonia due to Klebsiella pneumoniae: clinical and microbiological characteristics in Taiwan, 2001-2008. BMC Infect Dis. 2010;10:307.
38. Tseng C-P, Wu H-S, Wu T-H, et al. Clinical characteristics and outcome of patients with community-onset Klebsiella pneumoniae bacteremia requiring intensive care. J Microbiol Immunol Infect. 2013;46:217–23.
39. Decré D, Verdet C, Emirian A, et al. Emerging severe and fatal infections due to Klebsiella pneumoniae in two university hospitals in France. J Clin Microbiol. 2011;49:3012–4.
40. Inghammar M, Borand L, Goyet S, et al. Community-acquired pneumonia and Gram-negative bacilli in Cambodia-incidence, risk factors and clinical characteristics. Trans R Soc Trop Med Hyg. 2018;112:57–63.
41. Baker TM, Satlin MJ. The growing threat of multidrug-resistant Gram-negative infections in patients with hematologic malignancies. Leuk Lymphoma. 2016;57:2245–58.
42. Brooke JS. Stenotrophomonas maltophilia: an emerging global opportunistic pathogen. Clin Microbiol Rev. 2012;25:2–41.
43. Cha YK, Kim JS, Park SY, et al. Computed tomography findings of community-acquired Stenotrophomonas maltophilia pneumonia in an immunocompetent patient: a case report. Korean J Radiol. 2016;17:961–4.
44. Geller M, Nunes CP, Oliveira L, Nigri R. S. maltophilia pneumonia: a case report. Respir Med Case Rep. 2018;24:44–5.
45. Mori M, Tsunemine H, Imada K, et al. Life-threatening hemorrhagic pneumonia caused by Stenotrophomonas maltophilia in the treatment of hematologic diseases. Ann Hematol. 2014;93:901–11.
46. Falagas ME, Kastoris AC, Vouloumanou EK, Dimopoulos G. Community-acquired Stenotrophomonas maltophilia infections: a systematic review. Eur J Clin Microbiol Infect Dis. 2009;28:719–30.
47. Torres A, Lee N, Cilloniz C, et al. Laboratory diagnosis of pneumonia in the molecular age. Eur Respir J. 2016;48:1764–78.
48. Sibila O, Rodrigo-Troyano A, Shindo Y, et al. Multidrug-resistant pathogens in patients with pneumonia coming from the community. Curr Opin Pulm Med. 2016;22:219–26.
49. Gross AE, Van Schooneveld TC, Olsen KM, et al. Epidemiology and predictors of multidrug-resistant community-acquired and health care-associated pneumonia. Antimicrob Agents Chemother. 2014;58:5262–8.
50. Prina E, Ranzani OT, Polverino E, et al. Risk factors associated with potentially antibiotic-resistant pathogens in community-acquired pneumonia. Ann Am Thorac Soc. 2015;12:153–60.

51. Shindo Y, Ito R, Kobayashi D, et al. Risk factors for drug-resistant pathogens in community-acquired and healthcare-associated pneumonia. Am J Respir Crit Care Med. 2013;188: 985–95.
52. Cao B, Huang Y, She DY, et al. Diagnosis and treatment of community-acquired pneumonia in adults: 2016 clinical practice guidelines by the Chinese Thoracic Society, Chinese Medical Association. Clin Respir J. 2018;12:1320–60.
53. National Health and Medical Research Council. Therapeutic guidelines antibiotic version 15. In: Australian Clinical Practice Guidelines. Canberra: National Health and Medical Research Council; 2014.

Light and Shade of Antibiotics Recently Approved and in Advanced Development for Critically Ill Patients

37

M. Bassetti, E. Righi, and A. Carnelutti

37.1 Introduction

The progressive increase in antimicrobial resistance represents a major concern among critically ill patients, leading to prolonged length of hospital stay and increased mortality [1]. In this setting, prescription of adequate antibiotic treatment, which is of outstanding importance to reduce mortality rates and improve clinical outcomes, is frequently delayed, and the most commonly employed empiric antibiotic regimens are often inappropriate [2]. To confront the problem of antimicrobial resistance, many new antibiotics with activity against multidrug resistant (MDR) pathogens have recently been approved, and other agents are currently under investigation. Here we review the characteristics of the new therapeutic options for the treatment of serious infections caused by MDR pathogens, with a specific focus on the potential advantages of these drugs for the management of critically ill patients in everyday clinical practice.

Table 37.1 summarizes the spectrum of activity, dose, indications and current development phase of currently approved new antibiotics and those in an advanced stage of development for the treatment of infections due to MDR pathogens.

37.2 Ceftolozane/Tazobactam

Ceftolozane/tazobactam is the combination of a novel antipseudomonal cephalosporin with tazobactam, a β-lactamase inhibitor that inhibits most class A and some class C β-lactamases, providing enhanced activity against the majority of extended-spectrum β-lactamase (ESBL)-producing *Enterobacteriaceae* [3]. The

M. Bassetti (✉) · E. Righi · A. Carnelutti
Infectious Diseases Division, Santa Maria della Misericordia University Hospital, Udine, Italy
e-mail: matteo.bassetti@asuiud.sanita.fvg.it

J.-L. Vincent (ed.), *Annual Update in Intensive Care and Emergency Medicine 2019*, Annual Update in Intensive Care and Emergency Medicine,
https://doi.org/10.1007/978-3-030-06067-1_37

Table 37.1 Characteristics of new approved and in advanced phase of development new antibiotics for critically ill patients

Drug	Spectrum of activity	Approved dose	Approved indications	Investigational use	Development phase of approval
Ceftolozane/ tazobactam	Gram-negative pathogens, including MDR *P. aeruginosa* and ESBL-producing *Enterobacteriacae*. Limited activity against anaerobes, including *Bacteroides* spp. No activity against CPE, MRSA and enterococci.	1.5 g every 8 h (i.v.)	cUTIs cIAIs	Respiratory tract infections, including VAP	Approved
Ceftazidime/ avibactam	Gram negatives, including ESBL- and Ambler class A, C and some class D β-lactamase-producing Gram-negatives. Limited activity against anaerobes, including *Bacteroides* spp. No activity against MBL-CPE, MRSA and enterococci.	2.5 g every 8 h (i.v.)	cIAIs, cUTIs and HAP (including VAP) due to MDR Gram-negative pathogens	BSIs and sepsis due to MDR Gram-negative pathogens	Approved
Ceftaroline	Gram positive pathogens, including MRSA (no activity against enterococci). Gram negatives, with the exception of *P. aeruginosa*, *A. baumanii* and ESBL-producing *Enterobacteriacae* and CPE	600 mg every 12 h (i.v.); consider 600 mg every 8 h in patients with normal renal function and infections due to MRSA	ABSSTIs, CAP	HAP, BSIs, IE, CNS infections	Approved
Ceftobiprole	Gram positives, including MRSA and *E. faecalis* Gram negatives, including *P. aeruginosa*. No activity against ESBL-producing pathogens and CPE	500 mg every 8 h (i.v.)	cSSTIs, CAP, HAP (excluded VAP)	–	Approved
Tedizolid	Gram-positive pathogens, including MRSA and VRE	200 mg every 24 h (oral)	cSSTIs	Respiratory tract infections; osteomyelitis	Approved

Imipenem/ relebactam	Gram negatives, including ESBL- and Ambler class A and C β-lactamase-producing Gram negatives (both CPE and *P. aeruginosa*).	–	–	Severe infections (including HAP, VAP, cIAIs, cUTIs) due to MDR Gram negatives	Phase 3
Meropenem/ vaborbactam	Gram negatives, including ESBL- and Ambler class A and C β-lactamase-producing Gram negatives (both CPE and *P. aeruginosa*)	–	–	Severe infections (including BSIs, HAP, VAP, cIAIs, cUTIs) due to MDR Gram negatives	Phase 3
Cefiderocol	Gram negatives, including Ambler class A, B, C and class D β-lactamase-producing pathogens (both CPE and *P. aeruginosa*). Active against MDR *A. baumanii*. Limited activity against Gram positives and anaerobes.	–	–	Severe infections (including BSIs, HAP, VAP, cIAIs, cUTIs) due to MDR Gram negatives	Phase 3
Eravacycline	Gram positives, including MRSA and VRE. Gram negatives, including Ambler class A (both ESBL and KPC) and some class D CPE. Active against MDR *A. baumanii* and anaerobes. Not effective against *P. aeruginosa*.	1 mg/kg by i.v. infusion	cIAIs	Respiratory tract infections; infections due to MDR *A. baumanii*	Approved
Omadacycline	Similar to eravacycline	–	–	cSSTIs, cIAIs, respiratory tract infections	Phase 3
Plazomicin	Gram-negative pathogens, including MDR *Enterobacteriacae*, *P. aeruginosa* and *A. baumanii*. No activity against MBL-producing Gram negatives. Active against staphylococci. Limited activity against *S. pneumoniae* and enterococci.	15 mg/kg every 24 h (i.v.)	cUTIs	Infections due to MDR *Enterobacteriacae*	Approved

(continued)

Table 37.1 (continued)

Drug	Spectrum of activity	Approved dose	Approved indications	Investigational use	Development phase of approval
Ceftaroline/avibactam	Gram-positive pathogens, including MRSA; no activity against enterococci Gram negatives, including Ambler class A, C and some class D β-lactamase-producing *Enterobacteriacae*. Active against anaerobes. *P. aeruginosa* and *A. baumanii* are not susceptible.	–	–	Infections due to MDR *Enterobacteriacae*, particularly when concomitant coverage against MRSA is required	Phase 2
Aztreonam/avibactam	Gram negatives, including Ambler class A, B, C and some class D β-lactamase-producing *Enterobacteriacae*. Active against *P. aeruginosa* and *A. baumanii*. Limited activity against Gram positives and anaerobes.	–	–	Infections due to MDR *Enterobacteriacae*	Phase 3
Lefamulin	Gram positives (including MRSA and VRE) and intracellular pathogens (*Mycoplasma* spp., *Legionella pneumophila*, *Chlamydia* spp., *Neisseria gonorrhoeae*)	–	–	CAP	Phase 3
Murepavadin	MDR *P. aeruginosa*	–	–	Respiratory tract infections due to MDR *P. aeruginosa*	Phase 3

MDR multidrug resistant, *ESBL* extended spectrum β-lactamases, *CPE* carbapenemase-producing *Enterobacteriacae*, *VRE* vancomycin resistant *Enterococcus*, *MRSA* methicillin resistant *Staphylococcus aureus*, *cUTIs* complicated urinary tract infections, *cIAIs* complicated intra-abdominal infections, *VAP* ventilator-associated pneumonia, *HAP* hospital-acquired pneumonia, *MBLs* metallo β-lactamases, *BSIs* bloodstream infections, *ABSSSIs* acute bacterial skin and skin structure infections, *CAP* community-acquired pneumonia, *BSIs* bloodstream infections, *IE* infective endocarditis, *CNS* central nervous system, *i.v.* intravenous

most interesting characteristic of ceftolozane is the potent antipseudomonal activity, with a reported two- to eight-fold higher potency compared with ceftazidime and cefepime and retained activity also against ceftazidime- and meropenem-nonsusceptible strains [3]. This potent antipseudomonal activity is related to the greater affinity of ceftolozane for all essential penicillin-binding proteins (PBPs) (1b, 1c, 2, and 3) compared to ceftazidime and imipenem; moreover, ceftolozane is not affected by upregulation of efflux pumps or loss of porin channels, thus inhibiting all the three mechanisms of resistance displayed by *Pseudomonas aeruginosa* [3].

Adverse effects associated with the use of ceftolozane/tazobactam do not differ considerably from other cephalosporins; nausea, diarrhea, headache and pyrexia are the most commonly reported [4].

Ceftolozane/tazobactam is currently approved by the Food and Drug Administration (FDA) and the European Medical Agency (EMA) for the treatment of complicated urinary tract infections (cUTIs) and complicated intra-abdominal infections (cIAIs), at a dose of 1.5 g every 8 h. Due to lack of efficacy against *Bacteroides*, the addiction of metronidazole for the treatment of cIAIs is recommended. Pooled analyses of registration trials have demonstrated clinical efficacy of the drug against ESBL-producing *Enterobacteriaceae* [5]. However, apart from these data, published clinical experience remains limited against ESBL- and AmpC-producing organisms. The drug should also be used as an alternative to carbapenems for *Escherichia coli* urinary tract or intra-abdominal infections. However, we recommend caution in relation to ESBL-producing *Klebsiella* spp. and the drug should be avoided in the treatment of infections due to AmpC- or *Klebsiella pneumoniae* carbapenemase (KPC)-producing *Enterobacteriaceae.*

Because of the specific activity against MDR *P. aeruginosa*, which is frequently implicated in respiratory tract infections, and the good penetration into the epithelial lining fluid after parenteral administration, ceftolozane/tazobactam is currently under evaluation also in this setting [6]. Pharmacodynamic/pharmacokinetic (PK/PD) studies suggest that an increased dosage of 3 g every 8 h might be necessary for the treatment of pneumonia in patients with normal renal function to achieve a >90% probability of target attainment [7]. Some reports of respiratory tract infections sustained by MDR *P. aeruginosa* successfully treated with ceftolozane/tazobactam have been published recently [8], and a Phase III trial to assess the safety and efficacy of ceftolozane/tazobactam (3 g every 8 h) compared to meropenem (1 g every 8 h) for the treatment of ventilator-associated pneumonia (VAP) due to *P. aeruginosa* has recently been completed (ClinicalTrials.gov Identifier: NCT02070757). Ceftolozane/tazobactam is currently under evaluation also for the treatment of lower limb infections in diabetic patients [9] and a Phase 4 PK/PD study on the compound in patients with burns has recently been completed (ClinicalTrials.gov Identifier: NCT03002506). Moreover, an observational pharmacokinetic study of ceftolozane/tazobactam in critically ill patients with and without continuous renal replacement therapy (CRRT) is currently ongoing (ClinicalTrials.gov Identifier: NCT02962934).

37.3 Ceftazidime/Avibactam

Ceftazidime/avibactam is currently approved for the treatment of cIAIs (in combination with metronidazole because of limited antibacterial activity against *Bacteroides* spp.), cUTIs, hospital-acquired pneumonia (HAP) (including VAP) and difficult-to-treat infections caused by Gram-negative bacteria when other treatment options are limited. The compound is a fixed-combination drug containing ceftazidime, a third-generation cephalosporin, and avibactam, a new, semi-synthetic ß-lactamase inhibitor that *in vitro* inhibits the activity of Ambler class A (e.g., ESBL and KPC), class C and some class D enzymes. However, avibactam it is not active against metallo-ß-lactamases (MBLs: New Delhi MBL [NDM], Verona integrin-encoded MBL [VIM], imipenemase [IMP], Vietnam ESBL [VEB], *Pseudomonas* extended resistant [PER]) or against *Acinetobacter* OXA-type carbapenemases [10]. Thus, the combination with avibactam broadens the antibacterial activity of ceftazidime against the majority of *Enterobacteriacae*, resulting in susceptibility rates higher than 96%, also among ceftazidime-non-susceptible, colistin-resistant, MDR and meropenem-non-susceptible, MBL-negative isolates [11]. For this reason, ceftazidime/avibactam currently represents the most attractive therapeutic option for the treatment of infections due to MDR *Enterobacteriacae*, mainly represented by carbapenemase-producing *K. pneumoniae*. A recent review and meta-analysis including nine randomized controlled trials (RCTs) and three observational studies found improved clinical responses with reduced mortality in patients with carbapenem-resistant *Enterobacteriacae* (CRE) infections treated with ceftazidime/avibactam [12], and a recent retrospective study identified ceftazidime/avibactam as the only independent predictor of survival among patients with bacteremic KPC-producing *K. pneumoniae* (KPC-*Kp*) infections [13]. Whether ceftazidime/avibactam should be used as monotherapy or as combination therapy for the treatment of infections due to CRE, however, remains a matter of debate. The use of ceftazidime/avibactam, particularly when used as monotherapy, has been associated with the potential emergence of resistant strains in several reports [14]. For this reason, the use of ceftazidime-avibactam in combination with gentamicin, fosfomycin, tigecycline or colistin may be a good option to optimize efficacy while reducing the risk of resistance selection, although further studies specifically addressing this point are needed. Synergistic *in vitro* activity of ceftazidime/avibactam in combination with imipenem and meropenem against KPC-*Kp* has been reported recently, but the potential advantage of this combination in clinical practice is not established [15].

Globally, ceftazidime/avibactam is well tolerated, and the most common adverse events are headache, gastrointestinal symptoms (abdominal pain, vomiting, nausea and constipation), and infusion-site reactions [16]. Of note, administration of ceftazidime/avibactam is contraindicated in patients with known allergy to any penicillin antibiotic, limiting the use of the compound in this population.

37.4 Aztreonam/Avibactam

Aztreonam belongs to the family of monobactams and possesses broad-spectrum activity against Gram-negative pathogens (with the exception of *Enterobacter* spp.); conversely, aztreonam is not active against Gram-positive aerobic and anaerobic bacteria and *Bacteroides fragilis*. Aztreonam is easily hydrolyzed by class-A and class-C lactamases, but is the only β-lactam stable to hydrolysis by MBLs, thus representing an interesting option for the treatment of infections due to MBL-producing Gram-negative pathogens.

The combination of aztreonam with avibactam broadens the spectrum of activity of aztreonam, restoring antimicrobial activity against Gram-negative pathogens expressing Ambler class A, C and some class D β-lactamases [17]. Aztreonam/avibactam was active against up to 99.8% of *Enterobacteriaceae* isolates, including meropenem non-susceptible strains. Moreover, the compound has been reported to be 8- to 32-fold more potent than meropenem, with minimum inhibitory concentrations (MICs) of 8 g/mL and a MIC_{90} of 1 g/mL against MBL-producing *Enterobacteriaceae*. Conversely, the combination with avibactam does not confer enhanced activity against *Acinetobacter baumannii* or *P. aeruginosa* compared to aztreonam alone, resulting in a potential limited activity in infections due to non-fermenting MDR Gram-negative isolates [18]. The potential use of aztreonam/avibactam in clinical practice is currently under evaluation in Phase 1, 2 and 3 studies. Specifically, a Phase 1 study addressing the safety and tolerability of aztreonam/avibactam in healthy subjects (ClinicalTrials.gov Identifier: NCT01689207) and a Phase 2 study evaluating pharmacokinetic, safety and tolerability of aztreonam/avibactam for the treatment of cIAIs in hospitalized adults (REJUVENATE: ClinicalTrials.gov Identifier: NCT02655419) have been recently completed. A Phase 3 study to determine the efficacy, safety and tolerability of aztreonam/avibactam (with or without metronidazole) versus meropenem (with or without colistin) for the treatment of serious infections (including HAP and VAP) due to Gram-negative bacteria is currently ongoing (ClinicalTrials.gov Identifier: NCT03329092).

37.5 Ceftaroline

Ceftaroline is a new, fifth generation cephalosporin and is characterized by potent activity against methicillin-resistant *Staphylococcus aureus* (MRSA), including strains with reduced susceptibility to vancomycin, because of the high binding affinity for PBP-2a [19]. Compared to the other commonly used anti-MRSA agents (e.g., vancomycin, daptomycin and linezolid), an attractive characteristic of ceftaroline is its broad-spectrum activity, including both Gram-positive and Gram-negative bacteria. Ceftaroline is not active against enterococci, ESBL- and carbapenemase-producing *Enterobacteriaceae*, anaerobes and *P. aeruginosa*, thus limiting the use of the compound in infections where these pathogens are confirmed or suspected.

Ceftaroline is currently approved by the FDA and the EMA for the treatment of acute bacterial skin and soft tissue infections and community-acquired pneumonia (CAP). The use of ceftaroline in the setting of CAP is particularly attractive, because ceftaroline was found to be 16-fold more potent compared with ceftriaxone against methicillin-susceptible *S. aureus* (MSSA), *Streptococcus pneumoniae* and *Haemophilus influenzae*; moreover, enhanced activity of ceftaroline compared with ceftriaxone has also been reported against *Moraxella catharralis*, which is another pathogen commonly involved in community-acquired respiratory tract infections [20]. A recently published meta-analysis found that ceftaroline fosamil was superior to ceftriaxone in adult patients hospitalized with pneumonia (pneumonia outcomes research team [PORT] risk class 3–4) [21].

For the treatment of CAP and complicated skin and soft tissue infections (cSSTIs), ceftaroline is currently approved at the dose of 600 mg every 12 h. However, recent findings suggest that in patients with normal renal function, administration of higher doses of ceftaroline (600 mg every 8 h) may provide better clinical outcomes in MRSA infections [22]. A Phase 4 study evaluating ceftaroline (600 mg every 8 h) versus ceftriaxone (2 g every 24 h) plus vancomycin (15 mg/kg intravenously [i.v.] q12h initially and then dose adjusted based on trough concentrations) for the treatment of CAP in patients with risk factors for MRSA has recently been completed (ClinicalTrials.gov Identifier: NCT01645735). Despite the limited currently approved indications, there is increasing evidence supporting the use of ceftaroline for the treatment of a broad-spectrum of severe MRSA infections, such as bacteremia, infective endocarditis, nosocomial pneumonia and central nervous system (CNS) infections, as reported in a recently published systematic review [23]. Major advantages of ceftaroline compared with vancomycin are the broader spectrum of activity, higher potency against MSSA and the favorable tolerability profile, with low potential of renal toxicity. Moreover, ceftaroline does not require therapeutic drug monitoring. Overall, ceftaroline is well tolerated and only mild adverse effects are usually reported for treatment durations <7 days. However, agranulocytosis has been listed as a postmarket adverse event, occurring in up to 10% of patients, usually when treatment duration exceeds 7 days.

A potential concern in the use of ceftaroline is represented by the selection of resistant strains, due to alterations in the ceftaroline-binding site of PBP-2a [23]. Synergistic *in vitro* activity has been reported for ceftaroline in combination with daptomycin against MRSA, and potential *in vivo* efficacy is suggested by some case reports on severe MRSA infections (including persistent bacteremia) successfully treated with ceftaroline plus daptomycin; however, evidence is lacking and further studies are required to bring this strategy into wide clinical practice [24].

37.6 Ceftobiprole

Ceftobiprole, together with ceftaroline, belongs to the group of fifth generation cephalosporins, and is characterized by potent anti-MRSA activity. Unlike ceftaroline, ceftobiprole is also active against *Enterococcus faecalis* (but not *E.*

faecium) and exerts activity against *P. aeruginos*a superior to that of cefepime [25]. Ceftobiprole is currently approved by the FDA for the treatment of cSSTIs and by the EMA for the treatment of pneumonia (except VAP). In registrative clinical trials, ceftobiprole medocaril has been investigated for the treatment of CAP requiring hospitalization and HAP (including VAP) [25, 26]. Ceftobiprole (500 mg every 8 h, intravenously) was as effective as the comparator in CAP (ceftriaxone with or without linezolid) and in HAP (ceftazidime plus linezolid), providing cure rates of 86.6% and 59.6%, respectively. However, reported cure rates were only 23.1% in patients with VAP and for this reason the compound has not been approved by the EMA for use in this subset of patients [26, 27]. The approved dose of ceftobiprole is 500 mg every 8 h intravenously; however, an open-label study evaluating pharmacokinetics of ceftobiprole (1 g every 12 h versus 1 g every 8 h, both as 4-h infusions) among adult patients hospitalized in the intensive care unit (ICU) has recently been completed and results are pending (ClinicalTrials.gov Identifier: NCT00770978).

37.7 Ceftaroline/Avibactam

The combination of ceftaroline with avibactam broadens the antimicrobial spectrum of ceftaroline to include ESBL- and KPC-producing *Enterobacteriaceae* and anaerobes; conversely, no significantly enhanced activity against *P. aeruginosa* and *A. baumanii* has been reported [28]. Safety, tolerability and pharmacokinetics of ceftaroline/avibactam were evaluated in a Phase 1 study conducted in 60 healthy adult subjects. Ceftaroline/avibactam was well tolerated at total daily doses of up to 1800 mg of each compound, and all adverse events were mild-to-moderate in severity and were mainly represented by diarrhea, dry mouth and headache. Infusion-site reactions were the most common adverse events reported after multiple intravenous doses [29]. A Phase 1 study analyzing the pharmacokinetic profiles of ceftaroline and avibactam following intravenous administration of ceftaroline/avibactam in adults with augmented renal clearance has been completed (ClinicalTrials.gov Identifier: NCT01624246). A Phase 2 study comparing treatment with ceftaroline/avibactam versus doripenem for the treatment of adult patients with cUTIs has recently been completed and results are pending (ClinicalTrials.gov Identifier: NCT01281462). Because of its broad-spectrum activity, with a good tolerance profile, ceftaroline/avibactam might represent a potential option for the treatment of infections due to ESBL- or KPC-producing *Enterobacteriaceae*, particularly when a concomitant empiric or targeted treatment against MRSA is required.

37.8 Tedizolid

Tedizolid is a new oxazolidinone and is currently approved by FDA and EMA or the treatment of acute bacterial SSTIs, when a Gram-positive pathogen, including MRSA, is confirmed or suspected. Tedizolid is available both as oral and intravenous formulations and the recommended dosage is 200 mg every 24 h for 6 days. Tedizolid is characterized by potent *in vitro* activity against Gram-positive pathogens, including MRSA, with a four- to eight-fold greater activity than linezolid and retained activity against linezolid non-susceptible strains [30]. Major advantages of tedizolid over linezolid are the lower risk of myelotoxicity [31], the lower risk of drug–drug interactions with selective serotonin reuptake inhibitors (SSRIs) and other compounds with serotonergic activity, and adrenergic agents [32], and a higher bioavailability (>80%), with *in vivo* half-life value approximately two-fold greater compared with linezolid, allowing once daily administration [33]. PK/PD studies showed that tedizolid achieves approximately 40-fold higher concentrations in epithelial lining fluid relative to free plasma ones, making tedizolid an interesting option for the treatment of pneumonia [34]. Promising data come from murine models, showing tedizolid to be as effective as linezolid and more effective than vancomycin for the treatment of MRSA pneumonia [35]. A phase 3, randomized, double blind study comparing tedizolid (200 mg i.v. once daily for 7 days, or 14 days in bacteremia) versus linezolid (600 mg i.v. every 12 h for 10 days, or 14 days for bacteremia) for the treatment of ventilated patients with presumed Gram-positive HAP or VAP has recently been completed and results are pending (ClinicalTrials.gov Identifier: NCT02019420). A Phase 4 study designed to characterize the pharmacokinetics of intravenous and oral tedizolid in patients with cystic fibrosis in currently ongoing (ClinicalTrials.gov Identifier: NCT02444234).

37.9 Imipenem/Relebactam

Relebactam (formerly known as MK-7655) is a novel, intravenous, class A and class C β-lactamase inhibitor and is currently under evaluation in combination with imipenem/cilastatin for the treatment of resistant Gram-negative infections [36]. *In vitro* studies demonstrated that relebactam restored imipenem's activity against KPC-producing *Enterobacteriacae*, lowering imipenem MICs from 16–64 to 0.12–1 mg/L at a concentration of 4 mg/L. Moreover, relebactam is able to lower imipenem MICs for *P. aeruginosa*, particularly in strains with depressed OprD expression and increased AmpC expression [36]. Conversely, the addition of relebactam to imipenem does not seem to provide any adjunctive benefit against *A. baumanii* or *S. maltophilia* or against MBL-producing *Enterobacteriacae* [36]. A non-inferiority, Phase 3 trial evaluating the efficacy and safety of imipenem/relebactam compared to piperacillin/tazobactam for the treatment of HAP and VAP (ClinicalTrials.gov Identifier: NCT02493764) is currently recruiting. A Phase 3 study evaluating the efficacy and safety of imipenem/relebactam (200/100–500/250 mg depending on renal function) compared to colistimethate sodium plus imipenem/cilastatin for the treatment of imipenem-resistant bacterial infections, including HAP, VAP, cIAIs and cUTIs, has recently been completed and results are pending (ClinicalTrials.gov Identifier: NCT02452047). In Phase 2 trials, imipenem/relebactam was well tolerated, with diarrhea, nausea, vomiting and headache being the most commonly reported adverse events [37].

37.10 Meropenem/Vaborbactam

Vaborbactam (formerly known as RPX7009) is a new class A and class C β-lactamase inhibitor and is currently in Phase 3 clinical development in combination with meropenem for the treatment of infections due to resistant Gram-negative pathogens [38]. Similar to relebactam, vaborbactam broadens the spectrum of activity of meropenem against KPC-producing *Enterobacteriacae* and was found to be effective in lowering meropenem MIC_{50} from 32 to 0.06 g/mL and MIC_{90} from 32 to 1 g/mL in a study encompassing 991 isolates of KPC-producing *Enterobacteriaceae* [38]. In a Phase 1 study in healthy adult subjects, vaborbactam showed a favorable tolerability profile, with no serious reported adverse events. Mild adverse events were mainly represented by headache and catheter site complications [39]. Meropenem/vaborbactam was approved by the FDA on August 2017 for the treatment of cUTIs, based on the results of the TANGO1 trial, demonstrating the superiority of meropenem/vaborbactam (2/2 g every 8 h) over piperacillin/tazobactam (4/0.5 g every 8 h) for the treatment of cUTIs and acute pyelonephritis in adult patients [40]. A Phase 3 study evaluating the efficacy, safety and tolerability of meropenem/vaborbactam compared to best available therapy for the treatment of CRE infections has recently been completed. Meropenem/vaborbactam showed consistent improvement over best available therapy in efficacy endpoints, with improved safety and tolerability, as reported in preliminary data [41].

37.11 Cefiderocol

Cefiderocol (formerly known as S-649266), is a novel siderophore cephalosporin characterized by broad-spectrum activity against Gram-negative pathogens (including CRE and MDR *P. aeruginosa* spp., *A. baumanii* spp. and *Burkholderia* spp.) due to stability against class A, B, C and D carbapenemases. As for other cephalosporins, cefiderocol binds primarily to bacterial PBP3, but the catechol moiety at the 3-position side chain of the cephalosporin forms a chelated complex with ferric iron that promotes cefiderocol's crossing of the outer membrane of Gram-negative pathogens using the bacterial iron transport system. For this reason, although cefiderocol's activity is not impaired by the production of carbapenemases (including MBLs), the deficiency of iron-transporters in *P. aeruginosa* and in *E. coli* has been associated with a 16-fold increase in cefiderocol MICs. Only limited activity against Gram-positive pathogens and anaerobes has been described [42].

Population pharmacokinetic analysis based on plasma cefiderocol concentrations in healthy subjects, subjects with various degrees of renal function, and patients with cUTI or acute uncomplicated pyelonephritis caused by Gram-negative pathogens suggested that a cefiderocol standard dose of 2 g every 8 h may guarantee adequate exposure for the treatment of cUTI or acute pyelonephritis caused by Gram-negative pathogens [43]. A Phase 2 study comparing cefiderocol (2 g every 8 h) with imipenem/cilastatin (1 g every 8 h) for 7–14 days for the treatment of hospitalized adults with complicated urinary tract infections caused by Gram-negative pathogens has recently been completed (ClinicalTrials.gov Identifier: NCT02321800). A Phase 3, multicenter, randomized, open-label clinical study comparing cefiderocol with best available therapy for the treatment of severe infections (including healthcare-associated pneumonia [HCAP], HAP, VAP, bloodstream infections and sepsis) caused by carbapenem-resistant Gram-negative pathogens (ClinicalTrials.gov Identifier: NCT02714595) and another Phase 3 trial evaluating the role of cefiderocol for the treatment of HCAP, HAP and VAP caused by Gram-negative pathogens are currently recruiting (ClinicalTrials.gov Identifier: NCT0302380).

37.12 Eravacycline

Eravacycline is structurally related to tigecycline, but retains activity against tetracycline-resistant bacterial strains expressing both ribosomal protection and efflux resistance genes, exerting broad-spectrum activity against both Gram-positive and Gram-negative resistant pathogens, including MRSA, enterococci (including vancomycin-resistant enterococci [VRE]) and *Enterobacteriacae* expressing resistance genes from different classes of lactamases (particularly ESBL, KPC and OXA), with a two- to four-fold greater activity than tigecycline [44]. Moreover, eravacycline currently represents the most potent antibiotic against MDR *A. baumanii*, with a four-fold higher activity compared with tigecycline, including strains resistant to sulbactam, imipenem/meropenem, levofloxacin and amikacin/tobramycin [45]. Eravacycline also exerts potent activity against anaerobic pathogens [46]. As for tigecycline, eravacycline is not effective against *P. aeruginosa* [44].

Together with the broad-spectrum of activity, another attractive characteristic of eravacycline is the availability of both intravenous and oral formulations, making eravacycline a potential option for early oral de-escalation in patients with infections caused by MDR Gram-negative bacteria. However, the oral formulation failed the non-inferiority criteria in the treatment of cUTIs in one randomized controlled trial (RCT), suggesting that more data on oral formulation efficacy and bioavailability are required (ClinicalTrials.gov Identifier: NCT03032510). Eravacycline has been recently approved by the FDA for the treatment of cIAI at the dose of 1 mg/kg by i.v. infusion over approximately 60 min every 12 h, based on a recent Phase 3, randomized, double-blind, multicenter study reporting eravacycline to be non-inferior compared with ertapenem for the treatment of patients with cIAIs [47]. A Phase 1 study conducted in 20 healthy adult volunteers found that eravacycline achieved 6-fold and 50-fold higher concentrations in the epithelial lining fluid and alveolar macrophages than in plasma, respectively, supporting the potential role of eravacycline for the treatment of respiratory tract infections [48]. Moreover, eravacycline was as effective as linezolid in a neutropenic MRSA mouse lung infection model [49]. However, no studies evaluating the potential role of eravacycline for the treatment of respiratory tract infections are currently ongoing.

37.13 Omadacycline

Omadacycline is a semisynthetic antibiotic structurally related to tetracyclines, and, similar to eravacycline, is not affected by the two main mechanisms of tetracycline resistance, represented by efflux pumps and ribosomal protection proteins. Omadacycline is characterized by broad-spectrum activity including anaerobes and difficult-to-treat aerobic pathogens, in particular MRSA, VRE, ESBL- and carbapenemase-producing *Enterobacteriaceae*, MDR *Acinetobacter* spp. and *Stenotrophomonas maltophilia* [50]. Safety and pharmacokinetics of oral and i.v. formulations of omadacycline have been evaluated in a Phase 1 study including 24 healthy subjects. The absolute bioavailability of the tablets was approximately 34.5% compared with i.v. formulation (a 300 mg dose of the tablet formulation produced a total exposure equivalent to that of a 100 mg i.v. dose), with consistent intersubject variability. Overall, omadacycline was well tolerated, with dizziness, nausea and vomiting being the most frequently reported adverse events [51]. Omadacycline (100 mg i.v. once a day with an option to transition to 200 mg orally once a day) was non-inferior compared with linezolid (with or without aztreonam) for the treatment of cSSTIs in a Phase 2, randomized trial [52]. The efficacy of oral formulation in clinical practice is currently under investigation in a Phase 3 study comparing oral omadacycline with oral linezolid for the treatment of acute bacterial skin and skin structure infections (ClinicalTrial.gov Identifier: NCT02877927). Omadacycline concentrations in epithelial lining fluid have been reported to be similar to or even higher than the simultaneous total plasma concentrations, whereas concentrations in alveolar cells are significantly greater than those in plasma and epithelial lining fluid, with an overall magnitude of systemic exposure of omadacycline approximately three-fold higher than that of tigecycline in plasma, epithelial lining fluid and alveolar cells [53]. These data make omadacycline a potentially interesting option for the treatment of respiratory tract infections, and a Phase 3 study comparing omadacycline (both intravenous and oral formulations) with moxifloxacin for the treatment of CAP has been completed (ClinicalTrials.gov Identifier: NCT02531438). Moreover, a Phase 2 trial compering efficacy of oral omadacycline with oral nitrofurantoin for the treatment of cystitis is currently recruiting (ClinicalTrials.gov Identifier: NCT03425396).

37.14 Plazomicin

Plazomicin is a next-generation aminoglycoside that was approved by the FDA in June 2018 for the treatment of cUTIs, including pyelonephritis. Compared with the other aminoglycosides, plazomicin has been structurally modified to prevent inactivation by plasmid-borne aminoglycoside-modifying enzymes, which represent the main resistance mechanism impairing the activity of traditional aminoglycosides. For this reason, plazomicin exerts potent *in vitro* bactericidal activity against MDR *Enterobacteriacae*, including aminoglycoside-resistant pathogens that encode aminoglycoside-modifying enzymes. However, plazomicin's activity is impaired against strains with 16S ribosomal RNA-methyltransferases that confer pan-aminoglycoside resistance [54]. Plazomicin was tested against 4825 clinical isolates collected during 2014 and 2015 in 70 US hospitals as part of the ALERT (Antimicrobial Longitudinal Evaluation and Resistance Trends) program, and was found to be able to inhibit 99.2% of *Enterobacteriaceae* isolated at ≤4 μg/mL. Moreover, plazomicin, as well as other aminoglycosides, is effective against *P. aeruginosa* and *A. baumanni*. Regarding Gram-positive pathogens, plazomicin displays good activity against staphylococci, but possesses limited activity against *S. pneumoniae* and enterococci [54]. *In vitro* synergy between plazomicin and piperacillin/tazobactam or ceftazidime has been reported against MDR *Enterobacteriacae*, suggesting a potential role of plazomicin both as monotherapy and as combination therapy for the treatment of serious infections due to this class of pathogens [55]. Moreover, synergy with carbapenems for the treatment of MDR *A. baumanii* has been described [56]. Plazomicin at the dose of 15 mg/kg once daily for 5 days was effective in the treatment of adults with cUTIs and acute pyelonephritis (including patients with antibiotic-resistant *Enterobacteriaceae*) in a double-blind, Phase 2 study comparing plazomicin with levofloxacin [57]. A Phase 3 study comparing plazomicin (15 mg/kg daily) with meropenem (1 g every 8 h), with the option to switch to oral levofloxacin after at least 4 days, for the treatment of cUTIs has recently been completed (ClinicalTrials.gov Identifier: NCT02486627). A Phase 3 study comparing plazomicin with colistin, both in combination with tigecycline and meropenem, for the treatment of serious CRE infections (including HAP, VAP, bloodstream infections, cUTIs and acute pyelonephritis) has been completed and results are pending (ClinicalTrials.gov Identifier: NCT01970371). As for other aminoglycosides, ototoxicity, nephrotoxicity, neuromuscular blockade and fetal harm have been described, and therapeutic drug monitoring to minimize the risk of adverse effects developing is recommended, particularly in patients with creatinine clearance <90 mL/min.

37.15 Lefamulin

Lefamulin (formerly known as BC-3781) is the first-in-class pleuromutilin antibiotic and exhibits a unique mechanism of action through inhibition of protein synthesis by binding to the peptidyl transferase center of the 50S bacterial ribosome, thus preventing the binding of RNA for peptide transfer [58]. Lefamulin exerts potent activity against Gram-positive pathogens (including MRSA and VRE) and atypical organisms associated with CAP (e.g., *Mycoplasma pneumoniae*, *Legionella pneumophila* and *Chlamydophila pneumoniae*); moreover, lefamulin retains activity against MDR *Neisseria gonorrhoeae* and *Mycoplasma genitalium* [58]. Two Phase 3 studies assessing the safety and efficacy of lefamulin for the treatment of adult patients with CAP have recently been completed (ClinicalTrials.gov Identifier: NCT02559310 and ClinicalTrials.gov Identifier: NCT02813694) and results are pending.

37.16 Murepavadin

Murepavadin (formerly known as POL7080) represents the first-in-class of outer membrane protein targeting antibiotics (OMPTA) and acts by binding to the lipopolysaccharide (LPS) transport protein D (LptD), leading to LPS alterations in the outer membrane of the bacterium and inducing cell death [59]. *In vitro*, murepavadin exhibits specific and potent antimicrobial activity against *P. aeruginosa*, but was shown to be inactive against other Gram-negative species, including other *Pseudomonas* species (e.g., *P. luteola*, *P. oryzihabitans*), *Stenotrophomonas maltophilia*, *Burkholderia cepacia*, *Enterobacteriaceae*, *A. baumannii*, and against Gram-positive bacteria [59]. Due to good penetration into epithelial lining fluid, murepavadine is currently under investigation for the treatment of respiratory tract infections. In particular, a Phase 2 study investigating pharmacokinetics, safety and efficacy of murepavadine for the treatment of VAP caused by *P. aeruginosa* has recently been completed (ClinicalTrials.gov Identifier: NCT02096328), and a multicenter, Phase 3 study comparing murepavadin combined with one anti-pseudomonal antibiotic versus two anti-pseudomonal antibiotics in adult subjects with bacterial VAP suspected or confirmed to be caused by *P. aeruginosa* is currently ongoing (ClinicalTrials.gov Identifier: NCT03409679).

37.17 Conclusion

Many new drugs with broad-spectrum activity against MDR pathogens, which still represent a major challenge in clinical practice because of the lack of new therapeutic options, have been recently approved or are in an advanced stage of development. All these compounds represent promising options to enhance our antibiotic armamentarium, taking into account also their favorable toxicity profile and the availability of oral formulations. However, few data regarding the efficacy of these agents in real-life are currently available, and their role in therapy in many cases requires further investigation.

References

1. Tabah A, Koulenti D, Laupland K, et al. Characteristics and determinants of outcome of hospital-acquired bloodstream infections in intensive care units: the EUROBACT International Cohort Study. Intensive Care Med. 2012;38:1930–45.
2. Zilberberg MD, Shorr AF, Micek ST, Vazquez-Guillamet C, Kollef MH. Multi-drug resistance, inappropriate initial antibiotic therapy and mortality in Gram-negative severe sepsis and septic shock: a retrospective cohort study. Crit Care. 2014;18:596.
3. Sader HS, Flamm RK, Streit JM, Jones RN. Activity of novel antimicrobial ceftolozane/tazobactam tested against contemporary clinical strains from USA hospitals. Presented at the 52nd Interscience Conference on Antimicrobial Agents and Chemotherapy. 2011 (abst).
4. Wagenlehner FM, Umeh O, Steenbergen J, Yuan G, Darouiche RO. Ceftolozane/tazobactam compared with levofloxacin in the treatment of complicated urinary-tract infections, including pyelonephritis: a randomised, double-blind, phase 3 trial (ASPECT-cUTI). Lancet. 2015;385:1949–56.

5. Popejoy MW, Paterson DL, Cloutier D, et al. Efficacy of ceftolozane/tazobactam against urinary tract and intra-abdominal infections caused by ESBL-producing Escherichia coli and Klebsiella pneumoniae: a pooled analysis of Phase 3 clinical trials. J Antimicrob Chemother. 2017;72:268–72.
6. Chandorkar G, Huntington JA, Gotfried MH, Rodvold KA, Umeh O. Intrapulmonary penetration of ceftolozane/tazobactam and piperacillin/tazobactam in healthy adult subjects. J Antimicrob Chemother. 2012;67:2463–9.
7. Xiao AJ, Miller BW, Huntington JA, Nicolau DP. Ceftolozane/tazobactam pharmacokinetic/pharmacodynamic-derived dose justification for phase 3 studies in patients with nosocomial pneumonia. J Clin Pharmacol. 2016;56:56–66.
8. Castón JJ, De la Torre Á, Ruiz-Camps I, Sorlí ML, Torres V, Torre-Cisneros J. Salvage therapy with ceftolozane-tazobactam for multidrug-resistant Pseudomonas aeruginosa infections. Antimicrob Agents Chemother. 2017;61:e02136–16.
9. Monogue ML, Stainton SM, Baummer-Carr A, et al. Pharmacokinetics and tissue penetration of ceftolozane-tazobactam in diabetic patients with lower limb infections and healthy adult volunteers. Antimicrob Agents Chemother. 2017;61:e01449–17.
10. Keepers TR, Gomez M, Celeri C, Nichols WW, Krause KM. Bactericidal activity, absence of serum effect, and time-kill kinetics of ceftazidime-avibactam against b-lactamase-producing Enterobacteriaceae and *Pseudomonas aeruginosa*. Antimicrob Agents Chemother. 2014;58:5297–305.
11. Kazmierczak KM, de Jonge BLM, Stone GG, Sahm DF. In vitro activity of ceftazidime/avibactam against isolates of Enterobacteriaceae collected in European countries: INFORM global surveillance 2012–15. J Antimicrob Chemother. 2018;73:2782–8.
12. Zhong H, Zhao XY, Zhang ZL, et al. Evaluation of efficacy and safety of ceftazidime-avibactam in the treatment of Gram-negative bacterial infections: a systematic review and meta-analysis. Int J Antimicrob Agents. 2018;52:443–50.
13. Tumbarello M, Trecarichi EM, Corona A, et al. Efficacy of ceftazidime-avibactam salvage therapy in patients with infections caused by KPC-producing Klebsiella pneumoniae. Clin Infect Dis. 2018 (in press).
14. Gaibani P, Campoli C, Lewis RE, et al. In vivo evolution of resistant subpopulations of KPC-producing Klebsiella pneumoniaeduring ceftazidime/avibactam treatment. J Antimicrob Chemother. 2018;73:1525–9.
15. Gaibani P, Lewis RE, Volpe SL, et al. In vitro interaction of ceftazidime-avibactam in combination with different antimicrobials against KPC-producing Klebsiella pneumoniae clinical isolates. Int J Infect Dis. 2017;65:1–3.
16. Vazquez JA, González Patzán LD, Stricklin D, et al. Efficacy and safety of ceftazidime-avibactam versus imipenem-cilastatin in the treatment of complicated urinary tract infections, including acute pyelonephritis, in hospitalized adults: results of a prospective, investigator-blinded, randomized study. Curr Med Res Opin. 2012;28:1921–31.
17. Lahiri SD, Mangani S, Durand-Reville T, et al. Structural insight into potent broad-spectrum inhibition with reversible recyclization mechanism: avibactam in complex with CTX-M-15 and Pseudomonas aeruginosa AmpC b-lactamases. Antimicrob Agents Chemother. 2013;57:2496–505.
18. Karlowsky JA, Kazmierczak KM, de Jonge BLM, Hackel MA, Sahm DF, Bradford PA. In vitro activity of aztreonam-avibactam against Enterobacteriaceae and Pseudomonas aeruginosa isolated by clinical laboratories in 40 countries from 2012 to 2015. Antimicrob Agents Chemother. 2017;61:e00472-17.
19. Saravolatz LD, Stein GE, Johnson LB. Ceftaroline: a novel cephalosporin with activity against methicillin-resistant Staphylococcus aureus. Clin Infect Dis. 2011;52:1156–63.
20. Biedenbach DJ, Iaconis JP, Sahm DF. Comparative in vitro activities of ceftaroline and ceftriaxone against bacterial pathogens associated with respiratory tract infections: results from the AWARE surveillance study. J Antimicrob Chemother. 2016;71:3459–64.
21. Taboada M, Melnick D, Iaconis JP, et al. Ceftaroline fosamil versus ceftriaxone for the treatment of community-acquired pneumonia: individual patient data meta-analysis of randomized controlled trials. J Antimicrob Chemother. 2016;71:1748–9.

22. Canut A, Isla A, Rodríguez-Gascón A. Pharmacokinetic/pharmacodynamic analysis to evaluate ceftaroline fosamil dosing regimens for the treatment of community-acquired bacterial pneumonia and complicated skin and skin-structure infections in patients with normal and impaired renal function. Int J Antimicrob Agents. 2015;45:399–405.
23. Cosimi RA, Beik N, Kubiak DW, Johnson JA. Ceftaroline for severe methicillin-resistant Staphylococcus aureus infections: a systematic review. Open Forum Infect Dis. 2017;4:ofx084.
24. Lewis PO, Heil EL, Covert KL, Cluck DB. Treatment strategies for persistent methicillin-resistant Staphylococcus aureus bacteraemia. J Clin Pharm Ther. 2018;43:614–25.
25. Walkty A, Adam HJ, Laverdière M, et al. In vitro activity of ceftobiprole against frequently encountered aerobic and facultative Gram-positive and Gram-negative bacterial pathogens: results of the CANWARD 2007-2009 study. Diagn Microbiol Infect Dis. 2011;69: 348–55.
26. Nicholson SC, Welte T, File TM Jr, et al. A randomised, double-blind trial comparing ceftobiprole medocaril with ceftriaxone with or without linezolid for the treatment of patients with community-acquired pneumonia requiring hospitalisation. Int J Antimicrob Agents. 2012;39:240–6.
27. Awad SS, Rodriguez AH, Chuang YC, et al. A phase 3 randomized double-blind comparison of ceftobiprole medocaril versus ceftazidime plus linezolid for the treatment of hospital-acquired pneumonia. Clin Infect Dis. 2014;59:51–61.
28. Castanheira M, Sader HS, Farrell DJ, Mendes RE, Jones RN. Activity of ceftaroline-avibactam tested against Gram-negative organism populations, including strains expressing one or more β-lactamases and methicillin-resistant Staphylococcus aureus carrying various staphylococcal cassette chromosome mec types. Antimicrob Agents Chemother. 2012;56:4779–85.
29. Riccobene TA, Su SF, Rank D. Single- and multiple-dose study to determine the safety, tolerability, and pharmacokinetics of ceftaroline fosamil in combination with avibactam in healthy subjects. Antimicrob Agents Chemother. 2013;57:1496–504.
30. Li S, Guo Y, Zhao C, et al. In vitro activities of tedizolid compared with other antibiotics against Gram-positive pathogens associated with hospital-acquired pneumonia, skin and soft tissue infection and bloodstream infection collected from 26 hospitals in China. J Med Microbiol. 2016;65:1215–24.
31. Lodise TP, Fang E, Minassian SL, Prokocimer PG. Platelet profile in patients with acute bacterial skin and skin structure infections receiving tedizolid or linezolid: findings from the phase 3 ESTABLISH clinical trials. Antimicrob Agents Chemother. 2014;58:7198–204.
32. Shaw KJ, Barbachyn MR. The oxazolidinones: past, present, and future. Ann N Y Acad Sci. 2011;1241:48–70.
33. Flanagan S, Passarell J, Lu Q. Tedizolid population pharmacokinetics, exposure response, and target attainment. Antimicrob Agents Chemother. 2014;58:6462–70.
34. Lodise TP, Drusano GL. Use of pharmacokinetic/pharmacodynamic systems analyses to inform dose selection of tedizolid phosphate. Clin Infect Dis. 2014;58(Suppl 1):S28–34.
35. Tessier PR, Keel RA, Hagihara M, Crandon JL, Nicolau DP. Comparative in vivo efficacies of epithelial lining fluid exposures of tedizolid, linezolid, and vancomycin for methicillin-resistant Staphylococcus aureus in a mouse pneumonia model. Antimicrob Agents Chemother. 2012;56:2342–6.
36. Livermore DM, Warner M, Mushtaq S. Activity of MK-7655 combined with imipenem against Enterobacteriaceae and Pseudomonas aeruginosa. J Antimicrob Chemother. 2013;68: 2286–90.
37. Lucasti C, Vasile L, Sandesc D, et al. Phase 2, dose-ranging study of relebactam with imipenem-cilastatin in subjects with complicated intra-abdominal infection. Antimicrob Agents Chemother. 2016;60:6234–43.
38. Hackel MA, Lomovskaya O, Dudley MN, Karlowsky JA, Saham DF. In vitro activity of meropenem-vaborbactam against clinical isolates of KPC-positive Enterobacteriaceae. Antimicrob Agents Chemother. 2017;62:e01904-17.
39. Griffith DC, Loutit JS, Morgan EE, Durso S, Dudley MN. Phase 1 study of the safety, tolerability, and pharmacokinetics of the β-lactamase inhibitor vaborbactam (RPX7009) in healthy adult subjects. Antimicrob Agents Chemother. 2016;60:6326–32.

40. Kaye KS, Bhowmick T, Metallidis S, et al. Effect of meropenem-vaborbactam vs piperacillin-tazobactam on clinical cure or improvement and microbial eradication in complicated urinary tract infection: the TANGO I randomized clinical trial. JAMA. 2018;319:788–99.
41. Wunderink RG, Giamarellos-Bourboulis EJ, Rahav G, et al. Effect and safety of meropenem-vaborbactam versus best-available therapy in patients with carbapenem-resistant enterobacteriaceae infections: the TANGO II randomized clinical trial. Infect Dis Ther. 2018;7:439–55.
42. Hackel MA, Tsuji M, Yamano Y, Echols R, Karlowsky JA, Sahm DF. In vitro activity of the siderophore cephalosporin, cefiderocol, against carbapenem-nonsusceptible and multidrug-resistant isolates of Gram-negative bacilli collected worldwide in 2014 to 2016. Antimicrob Agents Chemother. 2018;62:e01968-17.
43. Kawaguchi N, Katsube T, Echols R, Wajima T. Population pharmacokinetic analysis of cefiderocol, a parenteral siderophore cephalosporin, in healthy subjects, subjects with various degrees of renal function, and patients with complicated urinary tract infection or acute uncomplicated pyelonephritis. Antimicrob Agents Chemother. 2018;62:e01391-17.
44. Abdallah M, Olafisoye O, Cortes C, Urban C, Landman D, Quale J. Activity of eravacycline against Enterobacteriaceae and Acinetobacter baumannii, including multidrug-resistant isolates, from New York City. Antimicrob Agents Chemother. 2015;59:1802–5.
45. Seifert H, Stefanik D, Sutcliffe JA, Higgins PG. In-vitro activity of the novel fluorocycline eravacycline against carbapenem non-susceptible Acinetobacte baumannii. Int J Antimicrob Agents. 2018;51:62–4.
46. Snydman DR, McDermott LA, Jacobus NV, Kerstein K, Grossman TH, Sutcliffe JA. Evaluation of the in vitro activity of eravacycline against a broad spectrum of recent clinical anaerobic isolates. Antimicrob Agents Chemother. 2018;62:e02206-17.
47. Solomkin J, Evans D, Slepavicius A, Lee P, et al. Assessing the efficacy and safety of eravacycline vs ertapenem in complicated intra-abdominal infections in the Investigating Gram-Negative Infections Treated with Eravacycline (IGNITE 1) trial: a randomized clinical trial. JAMA Surg. 2017;152:224–32.
48. Connors KP, Housman ST, Pope JS, et al. Phase I, open-label, safety and & pharmacokinetic study to assess bronchopulmonary disposition of intravenous eravacycline in healthy men and women. Antimicrob Agents Chemother. 2014;58:2113–8.
49. Grossman TH, Murphy TM, Slee AM, Lofland D, Sutcliffe JA. Eravacycline (TP-434) is efficacious in animal models of infection. Antimicrob Agents Chemother. 2015;59:2567–71.
50. Pfaller MA, Huband MD, Shortridge D, Flamm RK. Surveillance of omadacycline activity tested against clinical isolates from the United States and Europe as part of the 2016 SENTRY Antimicrobial Surveillance Program. Antimicrob Agents Chemother. 2018;62:e02327-17.
51. Sun H, Ting L, Machineni S, et al. Randomized, open-label study of the pharmacokinetics and safety of oral and intravenous administration of omadacycline to healthy subjects. Antimicrob Agents Chemother. 2016;60:7431–5.
52. Noel GJ, Draper MP, Hait H, Tanaka SK, Arbeit RD. A randomized, evaluator-blind, phase 2 study comparing the safety and efficacy of omadacycline to those of linezolid for treatment of complicated skin and skin structure infections. Antimicrob Agents Chemother. 2012;56:5650–4.
53. Gotfried MH, Horn K, Garrity-Ryan L, et al. Comparison of omadacycline and tigecycline pharmacokinetics in the plasma, epithelial lining fluid, and alveolar cells of healthy adult subjects. Antimicrob Agents Chemother. 2017;61:e01135-17.
54. Castanheira M, Davis AP, Mendes RE, Serio AW, Krause KM, Flamm RK. In vitro activity of plazomicin against gram-negative and gram-positive isolates collected from U.S. hospitals and comparative activities of aminoglycosides against carbapenem-resistant Enterobacteriaceae and isolates carrying carbapenemase genes. Antimicrob Agents Chemother. 2018;62:e00313-18.
55. Thwaites M, Hall D, Stoneburner A, et al. Activity of plazomicin in combination with other antibiotics against multidrug-resistant Enterobacteriaceae. Diagn Microbiol Infect Dis. 2018;92:338–45.

56. García-Salguero C, Rodríguez-Avial I, Picazo JJ, Culebras E. Can plazomicin alone or in combination be a therapeutic option against carbapenem-resistant Acinetobacter baumannii? Antimicrob Agents Chemother. 2015;59:5959–66.
57. Connolly LE, Riddle V, Cebrik D, Armstrong ES, Miller LG. A multicenter, randomized, double-blind, phase 2 study of the efficacy and safety of plazomicin compared with levofloxacin in the treatment of complicated urinary tract infection and acute pyelonephritis. Antimicrob Agents Chemother. 2018;62:e01989-17.
58. Veve MP, Wagner JL. Lefamulin: review of a promising novel pleuromutilin antibiotic. Pharmacotherapy. 2018;38:935–46.
59. Martin-Loeches I, Dale GE, Torres A. Murepavadin: a new antibiotic class in the pipeline. Expert Rev Anti Infect Ther. 2018;16:259–68.

Target Controlled Infusion in the ICU: An Opportunity to Optimize Antibiotic Therapy

38

P. Colin, K. Ferdinande, and J. J. De Waele

38.1 Introduction

Infection is a common yet important problem for patients admitted to intensive care units (ICUs) around the world and is a major cause of morbidity, mortality and costs [1]. Appropriate antibiotic therapy is a key element in the management of severe infections and it is important to achieve an adequate dose of the appropriate antibiotic at the site of infection. Treatment outcomes for severe infections remain poor, with critically ill patients having the highest mortality rates [2]. There are two important contributors to this worse outcome in critically ill patients. First, infection paradigms are largely based on infection models and clinical data that do not specifically compensate for the altered antimicrobial pharmacokinetics (PK) and severity of illness of these patients, which can lead to inadequate antibiotic dosing. Second, infections in ICU patients are increasingly caused by multidrug resistant (MDR) pathogens, which are associated with even worse outcomes [3]. This makes appropriate antibiotic therapy very challenging in critically ill patients and exemplifies the need for individualized antibiotic therapy in order to increase the accuracy of dosing and optimize outcomes [4].

In recent years, several solutions have been proposed to improve antibiotic dosing. Several studies have described the variability of antibiotic concentrations after standard dosing, and PK models have been described for many of the antibiotics commonly used in the ICU. These can help to improve antibiotic administration by

P. Colin
Department of Anesthesiology, University of Groningen, University Medical Center Groningen, Groningen, The Netherlands

Faculty of Pharmaceutical Sciences, Laboratory of Medical Biochemistry and Clinical Analysis, Ghent University, Ghent, Belgium

K. Ferdinande · J. J. De Waele (✉)
Department of Critical Care Medicine, Ghent University Hospital, Ghent, Belgium
e-mail: jan.dewaele@ugent.be

J.-L. Vincent (ed.), *Annual Update in Intensive Care and Emergency Medicine 2019*, Annual Update in Intensive Care and Emergency Medicine,
https://doi.org/10.1007/978-3-030-06067-1_38

adapting the dose of the antibiotic, the method of administration or the interval between doses. Although it is evident that dosing based on PK models results in improved target attainment, and software packages are available to be used at the bedside, individualized antibiotic dosing has not been adopted in most ICUs [5, 6].

One of the strategies to increase target attainment for β-lactam antibiotics has been the use of continuous infusion. β-lactam antibiotics are time-dependent antibiotics, which means that keeping the concentration above a target concentration increases the efficacy of the drug. Continuous infusion of selected β-lactam antibiotics is used widely in some countries, with meropenem, piperacillin/tazobactam and ceftazidime most frequently administered as continuous infusions. Other antibiotics are also increasingly administered continuously, for example, vancomycin and linezolid [6–8].

This alternative administration method offers an opportunity for the application of target-controlled infusion (TCI) for antibiotic dosing. Primarily developed as a method for improved dosing of sedatives and analgesics in anesthesia, we hypothesize that TCI may also be used to individualize and optimize antibiotic dosing. In this chapter, we will provide an overview of the current status of TCI in critical care, highlight the importance for individualized antibiotic therapy in critically ill patients and discuss potential for TCI and antibiotic therapy to optimize antibiotic exposure and maximize effectiveness.

38.2 Target-Controlled Infusion History and Current Applications

38.2.1 What is a TCI-System?

TCI is a technique of continuously infusing intravenous drugs and is mainly known in the field of anesthetics. TCI allows the clinician to target a predefined predicted concentration in a specific body compartment or tissue of interest. The computer then calculates the optimal infusion rate required to achieve this concentration as fast as possible without overshooting the target. An on-line coupled infusion pump then delivers this optimal infusion regimen to the patient. The TCI system calculates the optimal infusion rate considering several patient specific covariates (e.g., age, weight, estimated creatinine clearance and the predefined target plasma concentration). For so-called open-loop TCI systems, the infusion scheme is static, whereas in closed-loop TCI it considers feedback from (continuously) measured variables (e.g., somatosensory evoked potentials to assess the anesthetic depth, blood pressure, measured blood concentrations, exhaled drug concentrations). TCI infusion systems have been used clinically in anesthesia for over two decades with an estimated 2.6 million patients in Europe receiving drugs by TCI annually [9, 10].

38.2.2 History and Current Applications

TCI technology is based on more than 30 years of research and is commercially available for several drugs. In 1996, 'Diprifusor' was the first microprocessor target controlled system to be commercially available. Since its commercialization in 1996, more than 60,000 first- and second-generation TCI pumps have been sold worldwide. Nowadays, TCI is mainly used to administer propofol and opioids. For this purpose, an accurate PK/PD model is required. For the first commercialization of the TCI-pump there was only one PK/PD model available, namely the PK/PD model of Marsh et al. [11]. Because this PK/PD model is not the most suitable model for all patient subpopulations, new or expansions of the existing Marsh model have since been developed (e.g., the Shnider and Eleveld model). Most of the commercially available open-TCI pumps now also include an integrated PK/PD model published by Schnider et al., which offers more detailed covariate selection, such as age, sex, weight and height [12–16]. For an exhaustive overview of the history and development of currently used TCI systems the reader is referred to publications by Struys et al. and Absalom et al. [10, 17].

Propofol is the most well-known anesthetic drug for which the TCI concept is applied. In addition to the use of propofol, TCI is also used for other hypnotics, such as dexmedetomidine, and other drug classes, such as opioid and neuromuscular nondepolarizing agents [18].

38.3 Target-Controlled Infusion in Critical Care Medicine

Only a limited number of articles have described the use of TCI in critically ill patients and, so far, the focus has been on its use with hypnotics or analgesics. Propofol TCI has been used for sedating patients with respiratory failure with low tolerance to non-invasive ventilation (NIV) [19]. Arterial blood gases improved significantly in 10 patients who received TCI propofol during 85 NIV sessions. TCI enabled NIV to be well tolerated by all patients. During almost 99% of the infusion time, the sedation level was at the desired level, and patients recovered promptly [19]. Propofol TCI has been compared to midazolam for the treatment of refractory status epilepticus, and found to be equally effective, and associated with shorter hospital stays [20].

TCI has also been studied for the administration of dexmedetomidine in ICU patients. In patients after abdominal aortic aneurysm surgery, dexmedetomidine TCI requirements were much higher after remifentanil anesthesia than after fentanyl [18].

Chalumeau-Lemoine et al. evaluated remifentanil TCI in patients requiring fiberoptic bronchoscopy in a mixed ICU population. Fourteen patients received remifentanil TCI without severe hemodynamic or respiratory complications, and patients reported low pain levels [21]. Rezaiguia-Delclaux et al. also reported on the use of remifentanil TCI to facilitate fiberoptic bronchoscopy after postoperative thoracic surgery in non-intubated patients who had failed bronchoscopy by topical anesthesia. Remifentanil TCI was effective and acceptably safe [22].

In postoperative cardiac surgery patients, patient-controlled hydromorphone TCI offered satisfactory postoperative pain therapy with moderate side effects [23].

In summary, TCI is used only sparsely in the ICU and, when this is the case, it is used for the administration of hypnotics and/or analgesic drugs. Patient numbers are consistently small, and studies may be underpowered for many clinically relevant endpoints. Furthermore, studies are often non-comparative, and the advantage of TCI for critically ill patients has not been appropriately studied in the majority of them.

38.4 Target-Controlled Infusion for Antibiotic Therapy

38.4.1 Advantages of TCI for Antibiotics

In comparison to manually controlled infusions, TCI systems have several (theoretical) advantages. First, TCI systems achieve the target plasma concentration faster without a significant overshoot of the target. Whereas conventionally a loading dose followed by a maintenance dose are required to attain timely steady-state drug exposure, TCI systems automate this process by continuously adjusting the drug infusion rate to exactly match the disposition and elimination kinetics of the drug during treatment [24]. Second, treatment individualization is made easy via the use of population PK models and associated covariate models implemented in the TCI devices. In comparison to dosing nomograms, which are practicable for a limited number of patient characteristics only, there is no limit on the number of patient characteristics and the complexity of the covariate models used in population PK models. Moreover, dosage adjustments with TCI are continuous, unlike dosage adjustments described in nomograms, which are limited to discrete (practicable) changes in infusion rates, dose strengths, dosing intervals, etc.

TCI has the additional advantage of flexibility. Once adequately validated, it allows the selection of a patient-tailored target. This reduces the selection of an optimal dosing regimen for a specific patient to the selection of the appropriate target concentration for a specific patient, which is the true cornerstone of patient-tailored treatment. Moreover, the use of TCI guarantees that, once consensus has been reached on the optimal therapeutic target for a specific patient, the dosing regimen administered to reach this target will be identical across countries, hospitals, wards, etc.

Combined with the extensive experience in the field of anesthesia this offers, in our opinion, the opportunity to introduce model-informed personalized dosing of antibiotics via a dosing device that is already somewhat familiar to many practitioners. This familiarity might overcome some of the current resistance and could facilitate widespread implementation of model-informed precision dosing.

38.4.2 Available Data

Currently, data on the use of TCI in antibiotic therapy are scarce, and the aforementioned advantages of TCI over manually controlled infusions have been evaluated *in silico* by two groups of authors, in two pre-clinical studies and one clinical study. Below is an overview of available data on TCI in antibiotic therapy.

38.4.2.1 Piperacillin

Horton and Black simulated concentration time profiles following TCI, continuous infusions and intermittent bolus administrations (according to the drug label) for piperacillin. The simulations showed superior PK/pharmacodynamic (PK/PD) target attainment and a significant decrease (±30%) in total daily drug usage for the TCI group. Based on these results, the authors concluded that, for piperacillin, TCI appears to offer cost, efficacy and potential safety advantages over continuous infusions and intermittent bolus dosing [24].

38.4.2.2 Vancomycin

Colin et al. [25] conducted a clinical trial simulation based on published population PK models for vancomycin. Performance metrics, such as PK/PD target attainment and the attainment of potentially toxic concentrations, were compared between published (therapeutic drug monitoring [TDM]-based) dosing recommendations for continuous dosing and a virtual TCI system based on the Thomson model [26], with or without TDM-based Bayesian forecasting. The results showed superior performance of adaptive TCI (aTCI) (where TCI is combined with infrequent TDM sampling) over conventional dosing guidelines, most notably in the first 2 days of therapy. Moreover, the probability of attaining potentially toxic concentrations was negligible for aTCI compared to the second-best performing method (25% versus 65%). Finally, the authors found that the performance of aTCI, unlike conventional dosing strategies, was consistent across subgroups of patients within the population [25].

38.4.2.3 Amoxicillin and Fosfomycin

At present, practical experience with TCI for dosing antibiotics is very limited. In pre-clinical studies computer-controlled infusion has been used to achieve concentrations that approximate the concentration-time profile typically seen in humans following oral administration. Bugnon et al. [27] and Woodnutt and Berry [28] used this approach to deliver fosfomycin and amoxicillin in a rabbit endocarditis model and a respiratory tract infection model in rats. Although the intention in these experiments was not to target and maintain a user-defined plasma concentration target, they nicely demonstrate the versatility of computer-controlled continuous infusions and the steerability of antibiotic concentration time profiles when using TCI.

38.4.2.4 Cefepime

To the best of our knowledge, the only clinical study evaluating TCI performance with antibiotics was recently presented by Jonckheere et al. at the 2018 European Congress of Clinical Microbiology and Infectious Diseases (personal communication). Jonckheere et al. prospectively evaluated the performance of a TCI model for cefepime in a cohort of 21 ICU patients. In this study, a population PK model previously developed by the same authors, was used to target a cefepime plasma concentration of 16 mg/L for 1–5 days (median: 4.5 days). Three to fourteen (median: 10) blood samples were drawn per patient and performance metrics were characterized according to Varvel et al. [29]. The median absolute prediction error (MdAPE: a measure of accuracy) and the median prediction error (a measure of bias) were

28.7% and 20.3%, respectively. Except for the positive bias, which was caused by an overestimation of the central compartment (V1) in the tested TCI model, performance was acceptable (i.e., MdAPE <30%) and in line with the performance of current PK models used in TCI pumps in anesthesia.

38.4.3 Challenges for the Implementation of TCI for Antibiotic Therapy

At the moment, the use of TCI outside anesthesia is limited to a handful of specific applications. In our opinion, TCI is ideally suited for dosing of intravenous antibiotics (for reasons outlined earlier) and some evidence is available suggesting that patients might benefit from switching from manually controlled infusions to TCI. Nevertheless, we envision some specific challenges that should be addressed to expedite the use of TCI for antibiotic dosing.

38.4.3.1 PK Model Development

In anesthesia, data-sharing has led to the development of generic population PK models for propofol [16] and remifentanil [30]. These models have demonstrated superior predictive performance across patient subgroups compared to subgroup specific models. In the field of antibiotics, a plethora of subgroup- and context-specific population PK models derived from (very) small-sized patient cohorts exist. It was previously shown that when applied to external datasets, the performance of these PK models differs widely [31, 32]. Large scale data-sharing initiatives, such as the "Open TCI Initiative" (www.opentci.org) do not exist for antibiotics at the moment and we believe that data-sharing initiatives are necessary to develop robust and generically applicable population PK models to serve as input to antibiotic TCI systems.

38.4.3.2 Altered Pharmacokinetics in the Critically Ill Patient

An implicit assumption in current TCI systems for anesthetic drugs is that PK parameters within an individual are constant. In anesthesia, this assumption is reasonable as the length of TCI drug administration is usually restricted to (several) hours. However, appropriate antibiotic therapy often requires several days of drug dosing during which the (patho)physiological state of a patient (especially in the critically ill) might change dramatically. Hence, the assumption of constant within-individual PK parameters is likely inappropriate and TCI systems for antibiotics should therefore be able to account for dynamic (disease-related) changes during the course of treatment.

38.4.3.3 Use of Therapeutic Drug Monitoring to Enhance TCI Accuracy in the Individual Patient

In contrast to anesthetic agents where the effect of treatment is readily visible (sedation state) or easily monitored (electroencephalogram [EEG]-derived measures), no surrogate/clinical endpoints are available to guide antibiotic dosing. As a consequence, treatment individualization depends (solely) on measuring (local) antibiotic concentrations, and feedback control systems to individualize the patient's PK parameters during the drug infusion are likely needed to achieve clinically acceptable precision in PK/PD target attainment.

38.5 Future Perspectives

Opportunities for the application of TCI for antibiotic therapy in critical care are multiple. For the optimization of antibiotic treatment, dosing recommendations based on PK models and dosing simulations to identify optimized regimens are used for patients experiencing PK alterations, such as augmented renal clearance or patients infected with high-minimum inhibitory concentration (MIC) bacteria. While this approach is considered a form of therapeutic drug adaptation to improve target attainment, it is not individualized when used in a population. TDM of antibiotics on the other hand, is commonly seen as a highly individual strategy to overcome the variability in drug exposure amongst critically ill patients. Dose-adaptations based on TDM are commonly predicted and decided by the clinician, for example by increasing the dose or the dose-frequency by 25–50%; alternatively, doses could be predicted from PK software. This TDM-guided treatment individualization has been shown to increase clinical efficacy for vancomycin [33] and reduce mortality rates during aminoglycoside therapy [34]. We suggest that the same concept of TDM can be applied in the TCI system resulting in a closed-loop, adaptive, TCI system to further refine therapy (Fig. 38.1). In the case of antimicrobial drugs, feedback would ideally rely on the

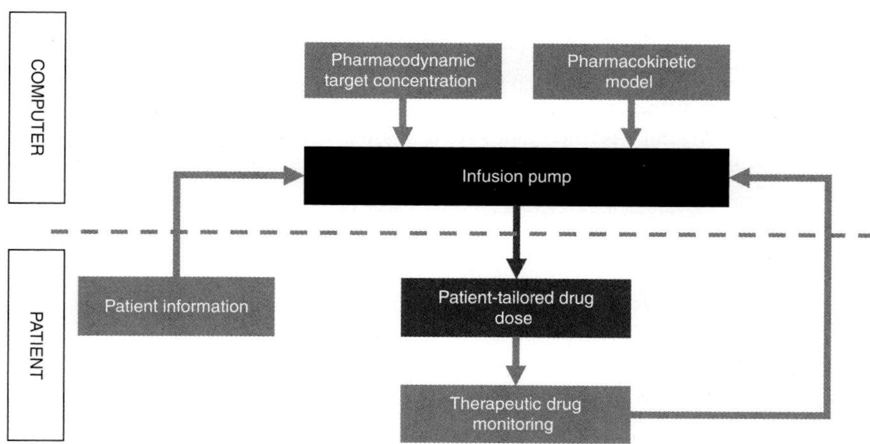

Fig. 38.1 Components of adaptive target controlled infusion of antibiotics

Table 38.1 Drugs of interest for adaptive target controlled infusion in critical care

Drug group	Drug name
Antibiotics	Piperacillin
	Ceftazidime
	Cefepime
	Meropenem
	Flucloxacillin
	Vancomycin
	Linezolid
Analgesics	Remifentanil
Hypnotics	Propofol
	Dexmedetomidine
	Pentobarbital
	Thiopental
	Ketamine
Anti-epileptics	Valproic acid
	Barbiturates

level of bacterial killing. However, in patients, it is not possible to continuously monitor the bacterial load. Therefore, we suggest that monitoring of plasma concentrations of antibiotics as a surrogate marker for (predicted) bacterial cell kill at the focus of infection can be used as feedback for the TCI pump. Closed-loop TCI has been explored mainly in the field of anesthetics, but for dose optimization of antimicrobial therapy this is a truly innovative and promising strategy to improve target attainment in critically ill patients.

The use of TCI in the ICU is not limited to the few antibiotics that have been studied so far. Apart from piperacillin, vancomycin and cefepime, the concept could also be applied to administer any drug that can be given as a continuous infusion (Table 38.1).

38.6 Conclusion

TCI has been adopted by many and is currently an established approach for administering anesthesia. In other specialties and for drugs other than those used in anesthesia, experience is very limited. As continuous infusion is also commonly used for many drugs in critical care, and as important PK variability is present for many of them, TCI can be considered an interesting concept for the ICU. More specifically, and although many challenges are present, TCI would offer a practical solution for improved administration of antibiotics. Research is needed to confirm that target attainment is better, and the role of TDM in an adaptive TCI approach also requires further investigation.

References

1. Vincent JL, Rello J, Marshall J, et al. International study of the prevalence and outcomes of infection in intensive care units. JAMA. 2009;302:2323–9.
2. Tängdén T, Ramos Martín V, Felton TW, et al. The role of infection models and PK/PD modelling for optimising care of critically ill patients with severe infections. Intensive Care Med. 2017;43:1021–32.

3. De Waele JJ, Akova M, Antonelli M, et al. Antimicrobial resistance and antibiotic stewardship programs in the ICU: insistence and persistence in the fight against resistance. A position statement from ESICM/ESCMID/WAAAR round table on multi-drug resistance. Intensive Care Med. 2018;44:189–96.
4. Roberts JA, Abdul-Aziz MH, Lipman J, et al. Individualised antibiotic dosing for patients who are critically ill: challenges and potential solutions. Lancet Infect Dis. 2014;14:498–509.
5. Wong G, Brinkman A, Benefield RJ, et al. An international, multicentre survey of β-lactam antibiotic therapeutic drug monitoring practice in intensive care units. J Antimicrob Chemother. 2014;69:1416–23.
6. Tabah A, De Waele J, Lipman J, et al. The ADMIN-ICU survey: a survey on antimicrobial dosing and monitoring in ICUs. J Antimicrob Chemother. 2015;70:2671–7.
7. Osthoff M, Siegemund M, Balestra G, Abdul-Aziz MH, Roberts JA. Prolonged administration of β-lactam antibiotics—a comprehensive review and critical appraisal. Swiss Med Wkly. 2016;146:w14368.
8. Buyle FM, Decruyenaere J, De Waele J, et al. A survey of beta-lactam antibiotics and vancomycin dosing strategies in intensive care units and general wards in Belgian hospitals. Eur J Clin Microbiol Infect Dis. 2013;32:763–8.
9. Kuizenga MH, Vereecke HE, Struys MM. Model-based drug administration: current status of target-controlled infusion and closed-loop control. Curr Opin Anaesthesiol. 2016;29:475–81.
10. Struys MM, De Smet T, Glen JI, Vereecke HE, Absalom AR, Schnider TW. The history of target-controlled infusion. Anesth Analg. 2016;122:56–69.
11. Marsh B, White M, Morton N, Kenny GN. Pharmacokinetic model driven infusion of propofol in children. Br J Anaesth. 1991;67:41–8.
12. Schnider TW, Minto CF, Struys MM, Absalom AR. The safety of target-controlled infusions. Anesth Analg. 2016;122:79–85.
13. Engbers FHM, Dahan A. Anomalies in target-controlled infusion: an analysis after 20 years of clinical use. Anaesthesia. 2018;73:619–30.
14. De Smet T, Struys MM, Greenwald S, Mortier EP, Shafer SL. Estimation of optimal modeling weights for a Bayesian-based closed-loop system for propofol administration using the bispectral index as a controlled variable: a simulation study. Anesth Analg. 2007;105:1629–38.
15. Glen JB. The development of 'Diprifusor': a TCI system for propofol. Anaesthesia. 1998;53(Suppl 1):13–21.
16. Eleveld DJ, Colin P, Absalom AR, Struys MMRF. Pharmacokinetic-pharmacodynamic model for propofol for broad application in anaesthesia and sedation. Br J Anaesth. 2018;120:942–59.
17. Absalom AR, Glen JI, Zwart GJ, Schnider TW, Struys MM. Target-controlled infusion: a mature technology. Anesth Analg. 2016;122:70–8.
18. Kunisawa T, Fujimoto K, Kurosawa A, et al. The dexmedetomidine concentration required after remifentanil anesthesia is three-fold higher than that after fentanyl anesthesia or that for general sedation in the ICU. Ther Clin Risk Manag. 2014;10:797–806.
19. Clouzeau B, Bui HN, Vargas F, et al. Target-controlled infusion of propofol for sedation in patients with non-invasive ventilation failure due to low tolerance: a preliminary study. Intensive Care Med. 2010;36:1675–80.
20. Masapu D, Gopala Krishna KN, Sanjib S, et al. A comparative study of midazolam and target-controlled propofol infusion in the treatment of refractory status epilepticus. Indian J Crit Care Med. 2018;22:441–8.
21. Chalumeau-Lemoine L, Stoclin A, Billard V, Laplanche A, Raynard B, Blot F. Flexible fiberoptic bronchoscopy and remifentanil target-controlled infusion in ICU: a preliminary study. Intensive Care Med. 2013;39:53–8.
22. Rezaiguia-Delclaux S, Laverdure F, Kortchinsky T, Lemasle L, Imbert A, Stéphan F. Fiber optic bronchoscopy and remifentanil target-controlled infusion in critically ill patients with acute hypoxaemic respiratory failure: a descriptive study. Anaesth Crit Care Pain Med. 2017;36:273–7.
23. Jeleazcov C, Ihmsen H, Saari TI, et al. Patient-controlled analgesia with target-controlled infusion of hydromorphone in postoperative pain therapy. Anesthesiology. 2016;124:56–68.

24. Horton MA, Black IH. Target controlled infusion versus traditional delivery of piperacillin: a computer model comparison. In: Proceedings of the 2009 annual meeting of the American Society Anesthesiologists. 2009. Available at: http://www.asaabstracts.com/strands/asaabstracts/abstract.htm?year=2009&index=7&absnum=43. Accessed 14 Nov 2018 (abst).
25. Colin PJ, Jonckheere S, Struys MMRF. Target-controlled continuous infusion for antibiotic dosing: proof-of-principle in an in-silico vancomycin trial in intensive care unit patients. Clin Pharmacokinet. 2018;57:1435–47.
26. Thomson AH, Staatz CE, Tobin CM, Gall M, Lovering AM. Development and evaluation of vancomycin dosage guidelines designed to achieve new target concentrations. J Antimicrob Chemother. 2009;63:1050–7.
27. Bugnon D, Potel G, Xiong YQ, et al. Bactericidal effect of pefloxacin and fosfomycin against Pseudomonas aeruginosa in a rabbit endocarditis model with pharmacokinetics of pefloxacin in humans simulated in vivo. Eur J Clin Microbiol Infect Dis. 1997;16:575–80.
28. Woodnutt G, Berry V. Two pharmacodynamic models for assessing the efficacy of amoxicillin-clavulanate against experimental respiratory tract infections caused by strains of Streptococcus pneumoniae. Antimicrob Agents Chemother. 1999;43:29–34.
29. Varvel JR, Donoho DL, Shafer SL. Measuring the predictive performance of computer-controlled infusion pumps. J Pharmacokinet Biopharm. 1992;20:63–94.
30. Eleveld DJ, Proost JH, Vereecke H, et al. An allometric model of remifentanil pharmacokinetics and pharmacodynamics. Anesthesiology. 2017;126:1005–18.
31. Wong G, Farkas A, Sussman R, et al. Comparison of the accuracy and precision of pharmacokinetic equations to predict free meropenem concentrations in critically ill patients. Antimicrob Agents Chemother. 2015;59:1411–7.
32. Felton TW, Roberts JA, Lodise TP, et al. Individualization of piperacillin dosing for critically ill patients: dosing software to optimize antimicrobial therapy. Antimicrob Agents Chemother. 2014;58:4094–102.
33. Ye ZK, Tang HL, Zhai SD. Benefits of therapeutic drug monitoring of vancomycin: a systematic review and meta-analysis. PLoS One. 2013;8:e77169.
34. Whipple JK, Ausman RK, Franson T, Quebbeman EJ. Effect of individualized pharmacokinetic dosing on patient outcome. Crit Care Med. 1991;19:1480–5.

Antimicrobial Stewardship in Sepsis

39

E. Plata-Menchaca, E. Esteban, and R. Ferrer

39.1 Introduction

Sepsis is a leading cause of death and life-threatening condition, affecting more than 19 million people each year, in which chances of survival mainly depend upon the effective accomplishment of timely, accurate, rational and protocolized treatment interventions [1, 2]. Current initiatives aimed to improve sepsis awareness and early treatment are intended to halt the catastrophic consequences of systemic errors occurring even within some experienced medical institutions where training programs promoting early sepsis diagnosis and management protocols are being encouraged [3].

In recent years, high-quality evidence has demonstrated the development of standardized approaches for protocolized care and early resuscitation in sepsis to be the best approach not only to reduce deaths, but also to prevent such systemic errors [4]. The Surviving Sepsis Campaign (SSC) guidelines established a set of recommendations, including the early administration of broad-spectrum antibiotics, preferably within 1 h from time of presentation [2, 5]. Furthermore, the current SSC bundle update [6] is an instrument in which authors simplified the 3- and 6-h bundles into the 1-h bundle as a means of providing health-care education and achieving improvements in sepsis management. A summary of the SSC bundles from 2012 to 2018 is provided in Box 39.1.

E. Plata-Menchaca
Research Department, Institut de Investigació Biomèdica de Bellvitge, L'Hospitalet de Llobregat, Barcelona, Spain

E. Esteban
Pediatric Intensive Care Unit, Hospital Sant Joan de Déu, Barcelona, Spain

R. Ferrer (✉)
Intensive Care Department, Hospital Universitario Vall d'Hebron, Barcelona, Spain

Shock, Organ Dysfunction and Resuscitation Research Group, Vall d'Hebron Research Institute, Barcelona, Spain
e-mail: r.ferrer@vhebron.net

J.-L. Vincent (ed.), *Annual Update in Intensive Care and Emergency Medicine 2019*, Annual Update in Intensive Care and Emergency Medicine,
https://doi.org/10.1007/978-3-030-06067-1_39

Box 39.1: Surviving Sepsis Campaign Bundles from 2012 to 2018

2012	2016	2018
6-h Resuscitation bundle: 1. Measure serum lactate. 2. Obtain blood cultures prior to antibiotic administration. 3. Administer broad-spectrum antibiotics within 3 h from time of presentation. 4. In the event of hypotension and/or lactate >4 mmol/L: (a) Deliver an initial minimum of 20 mL/kg of crystalloid (or colloid equivalent). (b) Apply vasopressors for hypotension not responding to initial fluid resuscitation to maintain mean arterial pressure (MAP) ≥65 mmHg. 5. In the event of persistent hypotension despite fluid resuscitation and/or lactate >4 mmol/L: (a) Achieve central venous pressure (CVP) of ≥8 mmHg. (b) Achieve central venous oxygen saturation ($ScvO_2$) of ≥70%. **24-h Management bundle:** 1. Administer low-dose steroids for septic shock in accordance with a standardized ICU policy. 2. Administer drotrecogin alfa (activated) in accordance with a standardized ICU policy. 3. Maintain glucose control ≥lower limit of normal, but <150 mg/dL. 4. Maintain inspiratory plateau pressures <30 cm H_2O for mechanically ventilated patients.	**3-h bundle:** 1. Measure serum lactate. 2. Obtain blood cultures prior to antibiotic administration. 3. Administer broad-spectrum antibiotics within 3 h from time of presentation. 4. Administer 30 mL/kg crystalloid for hypotension or lactate ≥4 mmol/L **6-h bundle:** 1. Apply vasopressors for hypotension not responding to initial fluid resuscitation to maintain MAP ≥65 mmHg. 2. In the event of persistent hypotension despite fluid resuscitation and/or lactate >4 mmol/L: (a) Measure CVP. (b) Measure $ScvO_2$ of ≥70%. 3. Re-measure lactate if initial lactate was elevated.	**1-h bundle:** 1. Measure lactate level. Re-measure if initial lactate is >2 mmol/L (Weak recommendation, low quality of evidence). 2. Obtain blood cultures prior to administration of antibiotics (Best practice statement). 3. Administer broad-spectrum antibiotics (Strong recommendation, moderate quality of evidence). 4. Rapidly administer 30 mL/kg crystalloid for hypotension or lactate ≥4 mmol/L (Strong recommendation, low quality of evidence). 5. Apply vasopressors if patient is hypotensive during or after fluid resuscitation to maintain MAP ≥65 mmHg (Strong recommendation, moderate quality of evidence).

As patient outcomes are time-dependent and first medical contact represents a crucial element initiating a series of actions, all healthcare professionals facing a suspected case of sepsis should be able to perform initial support interventions even while waiting for a clearer diagnosis and treatment [7]. Indeed, cases of suspected sepsis pose a great opportunity to apply the 1-h bundle when chances to survive are higher [8].

Substantial agreement exists among international experts regarding the establishment of earlier interventions to overcome barriers precluding definitive actions when facing a suspected case of sepsis. As such, novel concepts have recently been introduced, as significant delays in the time lapse from first medical contact to administration of antimicrobial therapy have been observed in pre- and in-hospital settings [9]. The 'door-to-needle' time of 60 min for antibiotic administration has been proposed, depicting global concerns regarding setting up a time-window for effective treatment after the onset of symptoms [10]. Nevertheless, attaining effective application of institutional protocols for antimicrobial administration within 1 h of presentation remains a challenge. Existing variations determining immediate medication availability [10], general beliefs regarding sepsis severity, institutional policies, etc., hinder initiatives aimed to encourage improvements in quality of care. Moreover, according to the Infectious Disease Society of America (IDSA), stipulating an aggressive, fixed-time period may lead to unintended consequences. There is an increased likelihood of prescribing broad-spectrum antibiotics to patients with sepsis-like syndromes in the rush to meet the fixed timeframe stipulated for infected patients.

Global concerns regarding the best antimicrobial stewardship interventions are being constantly recognized. As such, an outlook into the importance, recent evidence and current strategies regarding antimicrobial stewardship will be presented in this chapter.

39.2 Why Creating an Appropriate Antibiotic Stewardship Program is Crucial?

Sepsis is a time-dependent condition in which administration of early empirical antibiotic treatment and effective source control, improve changes in survival. Nevertheless, the frequency of multidrug resistance has been dramatically increasing worldwide, thus limiting our therapeutic arsenal. Some estimates suggest that antimicrobial resistance will be responsible for around 10 million deaths annually by 2050 [11]. The World Health Organization (WHO) reported more than 50% of strains of *Escherichia coli* and *Klebsiella pneumoniae* were resistant to third generation cephalosporins and quinolones in many areas worldwide [12]. Furthermore, an overwhelming increase in carbapenem-resistant microorganisms, and extended-spectrum β-lactamase (ESBL) producers have been reported. Multidrug resistant (MDR) microorganisms increase mortality, hospital length of stay and associated costs [13]. This latter situation turns especially dramatic in sepsis, where adequate empirical antibiotic therapy is critical for survival. Several initiatives have been adopted to fight against this phenomenon, in the way that governments and health agencies have taken over different policies stimulating the development of new antibiotics and optimizing the use of current agents. A judicious and optimal use of antimicrobials is the core objective of their efforts.

Antibiotic stewardship has been defined as "the optimal selection, dosage and duration of antimicrobial treatment that results in the best clinical outcome for the treatment or prevention of infection, with minimal toxicity to patients and minimal impact in subsequent resistance" [14]. The best antimicrobial therapy was defined by Joseph and Rodvold as the four Ds: "right drug, right dose, de-escalation and right duration" [15]. We may add that the best antimicrobial therapy should have minimal adverse effects and, under the best conditions, an acceptable cost. In addition, antibiotic stewardship implies de-escalation (substituting an initial antibiotic treatment for coverage with a narrower spectrum regimen), removing some agents in the case of multidrug therapies, and/or shortening treatment duration.

Despite the fact that antibiotic stewardship has been recognized as good practice by clinicians and healthcare institutions, its implementation has been observed to be widely variable in different settings. Niederman and Soulountsi [16] described how conductance of a de-escalation strategy in ventilator-associated pneumonia (VAP) varied from 23% to 74%. The authors also determined some barriers for undertaking such a strategy [16]. The main obstacles for performing adequate antibiotic stewardship were: fear of patient deterioration, fear of patients being colonized by microorganisms different from those initially isolated, unwillingness to reduce coverage when culture results are negative, and lack of local guidelines for de-escalation. The real concern of intensivists when taking care of patients with sepsis, is to determine whether antibiotic stewardship represents safe practice. This question seems crucial, considering that patient cure is our main goal. Different tools have been developed in order to ensure antibiotic stewardship is safe. These include the development of antibiotic stewardship programs, novel microorganism identification techniques and the use of biomarkers to guide decisions.

Combination antibiotic therapy is commonly required to ensure adequate empiric coverage, yet pathogen isolation or a favorable clinical response, even with negative culture results, allow "getting it right up front" treatment to be subsequently narrowed into a tailored therapy of the shortest acceptable duration [17]. The main purposes of antibiotic de-escalation programs are focused on reducing antimicrobial resistance and adverse drug-related events. However, the frequency of antibiotic de-escalation has been widely variable among studies. Mokart et al. [18] reported that de-escalation occurred in 40% of septic patients in an oncologic intensive care unit (ICU), although it had no impact on patient outcomes. Adequate empirical antibiotic treatment and compliance to guidelines for the use of empirical anti-pseudomonal antibiotics were independently associated with the frequency of de-escalation [18]. Several initiatives promoting streamlining of antimicrobial therapy have been implemented to increase the frequency of antibiotic de-escalation. The ABISS-Edusepsis project (AntiBiotic Intervention in Severe Sepsis, www.edusepsis.org), evaluated the impact of a quality improvement intervention focused on time-to-antibiotic in patients with severe sepsis. After the intervention, time-to-antibiotic in children was reduced from 60 (21.2–131.2) to 30 (21.1–60) min ($p < 0.001$). The percentage of patients who had antibiotic de-escalation was 50% and 48% before and after the intervention, respectively [19]. Similar results have been observed in adults. In Spain, an educational intervention consisting of a multifaceted educational program on sepsis care (with special emphasis on antimicrobial management) was performed. This intervention involved medical and nursing staff from different hospital departments (emergency department, medical and surgical wards, and ICU) [20]. In this trial, which included 2628 adult patients in 72 ICUs, a non-significant reduction in mortality was observed; however, the mean time from sepsis onset to empirical antibiotic therapy was reduced (2.5 ± 3.6 vs 2.0 ± 2.7 h, p = 0.002), the proportion of inappropriate empirical treatments was decreased (8.9% vs 6.5%, p = 0.024), and the proportion of patients in whom antibiotic treatment was de-escalated was increased (16.3% vs 20.1%, p = 0.004). Of note, the observed benefits after the intervention were maintained during the long-term follow-up period.

39.3 Antimicrobial Stewardship Programs

Antimicrobial stewardship programs have been created to support physicians' decisions, in order to ensure appropriate antimicrobial treatments (Fig. 39.1). Each hospital should create specialized teams addressed to organize such

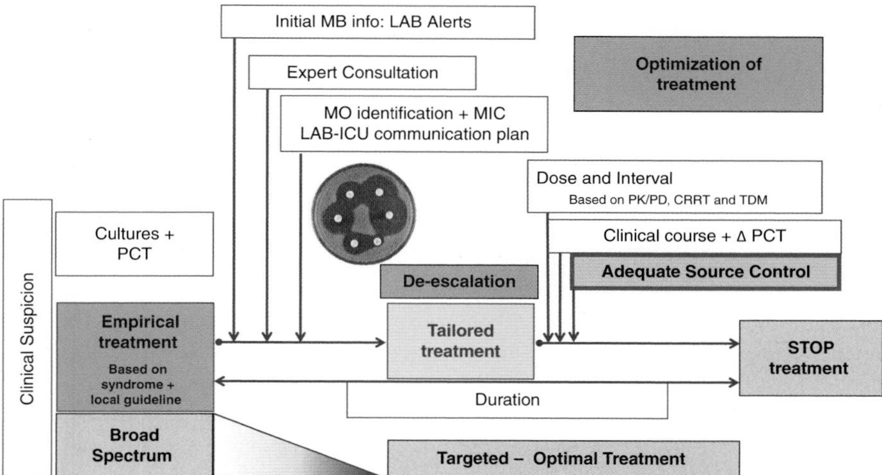

Fig. 39.1 Antibiotic stewardship for sepsis. Empirical treatment should be established within the first hour of diagnosis, according to clinical suspicion. De-escalation begins when narrowing antimicrobial spectrum: tailored treatment. Optimization of treatment doses and search for adequate source control are crucial steps for appropriate antimicrobial prescription. When achieving clinical improvement and completing treatment course, stop antimicrobials. Antibiotic oversight/expert consultations and closed-loop communications between laboratory (LAB) and the intensive care unit (ICU) should be encouraged. *PCT* procalcitonin, *MB* microbiological, *MO* microorganism, *MIC* minimum inhibitory concentration, *PK/PD* pharmacokinetics/pharmacodynamics, *CRRT* continuous renal replacement therapy, *TDM* therapeutic drug monitoring, *ΔPCT* change in procalcitonin concentration

Box 39.2: Stewardship Interventions to Improve Antimicrobial Use (Defined by the Centers for Disease Control and Prevention) [21]

a. Broad interventions	
Antibiotic "time-outs"	Reevaluation of the continuing need for or choice of antimicrobial 48 h after the onset of the therapy.
Prior authorization	Restrict the use of some antibiotics to ensure that use is reviewed with an expert.
Prospective audit and feedback	The audits are conducted by experts other than the treating team.
b. Pharmacy-driven interventions	
Automatic changes from intravenous to oral antibiotic	For selected antibiotics in adequate situations
Dose adjustments	In case of organ dysfunction
Dose optimization	Optimizing therapy for highly drug-resistant bacteria
Automatic alerts in situations where treatment might be unnecessarily duplicative	Simultaneous use of multiple antimicrobials with the same spectra
Time-sensitive automatic stop orders	Specially in case of surgical prophylaxis

programs, according to their available staff and budget [7]. There is no fixed mold for ideal team creation, therefore, each hospital should try to adapt its own program to surrounding circumstances. The Centers for Disease Control and Prevention (CDC) has identified seven core elements to obtain an efficacious model: leadership commitment, drug expertise, action, accountability, tracking, reporting and education. Interventions to improve antimicrobial use are summarized in Box 39.2 [21].

Most specialized teams include an infectious disease physician or pharmacist, microbiologist, hospital epidemiologist and clinicians in charge. In sepsis, intensivists with expertise in management of severe infections play a determinant role. Antimicrobial stewardship programs use several strategies, such as restrictive prescriptive authorities (their role is limited in sepsis, when antibiotics are emergently needed), prospective review and feedback, educational programs, decisions based on clinical guidelines, dose optimization based on drug pharmacokinetic/pharmacodynamic (PK/PD) properties and computer-assisted decision support programs. Yet, are antimicrobial stewardship programs useful? Zhang and Singh conducted a systematic review including studies assessing antimicrobial stewardship programs in different ICUs [22]. They found that 85% of studies had positive results for one or more of the following outcomes: the frequency of antibiotic use, ICU length of stay, antibiotic drug resistance and prescription-associated costs [22]. Of note, many studies have demonstrated the utility of antimicrobial stewardship programs in improving antibiotic prescription policies and reducing the economic burden of antibiotic prescription, albeit there are few data demonstrating that antimicrobial stewardship programs are effective to reduce antibiotic resistance.

39.4 Duration of Antimicrobial Therapy in Sepsis

Disregarding specific situations (e.g., infective endocarditis, Gram-negative meningitis), prolonged antimicrobial therapy has not been demonstrated to be beneficial. Indeed, it implies a higher risk of drug-associated adverse effects, higher economic costs and ICU/hospital length of stay and antimicrobial resistance. Fortunately, the general belief stipulating that 'the more severe the infection, the longer the therapy should be' has been increasingly substituted by shorter antibiotic courses while achieving the same effectiveness. In a review article on the duration of antimicrobial therapy in the ICU, Zilahi et al. concluded that shorter antibiotic courses were effective and safe, although they did not recommend a "one size fits all" approach for all situations [23]. Pugh et al. compared 8-day versus 5-day courses of antibiotic therapy for VAP and showed that shorter courses of therapy increased antibiotic-free days and reduced VAP infections caused by MDR microorganisms, while not adversely affecting mortality or treatment failure rates [24]. Chotiprasitsakul et al. demonstrated that shorter (6–10 days) versus longer regimens (11–16 days) for *Enterobacteriaceae* bacteremia had similar results on clinical outcomes; but a protective effect against MDR Gram-negative bacteria was observed [25]. Short courses of treatment for invasive meningococcal disease (4-day versus 7-day courses) were also successful without worsening the risk of recurrence [26].

Nevertheless, in some circumstances, duration of therapy cannot be well-defined, as adjustments of antimicrobial prescription mainly rely on effective source control [27]. Therefore, although initiation of antibiotics may represent a difficult decision, stopping antibiotic therapy often proves to be even more difficult in some situations. The clinical course of complicated intra-abdominal infections and infected necrotizing pancreatitis is often protracted, as timely effective control of infection cannot be achieved in some cases, favoring the emergence of antimicrobial resistance and making antimicrobial stewardship challenging.

39.5 Optimization of Antimicrobial Therapy in Sepsis: Pharmacokinetics and Pharmacodynamics

No specific dosing recommendations exist for antibiotics when treating septic patients, limiting applicability of conventional recommendations in this clinical setting, in which both PK and PD are significantly altered. Antimicrobial PK and PD are important considerations for antibiotic success, which may be particularly relevant in critically ill patients with sepsis and septic shock. Pathophysiologic changes in sepsis have major effects on PK by increasing volume of distribution and augmenting drug clearance, resulting in underdosing of antibiotics frequently administered at conventional doses [28]. Furthermore, important changes in drug metabolism are frequently observed in critically ill patients with sepsis. All of these changes may result in failure to achieve PD targets for antimicrobials and bacteriological cure, and emergence of antibiotic resistance. Alternative approaches to conventional antimicrobial management include the use of prolonged infusions of some antibiotics and/or higher doses.

39.6 Diagnostic Stewardship

Diagnostic stewardship is defined by the Global Antimicrobial Resistance Surveillance System, developed by the WHO, as the "coordinated guidance and interventions to improve appropriate use of microbiological diagnostics to guide therapeutic decisions". This system promotes appropriate and timely diagnostic testing, including specimen collection, pathogen identification and accurate and timely reporting of results [29]. The implementation of diagnostic stewardship takes into consideration different actions, such as regulatory laboratory policies allowing physicians to refuse requested diagnostic tests if not appropriate, and educational interventions to train practitioners in appropriate requesting and correct sampling. Morgan et al. pointed out the potential drawbacks of diagnostic stewardship: reducing diagnostic test requests, missed diagnoses and the need for close clinical monitoring of patients to ensure safety of actions [30]. In addition, clinicians should accurately interpret positive cultures, identifying those patients with colonization without infection.

One barrier to antimicrobial stewardship defined by Niederman and Soulountsi [16] was fear of not treating the causative microorganism in case of negative culture results. It is well-known that chances of positivity of microbiological cultures in the ICU setting are low. The international Extended Study on Prevalence of Infection in Intensive Care (EPIC II) reported a positivity rate of cultures of 51.4% [31]. When conventional methods for microbiological identification are used, the time required to obtain results often exceeds the critical decision time, precluding antimicrobial stewardship implementation. This situation becomes particularly relevant in sepsis, where delays from first medical contact to appropriate antibiotic therapy have been associated with an increased risk of death [9, 32].

Conversely, far-ranging opportunities are continuously arising for major innovations in antimicrobial stewardship when treating sepsis, as a consequence of continuous advances in diagnostic tools based on molecular microbiology. New technologies, such as the matrix-assisted laser desorption ionization-time of flight (MALDI-TOF), mass spectrometry and polymerase chain reaction (PCR)-assays, may improve appropriateness of therapy and favor antimicrobial stewardship [33, 34]. To date, these techniques might improve patient care and antibiotic streamlining, but effort is still needed to translate improvements in early microbiological diagnosis into fast and appropriate action by physicians. Rapid diagnostic tests must be interpreted with caution. The process of ordering and interpreting sophisticated diagnostic tests represents a complex and sometimes confounding task, favoring false-positive results. It is not uncommon that clinicians request unsuitable diagnostic tests without considering the whole picture of each clinical condition.

39.7 Biomarkers to Guide Antimicrobial Stewardship in Sepsis

Currently, there are several biomarkers being used as infection biomarkers. C-reactive protein (CRP) and procalcitonin (PCT) are the most widely studied. PCT is a biomarker of host response to bacterial infection. The half-life of PCT is around 24 h and a progressive decrease in PCT levels is commonly seen in well-controlled infections. Studies have shown how PCT-based algorithms have decreased antimicrobial consumption without adversely affecting clinical outcomes in some clinical situations [35, 36]. For treatment of low respiratory tract infections, a meta-analysis showed significant reductions in duration of therapy when implementing PCT-guided antibiotic treatment [37]. However, a recent randomized study did not show any reduction in antibiotics with PCT-guided antibiotic use than with standard care [38]; as such, a PCT-guided approach may not be adequate for this group of patients. In more severe infections, such as sepsis, PCT levels of <0.5 ng/mL or a decrease by 80% of the highest PCT peak concentration level have been observed to be useful to support the clinical decision of stopping antibiotics while also predicting favorable outcomes [35, 39]. Nevertheless, PCT is a non-specific biomarker of infection as it can be affected by other infection-like inflammatory conditions, making its interpretation challenging when treating surgical patients. The PCT-based algorithm was not observed to be useful in a single-center study of patients with intraabdominal infection and septic shock [40]. Jordan et al. demonstrated that PCT was useful to diagnose bacterial infection in children undergoing on-pump cardiac surgery; however, a higher PCT cut-off of 2 ng/mL was used, rather than the classic cut-off for medical patients [41]. CRP may also play a role in antibiotic stewardship. A recent trial of patients with sepsis found that CRP was as useful as PCT for reducing antibiotic use, with no associated harm [42].

Infection biomarkers are widely used in daily clinical practice as tools to support antibiotic discontinuation in sepsis, providing an opportunity to improve patient care; however, they do not substitute for clinical judgement. PCT-based algorithms have been incorporated in many antimicrobial stewardship programs. Of note, cut-off levels for each biomarker must be carefully interpreted according to the clinical condition of each patient.

39.8 The Impact of Antimicrobial Stewardship: Expectations and Concerns

According to Doron and Davidson, antimicrobial stewardship programs should consider the following three goals: help physicians to select the most appropriate antibiotic, avoid antibiotic overuse and minimize the spread of antimicrobial resistance [43]. During the last 15 years, antimicrobial stewardship programs incorporating these three goals have been developed in different institutions, and been promoted by governments and public health organizations as well.

So far, we have summarized antimicrobial stewardship definitions, institutions and settings in which antimicrobial stewardship occurs, and tools for its safe implementation. However, modification of antibiotic prescription dogmas is urgently needed. Despite the existing barriers and lack of evidence supporting the efficacy of antimicrobial stewardship programs in preventing drug-resistance, we can ascertain that we are moving in that direction. Until recently, most studies were observational and evidence was limited. Some recent studies have provided new data to support antimicrobial stewardship programs in terms of preventing drug-resistance. Molina et al. [44] conducted a quasi-experimental multifaceted educational intervention focused on antimicrobial stewardship programs in a tertiary-care hospital. The authors found a sustained reduction in antimicrobial consumption, a tendency to reduced candidemia and MDR bacteremia, and reduced mortality after the intervention [44]. Possibly, more time is needed for the effect of these initiatives to be noticed.

The major concern regarding increased antimicrobial stewardship programs is the phenomenon denominated 'squeezing the balloon': diminishing the use of one class of antimicrobials could result in an increased tendency to prescribe one antibiotic over another, favoring development of drug resistance. For example, the use of quinolones to treat *Pseudomonas aeruginosa* could result in resistance to both quinolones and carbapenems [45]. The use of clinical guidelines and close surveillance provided by antimicrobial stewardship programs could help counter this concern.

When treating suspicious or confirmed cases of sepsis, clinicians must prescribe a broad-spectrum antimicrobial within the first hour of diagnosis to reduce the risk of morbidity and mortality; yet, this is not the most challenging skill to learn. Beyond this, clinicians should try to optimize prescriptions when possible, being sensible regarding the responsibility broad-spectrum empirical antibiotic treatment involves. Not only will antimicrobial stewardship benefit our patients, it will also limit drug adverse effects and undesirable consequences of acquiring resistant infections. This latter issue represents a key point in order to protect patients against potential MDR infections.

Currently, antimicrobial stewardship programs are one of the best strategies to be introduced into a hospital setting. Leadership, team work, antimicrobial stewardship frameworks, clinical guideline recommendations on optimal duration of treatments, de-escalation, PCT-based algorithms and new diagnostic stewardship approaches will help us to improve quality of care.

39.9 Conclusion

Sepsis is a time-dependent medical emergency in which standardized approaches have been developed, using existing evidence, to provide recommendations for management in order to lessen heterogeneity and improve patient outcomes. Although antibiotic stewardship in sepsis should be assumed as inherent to this process, its global diffusion is still challenging.

Beyond advances in sepsis management, educational interventions can still improve the delivery of care and patient outcomes. Educational and training programs should be further assessed and encouraged in order to ensure effective application of current evidence on appropriate empirical antibiotic prescription, reduce the time from sepsis onset to antibiotic treatment, improve assessment of risk factors for MDR bacteria and ensure appropriate and timely de-escalation, along with ongoing maintenance of these skills. ICU staff training on the acquisition of core interventions focused on best practice standards while performing an antibiotic stewardship program should be advocated, in order to bring reasoning into antibiotic prescriptions in daily clinical practice.

References

1. Adhikari NK, Fowler RA, Bhagwanjee S, Rubenfeld GD. Critical care and the global burden of critical illness in adults. Lancet. 2010;376:1339–46.
2. Rhodes A, Evans LE, Alhazzani W, et al. Surviving sepsis campaign: international guidelines for management of sepsis and septic shock: 2016. Intensive Care Med. 2017;43:304–77.
3. Staunton O, Staunton C. The urgency of now: attacking the sepsis crisis. Crit Care Med. 2018;46:809–10.
4. Coz Yataco A, Jaehne AK, Rivers EP. Protocolized early sepsis care is not only helpful for patients: it prevents medical errors. Crit Care Med. 2017;45:464–72.
5. Ferrer R, Martin-Loeches I, Phillips G, et al. Empiric antibiotic treatment reduces mortality in severe sepsis and septic shock from the first hour: results from a guideline-based performance improvement program. Crit Care Med. 2014;42:1749–55.
6. Levy MM, Evans LE, Rhodes A. The surviving sepsis campaign bundle: 2018 update. Intensive Care Med. 2018;44:925–9283.
7. Vincent JL, Pereira AJ, Gleeson J, De Backer D. Early management of sepsis. Clin Exp Emerg Med. 2014;1:3.
8. Prescott HC, Cope TM, Gesten FC. Reporting of sepsis cases for performance measurement versus for reimbursement in New York State. Crit Care Med. 2018;46:666–73.
9. Seymour CW, Kahn JM, Martin-Gill C, et al. Delays from first medical contact to antibiotic administration for sepsis. Crit Care Med. 2017;45:759–65.
10. Laupland KB, Ferrer R. Is it time to implement door-to-needle time for "infection attacks"? Intensive Care Med. 2017;43:1712–3.
11. O'Neill J. Antimicrobial resistance: tackling a crisis for the health and wealth of nations. 2014. Available at: https://amr-review.org/sites/default/files/AMR Review Paper.pdf. Accessed 13 Nov 2018.
12. World Health Organization. Antimicrobial resistance global report on surveillance. 2014. Available at http://www.who.int/iris/bitstream/10665/112642/1/9789241564748_eng.pdf. Accessed 13 Nov 2018.
13. Cosgrove SE. The relationship between antimicrobial resistance and patient outcomes: mortality, length of hospital stay, and health care costs. Clin Infect Dis. 2006;42(Suppl 2): S82–9.
14. Gerding DN. The search for good antimicrobial stewardship. Jt Comm J Qual Improv. 2001;27:403–4.
15. Joseph J, Rodvold KA. The role of carbapenems in the treatment of severe nosocomial respiratory tract infections. Expert Opin Pharmacother. 2008;9:561–75.
16. Niederman MS, Soulountsi V. De-escalation therapy: is it valuable for the management of ventilator-associated pneumonia? Clin Chest Med. 2011;32:517–34.
17. Kollef MH. Broad-spectrum antimicrobials and the treatment of serious bacterial infections: getting it right up front. Clin Infect Dis. 2008;47:S3–S13.
18. Mokart D, Slehofer G, Lambert J, et al. De-escalation of antimicrobial therapy in neutropenic patients with severe sepsis: results from an observational study. Intensive Care Med. 2014;40:41–9.

19. Esteban E, Belda S, García-Soler P, et al. A multifaceted educational intervention shortened time to antibiotic administration in children with severe sepsis and septic shock: ABISS Edusepsis pediatric study. Intensive Care Med. 2017;43:1916–8.
20. Ferrer R, Martínez ML, Gomà G, et al. Improved empirical antibiotic treatment of sepsis after an educational intervention: the ABISS-Edusepsis study. Crit Care. 2018;22:167.
21. Pollack LA, Srinivasan A. Core elements of hospital antibiotic stewardship programs from the Centers for Disease Control and Prevention. Clin Infect Dis. 2014;59:S97–S100.
22. Zhang WZ, Singh S. Antibiotic stewardship programmes in intensive care units: why, how and where are they leading us. World J Crit Care Med. 2015;4:13–28.
23. Zilahi G, McMahon MA, Povoa P, Martin-Loeches I. Duration of antibiotic in the intensive care unit. J Thorac Dis. 2016;8:3774–80.
24. Pugh R, Grant C, Cooke RP, Dempsey G. Short-course versus prolonged-course antibiotic therapy for hospital-acquired pneumoniae in critically ill adults. Cochrane Database Syst Rev. 2015;2015:CD007577.
25. Chotiprasitsakul D, Jan JH, Cosgrove SE, et al. Comparing the outcomes of adults with Enterobacteriaceae bacteremia receiving short-course versus prolonged-course antibiotic therapy in a multicenter propensity score-matched cohort. Clin Infect Dis. 2018;66:172–7.
26. Cabellos C, Pelegrin I, Benavent E, et al. Invasive meningococcal disease: Impact of a short course therapy. A DOOR/RADAR study. J Infect. 2017;75:420–3.
27. Martínez ML, Ferrer R, Torrents E, et al. Impact of source control in patients with severe sepsis and septic shock. Crit Care Med. 2017;45:11–9.
28. Ulldemolins M, Vaquer S, Llaurado-Serra M, et al. Beta-lactam dosing in critically ill patients with septic shock and continuous renal replacement therapy. Crit Care. 2014;18:227.
29. World Health Organization. Global antimicrobial resistance surveillance system: manual for early implementation. 2015. Available at: http://www.who.int/antimicrobial-resistance/publications/surveillance-system-manual/en/. Accessed 13 Nov 2018.
30. Morgan DJ, Malani P, Diekema DJ. Diagnostic stewardship-leveraging the laboratory to improve antimicrobial use. JAMA. 2017;318:607–8.
31. Vincent JL, Rello J, Marshall J, et al. International study of prevalence and outcomes of infections in intensive care units. JAMA. 2009;302:2323–9.
32. Zaragoza R, Artero A, Camarena JJ, Sancho S, González R, Nogueira JM. The influence of inadequate empirical antimicrobial treatment in patients with bloodstream infections in an intensive care unit. Clin Microbiol Infect. 2003;9:412–8.
33. Beganovic M, Costello M, Wieczorkiewicz SM. Effect of Matrix-assisted laser desorption ionization-time of flight Mass spectrometry (MALDI-TOF MS) alone versus MALDI-TOF MS combined with real-time antimicrobial stewardship interventions on time to optimal antimicrobial therapy in patients with positive blood cultures. J Clin Microbiol. 2017;55:1437–45.
34. Frye AM, Baker CA, Rustvold DL, et al. Clinical impact of a real-time PCR-assay for rapid identification of staphylococcal bacteremia. J Clin Microbiol. 2012;50:127–33.
35. Bouadma L, Luyt CE, Tubach F, et al. Use of procalcitonin to reduce patient's exposure to antibiotics in intensive care units (PRORATA trial): a multicentre randomised controlled trial. Lancet. 2010;375:463–74.
36. de Jong E, van Oers JA, Beishuizen A, et al. Efficacy and safety of procalcitonin guidance in reducing the duration of antibiotic treatment in critically ill patients: a randomised, controlled open-label trial. Lancet Infect Dis. 2016;16:819–27.
37. Schuetz P, Wirz Y, Sager R, et al. Effect of procalcitonin-guided antibiotic treatment on mortality in acute respiratory infections: a patient level metaanalysis. Lancet Infect Dis. 2018;18:95–107.
38. Huang DT, Yealy DM, Filbin MR. Procalcitonin-guided use of antibiotics for lower respiratory tract infection. N Engl J Med. 2018;379:236–49.
39. Sager R, Kutz A, Mueller B, Schuetz P. Procalcitonin-guided diagnosis and antibiotic stewardship revisited. BMC Med. 2017;15:1–11.
40. Jung B, Molinari N, Nasri M, et al. Procalcitonin biomarker kinetics fails to predict treatment response in perioperative abdominal infections with septic shock. Crit Care. 2013;17:R255.

41. Garcia IJ, Gargallo MB, Torné EE, et al. Procalcitonin: a useful biomarker to discriminate infection after cardiopulmonary bypass in children. Pediatr Crit Care Med. 2012;13:441–5.
42. Oliveira CF, Botoni FA, Oliveira CR, et al. Procalcitonin versus C-reactive protein for guiding antibiotic therapy in sepsis: a randomized trial. Crit Care Med. 2013;41:2336–43.
43. Doron S, Davidson LE. Antimicrobial stewardship. Mayo Clin Proc. 2011;86:1113–23.
44. Molina J, Peñalva G, Gil-Navarro MV, et al. Long-term impact of an educational antimicrobial stewardship program on hospital acquired candidemia and multidrug-resistant bloodstream infections: a quasi-experimental study of interrupted time-series analysis. Clin Infect Dis. 2017;65:1992–9.
45. Livermore DM. Multiple mechanisms of antimicrobial resistance in Pseudomonas aeruginosa: our worst nightmare? Clin Infect Dis. 2002;34:634–40.

Part XII
Sepsis

Heterogeneity in Sepsis: New Biological Evidence with Clinical Applications

40

A. Leligdowicz and M. A. Matthay

40.1 Introduction

Since the first consensus definition of sepsis almost three decades ago [1], our understanding of the clinical characteristics that prognosticate the outcome of this complex syndrome has improved [2], resulting in a simpler classification scheme [3]. The existing definitions, however, remain imprecise and the clinical diagnosis of sepsis corresponds poorly with *post hoc* presence of infection [4]. Furthermore, the outcome of sepsis depends on factors beyond patient signs and symptoms [5], including age [6], the infection source [7], and the timing and appropriateness of therapeutic interventions [8] (Fig. 40.1). There is currently a promising shift from predicting outcome to a pathobiology-driven understanding of the heterogeneity in the host response to sepsis, utilizing novel translational high throughput tools and analytic methods to define distinct host response subgroups. It is now well recognized that biological markers improve the classification of sepsis and can facilitate identification of distinct patient subclasses, or endotypes.

A. Leligdowicz (✉)
Cardiovascular Research Institute, University of California-San Francisco, San Francisco, CA, USA

Interdepartmental Division of Critical Care Medicine, University of Toronto, Toronto, ON, Canada
e-mail: aleksandra.leligdowicz@uhn.ca

M. A. Matthay
Cardiovascular Research Institute, University of California-San Francisco, San Francisco, CA, USA

Division of Pulmonary, Critical Care, Allergy and Sleep Medicine, Department of Medicine, University of California-San Francisco, San Francisco, CA, USA

Departments of Medicine and Anesthesia, University of California-San Francisco, San Francisco, CA, USA

J.-L. Vincent (ed.), *Annual Update in Intensive Care and Emergency Medicine 2019*, Annual Update in Intensive Care and Emergency Medicine,
https://doi.org/10.1007/978-3-030-06067-1_40

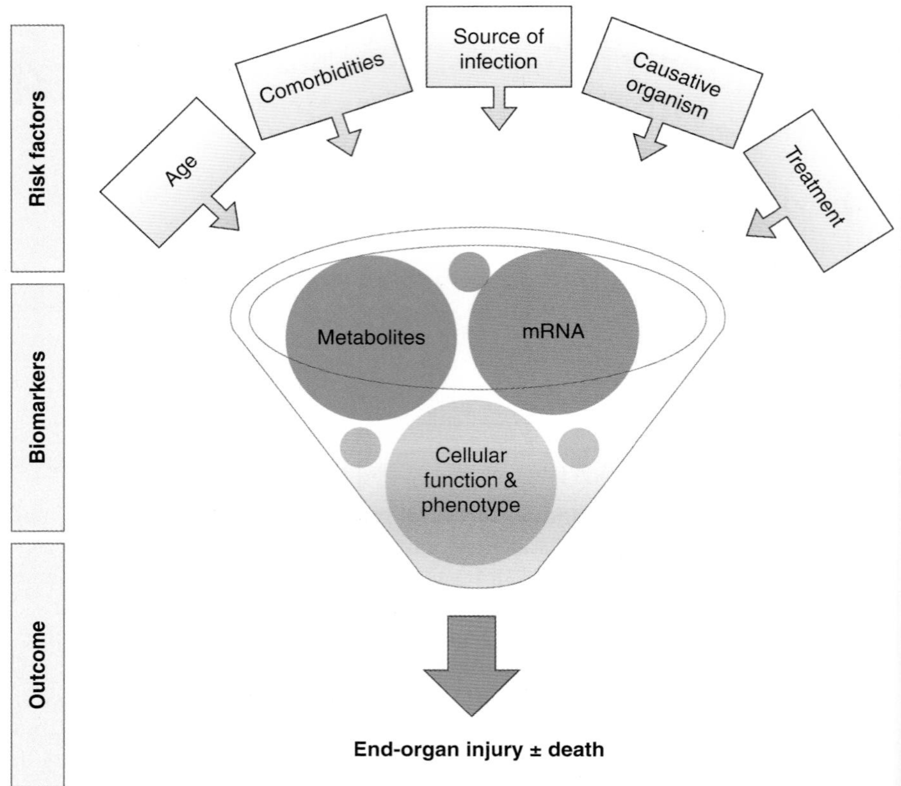

Fig. 40.1 Heterogeneity in critically ill patients with severe infection

Both excessive immune activation [9] and immunosuppression [10] are central to the pathophysiology of sepsis [11]. A clinical measure of immunosuppression is the acquisition of nosocomial infection. However, the development of intensive care unit (ICU)-acquired infection is not unique to patients with sepsis and, in fact, its incidence is comparable to patients admitted to the ICU without infectious conditions [12]. This finding suggests that mechanisms other than the immune response to infection are also contributory, with the key target pathways being (1) endothelial activation, (2) coagulopathy and (3) altered glucose and protein metabolism. Endotypes with derangements in all of these pathways have been identified, with divergent outcomes and differential response to therapies.

In this chapter, we highlight some of the most relevant recent advances in translational biology that assist in deconvoluting heterogeneity in patient response to sepsis. We focus on the use of molecular and metabolomic signatures as well as novel cellular function studies to identify distinct sepsis endotypes (Table 40.1). Identification of unique biological signatures in patients with sepsis could enable rational enrollment into clinical trials and, more importantly, enhance our approach to the diagnosis, prognosis, as well as individualized treatment to modulate the response to sepsis.

Table 40.1 Cohort studies of pathobiology-driven patient phenotypic classification

Endotypes	Cohort type (n)	Key biomarkers
Transcriptomic profiling		
Subclass A–C [13]	Pediatric septic shock (98)	44-gene classifier
SRS1 and SRS2 [14]	CAP (265)	7-gene classifier: *IDYRK2, DDNB1IP1, TDRD9, ZAP70, ARL14EP, MDC1 ADGRE3*
SRS1_FP and SRS2_FP [15]	Fecal peritonitis (117)	6-gene classifier: *CD163, CDHHC19, MME, FAM89A, ZBP1, B3GNT2*
Mars1-4 [16]	All-cause sepsis (306)	2-gene ratios: Mars1: *BPGM:TAP2,* Mars2: *GADD45A:PCGF5,* Mars3: *AHNAK:PDCD10,* Mars4: *IFIT5:GLTSCR2*
Inflammopathic, adaptive, coagulopathic [17]	Bacterial sepsis (700)	33-gene classifier
Neutrophil pathways [18]	Sepsis with (29) and without ARDS (28)	*OLFM4, LCN2 2, CD24, BPI*
Metabolomics		
Energy metabolism [27]	Septic shock (39), ICU controls (20)	↑Glucose, 3-hydroxybutyrate, *O*-acetylcarnitine, succinate, creatine, creatine phosphate ↓Branched-chain amino acids and arginine
Lipid homeostasis and tryptophan catabolism [28]	Septic shock (20)	↓Unsaturated long-chain PC and LPC, kynurenine
Defect in fatty acid-β-oxidation [29]	Community-acquired sepsis survivors (119) and nonsurvivors (31)	Acylcarnitine esters, amino/nucleic acid catabolites, glycolysis/citric acid cycle components
Lipid metabolism [30]	SIRS (29), Sepsis (30), sepsis-induced ARDS (31)	γ-glutamylphenylalanine, γ-glutamyltyrosine, 1-arachidonoyl-GPC (20:4), taurochenodeoxycholate, 3-(4-hydroxyphenyl) lactate, sucrose, kynurenine
Lipid metabolism [31]	SIRS (42), CAP (67), IAI (60), UTI (73) BSI (26)	SM C22:3 and, lysoPCaC24:0, lysoPCaC26:1, putrescine, lysoPCaC18:0, SM C16:1
Cellular function		
Immunophenotype [34]	Sepsis (148)	Neutrophil, monocyte, and T_{reg} phenotypes
Immunophenotype [35]	Sepsis (22)	Lymphocyte PD-1/PD-L1 expression
Immunophenotype [36]	Sepsis (505)	Monocyte and CD3, CD4, CD8 Tcell phenotypes
Endothelial permeability [37]	Sepsis (35)	Supernatants from whole blood treated with LPS
Endothelial permeability [38]	Primary (12) and secondary (6) sepsis	Neutrophils treated with fMLP

CAP community-acquired pneumonia, *PC* phosphatidylcholines, *LPC* lysophosphatidylcholines, *IAI* intraabdominal infection, *UTI* urinary tract infection, *BSI* bloodstream infection, *PD* programmed death, *LPS* lipopolysaccharide, *fMLP* formyl, methionyl-leucyl-phenylalanine, *SIRS* systemic inflammatory response syndrome

40.2 Transcriptomic Profiling

Interindividual transcriptome variation in sepsis has been recently evaluated in several large cohorts, with a dysfunctional immune response phenotype being a common theme. Clinical samples for these studies include peripheral blood leukocytes obtained within 24 h of ICU admission from patients with definite or probable infection. Unsupervised hierarchical clustering of approximately 25,000 genome-wide transcriptomic (gene expression microarray and RNA sequencing) profiles is then applied to identify distinct subgroups of patients in a derivation cohort and subsequently the findings are verified in at least one validation cohort. These sophisticated data-driven methods have identified patterns among expressed genes that define molecular subgroups representing different disease states without reference to clinical outcomes, but which could be associated to them. This approach could also define clusters indicative of the individual's premorbid state (age, comorbidities), illness stage and severity, mortality and genetic predisposition. However, subgroup membership cannot be distinguished on the basis of these clinical characteristics, as was the case for each of the studies summarized later.

One of the first studies to use unsupervised hierarchical clustering to study sepsis subgroups within the ICU population was done in a cohort of 98 children admitted to pediatric ICUs in the United States with septic shock [13]. Three subclasses were identified by differential genome-wide expression patterns: endotype A (29%), endotype B (46%), and endotype C (26%). These three classes differed significantly in clinical phenotypes including ICU mortality (highest in endotype A at 36% relative to 11% and 12% in endotypes B and C, respectively), illness severity and degree of organ failure (both highest in endotype A), and age (youngest in endotype A). The subclasses were also biologically plausible, with the most deranged signaling pathways in endotype A involving repression of genes key to the adaptive immune system, glucocorticoid receptor signaling, as well as to zinc homeostasis.

Similar methodology has recently been applied to the adult critically ill population. Among 265 patients admitted to 29 ICUs in the UK with sepsis due to community-acquired pneumonia (CAP) as part of the Genomic Advances in Sepsis (GAinS) study, transcriptomic profiles defined two sepsis response signatures (SRS1, 41% and SRS2, 59%) [14]. Relative to SRS2 patients, patients in the SRS1 group had a higher 14-day mortality (22% vs. 10%). SRS1 assignment was associated with relative immunosuppression, endotoxin-tolerance, T-cell exhaustion, human leukocyte antigen (HLA) class II downregulation, and metabolic derangements (switch from oxidative phosphorylation to glycolysis). Of the over 3000 differentially expressed genes, seven genes reliably predicted SRS membership. In future studies, patients prospectively assigned into SRS1 may benefit from therapies that boost their immune system and prevent nosocomial infection.

This analytical approach was subsequently used by the same investigators to study the gene expression patterns in 117 patients with fecal peritonitis (FP) [15]. Two distinct groups were again identified (SRS1_FP, 46% and SRS2_FP, 54%), with patients in the SRS1_FP group also having a higher 14-day mortality (19% vs. 4%). The findings were strongly correlated with the SRS groups identified in the

CAP study [14], again showing enrichment of endotoxin tolerance and T-cell activation but also in cell death, apoptosis and necrosis. Of the over 1000 differentially expressed genes, a simpler six-gene set was derived that predicted group membership. Of note, when gene expression patterns that distinguished SRS groups were tested in the pediatric cohort described above [13], the same enrichment was not observed (i.e., SRS1_FP [15] and endotype A [13]).

In a group of 306 patients admitted to two ICUs in the Netherlands as part of the Molecular Diagnosis and Risk Stratification of Sepsis (MARS) project, four molecular endotypes (Mars1-4) were identified [16]. Mortality at 28 days differed among the subgroups and was highest in the Mars1 group at 39%, compared to 22% in Mars2, 23% in Mars3 and 33% in Mars4. The Mars1 poor-prognosis endotype had a decrease in expression of genes involved in innate and adaptive immune functions (Toll-like receptor, nuclear factor-κB signaling [NF-κB], antigen presentation, and T-cell receptor signaling) and an increase in expression of cellular metabolic pathways (heme biosynthesis), processes which are both analogous to immune exhaustion. Mars2 and 4 endotype had upregulation of pattern recognition and cytokine pathways (interleukin [IL]-6, NF-κB, interferon signaling, inducible nitric oxide synthase), representing a hyperinflammatory state. Finally, Mars3 was a lower-risk endotype with increased expression of adaptive immune pathways (T-helper cells, natural killer cells, IL-4 signaling, B-cell development), which was highly correlated with the low-risk SRS2 endotype [14]. A two-gene expression ratio was derived to enable classification of each endotype at the time of ICU admission.

In the most recent and comprehensive attempt to identify sepsis subtypes, data from 14 transcriptomic datasets consisting of 700 patients revealed three robust host response clusters across the sepsis spectrum [17]. These were termed: (1) inflammopathic (increased innate and reduced adaptive immune signal marked by increased expression of IL-1 receptor, pattern recognition receptor activity, complement activation); (2) adaptive (reduced innate and high adaptive immune signal with lower mortality, marked by interferon signaling); and (3) coagulopathic (irregularities in the coagulation and complement systems, including platelet degranulation and glycosaminoglycan binding). Similar to the previous analyses, the three groups differed in 30-day mortality, with the highest mortality in the inflammopathic group at 30%, compared to 8% in the adaptive and 25% in the coagulopathic groups. A simplified 33-gene classifier was derived to facilitate cluster assignment. The assignment into the high-mortality inflammopathic cluster corresponded to SRS1 and the low-mortality adaptive cluster to SRS2 [14].

Early transcriptional changes may also have identified patients at risk of sepsis-associated complications at the time of ICU admission. One study from our research group that investigated 57 patients with sepsis found that the differential expression of key mediators of the initial neutrophil response to infection identified patients with acute respiratory distress syndrome (ARDS, n = 29) compared to those with sepsis who did not have ARDS (n = 28), a finding that could not be attributed to the neutrophil count [18].

To date, genome-wide expression studies in sepsis used whole leukocyte populations. However, distinct gene expression patterns are present among subsets of granulocytes and lymphocytes which represent the specialized function of each of these immune cells [19]. Since the transcriptome profile depends on the inflammatory cell type, it is possible that gene expression patterns that distinguish subclasses reflect different leukocyte populations instead of within-cell differences in gene expression. These findings also require validation in large cohorts spanning different countries as variation in ethnic background is a strong determinant of gene expression [20].

Nevertheless, these studies provide evidence of distinct categories of the host response to sepsis and potential novel therapeutic targets based on differentially expressed molecular pathways that distinguish patient endotypes. Furthermore, each study proposed potential 'downsizing' of the high-dimensional data into manageable predictive signals that could be incorporated into a simpler point-of-care test, assisting in translating the findings to the bedside.

40.3 mRNA and Protein Signatures

A more established and more feasible method of biological subclassification of patients with sepsis is plasma protein quantification and a vast number of studies have classified sepsis using this approach [21–23], which is beyond the scope of this review. A noteworthy method that could offer a novel way to derive sepsis subclasses is combining molecular and protein biomarkers to predict outcome in patients with septic shock. This approach was used to risk stratify pediatric septic shock using a previously validated risk score consisting of five plasma protein biomarkers (PERSEVERE decision tree) [23] and combining these with four top mortality assessment genes [24]. An improvement was noted in the performance of the risk score estimating the risk of 28-day mortality (PERSEVERE-XP, area under the receiver operating characteristic [AUROC] curve increase from 0.78 to 0.91). The plasma biomarkers were associated with dysfunctional inflammation and cellular injury whereas the genes were related to the tumor protein 53 (*TP53, p53*), a transcriptional factor functioning as a tumor suppressor, preventing the generation and persistence of cells with genomic damage. Taken together, this approach offers a plausible hypothesis regarding biological pathways that result in a poor outcome due to septic shock.

40.4 Metabolomics

Metabolomics is an expanding and less familiar method to decipher heterogeneity in sepsis. It refers to the global assessment of small metabolites in any biological sample, representing a composite 'snapshot' of gene expression, enzyme activity, and the physiological landscape [25]. More than 5000 metabolites can be detected in cells, tissues, or biofluids (blood components, urine) using nuclear magnetic resonance (NMR) spectroscopy or mass spectrometry, the latter of which is more sensitive and can detect low-abundant metabolites [26]. The metabolites can include both endogenous (lipids, carbohydrates, amino acids, nucleic acids) and exogenous (microbial components and byproducts) compounds. Alteration in endogenous metabolite concentration can be linked to biological pathways and the magnitude of change relates to the stage of illness, significantly magnifying transcriptome and proteome-level shifts. Studies so far included retrospective specimen collection with small sample sizes.

^{1}H NMR spectroscopy was used to analyze and compare serum samples derived from adults with septic shock and from ICU controls [27]. Sixty metabolites were recognized, 31 of which could distinguish between septic shock and ICU control patients, proposing a composite biomarker pattern that could differentiate between these patient groups. The metabolites were involved in energy metabolism and included glucose, 3-hydroxybutyrate, *O*-acetylcarnitine, succinate, creatine, creatine phosphate as well a decreased level of branched-chain amino acids and arginine. These results suggest that in early sepsis, metabolites involved in energy metabolism have a role in the pathophysiology of sepsis.

Alteration in metabolites involved in energy metabolism has also been recognized as key in distinguishing sepsis survivors from non-survivors using mass spectrometry to characterize lower concentration metabolites in plasma. In a substudy of the ALBIOS (Albumin Italian Outcome Sepsis) trial which enrolled 1818 patients with severe sepsis or septic shock, day 1 and 7 plasma samples were studied in 20 patients, 45% of whom died by day 28 [28]. The study identified 137 metabolites, many of which were significantly different between survivors and non-survivors. The most notable group of metabolites included a decrease in phosphatidylcholines and lysophosphatidylcholines as well as an increase in kynurenine. This decline in lipid species, particularly long-chain polyunsaturated fatty acids, may lead to increased T-cell activation and an excessive immune response.

The plasma metabolome was similarly studied using mass spectrometry in a subset of 150 patients who were among 1152 individuals with suspected sepsis enrolled in the Community Acquired Pneumonia and Sepsis Outcome Diagnostics (CAPSOD) study [29]. Of the 439 metabolites analyzed, 214 were detected at both day 0 (t_0) and at 24 h (t_{24}). Metabolites did not differ at either time point among infectious etiologies (*Streptococcus pneumoniae, Staphylococcus aureus or Escherichia coli*). There were 76 metabolites at t_0 and 128 metabolites at t_{24} that differed between sepsis survivors and non-survivors at 28 days. Acylcarnitine esters of all fatty acid length (medium- or short-chain) and branched-chain amino acid biochemical group differences were most pronounced between the two patient groups, suggesting that a defect in fatty acid-β-oxidation may occur at the level of the carnitine shuttle. Metabolites comprising fatty acid transport, gluconeogenesis and the citric acid cycle were also differentially deranged.

Another large cohort that used mass spectrometry for metabolomic profiling to study metabolite biomarkers in 60 ICU survivors and 30 ICU non-survivors found that of the 187 metabolites tested, 57 were associated with 28-day mortality [30] and 31 of them were replicated in the CAPSOD validation cohort [29]. These metabolites included diverse lipid, carbohydrate, amino acid and nucleotide products. Higher levels of tyrosine and phenylalanine catabolism products and lower levels of lipid metabolites were associated with mortality. Although this study used the same metabolomic datasets as the previously described study [29], a completely different network of metabolites was identified, which was also predictive of 28-day mortality, implying it is premature to focus on a single metabolite biomarker as several could be implicated in the pathobiology of different stages of sepsis.

The largest study to investigate metabolites using mass spectrometry in patients with sepsis included 406 patients, 268 of whom were included in a discovery cohort (42 patients with systemic inflammatory response syndrome [SIRS], 67 with CAP, 60 with intraabdominal infection, 73 with urinary tract infection and 26 with bloodstream infection) [31]. Again, acylcarnitines and lipids were altered in sepsis relative to SIRS. A sphingolipid SM C22:3 and glycerophospholipid lysoPCaC24:0 model discriminated between these two entities with an AUROC of 0.9. The analysis also indicated great heterogeneity in metabolite patterns depending on the anatomic source of infection and thus a one metabolite model was proposed to prognosticate unfavorable outcome for each infection type.

40.5 Cellular Function

While molecular, protein and metabolomic biomarkers provide associations between sepsis and its outcome, they cannot determine causality and mechanistic studies linking these associations to sepsis pathobiology are required. Two potentially high throughput techniques available to study *ex vivo* relationships between cell function and sepsis pathobiology include flow cytometry [32] and electric cell-substrate impedance sensing (ECIS) [33].

Immunophenotyping involves the use of flow cytometry and fluorescent-labeled monoclonal antibodies to simultaneously label multiple cell surface markers, such as those associated with immune dysfunction. In a group of 138 ICU patients recruited from four ICUs in the UK, leukocyte dysfunction defined by a combination of reduced neutrophil CD88 and monocyte HLA-DR as well as an elevated proportion of regulatory T cells ($CD4^{+}$, $CD25^{++}$, $CD127^{low}$) was associated with the development of nosocomial infection [34]. Lymphocyte dysfunction is also present in sepsis and can be quantified by the expression levels of programmed death protein 1 (PD1) and its ligand PDL1, which promote apoptosis. When peripheral blood mononuclear cells from 22 patients with sepsis were compared to healthy controls, both PD1 and PDL1 were higher on all lymphocyte subsets (CD4 T cells and B cells) in patients with sepsis [35]. Similar to transcriptome and metabolome analyses in sepsis, the early innate and adaptive immune status also vary according to infection type [36]. Therefore, the identification of patients with a prespecified source of infection who have an immunophenotype amendable to immunomodulatory therapy could allow for precision medicine-guided therapy.

The endothelium is one of the primary targets in sepsis. Measuring endothelial cell function *ex vivo* is challenging but our research group developed a novel assay (ECIS) that delineates the heterogeneity in endothelial cell response after exposure to different patient-derived samples. This assay is based on movement of current across a monolayer of endothelial cells, with a decrease in resistance indicative of an increase in vascular permeability. When pulmonary endothelial cells were exposed to lipopolysaccharide (LPS)-stimulated leukocyte supernatants derived from 35 ICU patients with sepsis, substantial heterogeneity in pulmonary endothelial permeability was observed [37]. The same method was used to test the ability of neutrophils from septic patients to induce endothelial damage, demonstrating that neutrophils from septic patients with compared to those without ARDS can induce greater endothelial damage [38]. This *in vitro* model of vascular permeability may be useful for testing therapeutic agents that could mitigate endothelial injury in early sepsis.

40.6 Challenges and Future Directions

Distinguishing consistent biological heterogeneity in sepsis will necessitate overcoming several technical hurdles. Inclusion criteria ought to be uniform across sites to minimize patient selection bias. The timing of sample collection is critical as endotype assignment is a dynamic process and nearly 50% of patients cross over from one endotype to another over the first 5 days of ICU admission, as demonstrated by serial sampling on sequential days [15]. Similarly, the duration of altered gene expression can vary between patients, and tends to normalize quicker in patients who recover faster [39], emphasizing that standardizing sample collection timing is crucial. Data collection will also need to be standardized to include common clinically meaningful outcomes as studies to date use ICU, hospital, 14-, 28-, 30-, or 90-day mortality. These outcomes represent different endpoints which could be measuring different biological processes. Early deaths are more likely to be directly attributed to the initial episode of sepsis whereas late deaths may represent complications of sepsis beyond nosocomial infections [40]. In the analysis phase, standardizing analytical methods will be important to determine whether sepsis can be categorized into two, three, four or potentially more endotypes.

It is plausible that the host response to sepsis may be nonspecific and could be elicited to different organisms, which invade different organs. Although there is evidence that there may be a shared host response at the transcriptome and metabolome level irrespective of the infection type (Gram-positive sepsis and Gram-negative sepsis) [29, 41] or the anatomic source of infection [15], the studies to date investigating these questions have been relatively small and when pooled data are used [42], there is a host gene expression signature that can discriminate sterile inflammation from bacterial or viral infections. For this reason, the largest transcriptomic analysis to date restricted analysis to only bacterial sepsis [17]. Also, when gene expression data for all-cause sepsis are re-analyzed including patients with only pneumonia and peritonitis, the two most common anatomic sources of infection [7], the proportion of patients assigned to an endotype varies depending on the infection source [16]. Metabolites also vary based on infection source, with CAP having a different metabolite pattern relative to other sites of infection [31]. A recent analysis of the plasma metabolome in H1N1 pneumonia successfully differentiated viral from bacterial culture-positive pneumonia and ventilated ICU controls [43]. Therefore, whether sepsis endotypes are truly independent of infection type and anatomical source will require large-scale prospective cohort studies with enough power to address this question.

In the future, it may be possible to treat distinct manifestations of the host response to sepsis based on signatures representing distinct biological pathways (Fig. 40.2). Assignment into endotypes could facilitate targeting appropriate therapies to the patient group with a pathway derangement endotype that would most benefit. It would also enable appropriate selection into clinical trials investigating pathway-driven therapeutics that to date have been unsuccessful largely due to the inclusion of a heterogenous group of patients with sepsis.

Validation in large, multicenter, and diverse cohorts is needed prior to transitioning from exploration and discovery to testing candidate mRNA, protein, and metabolite models. An overarching future collaborative study aim should include prospective validation in large cohorts to determine whether pathobiology biomarker-driven identification of sepsis endotype at the time of ICU admission can improve clinical outcomes and personalization of treatment.

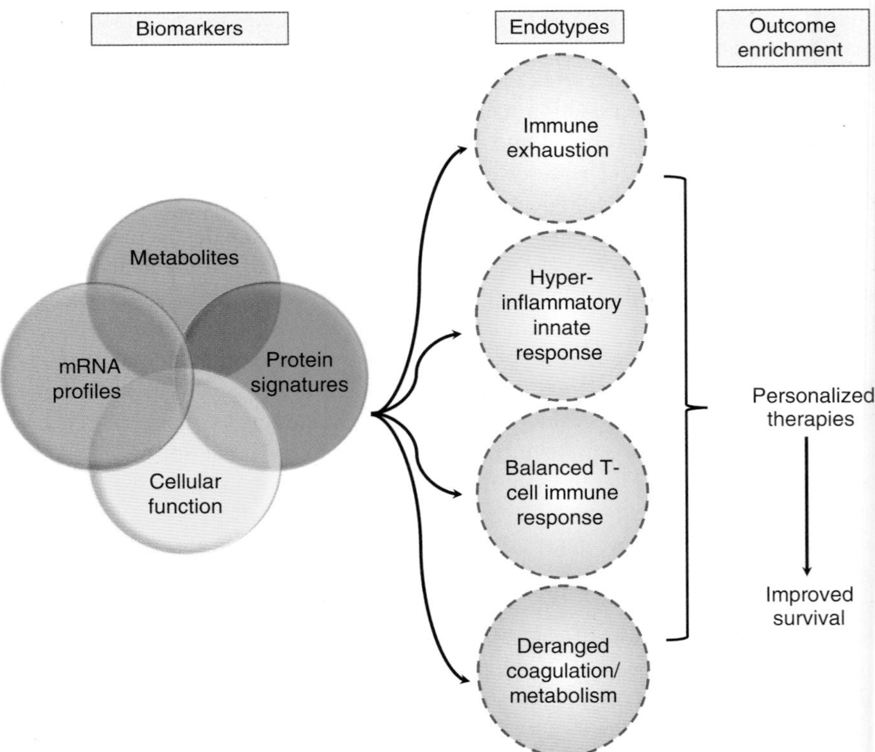

Fig. 40.2 Clustering into pathobiology-driven endotypes

40.7 Conclusion

Applying bioinformatics to integrate systems biology (transcriptomics, proteomics, metabolomics) in combination with functional cellular studies has the potential to identify biological endotypes, which cannot be predicted using clinical covariates alone. Optimizing these novel translational methods will require collaboration, expertise and standardization in patient sample collection, assay performance and data analysis. It is possible that the true nature of the heterogeneity of the host response to sepsis will require a combination of molecular, protein, metabolomic and functional signatures that will lead to an integrated, simple, and clinically useful diagnostic model that could be rapidly used at the time of ICU admission. Hopefully, a parsimonious set of biological markers will be useful to categorize patients into specific sub-groups that would be useful for testing specific new therapies. Ultimately, detection of key biological markers along with clinical indicators at the bedside could improve our approach to precision medicine-guided therapy and outcomes of patients with sepsis.

References

1. Bone RC, Balk RA, Cerra FB, et al. Definitions for sepsis and organ failure and guidelines for the use of innovative therapies in sepsis. Chest. 1992;101:1644–55.
2. Gotts JE, Matthay MA. Sepsis: pathophysiology and clinical management. BMJ. 2016;353:i1585.
3. Shankar-Hari M, Phillips GS, Levy ML, et al. Developing a new definition and assessing new clinical criteria for septic shock: For the Third International Consensus Definitions for Sepsis and Septic Shock (Sepsis-3). JAMA. 2016;315:775–87.
4. Klein Klouwenberg PM, Cremer OL, van Vught LA, et al. Likelihood of infection in patients with presumed sepsis at the time of intensive care unit admission: a cohort study. Crit Care. 2015;19:319.
5. Vincent JL, Opal SM, Marshall JC, Tracey KJ. Sepsis definitions: time for change. Lancet. 2013;381:774–5.
6. Brakenridge SC, Efron PA, Stortz JA, et al. The impact of age on the innate immune response and outcomes after severe sepsis/septic shock in trauma and surgical intensive care unit patients. J Trauma Acute Care Surg. 2018;85:247–55.
7. Leligdowicz A, Dodek PM, Norena M, et al. Association between source of infection and hospital mortality in patients who have septic shock. Am J Respir Crit Care Med. 2014;189:1204–13.
8. Ferrer R, Martinez ML, Goma G, et al. Improved empirical antibiotic treatment of sepsis after an educational intervention: the ABISS-Edusepsis study. Crit Care. 2018;22:167.
9. Delano MJ, Ward PA. The immune system's role in sepsis progression, resolution, and long-term outcome. Immunol Rev. 2016;274:330–53.
10. Boomer JS, To K, Chang KC, et al. Immunosuppression in patients who die of sepsis and multiple organ failure. JAMA. 2011;306:2594–605.
11. Hotchkiss RS, Monneret G, Payen D. Sepsis-induced immunosuppression: from cellular dysfunctions to immunotherapy. Nat Rev Immunol. 2013;13:862–74.
12. van Vught LA, Klein Klouwenberg PM, Spitoni C, et al. Incidence, risk factors, and attributable mortality of secondary infections in the intensive care unit after admission for sepsis. JAMA. 2016;315:1469–79.
13. Wong HR, Cvijanovich N, Lin R, et al. Identification of pediatric septic shock subclasses based on genome-wide expression profiling. BMC Med. 2009;7:34.

14. Davenport EE, Burnham KL, Radhakrishnan J, et al. Genomic landscape of the individual host response and outcomes in sepsis: a prospective cohort study. Lancet Respir Med. 2016;4:259–71.
15. Burnham KL, Davenport EE, Radhakrishnan J, et al. Shared and distinct aspects of the sepsis transcriptomic response to fecal peritonitis and pneumonia. Am J Respir Crit Care Med. 2017;196:328–39.
16. Scicluna BP, van Vught LA, Zwinderman AH, et al. Classification of patients with sepsis according to blood genomic endotype: a prospective cohort study. Lancet Respir Med. 2017;5:816–26.
17. Sweeney TE, Azad TD, Donato M, et al. Unsupervised analysis of transcriptomics in bacterial sepsis across multiple datasets reveals three robust clusters. Crit Care Med. 2018;46:915–25.
18. Kangelaris KN, Prakash A, Liu KD, et al. Increased expression of neutrophil-related genes in patients with early sepsis-induced ARDS. Am J Phys Lung Cell Mol Phys. 2015;308:L1102–13.
19. Palmer C, Diehn M, Alizadeh AA, Brown PO. Cell-type specific gene expression profiles of leukocytes in human peripheral blood. BMC Genomics. 2006;7:115.
20. Spielman RS, Bastone LA, Burdick JT, Morley M, Ewens WJ, Cheung VG. Common genetic variants account for differences in gene expression among ethnic groups. Nat Genet. 2007;39:226–31.
21. Hou PC, Filbin MR, Wang H, et al. Endothelial permeability and hemostasis in septic shock: results from the ProCESS trial. Chest. 2017;152:22–31.
22. van Vught LA, Wiewel MA, Hoogendijk AJ, et al. The host response in patients with sepsis developing intensive care unit-acquired secondary infections. Am J Respir Crit Care Med. 2017;196:458–70.
23. Wong HR, Salisbury S, Xiao Q, et al. The pediatric sepsis biomarker risk model. Crit Care. 2012;16:R174.
24. Wong HR, Cvijanovich NZ, Anas N, et al. Improved risk stratification in pediatric septic shock using both protein and mRNA biomarkers. PERSEVERE-XP. Am J Respir Crit Care Med. 2017;196:494–501.
25. Serkova NJ, Standiford TJ, Stringer KA. The emerging field of quantitative blood metabolomics for biomarker discovery in critical illnesses. Am J Respir Crit Care Med. 2011;184:647–55.
26. Eckerle M, Ambroggio L, Puskarich MA, et al. Metabolomics as a driver in advancing precision medicine in sepsis. Pharmacotherapy. 2017;37:1023–32.
27. Mickiewicz B, Duggan GE, Winston BW, et al. Metabolic profiling of serum samples by 1H nuclear magnetic resonance spectroscopy as a potential diagnostic approach for septic shock. Crit Care Med. 2014;42:1140–9.
28. Ferrario M, Cambiaghi A, Brunelli L, et al. Mortality prediction in patients with severe septic shock: a pilot study using a target metabolomics approach. Sci Rep. 2016;6:20391.
29. Langley RJ, Tsalik EL, van Velkinburgh JC, et al. An integrated clinico-metabolomic model improves prediction of death in sepsis. Sci Transl Med. 2013;5:195ra195.
30. Rogers AJ, McGeachie M, Baron RM, et al. Metabolomic derangements are associated with mortality in critically ill adult patients. PLoS One. 2014;9:e87538.
31. Neugebauer S, Giamarellos-Bourboulis EJ, Pelekanou A, et al. Metabolite profiles in sepsis: developing prognostic tools based on the type of infection. Crit Care Med. 2016;44:1649–62.
32. Venet F, Lepape A, Monneret G. Clinical review: flow cytometry perspectives in the ICU—from diagnosis of infection to monitoring of injury-induced immune dysfunctions. Crit Care. 2011;15:231.
33. Wegener J, Keese CR, Giaever I. Electric cell-substrate impedance sensing (ECIS) as a noninvasive means to monitor the kinetics of cell spreading to artificial surfaces. Exp Cell Res. 2000;259:158–66.
34. Conway Morris A, Datta D, Shankar-Hari M, et al. Cell-surface signatures of immune dysfunction risk-stratify critically ill patients: INFECT study. Intensive Care Med. 2018;44:627–35.
35. Wilson JK, Zhao Y, Singer M, Spencer J, Shankar-Hari M. Lymphocyte subset expression and serum concentrations of PD-1/PD-L1 in sepsis—pilot study. Crit Care. 2018;22:95.

36. Gogos C, Kotsaki A, Pelekanou A, et al. Early alterations of the innate and adaptive immune statuses in sepsis according to the type of underlying infection. Crit Care. 2010;14:R96.
37. Leligdowicz A, Chun LF, Jauregui A, et al. Human pulmonary endothelial cell permeability after exposure to LPS-stimulated leukocyte supernatants derived from patients with early sepsis. Am J Phys Lung Cell Mol Phys. 2018;315:L638–44.
38. Fox ED, Heffernan DS, Cioffi WG, Reichner JS. Neutrophils from critically ill septic patients mediate profound loss of endothelial barrier integrity. Crit Care. 2013;17:R226.
39. Cazalis MA, Lepape A, Venet F, et al. Early and dynamic changes in gene expression in septic shock patients: a genome-wide approach. Intensive Care Med Exp. 2014;2:20.
40. Goldenberg NM, Leligdowicz A, Slutsky AS, Friedrich JO, Lee WL. Is nosocomial infection really the major cause of death in sepsis? Crit Care. 2014;18:540.
41. Tang BM, McLean AS, Dawes IW, Huang SJ, Cowley MJ, Lin RC. Gene-expression profiling of gram-positive and gram-negative sepsis in critically ill patients. Crit Care Med. 2008;36:1125–8.
42. Sweeney TE, Wong HR, Khatri P. Robust classification of bacterial and viral infections via integrated host gene expression diagnostics. Sci Transl Med. 2016;8:346ra391.
43. Banoei MM, Vogel HJ, Weljie AM, et al. Plasma metabolomics for the diagnosis and prognosis of H1N1 influenza pneumonia. Crit Care. 2017;21:97.

The Role of Mitochondrial Dysfunction in Sepsis: What Is New?

41

Y. Wang, M. Chakraborty, and A. McLean

41.1 Introduction

Sepsis is a life-threatening disease caused by a dysregulated host response to infection, which leads to multiple organ failure (MOF). The mortality rate is 25% for uncomplicated sepsis and 80% in patients who develop MOF, making it the major cause of mortality in the intensive care unit (ICU). Despite decades of research dedicated to sepsis pathogenesis, the exact mechanisms contributing to sepsis-related MOF are yet to be elucidated.

Nearly 50 years ago in the 1970s, studies using experimental rat models of hemorrhagic hypovolemia and *Escherichia coli* endotoxin shock first demonstrated the inhibition of mitochondrial function in septic shock [1–3]. Subsequent studies produced conflicting results [4, 5] and it took another 20 years before the concept of mitochondrial dysfunction was established as an important mechanism contributing to the pathogenesis of sepsis [6, 7] supported by both animal and human studies [8–10]. Functional and ultrastructural abnormalities of mitochondria were found in liver, kidney and skeletal/heart muscle [9, 11] and later in blood cells [12]. Around the same period, mitochondrial dysfunction was found to be associated with oxidative stress, a state of redox imbalance involving overproduction of reactive species and/or free radicals and depletion of antioxidant [9, 13]. This association has since triggered more research into identifying potential therapeutic targets for sepsis [14, 15].

Y. Wang (✉)
Nepean Genomic Research Group, Sydney Medical School, Nepean Hospital, Kingswood, NSW, Australia

Centre for Immunology and Allergy Research, Westmead Institute for Medical Research, Westmead, NSW, Australia
e-mail: ya.wang@sydney.edu.au

M. Chakraborty · A. McLean
Department of Intensive Care Medicine, Nepean Hospital, Kingswood, NSW, Australia

J.-L. Vincent (ed.), *Annual Update in Intensive Care and Emergency Medicine 2019*, Annual Update in Intensive Care and Emergency Medicine, https://doi.org/10.1007/978-3-030-06067-1_41

This chapter highlights recent important findings and hypotheses that help to explain the role of mitochondrial dysfunction in the pathogenesis of sepsis with the focus on the role of oxidative stress. Furthermore the potential of putative therapies that target the mitochondrion or oxidative stress will be explored.

41.2 Mitochondria: The Powerhouse of Cells and More

Prior to reviewing mitochondrial dysfunction in sepsis, it is important to understand the physiological functions of mitochondria in healthy cells. Mitochondria are present in all cell types found in human bodies with the exception of erythrocytes, though the number of mitochondria per cell varies. Cells from liver and muscle tissues, which have higher energy demand, generally contain more mitochondria than cells from other tissue types. The main function of mitochondria is to produce adenosine triphosphate (ATP), the major energy currency essential for most cellular activities, such as cell division, cell signaling and muscle contraction. ATP is also generated in the cytosol through glycolysis but the majority of ATP is produced in mitochondria via oxidative phosphorylation, which is far more efficient than glycolysis. In the presence of oxygen, oxidative phosphorylation oxidizes nutrients to release energy used for ATP production. This process involves transfer of electrons from the tricarboxylic acid (TCA) cycle (also known as the Krebs cycle) to the electron transport chain consisting of a series of enzyme complexes (complex I–IV) located on the inner membrane of the mitochondria. As electrons move down the electron transport chain, protons are pumped across the membrane creating a proton gradient. This gradient provides energy for ATP synthase (complex V) to phosphorylate adenosine diphosphate (ADP) to ATP.

Oxygen consumption by mitochondrial oxidative phosphorylation accounts for over 90% of total body oxygen consumption. But not all the oxygen consumed by mitochondria is used for ATP production. Part of the oxygen consumed is uncoupled from energy production and used for producing reactive oxygen species (ROS) (approximately 1–2% of total oxygen) or generating heat. ROS generation mainly takes place at the electron transport chain where leakage of electrons at complex I and III leads to incomplete reduction of oxygen into superoxide. The level of ROS in healthy mitochondria is kept in check by endogenous antioxidant systems including manganese superoxide dismutase (MnSOD), glutathione and thioredoxin. The fine balance between ROS and antioxidant is crucial for the overall health of the mitochondria and the cells.

In addition to energy production, other roles of mitochondria in the cells include heat generation, intracellular calcium regulation, apoptosis and intracellular signaling, making the mitochondrion an important organelle in maintaining normal cell functions.

41.3 Sepsis and Mitochondrial Dysfunction: Survival of the Fittest

Sepsis is caused by a dysregulated host immune response to infections, which leads to systemic inflammatory response syndrome (SIRS) that can progress to MOF (severe sepsis) and septic shock (severe sepsis with hypotension). The cause of sepsis-related MOF is rather complex and involves the exaggerated inflammatory responses, microcirculation alterations and mitochondrial dysfunction. Therapies targeting pro-inflammatory mediators such as tumor necrosis factor-α (TNF-α) and interleukin-1 (IL-1) have however failed to show any benefits to sepsis patients [16, 17]. A healthy microcirculation is necessary for adequate tissue oxygenation and any disruption can therefore result in tissue hypoxia, thus directly impacting organ function. Although it has been shown that microcirculation alteration plays an important role in sepsis-related MOF [18], it is hard to assess this precisely in the context of affected organs. Postmortem examination revealed minimal cell death in organs like the heart, liver, brain and kidney [19, 20], which makes further validation hard.

In the early 1970s, studies measuring functions of mitochondria isolated from an endotoxic model suggested the inhibition of energy metabolism in liver, cardiac and skeletal muscle mitochondria. Reduction in mitochondrial oxidative respiration and swelling of mitochondria under electron microscopy were observed due to the effect of endotoxin (lipopolysaccharide [LPS]) extracted from *E. coli* [1, 3]. Mitochondrial dysfunction in sepsis has received more attention since the late 1990s when cytopathic hypoxia (decreased availability of oxygen at the cellular level) was first mentioned as a plausible mechanism contributing to tissue hypoxia and hence MOF in sepsis [6]. Tissue hypoxia in sepsis, first thought to result from microcirculatory disruption, does not however explain the increased tissue oxygen tensions [21, 22], minimal cell death observed in postmortem samples from various organs affected by sepsis [19], and more importantly the near-complete recovery of organ function in MOF survivors [23]. However, increased tissue oxygen tension seen in sepsis can be explained by cytopathic hypoxia or mitochondrial dysfunction which denotes reduced ATP production and oxygen consumption, despite normal or supranormal oxygen availability within the cells. Reduced ATP production, as evidenced by reduced ATP concentration in skeletal muscle and inhibited electron transport chain complex I activity, correlates with the severity and outcome of septic shock [9]. This is consistent with early findings in septic animal models. Further evidence has shown significant reduction in protein levels of complex I and complex IV subunits in critically ill patients as compared to controls. An overall reduction in oxidative phosphorylation transcript abundance was also observed in critically ill patients as compared to controls. In addition it has been shown that survivors have higher oxidative phosphorylation transcript abundance than non-survivors [24]. All this evidence suggests that cells from failed organs have reduced use of oxygen for ATP production probably as a result of impaired oxidative phosphorylation complexes.

However, questions such as why minimal cell death is detected in postmortem samples and why there is complete recovery of organ function in MOF survivors remain unanswered by cytopathic hypoxia or mitochondrial dysfunction. As mentioned earlier, mitochondria are the main source of ATP within the cells so, in theory, if mitochondrial dysfunction persists, it will eventually lead to cell death and then organ failure, which could be irreversible. An interesting hypothesis by Mervyn Singer suggests that reduced metabolic activity (low oxidative phosphorylation complex activity and low ATP production) as seen in sepsis patients can lead to reduced energy requirements. This creates a new steady-state that mimics hibernation [25]. So mitochondrial dysfunction is on the one hand associated with the development of MOF but on the other hand could well be an adaptive mechanism for cells to cope with the overwhelming systemic inflammatory response seen in sepsis. Survival therefore will rely on the recovery of respiratory function of mitochondria. Recovery of mitochondrial function via mitochondrial biogenesis (synthesis of new mitochondria) has been well demonstrated in several sepsis animal models induced by LPS or by *Staphylococcus aureus* [26, 27]. Genes that regulate mitochondrial biogenesis, such as peroxisome proliferator-activated receptor γ coactivator-1α (*PGC-1α*), mitochondrial transcription factor A (*Tfam*), and nuclear respiratory factor-1 (*NRF-1*), are upregulated prior to recovery of metabolic activity. PGC-1α is a transcription coactivator that plays a central role in regulating mitochondrial biogenesis through activation of NRF-1 and Tfam. *NRF-1* encodes a transcription factor that activates the expression of nuclear genes required for respiration, mitochondrial DNA transcription and replication. *Tfam* encodes a mitochondrial transcription factor that is a key activator of mitochondrial transcription and mitochondrial genome replication. Studies in critically ill patients also found increased PGC-1α mRNA in survivors but not in non-survivors. This further testifies to the importance of mitochondrial biogenesis in the recovery of organ function and eventual survival [24]. Whether or not patients survive MOF will depend on how quickly and how efficiently their cells switch on the recovery mechanism—the survival of the fittest.

41.4 Oxidative Stress and Mitochondrial Dysfunction

We have elaborated on the important role of mitochondrial dysfunction in the pathogenesis of sepsis-related MOF. Yet sepsis is well known to be caused by a dysregulated immune response to infection, which is characterized by a hyper-inflammatory phase and a subsequent immunosuppressive phase. How does the immune response in the case of sepsis impact mitochondrial function and organ function? Considering that various anti-inflammatory agents have failed to show any beneficial effects in sepsis patients, mediators other than cytokines need to be considered.

Along with exaggerated production of pro-inflammatory cytokines in sepsis, there is also overproduction of free radicals and reactive species by innate immune cells (oxidative burst) as part of the body's defense mechanisms for eradicating pathogens [28]. These include ROS and reactive nitrogen species (RNS), which act like antimicrobial agents and can destroy microbial pathogens directly. As mentioned earlier, ROS are produced as byproducts of oxidative phosphorylation in healthy mitochondria. ROS are also produced in the cytosol, peroxisomes, and endoplasmic reticulum and serve important roles in regulating cell growth, apoptosis, and signaling [29]. Similar to ROS, RNS also serve as a regulator of cell signaling and gene expression [30]. Despite the important roles of ROS and RNS as antimicrobial agents and regulators of cellular processes, overproduction of ROS or RNS can be detrimental to the cells if not controlled. Control of ROS level in healthy cells is by an endogenous antioxidant system consisting of enzymatic and non-enzymatic pathways. The enzymatic pathways include superoxide dismutase (SOD), glutathione peroxidase

(GPx) and catalase, which converts ROS into water or less reactive molecules. Non-enzymatic pathways include glutathione and thioredoxin. Control of RNS level is through regulation of nitric oxide synthase (NOS), the enzyme that catalyzes the production of nitric oxide (NO) from L-arginine.

Imbalance between ROS/RNS and antioxidant/NOS inhibition, as a result of ROS/RNS overproduction or deficiency in antioxidant/NOS inhibition, creates a state known as oxidative stress which is associated with several pathological conditions including sepsis [31]. Several studies have demonstrated the significance of oxidative stress in survival of sepsis patients. Sepsis survivors were shown to have higher antioxidant potential than non-survivors [32] and conversely deficiency in antioxidant capacity correlates with mortality [31]. ROS molecules implicated in sepsis pathogenesis include superoxide (O_2^-), hydrogen peroxide (H_2O_2), and hydroxyl radicals (HO). RNS molecules include NO and peroxynitrite ($ONOO^-$), the latter being formed by a reaction between NO and O_2^-. Among these, NO and its derivative $ONOO^-$ are the most well-studied in sepsis and therefore will be used as an example to illustrate the role of oxidative stress in mitochondrial dysfunction.

NO is produced from the amino acid L-arginine by NOS, which has different isoforms: neuronal NOS (nNOS), endothelial NOS (eNOS), mitochondrial NOS (mtNOS) and inducible NOS (iNOS). nNOS, eNOS and mtNOS are expressed constitutively, whereas iNOS expression is induced by infection, inflammation or trauma [33]. NO is produced both in and outside the mitochondria. Once formed, it can freely diffuse into mitochondria and exert its effects. Under physiological condition, NO reversibly binds to the oxygen binding site of cytochrome c oxidase (complex IV of the electron transport chain), serving as regulator of mitochondrial respiration. Under pathological conditions, such as sepsis, increased NO production via iNOS activation is induced by cytokines such as interferon γ (IFNγ), TNF-α, and IL-1β. This activation of iNOS is via the nuclear factor-κB (NF-κB) signaling pathway which leads to activation of several downstream genes including those responsible for NO and cytokine production [34]. Excess production of NO impairs mitochondrial function through several pathways: (1) binding of high concentration NO to complex IV interrupts the electron transport chain and hence inhibits mitochondrial respiration; (2) enhanced production of ROS, in particularly O_2^- and H_2O_2, as a result of interrupted electron transport chain and proton leak; (3) formation of $ONOO^-$ from interaction of NO and O_2^-. $ONOO^-$ is a powerful oxidant and nitrating agent that plays an important role in mediating mitochondrial dysfunction [35]. In fact, $ONOO^-$ accounts for most of the cytotoxic effects of NO, which include (1) peroxidation of the mitochondrial lipid cardiolipin, a phospholipid on the inner mitochondrial membrane that plays an important role in mitochondrial bioenergetics [36]; (2) inhibition of complex I, other enzyme complexes, and endogenous antioxidants, such as glutathione, by S-nitrosylation or tyrosine nitration [37]; (3) damage of mitochondrial DNA. These detrimental effects on mitochondrial lipids, proteins and DNA will lead to mitochondrial dysfunction and eventually organ failure. The effects of NO and $ONOO^-$ on mitochondria are illustrated in Fig. 41.1.

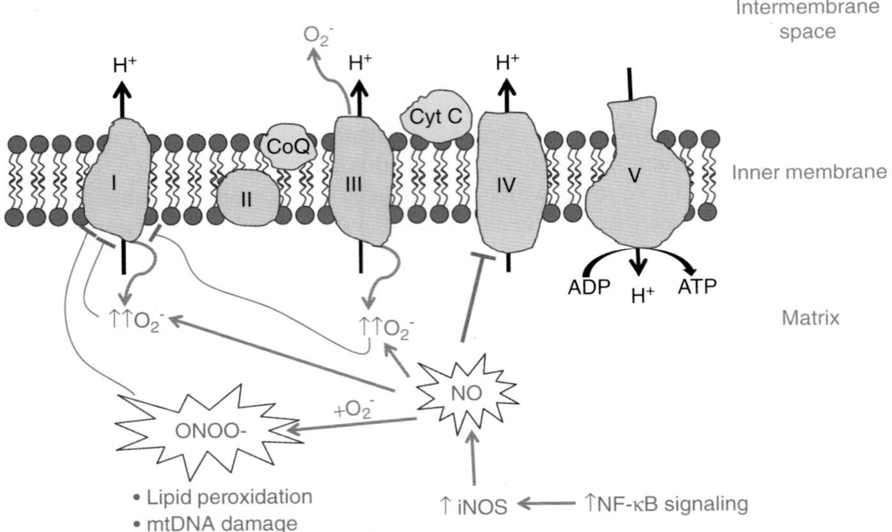

Fig. 41.1 Detrimental effects of nitric oxide (NO) overproduction on mitochondria. *I–V* electron transport chain complexes I–V, *NO* nitric oxide, *OHOO*$^-$ peroxynitrite, O_2^- superoxide, *iNOS* inducible nitric oxide synthase, *NF-κB* nuclear factor-κB, *CoQ* coenzyme Q10, *Cyt C* cytochrome c, *H+* proton, *ADP* adenosine diphosphate, *ATP* adenosine triphosphate

41.5 Potential Therapies for Sepsis: What the Future Holds for Mitochondria?

As discussed earlier in this chapter, mitochondrial dysfunction is associated with disease severity and outcome in septic patients. And oxidative stress has been shown to be one of the important factors contributing to mitochondrial dysfunction. Therefore, recovery of mitochondrial function, either by restoring balance between oxidants and antioxidants within mitochondria, or even better by boosting their biogenesis, could be the key towards better management of patients with sepsis. Recent studies have demonstrated the potential of several antioxidants or molecules to improve the outcome of patients with sepsis. Some of the promising therapies that have been tested in humans include ascorbic acid, NOS inhibitors, and melatonin [14]. Ascorbic acid, the redox form of vitamin C and a natural antioxidant, has passed a Phase I safety trial in patients with severe sepsis [38]. The NOS inhibitor, ketanserin, had beneficial effects in septic patients, with improved microcirculatory perfusion [39]. Melatonin, a hormone that is produced in the pineal gland in the brain, has both anti-inflammatory and antiapoptotic effects. Melatonin also acts as a ROS/RNS scavenger, and has been shown to reduce markers of inflammation and oxidative stress in human endotoxemia model [40]. Compared to targeting oxidative stress, strategies targeting mitochondria biogenesis are less developed due to the complexity of the biogenesis pathways. Several potential therapeutic targets, associated with mitochondrial biogenesis, include PGC-1α, Tfam and NRF-1 as mentioned earlier in this chapter. Another molecule, mitogen-activated protein kinase kinase 3 (MKK3), has also been shown to play an important role in mitochondrial biogenesis in a sepsis mouse model. Higher MKK3 activation has been detected in isolated peripheral blood mononuclear cells from septic patients compared to non-septic controls. In addition to biogenesis, MKK3 is also important for mitophagy (removal of dysfunctional mitochondria), an important process for recovery of mitochondrial function [41]. These molecules deserve further study to explore their therapeutic potential. Last but not least, mitochondrial transplantation, a novel way to replace dysfunctional mitochondria with viable and respiration competent ones, could potentially provide a kick-start to the recovery process of mitochondria, especially in patients with less capacity to initiate the biogenesis process. Mitochondrial transplantation has been tested in pediatric patients with congenital heart disease, resulting in improvement of myocardial function in a small group of the patients [42]. The therapeutic use of mitochondrial transplantation is still in its early days but definitely holds promise for recovering mitochondrial function and hence organ function in sepsis.

41.6 Conclusion

The role of mitochondrial dysfunction in sepsis pathogenesis has created much debate since the 1970s, with varying results likely due to differences in the choice of endotoxemia models (e.g., LPS vs. live bacteria, small animal vs. large animal models) as well as the variations in the generation of the models (e.g., doses of endotoxin or bacteria). Recent studies with the use of clinical samples, in conjunction with availability of more sensitive assays and better study designs, make studies on mitochondrial function more reproducible. This has led to a better understanding of the causes of mitochondrial dysfunction and its association with sepsis severity and outcomes. This is critical for the development of future therapies for sepsis, which is still the major cause of mortality in ICU patients. Antioxidants have been used clinically with some beneficial effects on septic patients; however targeting oxidative stress can be a double-edged sword. Considering the physiological functions of ROS/RNS as seen in healthy cells, it is crucial to achieve that fine balance between beneficial and harmful effects of any proposed therapy.

References

1. Schumer W, Dasgupta TK, Moss GS, Nyhus LM. Effect of endoxemia on liver cell mitochondria in man. Ann Surg. 1970;171:875–82.
2. Schumer W, Erve PR, Obernolte RP. Endotoxemia effect on cardiac and skeletal muscle mitochondria. Surg Gynecol Obstet. 1971;133:433–6.
3. Mela L, Bacalzo LV J, Miller LD. Defective oxidative metabolism of rat liver mitochondria in hemorrhagic and endotoxin shock. Am J Physiol. 1971;220:571–7.

4. Tanaka J, Kono Y, Shimahara Y, et al. A study of oxidative phosphorylative activity and calcium-induced respiration of rat liver mitochondria following living Escherichia coli injection. Adv Shock Res. 1982;7:77–90.
5. Geller ER, Jankauskas S, Kirkpatrick J. Mitochondrial death in sepsis: a failed concept. J Surg Res. 1986;40(5):514–7.
6. Fink M. Cytopathic hypoxia in sepsis. Acta Anaesthesiol Scand Suppl. 1997;110:87–95.
7. Singer M, Brealey D. Mitochondrial dysfunction in sepsis. Biochem Soc Symp. 1999;66:149–66.
8. Gellerich FN1, Trumbeckaite S, Opalka JR, et al. Mitochondrial dysfunction in sepsis: evidence from bacteraemic baboons and endotoxaemic rabbits. Biosci Rep. 2002;22:99–113.
9. Brealey D, Brand M, Hargreaves I, et al. Association between mitochondrial dysfunction and severity and outcome of septic shock. Lancet. 2002;360:219–23.
10. Crouser ED, Julian MW, Blaho DV, Pfeiffer DR. Endotoxin-induced mitochondrial damage correlates with impaired respiratory activity. Crit Care Med. 2002;30:276–84.
11. Porta F, Takala J, Weikert C, et al. Effects of prolonged endotoxemia on liver, skeletal muscle and kidney mitochondrial function. Crit Care. 2006;10:R118.
12. Belikova I, Lukaszewicz AC, Faivre V, Damoisel C, Singer M, Payen D. Oxygen consumption of human peripheral blood mononuclear cells in severe human sepsis. Crit Care Med. 2007;35:2702–8.
13. Galley HF. Oxidative stress and mitochondrial dysfunction in sepsis. Br J Anaesth. 2011;107:57–64.
14. Mantzarlis K, Tsolaki V, Zakynthinos E. Role of oxidative stress and mitochondrial dysfunction in sepsis and potential therapies. Oxidative Med Cell Longev. 2017;2017:5985209.
15. Prauchner CA. Oxidative stress in sepsis: pathophysiological implications justifying antioxidant co-therapy. Burns. 2017;43:471–85.
16. Abraham E, Laterre PF, Garbino J, et al. Lenercept (p55 tumor necrosis factor receptor fusion protein) in severe sepsis and early septic shock: a randomized, double-blind, placebo-controlled, multicenter phase III trial with 1,342 patients. Crit Care Med. 2001;29:503–10.
17. Fisher CJ Jr, Dhainaut JF, Opal SM, et al. Recombinant human interleukin 1 receptor antagonist in the treatment of patients with sepsis syndrome. Results from a randomized, double-blind, placebo-controlled trial. Phase III rhIL-1ra Sepsis Syndrome Study Group. JAMA. 1994;271:1836–43.
18. Ince C. The microcirculation is the motor of sepsis. Crit Care. 2005;9(Suppl 4):S13–9.
19. Hotchkiss RS, Swanson PE, Freeman BD, et al. Apoptotic cell death in patients with sepsis, shock, and multiple organ dysfunction. Crit Care Med. 1999;27:1230–51.
20. Takasu O, Gaut JP, Watanabe E, et al. Mechanisms of cardiac and renal dysfunction in patients dying of sepsis. Am J Respir Crit Care Med. 2013;187:509–17.
21. Rosser DM, Stidwill RP, Jacobson D, Singer M. Oxygen tension in the bladder epithelium rises in both high and low cardiac output endotoxemic sepsis. J Appl Physiol. 1995;79:1878–82.
22. Boekstegers P, Weidenhöfer S, Pilz G, Werdan K. Peripheral oxygen availability within skeletal muscle in sepsis and septic shock: comparison to limited infection and cardiogenic shock. Infection. 1991;19:317–23.
23. Noble JS, MacKirdy FN, Donaldson SI, Howie JC. Renal and respiratory failure in Scottish ICUs. Anaesthesia. 2001;56:124–9.
24. Carré JE, Orban JC, Re L, Felsmann K, et al. Survival in critical illness is associated with early activation of mitochondrial biogenesis. Am J Respir Crit Care Med. 2010;182:745–51.
25. Singer M. The role of mitochondrial dysfunction in sepsis-induced multi-organ failure. Virulence. 2014;5:66–72.
26. Suliman HB, Welty-Wolf KE, Carraway M, Tatro L, Piantadosi CA. Lipopolysaccharide induces oxidative cardiac mitochondrial damage and biogenesis. Cardiovasc Res. 2004;64:279–88.
27. Haden DW, Suliman HB, Carraway MS, et al. Mitochondrial biogenesis restores oxidative metabolism during Staphylococcus aureus sepsis. Am J Respir Crit Care Med. 2007;176:768–77.

28. Kaymak C, Basar H, Sardas S. Reactive oxygen species (Ros) generation in sepsis. FABAD J Pharm Sci. 2011;36:41–7.
29. Di Meo S, Reed TT, Venditti P, Victor VM. Role of ROS and RNS sources in physiological and pathological conditions. Oxidative Med Cell Longev. 2016;2016:1245049.
30. Bogdan C. Nitric oxide and the regulation of gene expression. Trends Cell Biol. 2001;11:66–75.
31. Karapetsa M, Pitsika M, Goutzourelas N, Stagos D, Tousia Becker A, Zakynthinos E. Oxidative status in ICU patients with septic shock. Food Chem Toxicol. 2013;61:106–11.
32. Cowley HC, Bacon PJ, Goode HF, Webster NR, Jones JG, Menon DK. Plasma antioxidant potential in severe sepsis: a comparison of survivors and nonsurvivors. Crit Care Med. 1996;24:1179–83.
33. Nathan C, Xie QW. Nitric oxide synthases: roles, tolls, and controls. Cell. 1994;78:915–8.
34. Perkins ND. Integrating cell-signalling pathways with NF-kappaB and IKK function. Nat Rev Mol Cell Biol. 2007;8:49–62.
35. Boczkowski J, Lisdero CL, Lanone S. Endogenous peroxynitrite mediates mitochondrial dysfunction in rat diaphragm during endotoxemia. FASEB J. 1999;13:1637–46.
36. Paradies G, Paradies V, De Benedictis V, Ruggiero FM, Petrosillo G. Functional role of cardiolipin in mitochondrial bioenergetics. Biochim Biophys Acta. 2014;1837:408–17.
37. Brown GC, Borutaite V. Inhibition of mitochondrial respiratory complex I by nitric oxide, peroxynitrite and S-nitrosothiols. Biochim Biophys Acta. 2004;1658:44–9.
38. Fowler AA, Syed AA, Knowlson S, et al. Phase I safety trial of intravenous ascorbic acid in patients with severe sepsis. J Transl Med. 2014;12:32.
39. Vellinga NA, Veenstra G, Scorcella C, et al. Effects of ketanserin on microcirculatory alterations in septic shock: an open-label pilot study. J Crit Care. 2015;30:1156–62.
40. Alamili M, Bendtzen K, Lykkesfeldt J, Rosenberg J, Gögenur I. Melatonin suppresses markers of inflammation and oxidative damage in a human daytime endotoxemia model. J Crit Care. 2014;29:184.e9–184.e13.
41. Mannam P, Shinn AS, Srivastava A, et al. MKK3 regulates mitochondrial biogenesis and mitophagy in sepsis-induced lung injury. Am J Physiol Lung Cell Mol Physiol. 2014;306:L604–19.
42. Emani SM, McCully JD. Mitochondrial transplantation: applications for pediatric patients with congenital heart disease. Transl Pediatr. 2018;7:169–75.

Potential Harm Related to Fluid Resuscitation in Sepsis

42

F. van Haren, L. Byrne, and E. Litton

42.1 Introduction

A liberal approach to fluid resuscitation in patients with sepsis and evidence of hypoperfusion is endorsed by international guidelines as an essential first-line intervention [1]. The use of this therapy is based in part on a long history and familiarity with fluid use in the resuscitation of other forms of shock and a "hypoperfusion centric" theory of the pathophysiology of sepsis [2]. The Surviving Sepsis Campaign recommendation for a fluid challenge given at a rate of 500–1000 mL of crystalloids or 300–500 mL of colloids over 30 min, is graded as Grade E, which means it is supported only by non-randomized historical controls, case series, uncontrolled studies and expert opinion [1]. In addition to a lack of high quality randomized controlled trials (RCTs), demonstrating benefit of standard volume fluid resuscitation for sepsis compared to a lower dose, the safety of standard doses of intravenous resuscitation has also been called into question. Data from experimental, observational and prospective randomized studies suggest improved outcomes with a restrictive approach to fluid resuscitation [2–5].

There are two main proposed mechanisms by which fluid resuscitation in sepsis may cause harm. The first relates to direct deleterious effects of fluid bolus therapy on several aspects of cardiovascular function. The second mechanism of harm is related to the consequences of fluid overload on end-organ function. The aim of this chapter is to describe the evidence supporting potential mechanisms by which the current standard, liberal approach to fluid resuscitation in patients with

F. van Haren (✉) · L. Byrne
Intensive Care Unit, Canberra Hospital, Woden, ACT, Australia

Medical School, Australian National University, Canberra, ACT, Australia
e-mail: fvanharen@me.com

E. Litton
Intensive Care Unit, Fiona Stanley Hospital, Perth, WA, Australia

J.-L. Vincent (ed.), *Annual Update in Intensive Care and Emergency Medicine 2019*, Annual Update in Intensive Care and Emergency Medicine,
https://doi.org/10.1007/978-3-030-06067-1_42

sepsis may be harmful. The risks and benefits of different types of resuscitation fluid (e.g., balanced fluids, colloids) have been addressed elsewhere and will not be reviewed.

42.2 Cardiovascular Dysfunction Associated with Bolus Fluid Therapy

Bolus fluid therapy is recommended as soon as sepsis-induced tissue hypoperfusion (hypotension or lactic acidosis) is recognized, and the goals of resuscitation should include central venous pressure (CVP), blood pressure, urine output and central venous oxygen saturation ($ScvO_2$) [1]. Improvement in these surrogate measures is presumed to indicate improved tissue perfusion which would then result in better outcomes. However, despite early signs of cardiovascular improvement after bolus fluid therapy, cardiovascular dysfunction and outcomes in fact seem to worsen.

In the Fluid Expansion As Supportive Therapy trial (FEAST), investigators randomized 3141 children with severe sepsis to receive fluid resuscitation with either 40 mL/kg of 0.9% saline, 4% albumin or no volume resuscitation [3]. The trial was stopped early for harm, demonstrating a 40% increase in mortality with fluid resuscitation irrespective of type. Much has been made with regard to the correct interpretation of these findings. It has been suggested that the findings are specific to the unique population, with a high incidence of malaria (57%), severe anemia <5 g/dL (32%) and acidosis (base deficit >8 mmol/L, 51%) and with saline and albumin causing disease-specific deterioration and worsening of both anemia and acidosis. However, the published subgroup analysis does not support these conclusions and shows similar point estimates for harm independent of prior malaria, baseline hemoglobin and base deficit [3]. Surprisingly, the increase in mortality did not appear to be related to complications of fluid overload but rather to delayed cardiovascular collapse causing refractory shock [6].

In another randomized clinical trial that included 209 adults with sepsis and hypotension presenting to an emergency department in Zambia, a 6-h sepsis protocol emphasizing administration of intravenous fluids, vasopressors, and blood transfusion was compared with usual care [4]. The sepsis protocol resulted in greater intravenous fluid administration use and, despite greater vasopressor (dopamine) use, similar systolic and diastolic blood pressure readings compared to patients in the standard care group. The sepsis protocol caused more frequent worsening of hypoxemia and tachypnea and higher rates of in-hospital and 28-day mortality (absolute differences 15% for in-hospital and 22% for 28-day mortality).

To investigate the mechanisms underlying the provocative findings of these clinical trials, a pre-clinical ovine study was conducted comparing an early fluid resuscitation strategy versus a no-fluid resuscitation strategy [7]. First, a hyperdynamic sheep model of sepsis reflective of human sepsis was established and validated [8]. Endotoxemic shock was induced after which the animals received either fluid resuscitation with 40 mL/kg of 0.9% saline (similar to the FEAST study) or commenced hemodynamic support with protocolized norepinephrine and vasopressin. As expected, the fluid resuscitated animals had a large increase in cardiac output immediately after the fluid bolus was administered. While mean arterial blood pressure (MAP) improved over the hour of resuscitation, the magnitude of the increase was modest compared to the increase in cardiac output because of a concurrent decrease in the systemic vascular resistance (SVR). Consistent with the findings of the two previously mentioned RCTs, animals that received fluid resuscitation required significantly more norepinephrine to maintain the same MAP in the 12 h after resuscitation, suggesting that fluid resuscitation induced vasodilation and resistance to vasopressor agents. Importantly, there were no differences between groups in effects on the microcirculation and on microvascular oxygen delivery, with similar brain, kidney, heart, and liver lactate/pyruvate ratios as measured by microdialysis.

The potential pathways that could contribute to the observed cardiovascular dysfunction following bolus fluid therapy for sepsis-induced tissue hypoperfusion are discussed below and summarized in Fig. 42.1.

42.2.1 Fluid Resuscitation-Induced Vasodilation

Fluid resuscitation-induced vasodilation has been reported in a number of experimental and clinical studies. It has been hypothesized that the use of fluid therapy to optimize cardiac preload could potentially contribute to impaired arterial load and ventriculo-arterial decoupling. Experimental studies have also suggested that the typical hemodynamic profile of vasodilatory shock (low SVR and high cardiac

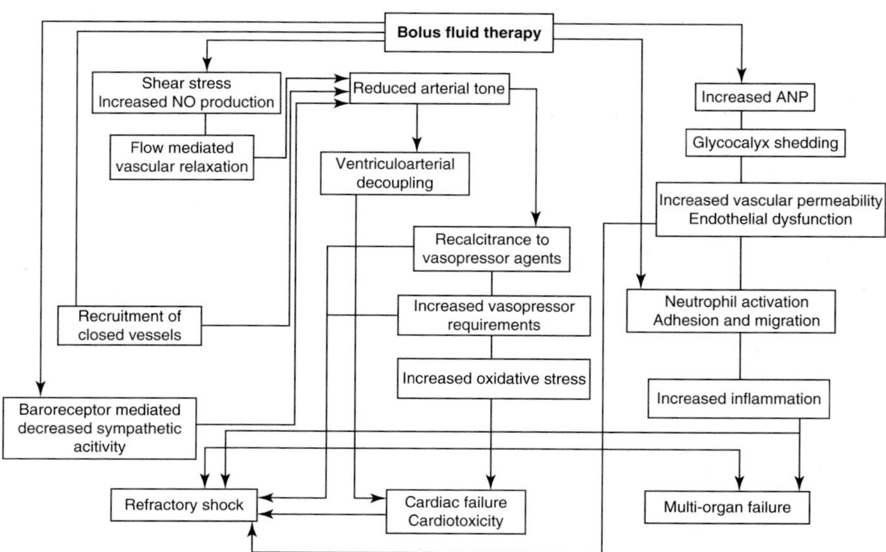

Fig. 42.1 Flow diagram of the proposed mechanisms of cardiovascular dysfunction associated with fluid bolus therapy in septic shock. *ANP* atrial natriuretic peptide, *NO* nitric oxide

output), could actually be induced by fluid administration, transforming the initial non-resuscitated hypodynamic profile into a hyperdynamic state [9–11]. Monge Garcia et al. described the immediate effects of fluid bolus resuscitation on arterial load in 81 patients with sepsis [12]. While 67% of the patients had an increase in cardiac output of at least 10% with fluid resuscitation, only 44% of those preload responsive patients also had an increase in MAP. Fluid resuscitation resulted in a decrease in SVR that was most marked amongst patients in whom cardiac output increased. The authors concluded that fluid administration significantly reduced arterial load in critically patients with septic shock and acute circulatory failure, even when increasing cardiac output. In a similar observational study in 51 patients with sepsis, Pierrakos et al. reported that for patients who had a significant increase in their cardiac output, fluid resuscitation resulted in a decrease in their SVR [13]. In another experimental study investigating the effects of arterial load variations, fluid bolus administration decreased the dynamic arterial elastance, with no relationship between changes in cardiac output and MAP after fluid administration [14].

The underlying mechanism of fluid resuscitation-induced vasodilation is unclear and several explanations have been suggested. Intravascular volume administration may blunt the baroreflex-mediated vasoconstriction in response to hypovolemia [12]. Fluid resuscitation could also recruit previously closed vessels, thereby reducing arterial resistance. Further, flow-mediated vascular relaxation secondary to endothelial shear stress and release of endothelial nitric oxide (NO) has been demonstrated to lead to a reduction in arterial tone. Intravital microscopic studies have suggested that large resistance vessels, which are responsible for 40–55% of the total network resistance, are under tight control of endothelial factors such as NO and endothelium-derived hyperpolarizing factor [15]. Fluid administration increases blood flow velocity and thus endothelial shear stress, causing the release of NO by the vascular endothelium [11]. Laminar shear stress also results in integrin-mediated release of fibroblast growth factor-2 (FGF-2), which is thought to be a stimulus in the endothelium-dependent control of vascular tone [16].

42.2.2 Fluid Resuscitation-Associated Cardiotoxicity

Another mechanism that could contribute to the observed cardiovascular collapse after bolus fluid resuscitation is through cardiotoxicity. In the abovementioned ovine study by Byrne and co-workers, animals that received fluid resuscitation also showed impaired myocardial contractility and increased troponin levels [7]. The observed increase in troponin suggests the additional vasopressors required to maintain hemodynamic stability may have important bystander effects and result in secondary cardiac injury.

The mechanism underlying this cardiotoxicity is unclear, but a number of potential mechanisms have been proposed. These include mitochondrial oxidative stress, microvascular thrombi and increased sarcolemma membrane permeability [17, 18]. Catecholamines have been shown to increase myocardial oxidative stress in experimental models and in a murine model of sepsis [19]. For example, using strain echocardiography, it was demonstrated that increased oxidative stress was a central factor in development of sepsis-induced myocardial dysfunction [20].

42.2.3 Effects of Fluid Resuscitation on the Glycocalyx

The effects of fluid infusion on the integrity of the glycocalyx remain poorly understood. Degradation of the glycocalyx on the vascular luminal cell membrane has been identified to be an early step in septic vascular endothelial cell disorder [21]. Fluid therapy has the potential to further damage the glycocalyx, especially when rapid infusions are used and when fluid infusion results in hypervolemia. Degradation of the glycocalyx barrier is often assessed by measuring plasma levels of glycocalyx breakdown products, such as hyaluronan. Hyaluronan is one of the main constituents of the glycocalyx barrier with plasma levels shown to correlate with glycocalyx thickness in humans [22] and the administration of hyaluronidase was shown to significantly reduce the size and volume of the glycocalyx [23]. Additionally, in experimental models of glycocalyx injury using ischemia/reperfusion models, increased levels of hyaluronan following injury have been shown to directly correlate with glycocalyx damage in subsequent imaging [24]. In clinical studies, increases in hyaluronan have been shown to occur in conjunction with other known glycocalyx products, such as syndecan and heparan sulphate [25].

A number of studies have found an increase in hyaluronan following intravenous fluid administration, suggesting that infusion of crystalloid fluids may cause damage to the glycocalyx. For example, following infusion of crystalloid solution in healthy volunteers, plasma hyaluronan levels increased [26]. This glycocalyx shedding may be mediated by release of atrial natriuretic peptide (ANP) in response to hypervolemia. Chappell et al. demonstrated experimentally that acute hypervolemia led to both ANP release and increased glycocalyx breakdown products in humans prior to undergoing surgery [25]. Others were able to demonstrate that administration of exogenous physiological levels of ANP led to glycocalyx shedding and increased vascular permeability in experimental models [23, 27]. In the study by Byrne et al., animals assigned to fluid resuscitation had prolonged endotoxemia-induced release of circulating ANP, followed by an increased rate of hyaluronic acid shedding into the blood [7].

42.2.4 Inflammatory Effects of Fluid Resuscitation

Different conventional hemodynamic optimization strategies in septic patients result in distinct biomarker patterns [28]. In experimental human endotoxemia, prehydration shifts the cytokine pattern toward a more anti-inflammatory state and results in fewer clinical sepsis symptoms, suggesting an association between the inflammatory response and the hydration or resuscitation status of patients with sepsis [29]. It has been suggested that resuscitation fluids have dose-related pro-inflammatory properties, relating to neutrophil activation and that there are differences between types of fluids [30, 31]. In patients with septic shock, hypertonic fluid administration compared with isotonic fluid may modulate expression of genes that are implicated in leukocyte-endothelial interactions and capillary leakage [32]. In the previously described study by Byrne et al., there was no evidence that treatment allocation affected the inflammatory response to endotoxemia, as assessed by levels of inflammatory and anti-inflammatory cytokines [7].

42.3 Harm Caused by Fluid Overload

It is now well established that fluid overload in patients with sepsis is associated with edema development and worse outcomes [5, 33–36]. The pathological sequelae of fluid overload in kidneys and other organ systems have been described in detail [37]. Fluid overload can be caused by initial or on-going fluid resuscitation by bolus fluid therapy, or by maintenance fluid therapy and fluid creep [38].

A conservative fluid strategy may therefore improve patient outcomes. This was shown in the ARDS Network Fluids and Catheters Treatment Trial (FACTT). In this study, 1000 patients with acute lung injury were randomized to a conservative or a liberal strategy of fluid management using explicit protocols that were applied for 7 days. Patients in the conservative strategy arm showed significantly improved lung function and shorter duration of mechanical ventilation and intensive care without increased non-pulmonary organ failures [39]. In a recently published Scandinavian RCT (the Conservative vs. Liberal Approach to fluid therapy of Septic Shock in Intensive Care [CLASSIC] trial), a protocol restricting resuscitation fluid successfully reduced volumes of resuscitation fluid compared with a standard care protocol in adult intensive care unit (ICU) patients with septic shock and showed that patient-centered outcomes all pointed towards benefit with fluid restriction [40]. Importantly, there were no indications of worsening of measures of circulatory efficacy in the first 24 h of restriction of resuscitation fluid as compared with standard care as assessed by urine output, lactate levels and norepinephrine requirements [41].

42.4 Bolus Fluid Therapy: Unresolved Issues

There are several important issues with the concept and use of bolus fluid therapy in clinical practice. First, there is no universally accepted definition of what bolus fluid therapy is and how it should be administered, and what physiological effects clinicians expect as a result of bolus fluid therapy. This was illustrated in a recent survey amongst acute care physicians in Australia and New Zealand [42]. This study showed that bolus fluid therapy is a poorly defined intervention with considerable variability in preferred fluid choice, volume given and speed of delivery. In addition, intensive care and emergency medicine specialists showed wide variation in what they expected the physiological response to bolus fluid therapy to be. Similar wide variability between individuals and countries was found when the researchers expanded their study to 3138 practitioners from 30 countries [43]. Another global inception cohort study, the Fluid challenges in Intensive Care (FENICE) study, concluded that current practice and evaluation of bolus fluid therapy in critically ill patients are highly variable [44].

Second, the physiological effects of bolus fluid therapy in critically ill patients have not been well studied. This was highlighted in a systematic review of contemporary data of physiological changes after bolus fluid therapy in sepsis [45]. No RCTs compared bolus fluid therapy with alternative interventions, such as vasopressors. Although 17 studies described the temporal course of physiological changes after bolus fluid therapy in 31 patient groups, only three studies described the physiological changes at 60 min, and only one study beyond this point. No studies related the physiological changes after bolus fluid therapy to clinically relevant outcomes. The authors concluded that there is a clear need to at least obtain randomized controlled evidence for the physiological effects of bolus fluid therapy beyond the period immediately after its administration. In addition, the most effective rate of bolus fluid therapy is unknown. The rate at which a fluid bolus is administered appears to influence hemodynamic variables. In a randomized crossover pilot study in a healthy volunteer model of compensated hemorrhagic shock, fast fluid resuscitation resulted in a higher blood pressure, but the cardiac index paradoxically decreased in most participants during the fast resuscitation phase; a finding not observed in the slow fluid resuscitation group [46].

Third, the hemodynamic response to a fluid bolus is usually small and short-lived, and the clinical relevance of this physiological effect is uncertain. In the previously mentioned systematic review of contemporary data of physiological changes after bolus fluid therapy, the MAP increased on average by 7.8 mmHg immediately after a fluid bolus, and returned close to baseline after 1 h, with no increase in urine output [45]. These results were confirmed in a well conducted prospective observational study, in which the duration of hemodynamic effects of crystalloids was assessed in patients with circulatory shock after their initial resuscitation [47]. The duration of the volume effect was found to be short in all patients, as well as in the subgroup of fluid responders, with cardiac output and blood pressure returning to baseline levels 60 min after the fluid bolus [47]. In a retrospective analysis of the ARDS Network FACTT, hemodynamic responses were investigated in a convenience sample of 127 patients. In this study, critically ill patients were given protocol-based crystalloid or albumin boluses for shock, low urine output, or low pulmonary artery occlusion pressure (PAOP). There were significant increases in mean CVP and mean PAOP following fluid boluses. However, there were no significant changes in urine output, and there were clinically small changes in heart rate, MAP and cardiac index [48]. These observations of clinically small and short-lived hemodynamic responses to bolus fluid therapy are not limited to patients who have already been fluid resuscitated. In shocked patients in the emergency department, the median increase in MAP was only 3 mmHg 1 h after bolus fluid therapy, with no effect on the heart rate [49].

Finally, bolus fluid therapy carries a significant potential for harm, especially if used indiscriminately. Alarmingly, clinicians do not appear to be particularly good at determining whether a patient will benefit from the administration of a fluid bolus, especially when basing this decision on clinical examination and static hemodynamic indices such as CVP. In studies summarized in a review by Michard and Teboul in 2002, around 50% of patients who received a fluid bolus based on clinical signs and static hemodynamic measurements such as CVP turned out to be not fluid responsive [50]. Unfortunately, clinicians do not widely use measures of fluid responsiveness in usual practice, as evidenced by the earlier referenced observational FENICE study [44]. Not only was prediction of fluid responsiveness not used routinely, safety limits for bolus fluid therapy were also rarely used. There was no statistically significant difference in the proportion of patients who received further fluids after the previous fluid bolus between those with a positive, with an uncertain or with a negatively judged response to fluids. In other words, patients who were proven to be not fluid responsive, continued to receive the same amount of subsequent fluid boluses as did fluid responsive patients [44]. This practice undoubtedly increases the risk of fluid overload-associated harm in critically ill patients.

42.5 Future Directions

Going forward, we need to focus on several important issues. First, we need to design rigorous experimental research to re-examine the effects of early fluid resuscitation in sepsis. The effects of fluid infusion in sepsis on the arterial load, the immune system, on endothelial function and on the integrity of the glycocalyx, remain poorly understood. Second, we need to perform adequately powered multicenter studies comparing limited or no fluid strategies to current standard care for the treatment of septic shock.

Next, we need to educate clinicians about the risks of fluid loading patients who are not fluid responsive. The potential of harm caused by bolus fluid therapy should more clearly feature in guidelines. Implementation of a physiologic, hemodynamically guided conservative approach to fluid therapy in patients with sepsis would possibly reduce the morbidity and improve outcomes. The safety, feasibility and efficacy of targeted fluid minimization strategies using protocol-guided assessments of fluid responsiveness holds promise but needs to be further investigated.

42.6 Conclusion

Fluid resuscitation has long been the cornerstone of the treatment of septic shock, albeit with a poor evidence base in terms of its effects on outcome. An increasing body of literature suggests that early bolus fluid therapy may cause harm. Potential mechanisms of harm include cardiovascular collapse associated with vasodilation, cardiotoxicity, endothelial glycocalyx damage and inflammatory effects. In addition, harm may be caused by the effects of fluid overload as a result of fluid administration.

Dr. Latta, in his landmark letter to the Lancet in 1831 when describing his experience with "the treatment of cholera by the copious injection of aqueous and saline fluids into the vein", wrote the following words: "..., and I have no doubt that it will be found, when judiciously applied, to be one of the most powerful, and one of the safest remedies yet used….." [51]. We still have some way to go to live up to Dr. Latta's expectations.

References

1. Rhodes A, Evans LE, Alhazzani W, et al. Surviving Sepsis Campaign: International Guidelines for Management of Sepsis and Septic Shock: 2016. Intensive Care Med. 2017;43:304–77.
2. Byrne L, Van Haren F. Fluid resuscitation in human sepsis: time to rewrite history? Ann Intensive Care. 2017;7:4.
3. Maitland K, Kiguli S, Opoka RO, et al. Mortality after fluid bolus in African children with severe infection. N Engl J Med. 2011;364:2483–95.
4. Andrews B, Semler MW, Muchemwa L, et al. Effect of an early resuscitation protocol on in-hospital mortality among adults with sepsis and hypotension: a randomized clinical trial. JAMA. 2017;318:1233–40.
5. Boyd JH, Forbes J, Nakada TA, Walley KR, Russell JA. Fluid resuscitation in septic shock: a positive fluid balance and elevated central venous pressure are associated with increased mortality. Crit Care Med. 2011;39:259–65.
6. Maitland K, George EC, Evans JA, et al. Exploring mechanisms of excess mortality with early fluid resuscitation: insights from the FEAST trial. BMC Med. 2013;11:1.
7. Byrne L, Obonyo NG, Diab SD, et al. Unintended consequences; fluid resuscitation worsens shock in an ovine model of endotoxemia. Am J Respir Crit Care Med. 2018;198:1043–54.
8. Byrne L, Obonyo NG, Diab S, et al. An ovine model of hyperdynamic endotoxemia and vital organ metabolism. Shock. 2017;49:99–107.
9. Cholley BP, Lang RM, Berger DS, Korcarz C, Payen D, Shroff SG. Alterations in systemic arterial mechanical properties during septic shock: role of fluid resuscitation. Am J Phys. 1995;269:H375–84.
10. Ricard-Hibon A, Losser MR, Kong R, Beloucif S, Teisseire B, Payen D. Systemic pressure-flow reactivity to norepinephrine in rabbits: impact of endotoxin and fluid loading. Intensive Care Med. 1998;24:959–66.
11. Losser MR, Forget AP, Payen D. Nitric oxide involvement in the hemodynamic response to fluid resuscitation in endotoxic shock in rats. Crit Care Med. 2006;34:2426–31.
12. Monge García IM, González PG, Romero MG, et al. Effects of fluid administration on arterial load in septic shock patients. Intensive Care Med. 2015;41:1247–55.
13. Pierrakos C, Velissaris D, Scolletta S, Heenen S, De Backer D, Vincent JL. Can changes in arterial pressure be used to detect changes in cardiac index during fluid challenge in patients with septic shock? Intensive Care Med. 2012;38:422–8.
14. Monge Garcia MI, Guijo Gonzalez P, Gracia Romero M, et al. Effects of arterial load variations on dynamic arterial elastance: an experimental study. Br J Anaesth. 2017;118:938–46.
15. Pohl U, De Wit C, Gloe T. Large arterioles in the control of blood flow: role of endothelium-dependent dilation. Acta Physiol Scand. 2000;168:505–10.
16. Hennig T, Mogensen C, Kirsch J, Pohl U, Gloe T. Shear stress induces the release of an endothelial elastase: role in integrin alpha(v)beta(3)-mediated FGF-2 release. J Vasc Res. 2011;48:453–64.
17. Maeder M, Fehr T, Rickli H, Ammann P. Sepsis-associated myocardial dysfunction: diagnostic and prognostic impact of cardiac troponins and natriuretic peptides. Chest. 2006;129:1349–66.
18. Bessière F, Khenifer S, Dubourg J, Durieu I, Lega J-C. Prognostic value of troponins in sepsis: a meta-analysis. Intensive Care Med. 2013;39:1181–9.
19. Neri M, Cerretani D, Fiaschi AI, et al. Correlation between cardiac oxidative stress and myocardial pathology due to acute and chronic norepinephrine administration in rats. J Cell Mol Med. 2007;11:156–70.

20. Haileselassie B, Su E, Pozios I, et al. Myocardial oxidative stress correlates with left ventricular dysfunction on strain echocardiography in a rodent model of sepsis. Intensive Care Med Exp. 2017;5:21.
21. Henrich M, Gruss M, Weigand MA. Sepsis-induced degradation of endothelial glycocalix. ScientificWorldJournal. 2010;10:917–23.
22. von Geldern TW, Budzik GP, Dillon TP, et al. Atrial natriuretic peptide antagonists: biological evaluation and structural correlations. Mol Pharmacol. 1990;38:771–8.
23. Bruegger D, Jacob M, Rehm M, et al. Atrial natriuretic peptide induces shedding of endothelial glycocalyx in coronary vascular bed of guinea pig hearts. Am J Physiol Heart Circ Physiol. 2005;289:H1993–9.
24. Chen C, Chappell D, Annecke T, et al. Sevoflurane mitigates shedding of hyaluronan from the coronary endothelium, also during ischemia/reperfusion: an ex vivo animal study. Hypoxia (Auckl). 2016;4:81–90.
25. Chappell D, Bruegger D, Potzel J, et al. Hypervolemia increases release of atrial natriuretic peptide and shedding of the endothelial glycocalyx. Crit Care. 2014;18:538.
26. Berg S, Engman A, Hesselvik JF, Laurent TC. Crystalloid infusion increases plasma hyaluronan. Crit Care Med. 1994;22:1563–7.
27. Jacob M, Saller T, Chappell D, Rehm M, Welsch U, Becker BF. Physiological levels of A-, B-and C-type natriuretic peptide shed the endothelial glycocalyx and enhance vascular permeability. Basic Res Cardiol. 2013;108:347.
28. Rivers EP, Kruse JA, Jacobsen G, et al. The influence of early hemodynamic optimization on biomarker patterns of severe sepsis and septic shock. Crit Care Med. 2007;35:2016–24.
29. Dorresteijn MJ, van Eijk LT, Netea MG, Smits P, van der Hoeven JG, Pickkers P. Iso-osmolar prehydration shifts the cytokine response towards a more anti-inflammatory balance in human endotoxemia. J Endotoxin Res. 2005;11:287–93.
30. Rhee P, Wang D, Ruff P, et al. Human neutrophil activation and increased adhesion by various resuscitation fluids. Crit Care Med. 2000;28:74–8.
31. Lee SH, Seo EH, Park HJ, et al. The effects of crystalloid versus synthetic colloid in vitro on immune cells, co-cultured with mouse splenocytes. Sci Rep. 2018;8:4794.
32. van Haren FM, Sleigh J, Cursons R, La Pine M, Pickkers P, van der Hoeven JG. The effects of hypertonic fluid administration on the gene expression of inflammatory mediators in circulating leucocytes in patients with septic shock: a preliminary study. Ann Intensive Care. 2011;1:44.
33. Malbrain ML, Marik PE, Witters I, et al. Fluid overload, de-resuscitation, and outcomes in critically ill or injured patients: a systematic review with suggestions for clinical practice. Anaesthesiol Intensive Ther. 2014;46:361–80.
34. Sadaka F, Juarez M, Naydenov S, O'Brien J. Fluid resuscitation in septic shock: the effect of increasing fluid balance on mortality. J Intensive Care Med. 2014;29:213–7.
35. Smith SH, Perner A. Higher vs. lower fluid volume for septic shock: clinical characteristics and outcome in unselected patients in a prospective, multicenter cohort. Crit Care. 2012;16:R76.
36. Samoni S, Vigo V, Resendiz LI, et al. Impact of hyperhydration on the mortality risk in critically ill patients admitted in intensive care units: comparison between bioelectrical impedance vector analysis and cumulative fluid balance recording. Crit Care. 2016;20:95.
37. Prowle JR, Echeverri JE, Ligabo EV, Ronco C, Bellomo R. Fluid balance and acute kidney injury. Nat Rev Nephrol. 2010;6:107–15.
38. Van Regenmortel N, Verbrugghe W, Roelant E, Van den Wyngaert T, Jorens PG. Maintenance fluid therapy and fluid creep impose more significant fluid, sodium, and chloride burdens than resuscitation fluids in critically ill patients: a retrospective study in a tertiary mixed ICU population. Intensive Care Med. 2018;44:409–17.
39. Wiedemann HP, Wheeler AP, Bernard GR, et al. Comparison of two fluid-management strategies in acute lung injury. N Engl J Med. 2006;354:2564–75.
40. Hjortrup PB, Haase N, Bundgaard H, et al. Restricting volumes of resuscitation fluid in adults with septic shock after initial management: the CLASSIC randomised, parallel-group, multicentre feasibility trial. Intensive Care Med. 2016;42:1695–705.

41. Hjortrup PB, Haase N, Wetterslev J, et al. Effects of fluid restriction on measures of circulatory efficacy in adults with septic shock. Acta Anaesthesiol Scand. 2017;61:390–8.
42. Glassford NJ, Jones SL, Martensson J, et al. Characteristics and expectations of fluid bolus therapy: a bi-national survey of acute care physicians. Anaesth Intensive Care. 2015;43:750–6.
43. Glassford NJ, Martensson J, Eastwood GM, et al. Defining the characteristics and expectations of fluid bolus therapy: a worldwide perspective. J Crit Care. 2016;35:126–32.
44. Cecconi M, Hofer C, Teboul JL, et al. Fluid challenges in intensive care: the FENICE study: a global inception cohort study. Intensive Care Med. 2015;41:1529–37.
45. Glassford NJ, Eastwood GM, Bellomo R. Physiological changes after fluid bolus therapy in sepsis: a systematic review of contemporary data. Crit Care. 2014;18:696.
46. Ho L, Lau L, Churilov L, et al. Comparative evaluation of crystalloid resuscitation rate in a human model of compensated haemorrhagic shock. Shock. 2016;46:149–57.
47. Nunes TS, Ladeira RT, Bafi AT, et al. Duration of hemodynamic effects of crystalloids in patients with circulatory shock after initial resuscitation. Ann Intensive Care. 2014;4:25.
48. Lammi MR, Aiello B, Burg GT, et al. Response to fluid boluses in the fluid and catheter treatment trial. Chest. 2015;148:919–26.
49. Bihari S, Teubner DJ, Prakash S, et al. Fluid bolus therapy in emergency department patients: indications and physiological changes. Emerg Med Australas. 2016;28:531–7.
50. Michard F, Teboul JL. Predicting fluid responsiveness in ICU patients: a critical analysis of the evidence. Chest. 2002;121:2000–8.
51. Latta T. Malignant cholera: documents communicated by the Central Board of Health, London, relative to the treatment of cholera by the copious injection of aqueous and saline fluids into the veins. Lancet. 1832;18:274–7.

Extracorporeal Cytokine Removal in Septic Shock

43

F. Hawchar, N. Öveges, and Z. Molnár

43.1 Introduction

The incidence of sepsis has increased over the decades and it seems to be the single most important cause of hospitalization, which makes it a serious health economic issue worldwide [1–3]. Despite recent advances in early recognition, adequate resuscitation, organ support, appropriate antibiotic therapy and source control, mortality rates are still around 20–50% depending on the source of the data [4, 5]. One of the more theoretical approaches to improve outcomes is the modulation of the immune system and the host response, which has been in the spotlight of research for decades. Hitherto, anti-inflammatory therapies, such as anti-cytokines, anti-oxidants, etc., have been tested, but the results disappointing [6, 7]. Nevertheless, modulating the "cytokine storm" that occurs in the early phase of septic shock as a result of a dysregulated immune response could provide some benefits by regaining the control between a pro-inflammatory and anti-inflammatory imbalance [8].

43.2 Pathophysiological Background

The immune system is a composite network that relies on both innate and adaptive components. The first line of defense against invaders consists of physical barriers, such as the skin [9, 10], and the mucous membranes of the respiratory [11], gastro-intestinal [12] and genitourinary tracts [13]. The second line of defense is the rapidly acting immune system that requires the co-production of the innate and adaptive immune systems [14].

By-and-large the role of the innate immune system is to kill invading pathogens by releasing pro-inflammatory mediators, cytokines, oxygen free radicals, etc. The role of

F. Hawchar · N. Öveges · Z. Molnár (✉)
Department of Anesthesiology and Intensive Care, University of Szeged, Szeged, Hungary
e-mail: molnar.lajos.zsolt@med.u-szeged.hu

J.-L. Vincent (ed.), *Annual Update in Intensive Care and Emergency Medicine 2019*, Annual Update in Intensive Care and Emergency Medicine,
https://doi.org/10.1007/978-3-030-06067-1_43

the adaptive immune system at this stage is to control this process by keeping the 'war' localized to the site of the infection, hence, not allowing the inflammatory response to become systemic. Normally, these two antagonistic forces are activated in a parallel manner.

It was a very important discovery that after trauma, burn injury, ischemia/reperfusion, pancreatitis, major surgery, hepatic cirrhosis etc., the same or at least a similar immune response is induced and similar molecules are released as in the case of infection, because of the common genetic background of mitochondria and bacteria [15]. These molecules are called damage-associated molecular patterns (DAMP) in the case of tissue and pathogen-associated molecular patterns (PAMP) in the case of infection.

Normally, the PAMP- and DAMP-induced pro- and anti-inflammatory forces work in parallel and in harmony with each other keeping an equilibrium for a certain period of time, then their activity returns to baseline and the infection is resolved (Fig. 43.1a). However, in patients with septic shock this balance becomes impaired

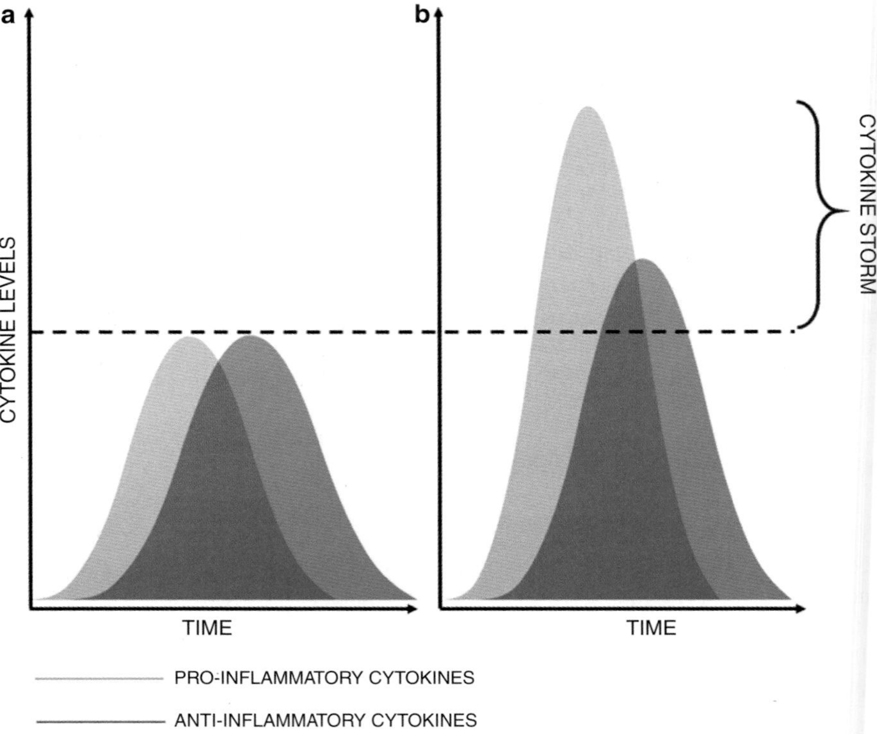

Fig. 43.1 Normal, and dysregulated pro- and anti-inflammatory response. (**a**) The 'normal' response for infection. In this case both the pro- and anti-inflammatory forces increase their activity in a parallel and more-or-less equal fashion. After a few days, infection is eradicated by the body's own defense, and the immune system's activity returns to baseline. A common scenario, which all of us have experienced a few times in our lives. (**b**) The dysregulated immune response. There is an overwhelming response on both sides, but the pro-inflammatory response is more pronounced. The area above the dotted line indicates the molecules that are in abundance and responsible for the "cytokine storm". For more explanation, see text

and the pro-inflammatory forces overwhelm the anti-inflammatory response (Fig. 43.1b). This overwhelming pro-inflammatory response can impair cellular function leading to increased vascular permeability, edema formation and subsequent organ dysfunction [16]. The overwhelming, acute release of pro-inflammatory cytokines and mediators is termed the "cytokine storm" [17]. As time goes by and pro-inflammatory activity is exhausted, anti-inflammatory forces may overwhelm pro-inflammatory forces, resulting in persistent immunoparalysis, leaving the patients prone to further infections.

In this chapter, our main interest is in modulation of the early dysregulated inflammatory response in septic patients. One of the key issues in this context is how to monitor the inflammatory response at the bedside? Which is the best biomarker to indicate a cytokine storm? Measuring all sorts of cytokines in a bundle-type fashion during daily practice is very costly, and there are limited data to explain how to interpret these results. The most frequently used clinical biomarkers of inflammation are: C-reactive protein (CRP), white blood cell (WBC) count, interleukin (IL)-6, soluble CD14-subtype (presepsin) and procalcitonin (PCT). Several studies, including ours, have shown that conventional markers of infection such as WBC count, body temperature and CRP are poor or unreliable, and are slowly acting indicators of inflammation [18]. In our daily routine, we use PCT to monitor the inflammatory response for several reasons, but explaining those are beyond the scope of this article; however they were discussed in detail in a recent review [19].

43.3 Cytokine Adsorption as Adjuvant Therapy

Given the pivotal role of cytokine production in sepsis, it seems logical that removal of these substances may attenuate the response and enhance recovery [20]. This is the basis of blood purification, which initially encompassed renal replacement therapies, in particular hemofiltration, to try and reduce the concentrations of inflammatory mediators in the circulation [20]. It was assumed that using these techniques would allow the mass removal of circulatory mediators in a non-specific manner [21–23]. Despite early promise, no multicenter randomized controlled studies have demonstrated a survival benefit. Following this, so-called high-volume hemofiltration, where higher flows may lead to increased removal, was tried (the immune modulation hypothesis), again with no success [8, 21, 24, 25]. Extracorporeal hemoadsorption with polymyxin B showed improvement in organ dysfunction and a survival benefit in small studies [26] including a small randomized trial [27], while larger trials could not confirm these beneficial effects [28, 29].

A relatively new alternative for extracorporeal blood purification is cytokine hemoadsorption. The only specifically approved device for this purpose is CytoSorb® (CytoSorbents, Corporation, New Jersey, USA), which consists of a single-use hemoadsorption cartridge that can be used with standard blood pumps, such as those found on devices routinely used for renal replacement therapy (RRT) [30–32].

CytoSorb contains biocompatible, porous polymer polystyrene beads in a cartridge of about 300 mL, which is able to adsorb a broad spectrum of molecules with molecular weights between the range of 5 and 60 kDa making it suitable to adsorb most pro- and anti-inflammatory cytokines. The cartridge has a filling blood volume of 120 mL and is pre-filled with 0.9% sodium chloride. The adsorber is gamma-sterilized and can be stored for 3 years. One device has an estimated active adsorption surface area of ~40,000 m^2 compared to conventional hemodialysis membranes with an average surface area of 2–2.5 m^2 [33]. Technically, it can be used either as stand-alone hemoperfusion treatment or in conjunction with RRT, heart-lung machines and extracorporeal membrane oxygenation (ECMO) devices.

During the onset of septic shock, because of the dysregulated immune response, both pro- and anti-inflammatory activity increases, but the pro-inflammatory response is more pronounced (Fig. 43.1b). CytoSorb is capable of adsorbing molecules irreversibly from the blood from both pro- and anti-inflammatory groups, but it follows simple logic that more molecules are adsorbed from the group that is most prevalent (i.e., mainly pro-inflammatory molecules during the cytokine storm). This is the postulated mechanism of how CytoSorb therapy helps to regain control by restoring the balance between pro- and anti-inflammatory cytokines and other PAMPs and DAMPs, bringing them closer to within a 'normal' range. This also explains why, in part, the treatment is reported to be most effective within the first 24 h after the onset of septic shock [34].

The potential clinical benefits of the treatment are all related to the attenuation of the inflammatory—mainly the pro-inflammatory—response. This may be reflected in the decreasing serum levels of certain cytokines and biomarkers, and in the reversal of vasoplegia resulting in reduced vasopressor requirements, as found in several case studies (see below).

Despite the fact that convincing evidence from large randomized trials showing benefit is not yet available, CytoSorb use has gained momentum over the last years. According to the manufacturer, to date more than 46,000 CytoSorb treatments have been reported in more than 700 medical centers around the world [32]. What we have learned so far about the treatment's effect is mainly based on the results of animal experiments, case reports, observational studies (including a registry) and a few clinical trials.

43.4 Current Data

43.4.1 Animal Experiments

In general, experimental data for cytokine adsorption therapy has shown positive results in its ability to reduce circulating cytokine levels, attenuate the inflammatory response of leukocytes and improve hemodynamics and sepsis-related survival [35]. In a recent sepsis animal model, rats were injected with endotoxin and underwent CytoSorb therapy resulting in up to 50% decreases in the levels of IL-6, IL-10 and tumor necrosis factor (TNF)-α, within 2 h of treatment initiation, with improved hemodynamic stability and increased short-term survival [32]. In another rat model of sepsis using cecal ligation and puncture, animals treated with hemoadsorption had trends to improved renal and hepatic function compared to the sham group [36].

43.4.2 Human Data

We have limited knowledge regarding extracorporeal cytokine adsorption in the context of clinical studies. The analysis of 1886 patients with presumed pneumonia by Kellum et al. found that elevated pro- and anti-inflammatory cytokine levels may predict the presence and mortality of severe sepsis [37]. Both pro- and anti-inflammatory cytokine levels were measured (IL-6, TNF, IL-10). Mean levels of all three cytokines were elevated on the first day. The highest cytokine levels were measured in fatal severe sepsis and the lowest in community-acquired pneumonia (CAP) with no sepsis. Combined high levels of the pro-inflammatory IL-6 and anti-inflammatory IL-10 was associated with the highest risk of death (hazard ratio 20.5; 95% confidence interval [CI] 10.8–39.0, $p < 0.001$).

Cytokine overproduction is frequently present in various life-threatening conditions such as sepsis, trauma, major surgery, viral infections, acute respiratory distress syndrome (ARDS), severe burn injury, acute pancreatitis and hepatic cirrhosis to name just a few. A handful of reports have been published about the use of CytoSorb treatment in some of these conditions, including in fulminant liver failure and hemophagocytic syndrome [38], β-hemolytic streptococcus-induced necrotizing fasciitis [39], septic shock with multiple organ dysfunction [40], and rhabdomyolysis [41]. As found in the aforementioned animal experiments, elevated cytokine levels have been reported during donor conditioning for organ transplantation, which were associated with dysfunction of donor organs before and after transplantation [42, 43]. In a recent clinical trial it was found that in addition to conventional treatment, attenuation of the inflammatory response by cytokine absorption could prolong graft survival [43].

A recently published, randomized, controlled trial by Schadler et al., investigated clinical outcomes in 97 mechanically ventilated patients with sepsis who underwent hemoadsorption therapy for 6 h per day for 7 consecutive days. Although the 6-h treatment did not result in an overall reduction in IL-6 compared to controls over a 24-h period, there was increased IL-6 elimination with the use of hemoadsorption [44].

We recently completed a prospective, randomized, controlled clinical proof-of-concept pilot study (Adsorbtion of Cytokines Early in Septic Shock [ACESS]). The aim was to investigate the effects of CytoSorb therapy applied as a 24-h standalone treatment in patients with septic shock. A total of 20 patients were involved and randomized into two groups: CytoSorb treated ($n = 10$) and control ($n = 10$) group. At the end of the 24-h treatment period, vasopressor requirements in the CytoSorb group were significantly lower than in the controls and PCT levels had also decreased significantly [45].

According to the latest published results of the CytoSorb Registry, there may also be survival benefit related to CytoSorb therapy [46]. Out of the 198 treated patients, 135 had septic shock. The predicted mortality of these patients on ICU admission was around 80% (mean APACHE II of 33) and the observed mortality was 65%.

Until we see the results of large trials, the message from the currently published human data indicates that: (1) CytoSorb therapy has been proved to be safe as no side effects have been reported thus far; (2) it seems to attenuate the inflammatory response especially as indicated by a series of measurements of IL-6 and PCT levels; (3) and it reduces vasopressor requirements dramatically.

43.5 How We Do It?

Adjunctive therapies in critically ill patients are by-and-large indicated in the case of persistent shock (high dose of vasopressor requirement and multiple organ failure) that shows no improvement after adequate resuscitation, appropriate antimicrobial therapy and source control, and when the levels of inflammatory mediators remain elevated or are increasing despite several hours of standard treatment [47]. This approach has been implemented in clinical practice and tested in a recently conducted proof-of-concept pilot trial, the ACESS study, as already mentioned in the previous paragraphs.

The inclusion criteria in the ACESS trial were the following: intubated, mechanically ventilated patients with suspected septic shock of medical origin; invasive hemodynamic monitoring-guided need for norepinephrine >10 μg/min; elevated lactate levels >2.0 mmol/L; and a PCT level ≥3 ng/mL. Inclusion had to take place after the first at least 6 h of resuscitation and antibiotic therapy, when there was no improvement as indicated by steady or increased norepinephrine requirement and confirmed by invasive hemodynamic measurements. CytoSorb treatment had to be commenced within the first 24 h after ICU admission or the onset of septic shock. As we specifically aimed to investigate the effects of stand-alone CytoSorb treatment, patients with acute or chronic renal insufficiency requiring RRT were excluded from the study.

This approach, based more-or-less on the inclusion criteria of the ACESS trial, has now been implemented into our daily routine. CytoSorb is either used on its own or in combination with RRT, in other words, RRT is not a pre-requisite of treatment, unlike in many other centers, where CytoSorb is only used in conjunction with RRT.

Regarding technical issues, we follow the company's recommendations and CytoSorb is placed in a blood pump circuit using an ordinary RRT device (MultiFiltrate, Fresenius Medical Care), with heparin anticoagulation and a blood flow rate of 250–400 mL/min. Alternatively, citrate or argatroban anticoagulation may also be used.

The broad details of the above-mentioned approach on 'which patient, when and how' to use CytoSorb are summarized in Fig. 43.2. The key elements of this are: (1) patients have to be in septic shock with two or more organ failures, but with a realistic chance of survival; (2) in terms of the patient's clinical progress, the most important element is vasopressor (norepinephrine) requirements; (3) in case of no improvement after a certain period of time of resuscitation, advanced hemodynamic monitoring is added to routine monitoring (which is a prerequisite before CytoSorb therapy), in order to prove sepsis-caused vasoplegia, and to exclude unrecognized, treatable causes of hemodynamic instability, such as hypovolemia, inotropic requirement, etc.; (4) finally, in case of no further improvement or in fact worsening

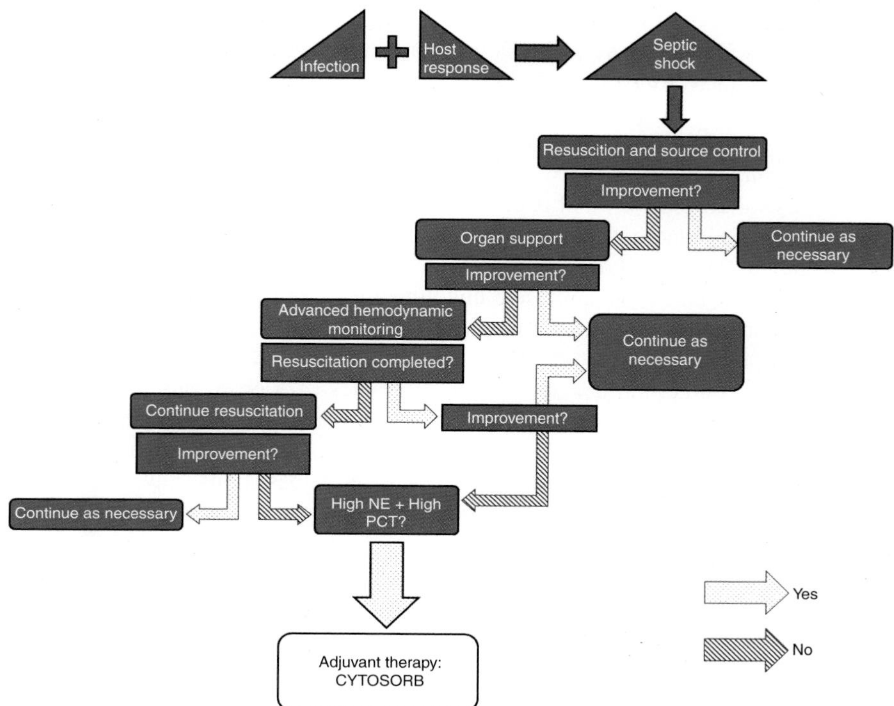

Fig. 43.2 Algorithm for use of CytoSorb therapy in our institute. Once septic shock is suspected, the first steps are basic resuscitation and source control: oxygen therapy, fluid resuscitation, empirical antibiotics with or without surgical removal or drainage of source. In case of improvement, management is 'continued as necessary', indicated by the patient's condition. In case of no improvement, 'organ support' is started, meaning: mechanical ventilation, vasopressor support, routine intensive monitoring (central venous, arterial and bladder catheters). If there is still no improvement, meaning increasing vasopressor requirements, lactate levels, worsening oxygenation, etc., then advanced hemodynamic monitoring-guided management is commenced in order to continue resuscitation. In cases where there is still no improvement and if procalcitonin (PCT) is elevated or shows an increasing trend, then CytoSorb therapy is considered. *NE* norepinephrine

in vasopressor requirements despite adequate fluid resuscitation and hemodynamic stabilization, PCT results are evaluated and if these are grossly elevated or tending to increase, CytoSorb treatment can be commenced.

43.6 Questions to Be Answered in the Future

43.6.1 Which Patients Would Benefit the Most?

CytoSorb therapy is not cheap and is invasive, requiring installation of an extracorporeal circuit be it a stand-alone treatment or in conjunction with RRT; hence, careful patient selection is mandatory. Therefore, the first question that has to be answered in the near future is: which patients benefit the most? In other words, on what basis should clinicians select the patient population and on what basis can the use of this adjunctive therapy be indicated?

As the working principle of CytoSorb is the concentration-dependent removal of substances, first patients with proven cytokine storm should be selected. This so-called biomarker-directed approach has also been recently suggested and recommended by others [32, 44] and is perfectly in line with the concept of the ACESS trial, which was based on a PCT-directed approach. The best biomarker to monitor the pro-inflammatory response in order to define the correct time point to intervene is yet to be determined, but at present undoubtedly the most experience and knowledge has been gathered from PCT studies [48].

However, it is important to note that making decisions based solely on biomarkers, especially on certain absolute or cut-off values of a given biomarker can be misleading. On the one hand, absolute values often reflect individual responses, hence they show a huge individual scatter, therefore, observing kinetics may be more beneficial [18]. On the other hand, biomarker values should always be put in the context of the clinical picture. Many patients will improve after standard resuscitation, source control and organ support, hence they do not need adjunctive therapy. But those who have received all the above, and do not deteriorate but do not improve either, may need some extra help in the form of adjunctive therapy, such as extracorporeal cytokine removal.

43.6.2 Timing of Treatment

There seems to be some sort of an agreement amongst those studying cytokine removal, and adjunctive therapies in general, that these should be commenced early, preferably within the first 24 h after the onset of septic shock [32, 34]. However, it is also important to acknowledge that treatment should not be started too early either. Many patients will have a positive response to initial standard treatment and commencing any adjuvant therapy in these patients would be unnecessary. The major challenge here is to define this optimal time frame within which extracorporeal cytokine removal would give the best results. Because of the heterogeneity in individual responses, this time frame cannot be generalized and should not be set as standard for every case. Appropriate indicators that help to assess the situation need to be further evaluated.

43.6.3 How Long Should Treatment Last?

Currently most centers apply the company's recommendations and give one treatment for 24 h [31]. However, this time frame is arbitrary, without clear evidence. In a recent study, we measured PCT levels before and after the CytoSorb cartridge in 20 patients (study is still ongoing). The interim analysis on the first 8 treatments clearly showed that shortly after commencing treatment the device had removed more than 90% of the PCT from the blood flowing through it, but after 12 h this was less than 10%, with no further change over the subsequent 12 h of therapy [45]. Although this can only be interpreted for PCT, these results suggest that it would be worthwhile to measure other important cytokines and molecules, and determine if this change in the removal rate over time can only be applied for PCT, or also to other molecules that may also behave in the same way? If the latter is true, then the cartridge should be changed every 12 h in general, but if the removal rate varies according to the given substance that we want to adsorb, then treatment time should be adjusted accordingly.

43.6.4 Assessing Treatment Efficacy and when to Stop?

To date, the most obvious effects reported by several authors are the reduction in vasopressor requirement and reduced levels of biomarkers and cytokines. There are also data from a recent case report that capillary integrity may be better preserved and capillary leakage reduced as an effect of CytoSorb therapy [49]. When human endothelial cells were treated *ex vivo* with the serum of the same septic patient before and 24 h after CytoSorb treatment, there was a dramatic improvement in transendothelial resistance. Taking this into account, measures such as extravascular lung water or other parameters suitable for evaluating capillary leakage, could be assessed in the future to see if they could be used as measures of treatment efficacy.

Regarding the length of treatment, it is also the company's recommendation to change the adsorber daily for up to 7 consecutive days [31]. As in the case of how long one treatment should last, the length of total therapy is arbitrary. Terminating CytoSorb therapy should be based on careful evaluation of the clinical picture and the behavior of the biomarkers used. It is important to bear in mind that since most cytokines are adsorbed by the cartridge, the change in cytokine/biomarker levels while on treatment may show a false positive signal of improvement.

Therefore, further trials should address this issue by testing different lengths of treatment with some time in between each treatment during which the patient's clinical progress and biomarker level changes are observed.

43.6.5 Removal of Other Substances

CytoSorb removes not only cytokines but several other molecules and substances, including myoglobin, free hemoglobin, bilirubin, bile acids and certain drugs such as venlafaxine, ticagrelor, meropenem and vancomycin [50]. In the context of septic shock, antibiotics are certainly the most important to consider and this effect raises the question whether drug serum levels should be monitored in patients who receive those antibiotics that are adsorbed by CytoSorb, while on treatment. This is another important issue to be investigated in the future.

43.7 Conclusion

Extracorporeal cytokine removal by CytoSorb has been tried and tested in tens of thousands of patients so far and has been proven to be a safe therapy in several critically ill conditions, which are assumed to be the result of a dysregulated host response caused cytokine storm. The continuous increase in the number of patients treated worldwide indicates that the positive results of case reports and observational studies can be repeated at the bedside. Time will tell whether these positive short-term effects of decrease in inflammatory biomarker levels, and reduction in vasopressor requirements, will eventually translate into longer term survival benefits for patients with septic shock.

References

1. Kaukonen KM, Bailey M, Suzuki S, Pilcher D, Bellomo R. Mortality related to severe sepsis and septic shock among critically ill patients in Australia and New Zealand, 2000–2012. JAMA. 2014;311:1308.
2. Gaieski DF, Edwards JM, Kallan MJ, Carr BG. Benchmarking the incidence and mortality of severe sepsis in the United States. Crit Care Med. 2013;41:1167–74.
3. Torio CM, Andrews RM (2013) National inpatient hospital costs: the most expensive conditions by payer. HCUP Statistical Brief #160. Agency for Healthcare Research and Quality, Rockville, MD. http://www.hcup-us.ahrq.gov/reports/statbriefs/sb160.pdf. Accessed 16 Nov 2018.
4. ProCESS Investigators. A randomized trial of protocol-based care for early septic shock. Process trial. N Engl J Med. 2014;370:1–11.
5. Thiel P, Schmidt K, Mueller F, Ludewig K, Brunkhorst F, Gensichen J. The Jena Sepsis Registry: a prospective observational registry for patients with severe sepsis or septic shock, supported by primary care. Infection. 2011;39:S138–9.
6. Alejandria M, Lansang M, Dans L, Mantaring JB III. Intravenous immunoglobulin for treating sepsis, severe sepsis and septic shock. Cochrane Database Syst Rev. 2013:CD001090.
7. Szakmany T, Hauser B, Radermacher P. N-acetylcysteine for sepsis and systemic inflammatory response in adults. Cochrane Database Syst Rev. 2012:CD006616.
8. Lukaszewicz AC, Payen D. Purification methods: a way to treat severe acute inflammation related to sepsis? Crit Care. 2013;17:3–4.
9. Harder J, Schröder JM, Gläser R. The skin surface as antimicrobial barrier: present concepts and future outlooks. Exp Dermatol. 2013;22:1–5.
10. Baroni A, Buommino E, De Gregorio V, Ruocco E, Ruocco V, Wolf R. Structure and function of the epidermis related to barrier properties. Clin Dermatol. 2012;30:257–62.
11. Rudraraju R, Jones BG, Surman SL, Sealy RE, Thomas PG, Hurwitz JL. Respiratory tract epithelial cells express retinaldehyde dehydrogenase ALDH1A and enhance IgA production by stimulated B cells in the presence of vitamin A. PLoS One. 2014;9:1–10.
12. Pelaseyed T, Bergström JH, Gustafsson JK, et al. The mucus and mucins of the goblet cells and enterocytes provide the first defense line of the gastrointestinal tract. Immunol Rev. 2014;260:8–20.
13. Ghosh M. Secreted mucosal antimicrobials in the female reproductive tract that are important to consider for HIV prevention. Am J Reprod Immunol. 2014;71:575–88.
14. Kompoti M, Michopoulos A, Michalia M, Clouva-Molyvdas PM, Germenis AE, Speletas M. Genetic polymorphisms of innate and adaptive immunity as predictors of outcome in critically ill patients. Immunobiology. 2015;220:414–21.

15. Zhang Q, Raoof M, Chen Y, et al. Circulating mitochondrial DAMPs cause inflammatory responses to injury. Nature. 2010;464:104–7.
16. Sompayrac l. How the immune system works. Chichester: Wiley-Blackwell; 2012.
17. Ferrara J, Abhyankar S, Gilliland D. Cytokine storm of graft-versus-host disease: a critical effector role for interleukin-1. Transplant Proc. 1993;25:1216–7.
18. Trásy D, Tánczos K, Németh M, et al. Early procalcitonin kinetics and appropriateness of empirical antimicrobial therapy in critically ill patients. A prospective observational study. J Crit Care. 2016;34:50–5.
19. László I, Trásy D, Molnár Z, Fazakas J. Sepsis: from pathophysiology to individualized patient care. J Immunol Res. 2015;2015:510436.
20. Nakada T, Oda S, Matsuda K, et al. Continuous hemodiafiltration with PMMA hemofilter in the treatment of patients with septic shock. Mol Med. 2008;14:257–63.
21. Honore PM, Jamez J, Wauthier M, et al. Prospective evaluation of short-term, high-volume isovolemic hemofiltration on the hemodynamic course and outcome in patients with intractable circulatory failure resulting from septic shock. Crit Care Med. 2000;28:3581–7.
22. Peng Z, Simon P, Rimmelé T, Clermont G, Kellum JA. Blood purification in sepsis: a new paradigm. Contrib Nephrol. 2010;65:322–8.
23. Rimmelé T, Kellum JA. Clinical review: blood purification for sepsis. Crit Care. 2011;15:1–10.
24. Cole L, Bellomo R, Journois D, Davenport P, Baldwin I, Tipping P. High-volume haemofiltration in human septic shock. Crit Care Med. 2001;27:978–86.
25. Joannes-Boyau O, Bagshaw SM, Dewitte A, Spapen HD, Ouattara A. High-volume versus standard-volume haemofiltration for septic shock patients with acute kidney injury (IVOIRE study): a multicentre randomized controlled trial. Intensive Care Med. 2013;39:1535–46.
26. Vincent J, Cohen J, Burchardi H, et al. A pilot-controlled study of a polymyxin B-immobilized hemoperfusion cartridge in patients with severe sepsis secondary to intra-abdominal infection. Shock. 2005;23:400–5.
27. Cruz DN, Antonelli M, Fumagalli R, et al. Early use of polymyxin b hemoperfusion in abdominal septic shock. JAMA. 2009;301:2445.
28. Payen DM, Lukaszewicz AC, Joannes-boyau O, Martin-lefevre L, Kipnis E. Early use of polymyxin B hemoperfusion in patients with septic shock due to peritonitis: a multicenter randomized control trial. Intensive Care Med. 2015;41:975–84.
29. Coudroy R, Payen D, Launey Y, et al. Modulation by polymyxin-B hemoperfusion of inflammatory response related to severe peritonitis. Shock. 2017;47:93–9.
30. Dellinger RP, Levy MM, Opal SM, et al. Surviving Sepsis Campaign: International Guidelines for Management of Severe Sepsis and Septic Shock, 2012. Intensive Care Med. 2013;39:165–228.
31. Cytosorbent Corporation. CytoSorb fields of application. http://cytosorb-therapy.com/the-therapy/fields-of-application. Accessed 18 Nov 2018.
32. Bonavia A, Karamchandani K. Clinical utility of extracorporeal cytokine hemoadsorption therapy : a literature review. Blood Purif. 2018;17033:337–49.
33. Taniguchi T. Cytokine adsorbing columns. Contrib Nephrol. 2010;166:134–41.
34. Kogelmann K, Jarczak D, Scheller M, Drüner M. Hemoadsorption by CytoSorb in septic patients: a case series. Crit Care. 2017;21:1–10.
35. Ronco C, Brendolan A, Dan M, et al. Adsorption in sepsis. Kidney Int. 2000;58:148–55.
36. Peng ZY, Wang HZ, Carter MJ, et al. Acute removal of common sepsis mediators does not explain the effects of extracorporeal blood purification in experimental sepsis. Kidney Int. 2012;81:363–9.
37. Kellum J, Kong L, Fink MP, et al. Understanding the inflammatory cytokine response in pneumonia and sepsis: results of the Genetic and Inflammatory Markers of Sepsis (GenIMS) Study. Arch Intern Med. 2007;167:1655–63.
38. Frimmel S, Schipper J, Henschel J, Tsui TY, Mitzner SR, Koball S. First description of single-pass albumin dialysis combined with cytokine adsorption in fulminant liver failure and hemophagocytic syndrome resulting from generalized herpes simplex virus 1 infection. Liver Transpl. 2014;20:1523–4.

39. Hetz H, Berger R, Recknagel P, Steltzer H. Septic shock secondary to β-hemolytic streptococcus-induced necrotizing fasciitis treated with a novel cytokine adsorption therapy. Int J Artif Organs. 2014;37:422–6.
40. Basu R, Pathak S, Goyal J, Chaudhry R, Goel RB, Barwal A. Use of a novel hemoadsorption device for cytokine removal as adjuvant therapy in a patient with septic shock with multi-organ dysfunction: a case study. Indian J Crit Care Med. 2014;18:822–4.
41. Wiegele M, Krenn CG. Cytosorb™ in a patient with legionella pneumonia—associated rhabdomyolysis: a case report. ASAIO J. 2015;61:18–20.
42. Wilhelm MJ, Pratschke J, Beato F, et al. Activation of the heart by donor brain death accelerates acute rejection after transplantation. Circulation. 2000;102:2426–33.
43. Kellum JA, Venkataraman R, Powner D, Elder M, Hergenroeder G, Carter M. Feasibility study of cytokine removal by hemoadsorption in brain-dead humans. Crit Care Med. 2008;36:268–72.
44. Schädler D, Pausch C, Heise D, et al. The effect of a novel extracorporeal cytokine hemoadsorption device on IL-6 elimination in septic patients: a randomized controlled trial. PLoS One. 2017;12:1–19.
45. Öveges N, Hawchar F, László I, et al. Early cytokine adsorption in septic shock (ACESS-trial): results of a proof concept, pilot study. Crit Care. 2018;22(Suppl 1):P113. (abst)
46. Friesecke S, Träger K, Schittek GA, et al. International registry on the use of the CytoSorb® adsorber in ICU patients: study protocol and preliminary results. Medi Klin Intensivmed Notfallmed. 2017; Sep 4. https://doi.org/10.1007/s00063-017-0342-5. [Epub ahead of print]
47. Becze Z, Molnár Z, Fazakas J. Can procalcitonin levels indicate the need for adjunctive therapies in sepsis ? Int J Antimicrob Agents. 2015;46:S13–8.
48. Trásy D, Molnár Z. Procalcitonin—assisted antibiotic strategy in sepsis. EJIFCC. 2017;28:104–13.
49. David S, Thamm K, Schmidt BMW, Falk CS, Kielstein JT. Effect of extracorporeal cytokine removal on vascular barrier function in a septic shock patient. J Intensive Care. 2017;5:1–5.
50. Morris C, Gray L, Giovannelli M. Early report: the use of Cytosorb TM haemabsorption column as an adjunct in managing severe sepsis: initial experiences, review and recommendations. J Intensive Care Soc. 2015;16:257–64.

Part XIII

Iron Metabolism

Iron Metabolism: An Emerging Therapeutic Target in Critical Illness

44

E. Litton and J. Lim

44.1 Introduction

Iron is required for erythropoiesis and is also essential for many other life-sustaining functions including deoxyribonucleic acid (DNA) and neurotransmitter synthesis, mitochondrial function and the innate immune response. Despite its importance in maintaining health, iron deficiency is the most common nutritional deficiency worldwide and many of the risk factors for iron deficiency are also risk factors for developing critical illness. The result is that iron deficiency is likely to be over-represented in critically ill patients, with an estimated incidence of up to 40% at the time of intensive care unit (ICU) admission [1].

Critical illness results in profound and characteristic changes to iron metabolism that are highly conserved from an evolutionary perspective. These changes are mediated predominantly by the polypeptide hepcidin, which acts to decrease the absorption and availability of iron, despite acute phase increases in iron-binding proteins, such as ferritin, which may suggest normal or increased iron stores. The result is a state of functional iron deficiency. This may be protective in the short term, providing a form of 'nutritional immunity' against invading microbes by diminishing access to free iron in response to infection. However, by reducing the capacity of the body to access iron for vital processes, persistent functional iron deficiency can become harmful. For patients with prolonged ICU admission, this may contribute to critical illness-associated cognitive, neuromuscular and cardio-pulmonary dysfunction.

E. Litton (✉)
Intensive Care Unit, Fiona Stanley Hospital, Perth, WA, Australia

School of Medicine, University of Western Australia, Perth, WA, Australia
e-mail: ed.litton@health.wa.gov.au

J. Lim
Intensive Care Unit, Fiona Stanley Hospital, Perth, WA, Australia

J.-L. Vincent (ed.), *Annual Update in Intensive Care and Emergency Medicine 2019*, Annual Update in Intensive Care and Emergency Medicine,
https://doi.org/10.1007/978-3-030-06067-1_44

Historically, the possibility of iron deficiency was largely unexplored in critically ill patients due to the confounding effects of acute inflammation on commonly available iron measures, the lack of safe and effective treatments and uncertainty as to the clinical significance of deranged iron metabolism. However, assays, including hepcidin, offer the potential to identify iron restriction despite the presence of inflammation and may be coupled with promising therapeutic options to address issues including nosocomial infection and functional recovery for patients admitted to the ICU.

These advances are timely as emerging data suggest that disordered iron metabolism is of substantial prognostic significance in critical illness. High serum transferrin saturation and iron concentration are independent predictors of mortality in patients admitted to the ICU [2]. These data are consistent with findings of increased infection risk and organ failure associated with deranged iron metabolism in studies of patients undergoing hematopoietic stem cell and renal transplantation [3, 4]. Failure to maintain iron homeostasis early after a profound insult may result in an accumulation of highly reactive free iron, or non-transferrin bound iron, inflicting further oxidative stress on vulnerable organs or scavenged by invading microorganisms. The requirement for tight homeostatic control of iron metabolism is further demonstrated by population data from Norway, suggesting an association between severe iron deficiency and risk of bloodstream infection [5].

In summary, the available evidence suggests that both iron deficiency and iron excess may be harmful for critically ill patients and that clinical assessment of iron status in the ICU is important and should include consideration of both possibilities. The risks related to different iron states and associated iron study patterns are provided in Fig. 44.1.

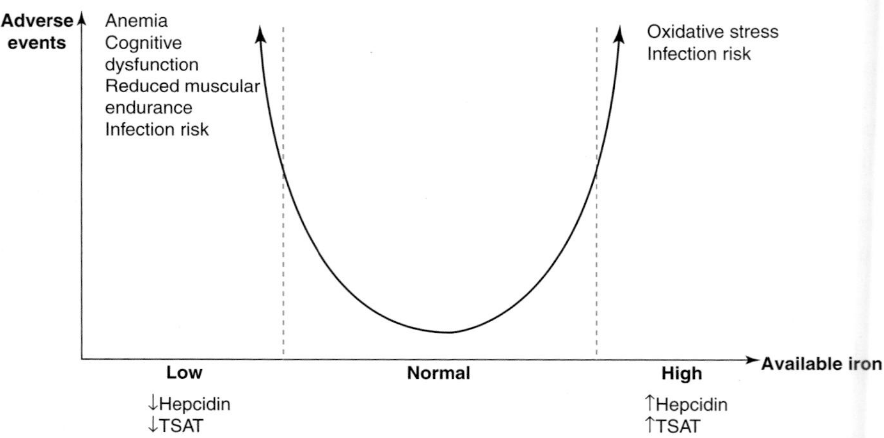

Fig. 44.1 Diagnostic patterns and risk of adverse effects related to different iron states. *TSAT* transferrin saturation

The advent of safe and effective intravenous iron preparations provides an opportunity to explore the potential benefits of treating patients diagnosed with functional iron deficiency in the ICU, when enteral iron is ineffective due to the actions of hepcidin. Intravenous iron therapies have largely been investigated in the context of erythropoiesis. There are high quality data that intravenous iron, compared to either oral iron or no iron, significantly decreases anemia and red blood cell (RBC) transfusion requirement in hospitalized patients, albeit with a potential increased risk of infection [6]. The evidence for patients admitted to the ICU is less clear. To date few randomized controlled trials (RCTs) have been conducted in critically ill patients, although a recent multicenter study suggested that intravenous iron is biologically active in this population, increasing hemoglobin without any signal of harm [7].

Whilst much of the focus of iron has been as a treatment for anemia, a risk factor for adverse outcomes in patients admitted to the ICU, non-anemic iron deficiency impairs aerobic metabolism and is associated with reduced maximal oxygen consumption (VO_{2max}), muscle endurance and cognitive performance [8–10]. It is plausible that interventions to address disrupted iron metabolism may have much wider benefit for reducing complications and improving functional recovery after critical illness, independent of erythropoiesis.

The similarities are striking between the pathological consequences of the alterations in iron metabolism during critical illness and many common and characteristic complications, particularly those associated with functional impairment, in patients requiring prolonged ICU admission. Exploring the role of iron dysmetabolism in nosocomial infection and cognitive, neuromuscular and cardiopulmonary dysfunction may uncover novel therapeutic targets to help to address the substantial public health burden of these conditions in survivors of critical illness.

44.2 Iron Metabolism and Critical Illness

Critical illness precipitates an inflammatory response that results in early and profound changes in iron metabolism. An acquired form of iron dysmetabolism can be said to occur when these changes are persistent and contribute to impaired end-organ function. Ferritin, a major repository of intracellular iron, and the iron-binding glycoprotein, lactoferrin, are acute phase reactants and are upregulated in proportion to the severity of the inflammatory response [11]. The higher affinity of ferritin and lactoferrin to bind iron relative to transferrin, the circulating iron transporter and a negative acute phase reactant, results in hypoferremia [11]. This pattern of low serum iron, low transferrin and high ferritin occurs in more than 75% of critically ill patients within 3 days of ICU admission [12, 13]. Akin to the partial uncoupling of intravascular volume status from total body water as a common consequence of ICU treatment in critical illness, total body iron stores may become uncoupled from available and circulating iron.

Although the immediate changes in ferritin and transferrin are initiated directly by cytokines, it is the effect of hepcidin, described as the master regulator of iron, that determines the severity and duration of an iron-restricted state. Hepcidin, a

25-amino acid peptide hormone synthesized predominantly by hepatocytes, is secreted in response to a variety of stimuli including inflammatory cytokines and iron excess. Hepcidin acts by binding to and degrading ferroportin, a cellular iron exporter found in duodenal cells, macrophages and hepatocytes. Increasing hepcidin secretion decreases the intestinal absorption of dietary iron, decreases the release of recycled heme iron by macrophages, increases the sequestration of iron stores in hepatocytes and reduces circulating free iron [14].

There are two key clinical consequences of the changes in iron metabolism associated with critical illness. The first is that diagnosis of functional iron deficiency is problematic and cannot be reliably excluded on the basis of standard iron study parameters. The second is that a persistent state of dysmetabolism predisposes a vulnerable population to the consequences of iron-restricted metabolism, a state most commonly considered in the context of erythropoiesis but with important implications for the risk and severity of nosocomial infection and critical illness-associated cognitive, neuromuscular and cardiopulmonary dysfunction.

44.2.1 Diagnosing Iron Deficiency

The inflammatory response that occurs in critical illness confounds the interpretation of commonly available assays to diagnose iron deficiency, including ferritin and transferrin. To address this, one approach has been to alter the threshold values of these markers to account for the acute phase response [15]. In patients with anemia requiring long term dialysis, a serum ferritin of <200 μg/L is highly suggestive of iron deficiency and predicts a good response to intravenous iron, whereas patients with a ferritin of between 500–1200 μg/L and a transferrin saturation <25% may also show an increase in hemoglobin in response to intravenous iron [15]. By applying similar criteria in critical illness, iron-restricted erythropoiesis has been reported to occur in more than a fourth of patients on admission to ICU [16]. However, validation studies against a gold standard of iron deficiency in critically ill patients are lacking and the accuracy of these criteria in predicting response to intravenous iron in this setting remains uncertain. Given the association between high transferrin saturation and adverse outcomes in critically ill patients, it may be that standard measures of iron metabolism are of greater use in identifying patients with potential iron overload, in whom intravenous iron therapy may pose greater risks, than in diagnosing functional iron deficiency *per se*.

In contrast, serum hepcidin concentration appears to provide a more reliable signal of iron-restricted erythropoiesis, decreasing in concentration with the onset of iron deficiency in patients admitted to the ICU even in the presence of inflammation [17]. In a recent study in critically ill patients with anemia, serum hepcidin concentration, but not ferritin or transferrin saturation, was able to identify patients in whom intravenous iron therapy was effective in reducing RBC transfusion requirement [18]. These findings require validation in further studies but are similar to findings in oncology, where hepcidin concentration appears to predict response to intravenous iron therapy in patients with chemotherapy-induced anemia [19]. In order for large validation studies to occur, accurate, clinically-available hepcidin assays are required.

A two-stage process may be of value, in which standard iron assays are first used to exclude patients at risk of iron excess and identify clear cases of iron deficiency. For patients not clearly overloaded or deficient, hepcidin concentration is then measured. As the evidence base grows and the role of hepcidin becomes more clearly defined, studies investigating its association with functional outcomes after ICU may also be of substantial interest.

44.2.2 Anemia

Anemia is associated with adverse outcomes and remains the most common indication for RBC transfusion in patients admitted to the ICU, even when adherence to a conservative transfusion threshold is high [20]. Preventing the onset and progression of anemia requires a multifaceted approach adapted to the specific clinical context. Major surgery requiring elective ICU admission represents a large patient cohort where a pre-emptive approach is preferable [21]. Approximately one in three patients scheduled to undergo major surgery is anemic, a potentially modifiable risk for perioperative adverse events, including myocardial infarction, stroke and mortality [22]. A recent international consensus statement recommends routine screening of all patients undergoing surgery with an expected blood loss >500 mL and consideration of intravenous iron for patients with anemia and evidence of iron deficiency when oral iron is inefficacious, not tolerated or surgery is planned to occur in less than 6 weeks [23]. In contrast, a Cochrane review on the use of preoperative iron therapy to correct anemia identified only three small RCTs and found no significant reduction in allogeneic RBC transfusion requirements [24]. The safety and efficacy of preoperative intravenous iron therapy is now the focus of several ongoing large scale RCTs in cardiac, abdominal and orthopedic surgery. A summary of major completed and ongoing RCTs of preoperative intravenous iron is provided in Table 44.1.

For patients admitted to the ICU there is some evidence to guide decisions on the use of intravenous iron therapy. A systematic review and meta-analysis on the efficacy of intravenous iron in the treatment of anemia in ICU patients did not demonstrate a significant decrease in anemia or RBC transfusion requirements but only included five relatively small studies [25]. More recently, a multicenter RCT including 140 patients demonstrated that intravenous iron administered within 48 h of ICU admission resulted in a significant increase in hemoglobin concentration at hospital discharge (107 g/L vs. 100 g/L, $p = 0.02$) without any infusion-related adverse event, but no difference in RBC transfusion rates, hospital length of stay or mortality [7]. Although these data suggest biological activity, the available evidence is currently insufficient to assess the effect of early intravenous iron administration on patient outcomes, or to exclude increased infection risk.

The timing of intravenous iron administration in patients admitted to the ICU may also be a strong determinant of whether the benefits outweigh the risks. The period of

Table 44.1 Randomized controlled trials of intravenous (i.v.) iron in major surgery

Study, year [ref], number (n) of patients	Population	Intervention	Outcomes
Kim, 2017 (FAIRY trial) [48] n = 454	Anemia post-radical gastrectomy	500–1000 mg i.v. FCM	Significantly more Hb responders No significant differences in QoL
Johansson, 2015 (PROTECT trial) [49] n = 60	Non-anemic patients undergoing cardiac surgery	100 mg i.v. iron isomaltoside	More non-anemic patients in i.v. iron group Higher Hb 1 month postoperative in i.v. iron group
Bernabeu-Wittel, 2016 [50] n = 306	Hip fracture surgery	1 g i.v. FCM+ 40,000 IU s.c. EPO	Higher Hb at discharge and 60-days post-discharge No significant differences in ABT, mortality, HRQoL, adverse events.
Froessler, 2016 [51] n = 72	Abdominal surgery with IDA	500–1000 mg i.v. FCM	Reduced ABT Improved preoperative Hb Improved postoperative Hb Reduced LOS
Intravenous iron for Treatment of Anemia before Cardiac Surgery (ITACS; ClincialTrials.gov Identifier: NCT02632760)	Anemic patients before elective cardiac surgery	1 g i.v. FCM (or similar product)	Primary outcome: Number of days alive and out of hospital from surgery to 30 days post-surgery
Preoperative Intravenous Iron to Treat Anemia in Major Surgery (PREVENTT; ClinicalTrials.gov Identifier: NCT01692418)	Anemic patients before major open abdominal surgery	1 g i.v. FCM	Primary outcome: ABT requirement
Intravenous Iron, Functional Recovery and Delirium in Patients with Hip Fracture (FEDEREF; EudraCT: 2014-001923-53)	Hip fracture patients	200 mg iron sucrose on days 1, 3 and 5 from admission	Primary outcome: Functional variables, including ability to perform activities of daily living and walking. Cognitive variables, including cognitive status and incidence of delirium ABT requirement

ABT allogeneic blood transfusion, *EPO* erythropoietin, *FCM* ferric carboxymaltose, *Hb* hemoglobin, *HRQoL* health-related quality of life, *IDA* iron-deficiency anemia, *LOS* length of stay, *QoL* quality of life, *s.c.* subcutaneous

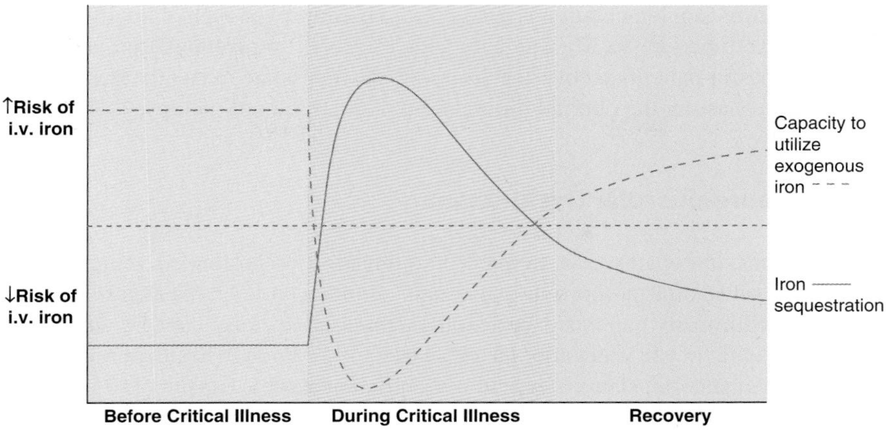

Fig. 44.2 Changes in iron storage and capacity to use iron over time in critical illness

greatest physiological stress generally occurs early after ICU admission. The effects of critical illness and related treatments, such as RBC transfusion and catecholamine infusions, increase the risks and also exacerbate the consequences of iron dysmetabolism and excess free iron. A diminished capacity to process exogenous parenteral iron may worsen this situation. *In vitro* data suggest dose-dependent and formulation-dependent effects of intravenous iron compounds on macrophage handling and the extent of oxidative stress [26]. Early initiation of intravenous iron provides time to develop an erythropoietic response. However, this neglects a wider therapeutic window after the most acute period of critical illness has abated when the risk benefit ratio may be more favorable and addressing the functional outcomes of prolonged ICU admission can be prioritized. The temporal changes in iron metabolism and response to intravenous iron therapy in critical illness are summarized in Fig. 44.2.

44.2.3 Cognitive Dysfunction

Cognitive dysfunction is common in survivors of critical illness, affecting more than one in four patients and often persisting after physical recovery [27]. The pathophysiology is multifactorial and characterized by new deficits or deterioration of pre-existing mild deficits in global cognition or executive function. However, the underlying causes remain poorly understood and there are no established treatments [27].

Iron is essential for neurotransmitter synthesis, uptake and degradation and is necessary for mitochondrial function in metabolically active brain tissue [28]. Iron deficiency has cerebral and behavioral effects consistent with dopaminergic dysfunction, manifesting as poor inhibitory control and diminished executive and motor function [29]. In both children and pre-menopausal women with non-anemic iron deficiency, iron supplementation is associated with improved mental quality-of-life and cognitive function [9, 30]. Studies on the effects of intravenous iron on cognitive outcomes in patients recovering from critical illness are currently lacking and will need to consider the optimal timing, dose and duration of therapy.

44.2.4 Neuromuscular Dysfunction

Critical illness myopathy is a frequent complication of prolonged acute illness, affecting a substantial proportion of patients admitted to ICU. Weakness is often prolonged with many patients experiencing decreased exercise capacity and compromised quality of life years after the acute event [31]. Even in healthy non-anemic subjects, adequate iron status is essential for efficient aerobic capacity [10]. Fatigue is also a significant factor in recovery after critical illness, influencing a patient's ability to engage with rehabilitation. Iron deficiency persisted in more than one in three patients at 6 months after prolonged ICU admission and is associated with increased fatigue independent of anemia [32]. Given the catabolic state conferred by critical illness and role of iron in myoglobin and muscle oxidative metabolism, further evaluation of the relationship between iron deficiency and critical illness myopathy may provide insight into the role of iron supplementation in improving physical recovery after acute severe illness.

44.2.5 Cardiopulmonary Dysfunction

Iron is an essential component of structural proteins in cardiomyocytes and an obligate co-factor for hypoxia-inducible factor (HIF), a mediator of the systemic cardiovascular response to hypoxia. As a consequence, iron plays an important role in systolic heart function and hypoxic pulmonary vasoconstriction.

Independent of anemia, iron deficiency is associated with increased risk of death in patients with heart failure [33]. High quality evidence suggests that intravenous iron for patients with systolic heart failure improves exercise capacity, survival and quality of life [34]. Critical illness may impair myocardial iron use through a number of mechanisms including catecholamine-induced downregulation of myocardial transferrin receptor 1 (TfR1) and upregulation of hepcidin [35]. Emerging data also suggest disrupted iron metabolism may be important in various subtypes of pulmonary artery hypertension and that altitude-associated pulmonary artery hypertension is improved by intravenous iron therapy [36]. Pulmonary artery hypertension, and associated right ventricular dysfunction, is common in patients admitted to the ICU with severe acute respiratory distress syndrome (ARDS) and is a poor prognostic indicator [37]. Whether the beneficial effects of intravenous iron for patients with isolated systolic heart failure and pulmonary artery hypertension are translatable to patients being treated in the ICU requires further investigation, but assessment of iron status and potential initiation of iron therapy in patients with severe cardiac failure and markers of iron deficiency should be considered on an individual patient basis.

44.2.6 Infection

The term 'nutritional immunity' describes the changes in iron metabolism of the mammalian host during infection, in which the acute phase response acts to limit the availability of free iron for microbes including invasive fungi and avid iron-binding bacteria [38, 39]. Hereditary iron overload disorders increase the risk and severity of infection with siderophilic bacteria, such as *Vibrio vulnificus* and *Yersinia enterocolitica*, although these bacteria are only moderately pathogenic in other settings [39]. Iron overload not only predisposes to infection from particular organisms, but also then impairs components of the innate immune response including chemotaxis, phagocytosis, lymphocyte and macrophage function [40].

Investigating a potential causal link between iron supplementation and infection risk is complex. The relationship is likely to depend on a large range of factors, including the setting, participant population and particular iron dosing strategy. For example, oral iron supplementation for children in malaria endemic areas does not appear to increase the risk of malaria overall, but may increase the risk where malaria prevention strategies are unavailable and decrease the risk where they are available [41]. Although an increased risk of infection has been suggested in a systematic review of RCTs investigating hospitalized patients treated with intravenous iron, infection was only reported in a minority of trials and the risk, including in critically ill patients, remains uncertain [6]. A RCT of intravenous iron sucrose compared with oral iron in patients with chronic kidney disease was stopped early due to increased serious adverse events, including infection requiring hospitalization, in the intravenous iron group [42]. On the other hand a RCT of intravenous ferric carboxymaltose for patients with cardiac failure demonstrated improved functional capacity and quality of life with no significant between-group differences in serious adverse events, including infection [43]. These contrasting findings demonstrate the need for context-specific assessment of infection risk and the potential for dose and formulation-dependent differences [26]. For patients admitted to the ICU, it is plausible that the risk of infection related to parenteral supplementation is not uniform, but may vary between patients and within a patient over time (see Fig. 44.2).

Whilst uncertainty regarding the risk of infection may still limit widespread use of intravenous iron in the acute phase of critical illness, the relationship between changes in iron metabolism and infection also provides therapeutic opportunities. Nosocomial infection remains a major source of morbidity in patients admitted to the ICU. Oral supplementation with the iron-binding glycoprotein, lactoferrin, appears to reduce nosocomial infection in preterm infants, although the results of large studies are awaited; results have not been replicated in the adult ICU setting [44, 45].

Other potential therapeutic targets of iron metabolism exist or are in development that may also be of relevance to reducing nosocomial infection. For example, the nutritional immunity conferred by reducing iron availability during infection is mediated by hepcidin, secreted in response to inflammatory mediators. However, inhibitors of hepcidin secretion, including anemia and hypoxia, may exert a counterbalancing effect in critically ill patients resulting in relative hepcidin deficiency and increased free iron available for invading microbes. For critically ill patients with early sepsis and low hepcidin concentrations, hepcidin agonists currently in development may attenuate the severity of the infective insult [46]. Likewise, iron chelators are known to be synergistic with some antifungal therapies in managing a range of fungal infections and may be beneficial in the prevention and treatment of nosocomial infections [47].

44.3 Conclusion

Iron deficiency is common in the general population and likely to be over-represented in patients admitted to the ICU. Critical illness exacerbates this situation by initiating a form of functional iron deficiency in which iron absorption and recycling is diminished and stored iron is less accessible for use. Although there may be beneficial short-term effects from this process by conferring a form of nutritional immunity against invading microbes, there are also risks. Homeostatic control of iron may be lost leading to the risk of iron excess, as suggested by emerging evidence that high transferrin saturation is a poor prognostic marker early after ICU admission. Perhaps most importantly, whether or not critical illness is initiated by an infection, it is often prolonged. Persistent functional iron deficiency may lead to iron dysmetabolism in which reduced iron availability contributes to impaired end-organ function.

The reduced availability of iron in critical illness is often considered in the context of anemia, but the consequences are much broader than this and overlap extensively with many of the issues faced by ICU survivors. Correction of non-anemic iron deficiency improves cognitive and cardiopulmonary dysfunction and aerobic performance and reduces fatigue. Recent data suggest that hepcidin measurement may be useful in targeting intravenous iron therapy at those most likely to benefit. For patients requiring prolonged ICU admission, considering iron dysmetabolism may be of substantial therapeutic benefit in improving functional recovery after critical illness.

References

1. Bellamy MC, Gedney JA. Unrecognised iron deficiency in critical illness. Lancet. 1998;352:1903.
2. Tacke F, Nuraldeen R, Koch A, et al. Iron parameters determine the prognosis of critically ill patients. Crit Care Med. 2016;44:1049–58.
3. Bazuave GN, Buser A, Gerull S, Tichelli A, Stern M. Prognostic impact of iron parameters in patients undergoing allo-SCT. Bone Marrow Transplant. 2011;47:60.
4. Fernández-Ruiz M, López-Medrano F, Andrés A, et al. Serum iron parameters in the early post-transplant period and infection risk in kidney transplant recipients. Transpl Infect Dis. 2013;15:600–11.
5. Mohus RM, Paulsen J, Gustad L, et al. Association of iron status with the risk of bloodstream infections: results from the prospective population-based HUNT Study in Norway. Intensive Care Med. 2018;44:1276–83.

6. Litton E, Xiao J, Ho KM. Safety and efficacy of intravenous iron therapy in reducing requirement for allogeneic blood transfusion: systematic review and meta-analysis of randomised clinical trials. BMJ. 2013;347:f4822.
7. Litton E, Baker S, Erber WN, et al. Intravenous iron or placebo for anaemia in intensive care: the IRONMAN multicentre randomized blinded trial: a randomized trial of IV iron in critical illness. Intensive Care Med. 2016;42:1715–22.
8. Abbaspour N, Hurrell R, Kelishadi R. Review on iron and its importance for human health. J Res Med Sci. 2014;19:164–74.
9. Bruner AB, Joffe A, Duggan AK, Casella JF, Brandt J. Randomised study of cognitive effects of iron supplementation in non-anaemic iron-deficient adolescent girls. Lancet. 1996;348:992–6.
10. Brutsaert TD, Hernandez-Cordero S, Rivera J, Viola T, Hughes G, Haas JD. Iron supplementation improves progressive fatigue resistance during dynamic knee extensor exercise in iron-depleted, nonanemic women. Am J Clin Nutr. 2003;77:441–8.
11. Weiss G, Goodnough LT. Anemia of chronic disease. N Engl J Med. 2005;352:1011–23.
12. Bobbio-Pallavicini F, Verde G, Spriano P, et al. Body iron status in critically ill patients: significance of serum ferritin. Intensive Care Med. 1989;15:171–8.
13. Hobisch-Hagen P, Wiedermann F, Mayr A, et al. Blunted erythropoietic response to anemia in multiply traumatized patients. Crit Care Med. 2001;29:743–7.
14. Ganz T. Hepcidin, a key regulator of iron metabolism and mediator of anemia of inflammation. Blood. 2003;102:783–8.
15. Thomas DW, Hinchliffe RF, Briggs C, et al. Guideline for the laboratory diagnosis of functional iron deficiency. Br J Haematol. 2013;161:639–48.
16. Litton E, Xiao J, Allen CT, Ho KM. Iron-restricted erythropoiesis and risk of red blood cell transfusion in the intensive care unit: a prospective observational study. Anaesth Intensive Care. 2015;43:612–6.
17. Lasocki S, Baron G, Driss F, et al. Diagnostic accuracy of serum hepcidin for iron deficiency in critically ill patients with anemia. Intensive Care Med. 2010;36:1044–8.
18. Litton E, Baker S, Erber WN, et al. Hepcidin predicts response to IV iron therapy in patients admitted to the Intensive Care Unit: a nested cohort study. J Intensive Care. 2018;6:60.
19. Steensma DP, Sasu BJ, Sloan JA, Tomita DK, Loprinzi CL. Serum hepcidin levels predict response to intravenous iron and darbepoetin in chemotherapy-associated anemia. Blood. 2015;125:3669–71.
20. Westbrook A, Pettila V, Nichol A, et al. Transfusion practice and guidelines in Australian and New Zealand ICUs. Intensive Care Med. 2010;36:1138–46.
21. Lim J, Miles L, Litton E. Intravenous iron therapy in patients undergoing cardiovascular surgery: a narrative review. J Cardiothorac Vasc Anesth. 2018;32:1439–51.
22. Klein AA, Collier T, Yeates J, et al. The ACTA PORT-score for predicting perioperative risk of blood transfusion for adult cardiac surgery. Br J Anaesth. 2017;119:394–401.
23. Munoz M, Acheson AG, Auerbach M, et al. International consensus statement on the perioperative management of anaemia and iron deficiency. Anaesthesia. 2017;72:233–47.
24. Ng O, Keeler BD, Mishra A, Simpson A, Neal K, Brookes MJ, Acheson AG. Iron therapy for pre-operative anaemia. Cochrane Database Syst Rev. 2015:CD011588.
25. Shah A, Roy NB, McKechnie S, Doree C, Fisher SA, Stanworth SJ. Iron supplementation to treat anaemia in adult critical care patients: a systematic review and meta-analysis. Crit Care. 2016;20:306.
26. Connor JR, Zhang X, Nixon AM, Webb B, Perno JR. Comparative evaluation of nephrotoxicity and management by macrophages of intravenous pharmaceutical iron formulations. PLoS One. 2015;10:e0125272.
27. Pandharipande PP, Girard TD, Jackson JC, et al. Long-term cognitive impairment after critical illness. N Engl J Med. 2013;369:1306–16.
28. Youdim MB, Yehuda S. The neurochemical basis of cognitive deficits induced by brain iron deficiency: involvement of dopamine-opiate system. Cell Mol Biol. 2000;46:491–500.
29. Lozoff B. Early iron deficiency has brain and behavior effects consistent with dopaminergic dysfunction. J Nutr. 2011;141:740S–6S.

30. Favrat B, Balck K, Breymann C, et al. Evaluation of a single dose of ferric carboxymaltose in fatigued, iron-deficient women—PREFER a randomized, placebo-controlled study. PLoS One. 2014;9:e94217.
31. Guarneri B, Bertolini G, Latronico N. Long-term outcome in patients with critical illness myopathy or neuropathy: the Italian multicentre CRIMYNE study. J Neurol Neurosurg Psychiatry. 2008;79:838–41.
32. Lasocki S, Chudeau N, Papet T, et al. Prevalence of iron deficiency on ICU discharge and its relation with fatigue: a multicenter prospective study. Crit Care. 2014;18:542.
33. Jankowska EA, Kasztura M, Sokolski M, et al. Iron deficiency defined as depleted iron stores accompanied by unmet cellular iron requirements identifies patients at the highest risk of death after an episode of acute heart failure. Eur Heart J. 2014;35:2468–76.
34. Jankowska EA, Tkaczyszyn M, Suchocki T, et al. Effects of intravenous iron therapy in iron-deficient patients with systolic heart failure: a meta-analysis of randomized controlled trials. Eur J Heart Fail. 2016;18:786–95.
35. Maeder MT, Khammy O, dos Remedios C, Kaye DM. Myocardial and systemic iron depletion in heart failure: implications for anemia accompanying heart failure. J Am Coll Cardiol. 2011;58:474–80.
36. Ramakrishnan L, Pedersen SL, Toe QK, Quinlan GJ, Wort SJ. Pulmonary arterial hypertension: iron matters. Front Physiol. 2018;9:641.
37. Zochios V, Parhar K, Tunnicliffe W, Roscoe A, Gao F. The right ventricle in ARDS. Chest. 2017;152:181–93.
38. Cassat JE, Skaar EP. Iron in infection and immunity. Cell Host Microbe. 2013;13:509–19.
39. Ganz T. Iron and infection. Int J Hematol. 2018;107:7–15.
40. Puntarulo S. Iron, oxidative stress and human health. Mol Asp Med. 2005;26:299–312.
41. Neuberger A, Okebe J, Yahav D, Paul M. Oral iron supplements for children in malaria-endemic areas. Cochrane Database Syst Rev. 2016:CD006589.
42. Agarwal R, Kusek JW, Pappas MK. A randomized trial of intravenous and oral iron in chronic kidney disease. Kidney Int. 2015;88:905–14.
43. Anker SD, Comin Colet J, Filippatos G, et al. Ferric carboxymaltose in patients with heart failure and iron deficiency. N Engl J Med. 2009;361:2436–48.
44. Pammi M, Suresh G. Enteral lactoferrin supplementation for prevention of sepsis and necrotizing enterocolitis in preterm infants. Cochrane Database Syst Rev. 2017:CD007137.
45. Muscedere J, Maslove DM, Boyd JG, et al. Prevention of nosocomial infections in critically ill patients with lactoferrin: a randomized, double-blind, placebo-controlled study. Crit Care Med. 2018;46:1450–6.
46. Sebastiani G, Wilkinson N, Pantopoulos K. Pharmacological targeting of the hepcidin/ferroportin axis. Front Pharmacol. 2016;7:160.
47. Balhara M, Chaudhary R, Ruhil S, et al. Siderophores; iron scavengers: the novel & promising targets for pathogen specific antifungal therapy. Expert Opin Ther Targets. 2016;20:1477–89.
48. Kim YW, Bae JM, Park YK, et al. Effect of intravenous ferric carboxymaltose on hemoglobin response among patients with acute isovolemic anemia following gastrectomy: the FAIRY randomized clinical trial. JAMA. 2017;317:2097–104.
49. Johansson PI, Rasmussen AS, Thomsen LL. Intravenous iron isomaltoside 1000 (Monofer®) reduces postoperative anaemia in preoperatively non-anaemic patients undergoing elective or subacute coronary artery bypass graft, valve replacement or a combination thereof: a randomized double-blind placebo-controlled clinical trial (the PROTECT trial). Vox Sang. 2015;109:257–66.
50. Bernabeu-Wittel M, Romero M, Ollero-Baturone M, et al. Ferric carboxymaltose with or without erythropoietin in anemic patients with hip fracture: a randomized clinical trial. Transfusion. 2016;56:2199–211.
51. Froessler B, Palm P, Weber I, Hodyl NA, Singh R, Murphy EM. The important role for intravenous iron in perioperative patient blood management in major abdominal surgery: a randomized controlled trial. Ann Surg. 2016;264:41–6.

Transferrin as a Possible Treatment for Anemia of Inflammation in the Critically Ill

45

M. Boshuizen, G. Li Bassi, and N. P. Juffermans

45.1 Introduction

Previously termed 'anemia of chronic diseases', anemia developing as a consequence of inflammation is now called anemia of inflammation. In this chapter, we describe the prevalence and etiology of anemia of inflammation. Therapeutic strategies for anemia of inflammation that are currently under development are discussed, with a special emphasis on the rationale of transferrin as a novel therapy for anemia of inflammation.

45.2 Prevalence of Anemia of Inflammation

Anemia is very common in patients in the intensive care unit (ICU). At ICU admission, the mean hemoglobin concentration is between 10.5–11.3 g/dL [1, 2]. By 3 days after ICU admission, 95% of patients are anemic [3]. Thereby, anemia can be considered a hallmark of critical illness. The cause of the anemia is often multifactorial, including insufficient dietary intake, blood loss, hemolysis and iatrogenic factors, including frequent blood sampling, hemodilution and bleeding as a result of invasive procedures [4]. The most common cause of anemia however, is thought to be inflammation, which constitutes another central process in critical illness.

M. Boshuizen (✉) · N. P. Juffermans
Department of Intensive Care Medicine, Amsterdam UMC, University of Amsterdam, Amsterdam, The Netherlands

Laboratory of Experimental Intensive Care and Anesthesiology, Amsterdam UMC, University of Amsterdam, Amsterdam, The Netherlands
e-mail: m.boshuizen@amc.uva.nl

G. Li Bassi
Department of Pulmonary and Critical Care Medicine, Thorax Institute, Hospital Clinic, Barcelona, Spain

J.-L. Vincent (ed.), *Annual Update in Intensive Care and Emergency Medicine 2019*, Annual Update in Intensive Care and Emergency Medicine,
https://doi.org/10.1007/978-3-030-06067-1_45

Although differentiating between absolute iron deficiency and low iron availability due to anemia of inflammation (functional iron deficiency) is difficult, and these syndromes may also overlap, novel diagnostic modalities suggest that anemia of inflammation may contribute to the development of anemia in the majority of anemic patients [5, 6].

45.3 Etiology of Anemia of Inflammation

Anemia of inflammation results from the inhibitory effects of inflammatory cytokines on erythropoiesis. Interleukin (IL)-1 and tumor necrosis factor (TNF) inhibit erythropoietin (EPO) synthesis and activity [7]. These cytokines also inhibit release of iron from the reticuloendothelial system and incorporation of iron into red blood cells (RBCs). In addition, IL-6 induces the production of hepcidin. Hepcidin is a peptide that is secreted by the liver and causes degradation of ferroportin, which is the iron exporter of macrophages, hepatocytes and enterocytes. Thereby, hepcidin results in sequestration of iron in these cells, further lowering plasma iron levels [8]. Another response to inflammation is that increased levels of IL-1 and TNF induce upregulation of ferritin as an acute phase reactant. As ferritin is an intracellular protein that stores iron atoms in an inactive form, a high ferritin level contributes to sequestration of iron within cells [9]. Simultaneously, transferrin, which is the main transporter of iron, is a negative acute phase reactant and as such is downregulated during inflammation. Because of a decreased production of transferrin by the liver in response to inflammatory cytokines, transferrin levels are decreased during inflammation [10]. Together, these changes alter iron trafficking and lower iron availability (Fig. 45.1). These combined synergistic pathologic processes of altered iron

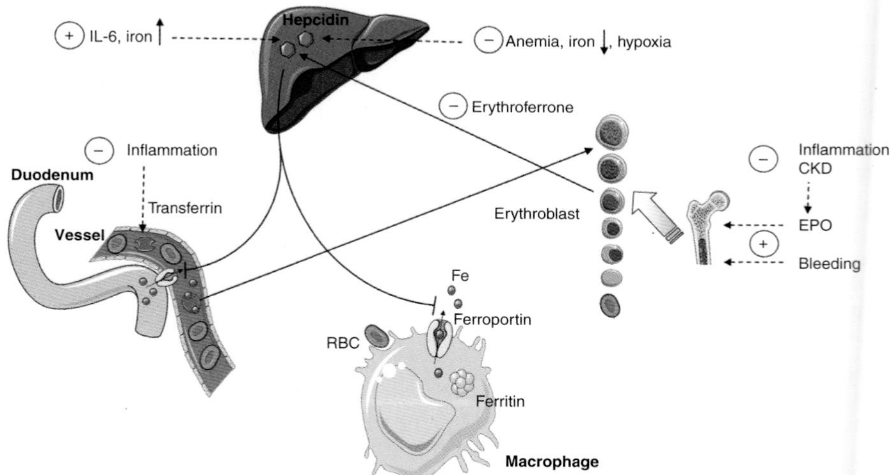

Fig. 45.1 Iron metabolism in anemia of inflammation. *IL* interleukin, *EPO* erythropoietin, *CKD* chronic kidney disease

availability and impaired EPO synthesis and function, result in decreased availability of iron to erythroid progenitor cells, with subsequent iron-deficient erythropoiesis. In addition to this impaired erythropoiesis, inflammation causes erythrophagocytosis, resulting in a shortened RBC lifespan [11].

45.4 Consequences of Anemia of Inflammation

During inflammation, there seems to be a strong evolutionary response of the body to lower iron availability. As a result, the development of anemia during severe inflammation is a rapid process. In patients with sepsis, half of the patients require RBC transfusion within the first 24 h of ICU admission [12]. It has been suggested that these alterations in iron metabolism have evolved as an endogenous protective response to infection. As most invading microorganisms feed on iron, low iron levels may reduce bacterial outgrowth and reproduction [13]. This theory infers that low iron levels, and possibly even ensuing anemia, may be protective against infection and that these conditions should not be 'corrected' by interventions, but rather ought to be accepted in clinical practice for an optimal response to an ongoing infection. Although these theories are appealing, the presence of functional iron deficiency and anemia negatively impacts outcome in the critically ill [1]. Randomized controlled trials (RCTs) in specific patient populations suggest that a restrictive transfusion trigger is associated with adverse outcomes compared to a more liberal transfusion trigger, which may be true for patients with active coronary disease and elderly patients [14–16]. This would suggest that anemia is detrimental and that transfusion to correct anemia may improve outcome. Data from Jehovah's witnesses show that at a certain nadir, anemia results in death. Thereby, correction of anemia is currently still common clinical practice.

45.5 Current Therapy of Anemia of Inflammation

45.5.1 Iron

As argued, there is not absolute iron deficiency in anemia of inflammation, but rather decreased iron availability. Consequently, supplementation of iron to support erythropoiesis in critically ill patients with anemia has not been unequivocally successful [17–19]. Several clinical studies have investigated the effect of oral [20, 21] or intravenous iron therapy for anemia in the critically ill [17–19, 22]. Oral iron was shown to decrease the number of transfusions in surgical critically ill patients with baseline iron deficiency anemia [20]. However, these positive findings were not confirmed in another similar study [23]. Uptake of iron administered orally may be reduced due to hepcidin, which inhibits the enteral uptake of iron during inflammation. Thereby, intravenous iron may be more effective. However, studies with intravenous iron therapy also showed conflicting results. An increase in hemoglobin concentrations was found in the IRONMAN study [19]; however, studies did not show a reduction in the need for transfusions [17, 18, 22].

45.5.2 Erythropoietin

In anemia of inflammation, inflammatory cytokines lower the endogenous synthesis of EPO. The bone marrow of these patients is also hyporesponsive to EPO [4]. Thereby, higher doses of EPO are required for the production of RBCs, suggesting a rationale for exogenous EPO. In line with this, EPO supplementation reduced the number of transfusions and increased hemoglobin levels in the critically ill [24]. However, there are also increased thromboembolic events in patients treated with EPO compared to placebo [25, 26]. Currently, EPO is not recommended for correction of anemia in the critically ill.

45.5.3 Red Blood Cell Transfusions

In anemia of inflammation, correction of anemia is usually achieved by blood transfusion. Approximately 40% of all critically ill patients receive RBC transfusions during the ICU stay, with a mean of five RBC units [4]. In patients with an ICU stay of more than 1 week, the proportion of patients who receive a transfusion increases even to 85% [3]. However, RBC transfusions are an independent risk factor for morbidity, including nosocomial infections [23], acute respiratory distress syndrome (ARDS) [27] and a prolonged length of stay in the ICU and in the hospital [3]. RBC transfusion is also an independent risk factor for mortality in the critically ill [1, 3, 27]. Thereby, as both anemia and transfusion are associated with adverse outcome, novel therapies are warranted.

45.6 Development of Novel Therapies for Anemia of Inflammation

45.6.1 Iron Modulating Therapies

Several new therapies are in development to treat anemia of inflammation by targeting iron metabolism. IL-6 inhibitor [28], IL-6 receptor blocker [29–31], inactivators of hepcidin [32–34] and hepcidin production inhibitors [35, 36] proved to be effective in animal models and some of these agents are being tested in clinical trials. Tocilizumab, an IL-6 receptor inhibitor, normalized iron parameters and increased hemoglobin concentrations in patients with rheumatoid arthritis with anemia of inflammation [29–31]. NOX-94, a molecule that binds hepcidin and blocks its biological function, has been shown to reverse hypoferremia and to inhibit the development of anemia in monkeys with IL-6-induced anemia of inflammation [32]. In a model of human endotoxemia, NOX-94 abrogated a fall in serum iron levels [33]. Furthermore, *in vitro* and *in vivo* studies have shown that hepcidin production can be inhibited by blocking the activity of bone morphogenetic protein (BMP) [35, 36]. BMP signaling has an important role in hepatic hepcidin expression and blocking this protein attenuated anemia and hypoferremia in mice with IL-6-induced anemia of inflammation [33]. By targeting cytokines and hepcidin, these experimental therapies may enable redistribution of iron from storage sites and allow for dietary iron absorption. Thereby, iron availability for erythropoiesis would increase and anemia of inflammation may not evolve or would be corrected. However, follow-up studies are warranted to ensure safety, as well as efficacy, of such strategies.

45.6.2 Transferrin Supplementation

Transferrin is a glycosylated glycoprotein of 76 kDa molecular weight [37]. Transferrin is mainly synthesized in the liver and has a half-life of 8–10 days. This plasma protein is the major iron binding and transporting protein in the bloodstream. It has the capacity to bind two atoms of iron and thus prevents the participation of iron in redox reactions with ensuing formation of toxic reactive oxygen species (ROS). Transferrin is present in the circulation in two forms: not bound to iron, termed apotransferrin; and bound to iron, termed holotransferrin. Holotransferrin is taken up by cells that express the transferrin receptor via receptor mediated endocytosis. There are two transferrin receptors: transferrin receptor 1 (TfR1) and transferrin receptor 2 (TfR2). TfR1 is expressed by all cell types and TfR2 is expressed by erythroblasts, hepatocytes and peripheral blood mononuclear cells. Upon binding to its receptor, iron is released from holotransferrin. The complex formed by apotransferrin and the receptor is then transported to the cell membrane, where apotransferrin is released in the circulation for re-use and the receptor can bind another holotransferrin [38]. When serum iron levels increases and the iron binding capacity of transferrin is exceeded, this can result in the appearance of toxic free iron. This non-transferrin bound iron may catalyze the formation of ROS, causing oxidative stress and tissue damage [39, 40].

45.6.3 Rationale for Supplementing Transferrin in Anemia of Inflammation

Transferrin can be purified relatively simple from human plasma by Cohn fractionation, ion exchange chromatography and ultrafiltration [41]. Currently, supplementation of transferrin is only used in patients with the rare condition of atransferrinemia [42]. However, transferrin supplementation could be beneficial in several other conditions, by acting as a sword that cuts both ways. First, transferrin supplementation may correct anemia by modulating the level of iron available for erythropoiesis. Second, (apo)-transferrin supplementation may reduce inflammatory reactions by inhibiting oxidative stress via binding of free iron.

45.7 Transferrin Supplementation to Correct Anemia

45.7.1 Patients with Transferrin Deficiency

Atransferrinemia or hypotransferrinemia is a rare, hereditary disorder characterized by anemia, very low or undetectable transferrin levels and increased ferritin levels [42]. These patients suffer from severe anemia, growth retardation and cognitive impairment, causing death at a young age. Since 1972, patients with atransferrinemia have been treated with purified apotransferrin. Treatment with apotransferrin injections corrects the anemia and improves mental development [43]. Currently, there is a clinical trial running since 2010 in which apotransferrin has been given to patients in Europe with atransferrinemia to further investigate the efficacy and safety of apotransferrin therapy in atransferrinemia patients (ClincialTrials.gov Identifier: NCT01797055).

45.7.2 Model of β-Thalassemia

β-thalassemia is characterized by ineffective erythropoiesis, extramedullary erythropoiesis and subsequent splenomegaly. The erythroid progenitor precursors do not mature and either go into apoptosis, or develop into abnormal RBCs with a shortened lifespan. As a result, these patients are anemic, which is treated with repeated RBC transfusions, often resulting in iron overload. In animal models of thalassemia, transferrin supplementation corrected anemia, reduced levels of non-transferrin bound iron and prevented iron loading in tissues. Hemoglobin concentrations increased by approximately 40%, reticulocyte counts decreased and the mean corpuscular volume and mean corpuscular hemoglobin decreased. It was postulated that exogenous transferrin binds non-transferrin bound iron in the circulation and that a decrease in extramedullary erythropoiesis may lead to a marked reduction in spleen size combined with improved organized splenic architecture. Transferrin was also associated with decreased iron deposition in liver, spleen and kidney. The reduction in tissue iron content and the increase in the number of RBCs shows that transferrin results in a shift of iron from the organs into the circulation, thereby removing iron from the parenchyma, where it is potentially harmful [43]. A clinical trial with transferrin in thalassemia patients is under development (personal communication).

45.7.3 Model of Pulmonary Sepsis

More relevant to the field of critical care medicine is the effect of transferrin on anemia of inflammation caused by sepsis. In a model of mechanically ventilated pigs with pulmonary sepsis induced by intrabronchial inoculum of 10^{7-8} colony forming units/mL of *Pseudomonas aeruginosa* (Fig. 45.2), severe septic shock develops 8–12 h after inoculum, characterized by hypotension not responsive to

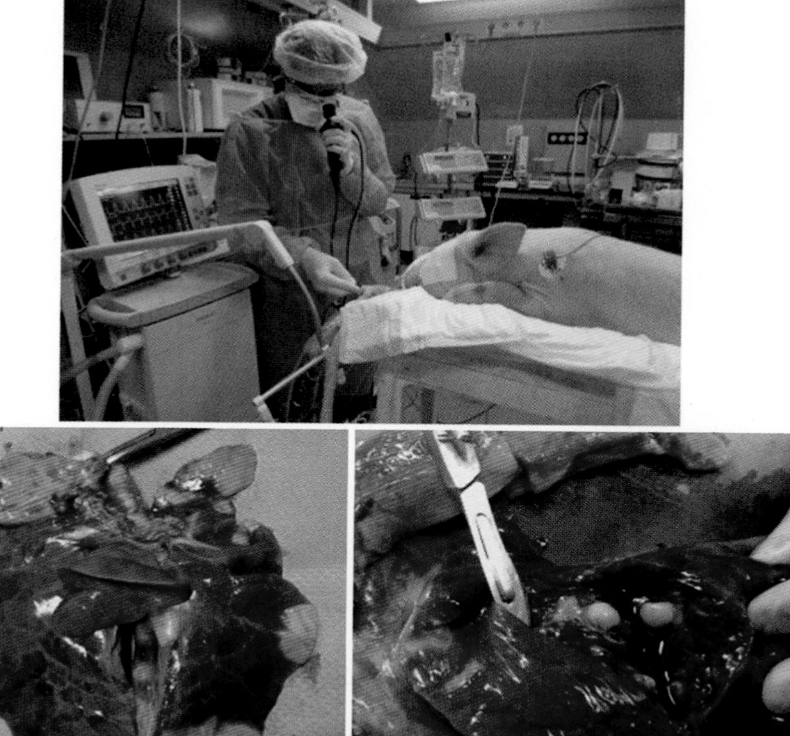

Fig. 45.2 Pulmonary challenge: animals challenged with *P. aeruginosa*, instilled into each pulmonary lobe of the animals (upper panel). Following inoculum, diagnosis of pneumonia is established based on a decline in arterial partial pressure of oxygen/inspiratory fraction of oxygen ratio (PaO_2/FiO_2) to ≤100, plus one of the following signs of infection: a temperature of ≥39.5 °C, leukocytosis of ≥20,000 × 10^9 cells/L and purulent secretions. The figure depicts lungs retrieved from an infected pig 68 h after bacterial inoculum and highlights multi-lobar pneumonia (lower left) and regions highly congested with copious intrabronchial amounts of purulent secretions (lower right)

fluid challenges, need for vasoactive drugs and reduced urine output [44–46]. Importantly, this animal model of pulmonary sepsis is also characterized by severe anemia that progressively worsens during the course of the 72-h study. In a recently conducted pilot study from our group (unpublished data), pigs were randomized to receive either iron or apotransferrin combined with iron. A control animal received no therapy. In the control animal, the drop in hemoglobin concentration from 16 to 11 g/dL was partly prevented by iron, but completely prevented by administration of transferrin with iron (Fig. 45.3).

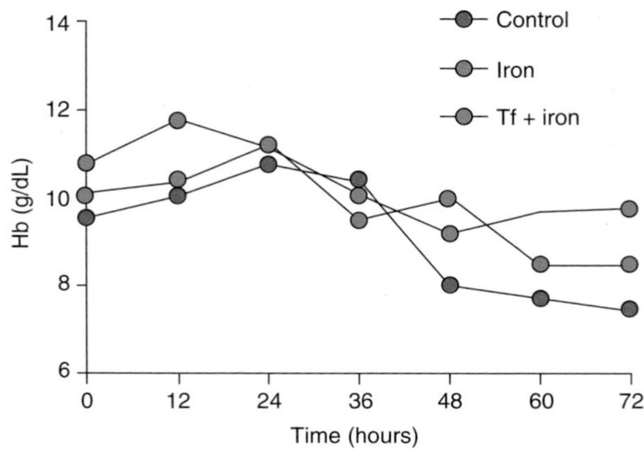

Fig. 45.3 Effect of iron and transferrin (Tf) on hemoglobin (Hb) concentrations in a pig model of pulmonary sepsis

45.8 Transferrin Supplementation to Decrease Free Iron-Mediated Organ Damage

45.8.1 Patients Undergoing High-Dose Chemotherapy

Patients who receive high-dose chemotherapy prior to receiving stem cell transplantation can have increased serum iron levels, as well as very high non-transferrin bound iron levels. The chemotherapy causes a pause in erythrocyte production and damages hepatocytes, resulting in the release of iron deposits, which exceeds the iron binding capacity of serum transferrin. The iron thus remains in the circulation of these patients as non-transferrin bound iron, which contributes to organ failure. In patients with iron overload after high-dose chemotherapy and stem cell transplantation, a single injection of 100 mg/kg of apotransferrin resulted in a decrease in non-transferrin bound iron levels. Serum iron levels also showed a dose-dependent increase. This may indicate that transferrin either causes iron release from tissue or that transferrin increases serum iron by binding of non-transferrin bound iron [43].

As high levels of non-transferrin bound iron are associated with infections caused by pathogens that depend on free iron for growth, the use of transferrin therapy could decrease the risk of infections in these patients as well. Indeed, transferrin reduced the number of days with fever, C-reactive protein (CRP) elevation and need for antibiotics, in patients undergoing chemotherapy. Also, in an *ex vivo* setting, exogenous apotransferrin prevented *Staphylococcus epidermidis* growth in plasma of stem cell transplantation patients compared to controls [43]. However, whether transferrin decreases risk of infection in this population is as yet unclear.

45.8.2 Model of Hyperoxic Lung Injury

Oxygen therapy can contribute to alveolar hyperoxia with subsequent ROS production in the lungs. ROS can cause lung injury by inhibiting the function of lung surfactant. In rabbit models of preterm lung injury induced by hyperoxia and successive bronchoalveolar lavages, a single injection of intratracheal or intravenous apotransferrin increases surfactant activity and decreases alveolar-capillary permeability. In addition, fewer peroxidation products and extravascular lung water were found after apotransferrin administration. In contrast, administration of holotransferrin resulted in a dose-dependent increase in respiratory failure suggesting that iron can counteract the protective effect of transferrin [43]. Thereby, transferrin might contribute to the recovery and prevention of respiratory failure caused by hyperoxia by the binding of free iron.

45.8.3 Model of Ischemia/Reperfusion Injury

Renal ischemia/reperfusion injury plays an important role in acute renal failure caused by shock or major surgery. The pathophysiology of ischemia/reperfusion injury includes oxidative stress formation, which leads to vascular and epithelial injury. In a mouse model of ischemia/reperfusion injury, a single dose of apotransferrin lowered circulating redox-active iron and superoxide formation and improved renal function. In contrast, holotransferrin did not prevent ischemia/reperfusion injury. In a cat model of intestinal ischemia/reperfusion injury, apotransferrin decreased the intestinal vascular permeability. Again, holotransferrin had no protective effect [43]. An ongoing clinical study is appraising the effectiveness of a combined drug approach including apotransferrin to reduce ischemia/reperfusion injury during liver transplantation in patients with liver failure (ClincialTrials.gov Identifier: NCT02251041).

45.8.4 Model of Pulmonary Sepsis

As discussed, sepsis patients frequently receive RBC transfusions [12]. Transfusion however can contribute to accumulation of iron, exceeding the binding capacity of transferrin, leading to free iron, which can induce inflammation and promote bacterial outgrowth [47]. Currently, we are investigating the impact of apotransferrin as an adjunct therapy to transfusion in a rat model of pulmonary sepsis on various clinically relevant outcomes, including the inflammatory response, organ injury and bacterial outgrowth.

45.9 Conclusion

Supplementation of transferrin may be beneficial for treatment of anemia of inflammation in two distinct ways that are both relevant to the critically ill. Transferrin may improve iron availability for erythropoiesis, thereby preventing the development of anemia. Also, transferrin scavenges free iron, thereby preventing ROS-mediated inflammation and improving organ failure. Although mostly experimental, data hitherto suggest that supplementation with apotransferrin has promising therapeutic properties. Transferrin corrects anemia in patients with hypotransferrinemia and in models of β-thalassemia. Also, transferrin decreases non-transferrin bound iron levels in patients receiving chemotherapy, and reduces organ injury by reducing oxidative stress and iron overload in tissues. Taken together, transferrin is a promising therapy in conditions characterized by anemia and oxidative stress related to iron overload. Currently, transferrin isolated from human plasma is an approved therapy for atransferrinemia. A clinical trial is ongoing to determine the efficacy and safety of repeated transferrin infusions. More clinical trials are needed to investigate the efficacy and safety of transferrin therapy in other disorders characterized by altered iron metabolism.

References

1. Vincent JL, Baron JF, Reinhart K, et al. Anemia and blood transfusion in critically ill patients. JAMA. 2002;288:1499–507.
2. Walsh TS, Lee RJ, Maciver CR, et al. Anemia during and at discharge from intensive care: the impact of restrictive blood transfusion practice. Intensive Care Med. 2006;32:100–9.
3. Corwin HL, Gettinger A, Pearl RG, et al. The CRIT Study: anemia and blood transfusion in the critically ill—current clinical practice in the United States. Crit Care Med. 2004;32:39–52.
4. Sihler KC, Napolitano LM. Anemia of inflammation in critically ill patients. J Intensive Care Med. 2008;23:295–302.
5. Lasocki S, Baron G, Driss F, et al. Diagnostic accuracy of serum hepcidin for iron deficiency in critically ill patients with anemia. Intensive Care Med. 2010;36:1044–8.
6. Prakash D. Anemia in the ICU: anemia of chronic disease versus anemia of acute illness. Crit Care Clin. 2012;28:333–43.
7. Pieracci FM, Barie PS. Diagnosis and management of iron-related anemias in critical illness. Crit Care Med. 2006;34:1898–905.
8. Ganz T. Hepcidin, a key regulator of iron metabolism and mediator of anemia of inflammation. Blood. 2003;102:783–8.
9. Truman-Rosentsvit M, Berenbaum D, Spektor L, et al. Ferritin is secreted via 2 distinct non-classical vesicular pathways. Blood. 2018;131:342–52.
10. Ritchie RF, Palomaki GE, Neveux LM, et al. Reference distributions for the negative acute-phase serum proteins, albumin, transferrin and transthyretin: a practical, simple and clinically relevant approach in a large cohort. J Clin Lab Anal. 1999;13:273–9.
11. Weiss G, Goodnough LT. Anemia of chronic disease. N Engl J Med. 2005;352:1011–23.
12. Holst LB, Haase N, Wetterslev J, et al. Lower versus higher hemoglobin threshold for transfusion in septic shock. N Engl J Med. 2014;371:1381–91.
13. Cassat JE, Skaar EP. Iron in infection and immunity. Cell Host Microbe. 2013;13:509–19.
14. Hébert PC, et al. TRICC Trial—a multicenter, randomized, controlled clinical trial of transfusion requirements in critical care. N Engl J Med. 1999;340:409–17.
15. Murphy GJ, Pike K, Rogers CA, et al. Liberal or restrictive transfusion after cardiac surgery. N Engl J Med. 2015;372:997–1008.
16. Carson JL, Terrin ML, Noveck H, et al. Liberal or restrictive transfusion in high-risk patients after hip surgery. N Engl J Med. 2011;365:2453–62.
17. Pieracci FM, Stovall RT, Jaouen B, et al. A multicenter, randomized clinical trial of IV iron supplementation for anemia of traumatic critical illness. Crit Care Med. 2014;42:2048–57.

18. Shah A, Roy NB, McKechnie S, et al. Iron supplementation to treat anaemia in adult critical care patients: a systematic review and meta-analysis. Crit Care. 2016;20:306.
19. Litton E, Baker S, Erber WN, et al. Intravenous iron or placebo for anaemia in intensive care: the IRONMAN multicentre randomized blinded trial. Intensive Care Med. 2016;42:1715–22.
20. Pieracci FM, Henderson P, Rodney JRM, et al. Randomized, double-blind, placebo-controlled trial of effects of enteral iron supplementation on anemia and risk of infection during surgical critical illness. Surg Infect. 2009;10:9–19.
21. Garrido-Martín P, Nassar-Mansur MI, de la Llana-Ducrós R, et al. The effect of intravenous and oral iron administration on perioperative anaemia and transfusion requirements in patients undergoing elective cardiac surgery: a randomized clinical trial. Interact Cardiovasc Thorac Surg. 2012;15:1013–8.
22. Madi-Jebara SN, Sleilaty GS, Achouh PE, et al. Postoperative intravenous iron used alone or in combination with low-dose erythropoietin is not effective for correction of anemia after cardiac surgery. J Cardiothorac Vasc Anesth. 2004;18:59–63.
23. Rohde JM, Dimcheff DE, Blumberg N, et al. Health care-associated infection after red blood cell transfusion: a systematic review and meta-analysis. JAMA. 2014;311:1317–26.
24. Corwin HL, Gettinger A, Pearl RG, et al. Efficacy of recombinant human erythropoietin in critically ill patients a randomized controlled trial. JAMA. 2002;288:2827–35.
25. Drueke TB, Locatelli F, Clyne N, et al. Normalization of hemoglobin level in patients with chronic kidney disease and anemia. N Engl J Med. 2006;355:333–40.
26. Tonia T, Mettler A, Robert N, et al. Erythropoietin or darbepoetin for patients with cancer. Cochrane Database Syst Rev. 2012;2012:CD003407.
27. Marik PE, Corwin HL. Efficacy of red blood cell transfusion in the critically ill: a systematic review of the literature. Crit Care Med. 2008;36:2667–74.
28. Schipperus M, Rijnbeek B, Reddy M, et al. CNTO328 (Anti-IL-6 mAb) Treatment is associated with an increase in hemoglobin (Hb) and decrease in hepcidin levels in renal cell carcinoma (RCC). Blood. 2009;114:1551 (abst).
29. Song S-NJ, Iwahashi M, Tomosugi N, et al. Comparative evaluation of the effects of treatment with tocilizumab and TNF-a inhibitors on serum hepcidin, anemia response and disease activity in rheumatoid arthritis patients. Arthritis Res Ther. 2013;15:1.
30. Song SNJ, Tomosugi N, Kawabata H, et al. Down-regulation of hepcidin resulting from long-term treatment with an anti-IL-6 receptor antibody (tocilizumab) improves anemia of inflammation in multicentric Castleman disease. Blood. 2010;116:3627–34.
31. Isaacs JD, Harari O, Kobold U, et al. Effect of tocilizumab on haematological markers implicates interleukin-6 signalling in the anaemia of rheumatoid arthritis. Arthritis Res Ther. 2013;15:R204.
32. Schwoebel F, van Eijk LT, Zboralski D, et al. The effects of the anti-hepcidin Spiegelmer NOX-H94 on inflammation-induced anemia in cynomolgus monkeys. Blood. 2013;121:2311–5.
33. Van Eijk LT, John ASE, Schwoebel F, et al. Effect of the antihepcidin Spiegelmer lexaptepid on inflammation-induced decrease in serum iron in humans. Blood. 2014;124:2643–6.
34. Sasu BJ, Cooke KS, Arvedson TL, et al. Antihepcidin antibody treatment modulates iron metabolism and is effective in a mouse model of inflammation-induced anemia. Blood. 2010;115:3616–24.
35. Poli M, Girelli D, Campostrini N, et al. Heparin: a potent inhibitor of hepcidin expression in vitro and in vivo Heparin: a potent inhibitor of hepcidin expression in vitro and in vivo. Blood. 2010;117:997–1004.
36. Steinbicker AU, Sachidanandan C, Vonner AJ, et al. Inhibition of bone morphogenetic protein signaling attenuates anemia associated with inflammation. Blood. 2011;117:4915–24.
37. Chung MCM. Stucture and function of transferrin. Biochem Educ. 1984;12:146–54.
38. Crichton RR, Charloteaux-wauters M. Iron transport and storage. Eur J Biochem. 1987;164:485–506.
39. Parkkinen J, von Bonsdorff L, Ebeling F, Sahlstedt L. Function and therapeutic development of apotransferrin. Vox Sang. 2002;83(Suppl 1):321–6.

40. Prakash M. Role of non-transferrin-bound iron in chornic renal failure and other disease conditions. Ren Physiol. 2007;17:188–93.
41. von Bonsdorff L, Tölö H, Lindeberg E, et al. Development of a pharmaceutical apotransferrin product for iron binding therapy. Biologicals. 2001;29:27–37.
42. Hayashi A, Wada Y, Suzuki T, Shimizu A. Studies on familial hypotransferrinemia: unique clinical course and molecular pathology. Am J Hum Genet. 1993;53:201–13.
43. Boshuizen M, van der Ploeg K, von Bonsdorff L, et al. Therapeutic use of transferrin to modulate anemia and conditions of iron toxicity. Blood Rev. 2017;31:400–5.
44. Li Bassi G, Rigol M, Marti JD, et al. A novel porcine model of ventilator-associated pneumonia caused by oropharyngeal challenge with Pseudomonas aeruginosa. Anesthesiology. 2014;120:1205–15.
45. Sibila O, Agustí C, Torres A, et al. Experimental Pseudomonas aeruginosa pneumonia: evaluation of the associated inflammatory response. Eur Respir J. 2007;30:1167–72.
46. Luna CM, Baquero S, Gando S, et al. Experimental severe Pseudomonas aeruginosa pneumonia and antibiotic therapy in piglets receiving mechanical ventilation. Chest. 2007;132:523–31.
47. Hod EA, Zhang N, Sokol SA, et al. Transfusion of red blood cells after prolonged storage produces harmful effects that are mediated by iron and inflammation. Blood. 2015;115:4284–93.

Part XIV

Extremes of Age

Functional Impairments in Pediatric Critical Illness Survivors

46

C. S. Ong and Z. A. Puthucheary

46.1 Introduction

With decreasing mortality rates, the world of critical care is becoming increasingly focused on not only maximizing survival, but maximizing survival with good function. Functional status has been suggested as a more meaningful outcome measure than mortality, and the push to report functional status as an outcome for pediatric intensive care unit (PICU) studies has recently translated to action [1, 2]. The PICU community is currently in the process of trying to understand the prevalence and pathophysiology of the problem, as well as interventions with the goal of improving or restoring a patient's functional status to baseline.

In adult critical illness literature, a major finding in survivors is that of impaired physical function persisting up to years after discharge from the intensive care unit (ICU), attributed to significant muscle wasting and dysfunction [3, 4]. This persistent impairment contributes a significant burden to the patient, their families and the economy [3]. Extensive study has since been undertaken to further understand the pathophysiology in order to prevent or reverse the impairment [4]. A recent systematic review mapped the physical impairments observed in adult post-intensive care

C. S. Ong
Department of Biochemistry, Yong Loo Lin School of Medicine,
National University of Singapore, Singapore, Singapore

Department of Nutrition and Dietetics, KK Women's and Children's Hospital,
Singapore, Singapore

Z. A. Puthucheary (✉)
William Harvey Research Institute, Barts Health NHS Trust, London, UK

The London School of Medicine and Dentistry, Queen Mary University of London, London, UK

Adult Critical Care Unit, Royal London Hospital, Barts Health NHS Trust, London, UK
e-mail: Zudin.puthucheary.09@ucl.ac.uk

J.-L. Vincent (ed.), *Annual Update in Intensive Care and Emergency Medicine 2019*, Annual Update in Intensive Care and Emergency Medicine,
https://doi.org/10.1007/978-3-030-06067-1_46

syndrome (PICS) to the world health organization (WHO) International Classification of Functioning, Disability and Health (ICF) [5]. The authors demonstrated that the physical impairments are extensive, affecting not just impairments in body structure and function, but also restricting activities of daily living and one's participation within the society. Physical and nutritional interventions are being actively studied in an effort to reduce this impairment [6, 7].

The existence of the PICS in pediatric survivors has also recently been recognized [8]. The proposed framework of the PICS in pediatrics (PICS-p) includes four constructs of physical, cognitive, emotional and social function. These functional areas are by no means isolated; impairment in one aspect of function can and often does affect the others. Central to the PICS-p is the PICU patient, but it is recognized that family members such as siblings and caregivers may be similarly affected by these impairments.

However, unlike in adult critical illness, understanding of the prevalence and pathophysiology of physical impairments within the PICS-p is currently limited. Children similarly experience a catabolic state during critical illness, suggesting the possibility of significant physical function impairments in PICU survivors [9]. In this chapter, we review the existing evidence regarding acquired impairments in physical function following pediatric critical illness, and discuss future steps to improve our knowledge and understanding of this problem.

46.2 Current Knowledge

46.2.1 Measurement Tools and Rates of Physical Function Impairment

Rates of acquired functional impairments as a result of pediatric critical illness vary with population type, measurement tool and time point (Table 46.1). Two main types of measurement tools have typically been used in the reporting of functional impairments in pediatric critical illness. The first are global measures of overall function or health state, often on a spectrum from good to poor function. The second are more detailed, multi-dimensional assessments of function, which commonly explore various domains within the different components of cognitive, physical, emotional and social functioning, with significant degree of overlap in the constructs across tools (Fig. 46.1). However, the degree of detail within each multidimensional domain can vary. Both types of measures can be either assessed by a healthcare professional or patient-reported.

The first widely used global assessment tool was the pediatric overall performance category (POPC) and the pediatric cerebral performance category (PCPC), developed by Fiser [10]. The POPC and PCPC are typically used together to assess general neurological function as well as overall function with consideration of non-neurological functional deficits, and each is scored by the clinician using a semi-objective assessment tool on a scale of 1–6. Similar to the POPC, the modified Glasgow Outcome Scale (mGOS) allows the clinician to rate the overall functional

Table 46.1 Trajectories of overall functional status reported in different studies

			Acquired rates of overall impairment in survivors (%)					
Study author [ref]	Tool used	Population	PICU discharge	Hospital discharge	3 months	6 months	1 year	>1 year
Alievi [13]	POPC	General	36					
Mestrovic [14]	POPC	General	25					
Fiser [35]	POPC	General	24					
Bone [15]	POPC	General	10					
Farris [16]	POPC	Sepsis	34					
de Mos [17]	POPC	In PICU cardiac arrest		36				
Knoester [19]	POPC	Previously healthy	91		50			
Butt [11]	mGOS	General						7.8 (3 years)
Taylor [18]	mGOS	General						17.3 (3.5 years)
Namachivayam [20]	mGOS	Long stayers						33 (4 years)
Polic [12]	RAHC MOF	General				26		19 (2 years)
Pollack [36]	FSS	General		5				
Pinto [23]	FSS	General		5.2		6.5		10.4 (3 years)
Bennett [26]	FSS	TBI		37				
Berger [24]	FSS	Cardiac surgery		5				
Beshish [25]	FSS	eCPR		50				
Gemke [30]	HUI2	General					27	
Cunha [31]	HUI3	General				41		
Choong [32]	PEDI-CAT	General	81.5		>29.1	>24.4		

eCPR extracorporeal cardiopulmonary resuscitation, *FSS* functional status scale, *HUI* health utilities index, *mGOS* modified Glasgow Outcome Scale, *PEDI-CAT* pediatric evaluation of disability inventory-computer adaptive test, *PICU* pediatric intensive care unit, *POPC* pediatric overall performance category, *RAHC MOF* Royal Alexandra Hospital for children measure of function, *TBI* traumatic brain injury

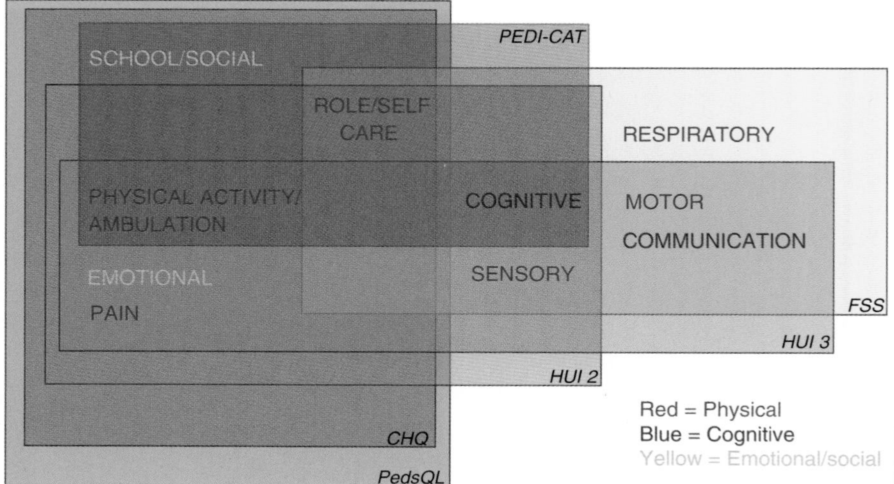

Fig. 46.1 Overlapping constructs in multi-dimensional functional status tools used in critically ill children. *CHQ* child health questionnaire 28-item short form, *FSS* functional status scale, *HUI 2* health utilities index mark 2, *HUI 3* health utilities index mark 3, *PedsQL* Pediatric Quality of Life inventory 4.0, *PEDI-CAT* pediatric evaluation of disability inventory-computer adaptive test

status using a 5-point scale from normal to severe disability [11], whereas the Royal Alexandra Hospital for Children Measure of Function (RAHC MOF) allows a patient-reported global health score from 0–100 [12]. Using these global measurement tools, rates of acquired impairment in overall function in general PICU populations ranged from 10–36% at PICU discharge, to approximately 26% at 6 months, and 8–19% at follow-ups between 2 and 4 years post-discharge [10–18]. In select patient populations (sepsis, in PICU cardiac arrest, those with prolonged stays and previously healthy children), rates of global impairment are higher, up to 91% at PICU discharge and 33% at 4 years post-discharge [19, 20]. Interestingly, comparison of the POPC scores with the PCPC scores revealed that more children had abnormal POPC compared to PCPC scores at 3 months post-discharge, suggesting that the differences were attributable to physical impairments, and were more prevalent and persistent than cognitive impairments in previously healthy children [19]. However, while easy to administer and indicative of the presence of functional impairment, these global assessment tools were unable to provide further information regarding types of physical or other function.

To introduce greater objectivity and granularity, the functional status scale (FSS) was developed and published by Pollack et al. and the Collaborative Pediatric Critical Care Research Network (CPCCRN) in 2009 as an outcome measurement tool specific to the PICU [21]. The FSS consists of a 5-point scale across six domains of function: mental, sensory, communication, motor, feeding and respiratory, and has been validated against more comprehensive measures of function, such as the Vineland Adaptive Behavior Scale (VABS-2) [21]. An increase in total score of ≥3 points is recognized as a clinically significant new functional morbidity [21]. Using this definition, rates of overall functional impairment in survivors at hospital discharge range from 5% in a general PICU population, to 37% in traumatic brain injury (TBI), and 50% in children requiring extracorporeal cardiopulmonary resuscitation (eCPR) [22–25]. The FSS demonstrated that the most severely affected domains included the motor and respiratory function in general PICU patients, and the motor and feeding domains in TBI patients [19, 26].

By retaining the relative ease of scoring with added granularity, the FSS score has enabled quantification of functional impairment in large PICU cohort studies as well as smaller exploratory studies in specific PICU cohorts. However, given the complexity of the PICS-p, the FSS still lacks a degree of sensitivity in sufficiently characterizing functional impairments. Specifically, the FSS is unable to capture detailed aspects of functional capacity beyond that of its six domains. In addition, during the development of FSS, a significant percentage of patients (18%) had the best possible score of 6 at PICU discharge [21], which suggests a possible ceiling effect and limitations of the FSS in determining changes beyond the PICU.

Health-related quality of life (HRQoL) is increasingly used to drive patient-centered care. Many multi-dimensional HRQoL tools incorporate questions that address body function, activity and participation according to the WHO ICF for Children and Youth (WHO ICF-CY), and can provide some information regarding physical function and impairment [27]. A review of all HRQoL tools that have been used in PICU patients concluded that the pediatric quality of life inventory (PedsQL) 4.0, the KIDSCREEN-27, the 28-item child health questionnaire (CHQ-28) and the KINDL perform best in terms of validity, administration burden and sensitivity [28]. Of these, the PedsQL 4.0 and the CHQ-28 appear to cover more areas of physical function (mobility, neuromusculoskeletal and movement function) within the WHO ICF-CY framework [27], and the construct validity and responsiveness of the PedsQL 4.0 has been specifically demonstrated in PICU patients [29]. Two studies measured functional impairment using the health utilities index (HUI) mark 2 and three HRQoL questionnaires, and reported acquired impairment rates of 41% and 27% at 6 and 12 months, respectively, post-discharge [30, 31].

The recently published "WeeCover" PICU survivorship study used the pediatric disability inventory-computer adaptive test (PEDI-CAT) to detect changes in functional abilities at baseline, PICU discharge, 3 and 6 months [32]. The PEDI-CAT consists of questions regarding four functional domains—daily activity, mobility, social/cognitive and responsibility—and was designed to be aligned with the WHO ICF-CY framework [33, 34]. The advantage of the PEDI-CAT is the ability to measure age-appropriate functional performance, providing a more meaningful representation of the child's function in the context of social and community participation. In addition, the computer-adaptive nature of the test also allows for an abbreviated assessment that maximizes the tool's precision while minimizing time required. The "WeeCover" study was the first to demonstrate the trajectory of functional impairment in various domains from baseline until 6 months post-PICU discharge. Of note, the greatest impairments at PICU discharge and the slowest recovery at 6 months post-discharge were observed in the mobility domain [32].

Considering all of the above studies, rates of PICU-acquired functional impairments appear to be greatest at PICU discharge, with greatest recovery observed in the first 3 months, slowing down thereafter up to 6 months post-PICU discharge [32]. Despite the use of different measurement tools, significant physical functional impairments have been reported. However, rates differ, with higher rates reported using multi-dimensional measures. There is also a lack of longitudinal studies with sufficient follow-up duration, making it difficult to determine the trajectory of function beyond. Whether physical function persists beyond the 3–6 months post PICU discharge is unclear from the current evidence.

46.2.2 Risk Factors

Knowledge of risk factors for functional impairment can provide more targeted research to elucidate pathophysiology. From the various studies, several risk factors have been associated with acquired functional impairment, of which three are repeated in several studies (Box 46.1).

Several illness severity scores, such as the pediatric risk of mortality (PRISM) and the pediatric index of mortality (PIM), have been developed to predict mortality risk within the PICU. Higher illness severity calculated by these scores was associated with acquired overall functional impairment in several studies [12–16, 32, 35]. However, the association between illness severity and morbidity risk does not appear to follow a linear relationship [22]. Using data from over 10,000 patients, Pollack et al. demonstrated that the risk of mortality and morbidity could be simultaneously predicted using PRISM III scores [22]. With increasing PRISM scores, the risk of morbidity and mortality initially increased proportionally; however above a certain PRISM score, the risk of morbidity decreased while mortality risk continued to increase. The authors suggest that morbidity and mortality are closely interlinked and are in fact different end-points within the same trajectory, dependent on the level of physiological dysfunction. The increased risk of functional impairment has also been demonstrated in those with high PIM 2 scores [12, 15]. Unfortunately, these studies used global function measures, precluding further

Box 46.1: Risk Factors for Acquired Overall Functional Impairment from Published Studies

Pre-PICU	Intra-PICU
• Better baseline function [32] • Younger age <1 year [36] • Neurological injury on admission [32, 36]	• Illness severity scores: PIM2, PRISM [12–16, 35] • Need for mechanical ventilation [23] • PICU length of stay [15, 35]

PICU pediatric intensive care unit, *PIM* pediatric index of mortality, *PRISM* pediatric risk of mortality

analysis on risk factors specific to physical impairment. However, in the "WeeCover" study, multivariable regression analyses were conducted for change in each functional domain. Higher PRISM III scores were significantly associated with impairment in social/cognitive function, but not daily activities, mobility or responsibility domains [32]. More studies are needed to determine whether increasing disease severity is associated with decline in physical function.

Certain admission diagnoses appear to be associated with risk of new functional impairment. Specifically, in a large cohort study using the FSS, Pollack et al. found that neurological diagnoses as the primary system of dysfunction were associated with the highest rates of new global functional impairment [36]. Choong et al. similarly found that neurological injury (e.g., status epilepticus, TBI, hemorrhage) at PICU admission was significantly associated with greater impairment in all aspects of function at PICU discharge, including mobility and daily activities [32]. Neurological injury was also significantly associated with slower recovery of daily activities and mobility at 6-month follow-up, suggesting that children admitted with primary neurological injuries should be closely monitored for physical function impairments.

Two studies have reported greater rates of acquired global functional impairment in patients with longer PICU length of stay [15, 35]. Longer PICU stay is typically a result of increased disease severity, but is also associated with longer periods of sedation, immobility and malnutrition—possible factors that could contribute to muscle wasting and physical impairments. However, a recent randomized controlled trial (RCT) of protocolized-sedation in critically ill children found that reduced sedation did not seem to impact acquired global functional impairment at 6 months post-discharge [1].

46.3 Future Directions

46.3.1 Gaps and Considerations

It is evident that the problem of physical function impairment in survivors of pediatric critical illness is still not sufficiently understood, likely stemming in part from the poor recognition and reporting of functional status as a main PICU outcome until recently. Two main obstacles currently lie in the way of our better understanding of physical impairment. The first is the limited availability of tools to measure physical impairments in the pediatric population, while taking into consideration age-appropriate developmental milestones. Second, and in part related to the first, is the lack of standardization of assessment time points across studies. Appropriate measurement tools at critical time points are necessary to enable the early identification of physical impairments, guide therapy and monitor recovery in these patients.

In adult survivors of critical illness, reported impairments in body function and structure include those of reduced limb muscle and handgrip strength, as well as respiratory function [5], while limitations in activity and participation involve reduced physical endurance as measured by the 6-minute walk test (6MWT) and dependence in activities of daily living. It is recommended that assessment of physical function in adult ICU patients begins with determination of baseline abilities, followed by a combination of strength, range of motion, mobility and endurance within the ICU [37]. Following ICU discharge, patient reported outcomes via the short-form 36 (SF-36) HRQoL questionnaire is considered a core outcome of adult ICU studies [38].

From the available evidence in PICU survivors, physical limitations in motor function, respiration and mobility are present at hospital discharge [19, 32]. However, measurement tools to determine limb and respiratory muscle strength and physical activity in PICU survivors are not widely used, mainly limited to the burn injury population [39, 40]. Granted, some of these measures are only valid and applicable to older children (>6 years); in the young, a more meaningful assessment may concern that of age-appropriate developmental milestones. Understanding which short- and long-term outcomes matter most to families and caregivers is also necessary to provide patient-centered care [2]. Indeed, the PICU community is conscious of these considerations, and tools designed for use in the adult ICU are currently being revised and tested within the PICU population [2, 41]. Determination of their clinimetric properties, including reliability, validity, responsiveness, floor and ceiling effects, will hopefully guide research and clinical practice in the future.

Along with these assessment tools, time points for measurement of functional status need to be standardized. Baseline assessment is critical to determine the presence of acquired impairment, but this could be challenging depending on the type of tool being used. Baseline assessment would most often require a proxy report, and can be subject to recall bias [42]. Within the PICU, early identification of physical function impairments may allow more conscious efforts to reduce offending interventions and provide rehabilitative care. Unfortunately, in young children the lack of cooperation or inability to understand instructions suggests the need for non-volitional assessment methods. Assessment at PICU or hospital discharge is also important for determining the need for follow-up care and monitoring in the sub-acute or community setting. Finally, follow-ups within the first year would help inform the trajectory of recovery or subsequent impairment.

While desirable, it is unlikely that a single tool would be sufficient to adequately capture physical function impairments throughout the entire spectrum of illness and recovery. A combination of tools—global vs. multi-dimensional, clinician-assessed vs. patient-reported—may be the most practical solution at present.

46.4 Conclusion

Functional status is now recognized as an important outcome measure in pediatric critical care survivorship. Acquired impairments in physical function appear significant to these children and seems to persist beyond hospital discharge, although the complete trajectory is unclear. Patients with high illness severity scores and neurological injuries at baseline appear to be at greater risk of physical function impairments.

Understanding of the acquired physical impairments following pediatric critical illness remains poor, in part due to the limitations of currently available tools that have been validated in this population and insufficiencies in longitudinal monitoring. There is a need for more study into domain-specific functional assessments with proper testing of validity, reliability, responsiveness, and floor and ceiling effects. Follow-up time points in PICU survivors should also be standardized, minimally within the first year of PICU discharge. This would provide a better understanding of the problem of acquired functional impairment in pediatric critical illness survivors such as to guide measurement of future interventions.

References

1. Watson RS, Asaro LA. Long-term outcomes after protocolized sedation versus usual care in ventilated pediatric patients. Am J Respir Crit Care Med. 2018;197:1457–67.
2. Merritt C, Menon K, Agus MSD, et al. Beyond survival: pediatric critical care interventional trial outcome measure preferences of families and healthcare professionals. Pediatr Crit Care Med. 2018;19:e105–11.
3. Herridge MS, Tansey CM, Matté A, et al. Functional disability 5 years after acute respiratory distress syndrome. N Engl J Med. 2011;364:1293–304.
4. Puthucheary ZA, Rawal J, McPhail M, et al. Acute skeletal muscle wasting in critical illness. JAMA. 2013;310:1591–600.
5. Ohtake PJ, Lee AC, Scott JC, et al. Physical impairments associated with post-intensive care syndrome: systematic review based on the World Health Organization's International Classification of Functioning, Disability and Health Framework. Phys Ther. 2018;98:631–45.
6. Fetterplace K, Deane AM, Tierney A, et al. Targeted full energy and protein delivery in critically ill patients: a study protocol for a pilot randomised control trial (FEED Trial). Pilot Feasibility Stud. 2018;4:52.
7. Kho ME, Molloy AJ, Clarke F, et al. CYCLE pilot: a protocol for a pilot randomised study of early cycle ergometry versus routine physiotherapy in mechanically ventilated patients. BMJ Open. 2016;6:e011659.
8. Manning JC, Pinto NP, Rennick JE, Colville G, Curley MAQ. Conceptualizing post intensive care syndrome in children—the PICS-p framework. Pediatr Crit Care Med. 2018;19:298–300.
9. Coss-Bu JA, Klish WJ, Walding D, Stein F, Smith EOB, Jefferson LS. Energy metabolism, nitrogen balance, and substrate utilization in critically ill children. Am J Clin Nutr. 2001;74:664–9.
10. Fiser DH. Assessing the outcome of pediatric intensive care. J Pediatr. 1992;121:68–74.
11. Butt W, Shann F, Tibballs J, et al. Long-term outcome of children after intensive care. Crit Care Med. 1990;18:961–5.
12. Polic B, Mestrovic J, Markic J, et al. Long-term quality of life of patients treated in paediatric intensive care unit. Eur J Pediatr. 2013;172:85–90.
13. Alievi PT, Carvalho PR, Trotta EA, Mombelli Filho R. The impact of admission to a pediatric intensive care unit assessed by means of global and cognitive performance scales. J Pediatr. 2007;83:505–11.
14. Mestrovic J, Polic B, Mestrovic M, Kardum G, Marusic E, Sustic A. Functional outcome of children treated in intensive care unit. J Pediatr. 2008;84:232–6.
15. Bone MF, Feinglass JM, Goodman DM. Risk factors for acquiring functional and cognitive disabilities during admission to a PICU. Pediatr Crit Care Med. 2014;15:640–8.
16. Farris RW, Weiss NS, Zimmerman JJ. Functional outcomes in pediatric severe sepsis: further analysis of the researching severe sepsis and organ dysfunction in children: a global perspective trial. Pediatr Crit Care Med. 2013;14:835–42.

17. de Mos N, van Litsenburg RR, McCrindle B, Bohn DJ, Parshuram CS. Pediatric in-intensive-care-unit cardiac arrest: incidence, survival, and predictive factors. Crit Care Med. 2006;34:1209–15.
18. Taylor A, Butt W, Ciardulli M. The functional outcome and quality of life of children after admission to an intensive care unit. Intensive Care Med. 2003;29:795–800.
19. Knoester H, Bronner MB, Bos AP. Surviving pediatric intensive care: physical outcome after 3 months. Intensive Care Med. 2008;34:1076–82.
20. Namachivayam P, Taylor A, Montague T, et al. Long-stay children in intensive care: long-term functional outcome and quality of life from a 20-yr institutional study. Pediatr Crit Care Med. 2012;13:520–8.
21. Pollack MM, Holubkov R, Glass P, et al. Functional Status Scale: new pediatric outcome measure. Pediatrics. 2009;124:e18–28.
22. Pollack MM, Holubkov R, Funai T, et al. Simultaneous prediction of new morbidity, mortality, and survival without new morbidity from pediatric intensive care: a new paradigm for outcomes assessment. Crit Care Med. 2015;43:1699–709.
23. Pinto NP, Rhinesmith EW, Kim TY, Ladner PH, Pollack MM. Long-term function after pediatric critical illness: results from the survivor outcomes study. Pediatr Crit Care Med. 2017;18:e122–30.
24. Berger JT, Holubkov R, Reeder R, et al. Morbidity and mortality prediction in pediatric heart surgery: Physiological profiles and surgical complexity. J Thorac Cardiovasc Surg. 2017;154:620–628.e626.
25. Beshish AG, Baginski MR, Johnson TJ, Deatrick BK, Barbaro RP, Owens GE. Functional status change among children with extracorporeal membrane oxygenation to support cardiopulmonary resuscitation in a pediatric cardiac ICU: a single institution report. Pediatr Crit Care Med. 2018;19:665–71.
26. Bennett TD, Dixon RR, Kartchner C, et al. Functional status scale in children with traumatic brain injury: a prospective cohort study. Pediatr Crit Care Med. 2016;17:1147–56.
27. Janssens A, Rogers M, Thompson Coon J, et al. A systematic review of generic multidimensional patient-reported outcome measures for children, part II: evaluation of psychometric performance of English-language versions in a general population. Value Health. 2015;18:334–45.
28. Aspesberro F, Mangione-Smith R, Zimmerman JJ. Health-related quality of life following pediatric critical illness. Intensive Care Med. 2015;41:1235–46.
29. Aspesberro F, Fesinmeyer MD, Zhou C, Zimmerman JJ, Mangione-Smith R. Construct validity and responsiveness of the Pediatric Quality of Life Inventory 4.0 generic core scales and infant scales in the PICU. Pediatr Crit Care Med. 2016;17:e272–9.
30. Gemke RJ, Bonsel GJ, van Vught AJ. Long-term survival and state of health after paediatric intensive care. Arch Dis Child. 1995;73:196–201.
31. Cunha F, Mota T, Teixeira-Pinto A, et al. Factors associated with health-related quality of life changes in survivors to pediatric intensive care. Pediatr Crit Care Med. 2013;14:e8–15.
32. Choong K, Fraser D, Al-Harbi S, et al. Functional recovery in critically ill children, the "WeeCover" multicenter study. Pediatr Crit Care Med. 2018;19:145–54.
33. Haley SM, Coster WJ, Dumas HM, et al. Accuracy and precision of the Pediatric Evaluation of Disability Inventory computer-adaptive tests (PEDI-CAT). Dev Med Child Neurol. 2011;53:1100–6.
34. World Health Organization. International classification of functioning, disability, and health: children & youth version: ICF-CY. 2007. Available at: apps.who.int/iris/bitstream/10665/43737/1/9789241547321_eng.pdf. Accessed Aug 2018.
35. Fiser DH, Tilford JM, Roberson PK. Relationship of illness severity and length of stay to functional outcomes in the pediatric intensive care unit: a multi-institutional study. Crit Care Med. 2000;28:1173–9.
36. Pollack MM, Holubkov R, Funai T, et al. Pediatric intensive care outcomes: development of new morbidities during pediatric critical care. Pediatr Crit Care Med. 2014;15:821–7.
37. Parry SM, Huang M, Needham DM. Evaluating physical functioning in critical care: considerations for clinical practice and research. Crit Care. 2017;21:249.

38. Needham DM, Sepulveda KA, Dinglas VD, et al. Core outcome measures for clinical research in acute respiratory failure survivors. An international modified delphi consensus study. Am J Respir Crit Care Med. 2017;196:1122–30.
39. Cucuzzo NA, Ferrando A, Herndon DN. The effects of exercise programming vs traditional outpatient therapy in the rehabilitation of severely burned children. J Burn Care Rehabil. 2001;22:214–20.
40. Rontoyanni VG, Malagaris I, Herndon DN, et al. Skeletal muscle mitochondrial function is determined by burn severity, sex, and sepsis, and is associated with glucose metabolism and functional capacity in burned children. Shock. 2018;50:141–8.
41. Ferguson A, Wright S, Long D, Stockton K, Stocker C. The children's Chelseaa Critical Care Physical Assessment Tool: modification of a validated adult assessment tool using delphi method. Pediatr Crit Care Med. 2018;19:255 (abst).
42. Scholten AC, Haagsma JA, Steyerberg EW, van Beeck EF, Polinder S. Assessment of pre-injury health-related quality of life: a systematic review. Popul Health Metrics. 2017;15:10.

Care of the Critically Ill Older Adult

47

C. A. Gao and L. E. Ferrante

47.1 Introduction: An Aging Population

As the population ages, so too does the intensive care unit (ICU) population. Already, it is estimated that greater than 50% of ICU admissions are patients aged 65 years and older, and this percentage is only expected to grow over time [1]. The growth of the 'oldest old', those above 80 years of age, is also expected to increase dramatically over the next three decades; in a study of European ICU admissions, some countries have seen the admission rate of patients in this demographic increase from 11% to 15% in a decade [2]. Older adults represent a unique population, with higher rates of preexisting comorbidities and vulnerabilities, and greater risk for developing ICU complications such as delirium. In this chapter, we discuss topics pertaining to care of the critically ill older patient, with a focus on new advancements in the last decade since Wunsch et al.'s excellent review published in 2009 [3], and a look to future studies that will help inform our day-to-day care of this sizeable, growing, and vulnerable population.

47.2 Getting to the ICU

Envision Mrs. L, an 80-year-old woman with diabetes and hypertension who lives alone. She is independent in all activities of daily living (ADLs). She drives to the store to shop for groceries every week, though her son comes by once a week to help her clean the house.

C. A. Gao
Department of Internal Medicine, Yale School of Medicine, New Haven, CT, USA

L. E. Ferrante (✉)
Section of Pulmonary, Critical Care, and Sleep Medicine, Department of Internal Medicine, Yale School of Medicine, New Haven, CT, USA
e-mail: lauren.ferrante@yale.edu

J.-L. Vincent (ed.), *Annual Update in Intensive Care and Emergency Medicine 2019*, Annual Update in Intensive Care and Emergency Medicine, https://doi.org/10.1007/978-3-030-06067-1_47

She walks around the neighborhood daily for exercise and has not had any falls. One day, she develops a cough and fever and is found confused and lethargic by her son. He calls 911 and she is taken to a local emergency room, where she remains hypotensive despite fluid resuscitation. The ICU team is notified.

47.2.1 Triage, Ageism and Mortality Benefit

ICU triage is difficult, and especially so in a vulnerable older population. Interviews with physicians have revealed that providers hold both positive and negative stereotypes of elderly patients, and ageism has been linked to poorer quality care in multiple reports [4]. Currently there is no standardized approach to ICU triage of older adults, and great variability in physician decisions regarding ICU admission for life-sustaining treatments among the oldest old [5].

The French ICE-CUB study of 2646 patients >80 years demonstrated that older patients may be less likely to be admitted to the ICU [6]. Despite 1426 of these patients meeting "definite admission criteria" according to the most recent Society of Critical Care Medicine guidelines, only 441 (31%) were referred for ICU admission and, of these, only 231 were actually admitted (16%). Among the 1041 patients with "equivocal" admission criteria, only 181 (17%) were referred for ICU evaluation and only 79 (7.6%) were admitted to the ICU. Older age and lower ADL score were among several factors associated with increased odds of not receiving an ICU referral. Although this study did not include information on bed availability or treatment preferences, it is an informative illustration of the ICU referral process for the oldest old.

The Eldicus trial (Part II) evaluated the benefit of ICU admission for older adults, reviewing 8472 triages in 11 European ICUs [7]. Rejection of admission to the ICU was higher with older patients (36% rejection rate for patients >84 years vs. an 11% rejection rate for patients aged 18–44). The mortality difference between those accepted versus refused widened with age: among patients aged 18–44, the mortality difference between accepted vs. rejected patients was just over 2% (10.2% vs. 12.5%), whereas the mortality difference for those over 84 years of age was 41.5% vs. 58.5%. Although these mortality differences are compelling, this study did not include information about treatment preferences and may have also been limited by the use of the Simplified Acute Physiology Score II (SAPS II) without age points.

Given that the aforementioned studies were limited by their observational methods, the ICE-CUB 2 study, a cluster-randomized trial of ICU admission for patients aged >75 years, was conducted at 24 French hospitals [8]. The investigators enrolled 3037 patients with preserved functional and nutritional status and without cancer, and randomized centers to use either standard practice or a program of "systematic ICU admission". Patients in the intervention arm were more likely to be admitted to the ICU (61% versus 34% in the control arm) but there was no difference at 6-month follow-up in death, functional status, or physical quality of life. Of note, more than one third of older patients recommended for admission in the intervention arm were not admitted to the ICU because the final decision rested with the clinical team. Although patients in the intervention arm had a higher risk of in-hospital death (relative risk [RR] 1.18, 95% confidence interval [CI] 1.03–1.33), it is important to note that data on withdrawal of life-sustaining therapies were not collected, so this finding may be due to earlier or more frequent discussions regarding treatment preferences that led to withdrawal of life-sustaining therapies.

Other studies have clearly demonstrated improved outcomes after ICU admission among older adults. Recently, a large study evaluating over one million Medicare patients with pneumonia found that ICU admission for "discretionary" patients (for whom the decision varied depending on distance from the hospital, rather than an absolute need for critical care) was associated with an absolute reduction in 30-day mortality of 5.7% compared with patients admitted to the general wards [9]. ICU admission was not associated with significant differences in Medicare spending or hospital costs. Although additional studies are warranted, these results suggest that older adults with pneumonia may benefit from increased access to the ICU.

47.2.2 The Importance of Preexisting Vulnerability Factors Over Chronological Age

Older adults are more likely to develop comorbidities, geriatric syndromes, and other risk factors that confer increased vulnerability to adverse outcomes after an acute insult such as an ICU admission. Although age is often a focus in decisions about ICU triage, a large body of work has revealed that other preexisting factors may be more informative predictors of post-ICU outcomes.

Pre-ICU functional status is an important determinant of post-ICU outcomes among older adults. In a recent prospective cohort study of older adults admitted to the ICU, the pre-ICU functional trajectory (a monthly measure of function in 13 basic, instrumental, and mobility activities measured over the year prior to ICU admission) was strongly associated with post-ICU functional outcomes and mortality [10]. Those with a pre-ICU trajectory of severe disability had more than three times the risk of dying by 1 year compared to those with minimal to mild disability (68% versus 19%). Another recent study of the oldest old determined that a poor premorbid functional status predicted an increased risk of in-hospital death (odds ratio [OR] 1.50, 95% CI 1.07–2.10) and 1-year mortality (OR 2.18, 95% CI 1.67–2.85) [11].

Frailty, a multidimensional syndrome of decreased reserve that confers greater vulnerability to adverse outcomes, is increasingly prevalent with advancing age [12]. The most widely used frailty assessment tool is the Fried phenotype, a score (0–5) based on weight loss, exhaustion, muscle weakness, slow gait speed, and low physical activity; a person is frail when they meet 3–5 of these criteria and pre-frail when they meet 1–2 of these criteria. One recent prospective cohort study evaluated the association of frailty (measured prior to the critical illness, when the participant was at their baseline) with post-ICU disability, new nursing home admission and mortality [13]. Frailty was associated with 41% greater disability over 6 months (adjusted risk ratio 1.41, 95% CI 1.12–1.78) and increased new nursing home admission; each one-point increase in frailty was associated with double the likelihood of death through 6 months of follow-up. Because the Fried phenotype cannot be administered to non-participatory critically ill patients, other frailty assessment tools that can be administered to proxies have been used in the ICU. One example of this is the Clinical Frailty Scale (CFS), a measure that uses clinical descriptions and pictographs to help clinicians stratify older adult vulnerability [14]. One multicenter cohort study assessed 421 patients aged 50 and older with the CFS and found that frail ICU survivors had greater difficulty with mobility (71% versus 45%), self-care (49% versus 15%) and usual activities (80% versus 52%) compared with not-frail patients; frail ICU survivors also described lower health-related quality of life (HRQoL) on both the physical and mental component scores [15]. A recent meta-analysis of 10 observational studies with a total of 3030 ICU patients demonstrated that frailty (using any of these measures) was associated with higher in-hospital mortality (RR 1.71, 95% CI 1.43–2.05) and long-term mortality (RR 1.53, 95% CI 1.40, 1.68) [16].

Other vulnerability factors, such as pre-ICU cognitive function, have been shown to be associated with post-ICU outcomes among older adults. In one prospective cohort study, minimal cognitive impairment (defined as a mini-mental status exam score [MMSE] of 24–27) was associated with increased post-ICU disability (relative to intact cognitive status); moderate cognitive impairment (MMSE <24) was associated with a slightly larger increase in disability over the 6-month follow up period [17]. Moderate impairment was also associated with double the likelihood of nursing home admission. While survival differed across the three cognitive groups, there was no association with mortality upon multivariable analysis. Importantly, the proportion of participants with moderate cognitive impairment was smaller than expected given the age of the population, suggesting that participants with more severe cognitive impairment may not have been admitted to the ICU, which may have attenuated the magnitude of the post-ICU outcomes.

It is clear that a more complex evaluation of the older patient (including an assessment of pre-ICU functional status, frailty and cognitive function) is necessary for more accurate risk stratification in the ICU. Some data on potentially stratifying factors exist as discussed earlier, but further studies should focus on the development and validation of a prognostic severity scoring system incorporating functional status to help risk-stratify critically ill older adults.

47.3 Optimizing Care of Older Patients While in the ICU

Mrs. L is hypotensive despite fluid resuscitation in the ED and her chest X-ray has an infiltrate; her respiratory status becomes progressively worse. Given her son's description of her excellent pre-morbid functional status, she is admitted to the ICU for septic shock and respiratory failure. In the rush to get to the hospital, her son forgot to bring her medication list (which she managed independently), her hearing aids, and her glasses.

Caring for the critically ill older adult can pose unique challenges. Older adults are at especially high risk of critical illness neuropathy and myopathy [18]. They are more prone to delirium and are more likely to present to the ICU with sensory impairment than younger patients. They may also have different pharmacokinetics and slower metabolism of commonly used ICU sedatives. Historically, ICU clinical practice has rarely considered geriatric concepts that may improve patient outcomes [19]. The critical care clinician should consider the following areas to optimize care of older patients.

47.3.1 The Dangers of Delirium

Delirium is defined as an acute and fluctuating change in cognition, with a reduced ability to focus. It is common in the ICU, particularly in older patients: one study of 614 patients in the medical ICU detected delirium in 71.8% of patients aged 65 years and older [20]. Days of delirium are associated with increased 1-year mortality, as demonstrated in a pivotal study following 304 patients aged 60 years and older; even after adjustment for age, comorbidities, and severity of illness, the number of days of ICU delirium was significantly associated with time to death within 1 year after ICU admission (hazard ratio [HR] 1.10; 95% CI 1.02–1.18) [21].

Delirium is also strongly associated with long-term cognitive impairment among ICU survivors. The BRAIN-ICU study followed 821 patients (median age 61) after their ICU stays for 12 months [22]. Delirium occurred in 74% of the patients. A longer duration of delirium was an independent risk factor for worse global cognition scores and worse executive function. At 3-month follow-up, 40% of the patients had global cognition scores that were comparable to those seen with moderate traumatic brain injury (TBI) and 26% had scores comparable to patients with mild Alzheimer's. Many of these deficits persisted to follow-up at 12 months.

Hypoactive delirium especially is more common in older patients and can be difficult to pick up on routine examination. The Confusion Assessment Method for the Intensive Care Unit (CAM-ICU) is a quick and validated tool to evaluate for delirium [23] and should be part of routine care in the ICU to detect delirium.

47.3.2 Prevention of Delirium

It is well established that benzodiazepines and opioids are harmful. A prospective cohort study of 304 patients aged 60 and older demonstrated that use of benzodiazepine or opioid was associated with increased delirium duration [24]. Receipt of lorazepam in particular has been shown to be independently associated with increased next-day delirium in a dose-dependent manner [25].

The data on prophylactic haloperidol were mixed, so the randomized, placebo-controlled REDUCE trial of prophylactic haloperidol was conducted [26]. The investigators randomized 1789 critically ill patients and found no difference in delirium incidence, duration of mechanical ventilation, ICU or hospital length of stay, or 28-day survival. Thus, the Society of Critical Care Medicine recommends against the administration of prophylactic haloperidol in critically ill patients [27].

Dexmedetomidine may be a promising agent for delirium prevention. In a double-blind, placebo-controlled trial, 100 delirium-free patients were randomized to receive either nocturnal dexmedetomidine or placebo until ICU discharge [28]. Patients who received nocturnal dexmedetomidine were more likely to be delirium-free than patients who received placebo (RR 0.44, 95% CI 0.23–0.82). The two arms had similar sleep quality and rates of bradycardia and hypotension. The group receiving dexmedetomidine also required less fentanyl, potentially because of some analgesic benefit from dexmedetomidine. However, prophylactic dexmedetomidine has not yet been studied in the older adult population, and more studies are needed before it can be considered for routine use in this demographic.

In the geriatrics literature, a multicomponent intervention to reduce the incidence of delirium among older adults on the general wards has been studied extensively. In a landmark study of 852 hospitalized patients aged 70 and older, a multicomponent intervention decreased the incidence of delirium and decreased the total number of days and episodes with delirium [29]. This intervention targeted six risk factors for delirium (cognitive impairment, sleep deprivation, immobility, visual impairment, hearing impairment and dehydration) with multidisciplinary teams and standardized intervention protocols. The protocols included an emphasis on orientation, cognitive-stimulating activities, non-pharmacologic sleep protocols, unit-wide noise reduction strategies, visual and hearing aids, and early mobilization. Many of these principles can be integrated into current ICU care by building on existing bundles, such as the Awakening and Breathing Coordination, Choice of drugs, Delirium monitoring and management, Early mobility and Family engagement (ABCDEF) bundle, which has been shown to reduce delirium and improve survival [30].

It is important to note that the aforementioned geriatric intervention targeted sensory impairment, which is common among older adults but rarely considered in the course of ICU clinical practice. However, a recent ICU study in older adults demonstrated that sensory impairment in both hearing and vision was strongly associated with a lack of functional recovery after a critical illness (HR for hearing impairment 0.38, 95% CI 0.22–0.66; HR for vision impairment 0.59, 95% CI 0.37–0.95) [31]. This finding is consistent with studies in (non-ICU) hospitalized older patients, where hearing and visual aids have been shown to reduce delirium, reduce the rate of functional decline, increase mobilization, and reduce the use of physical restraints [32]. Use of visual aids in the ICU is low: in one quality improvement study of ICU patients with known vision impairment, only 20% of patients had visual aids available for use; however, this improved to 97% after two cycles of intervention [33]. It can be difficult to assess sensory impairment among critically ill patients, emphasizing the importance of family involvement. Fortunately, it is easy to provide magnifiers and portable amplifying devices in the ICU to any patient who may potentially have vision or hearing impairment. While more ICU-focused studies on sensory impairment are needed, the data from hospitalized older adults are compelling, and implementing these interventions now is low-risk and potentially high-impact.

Optimizing sleep quality for older adults in the ICU is an understudied area that has the potential to improve outcomes by reducing the incidence of delirium. With age, total sleep time decreases considerably, and sleep architecture changes to have less time spent in slow wave stage 3 sleep and more frequent wakefulness after sleep onset [34]. Older adults are thus especially vulnerable to sleep disturbances, which happen commonly in the ICU. A complicating factor is a lack of standardized sleep assessment; polysomnography remains the gold standard, but is difficult to obtain in the ICU [35]. There is some evidence, though of low quality, that earplugs or eye masks may have benefits on improving sleep and reducing delirium [36], but more studies need to be done.

47.3.3 Early Mobilization

Older adults are especially vulnerable to decline in mobilization ability, especially after critical illness [37]. Preventing this deterioration with early mobilization interventions may help prevent post-discharge decline. A landmark 2009 study randomized intubated patients to early mobilization and found they had a higher return to independent functional status at discharge (59% versus 35%) and shorter duration of delirium and ventilation; only one adverse event of a desaturation occurred in the 498 therapy sessions [38]. Since that time, many early mobilization studies have been conducted; one study of 12,490 older patients (mean age 80 years old) in hospitals implementing an early mobilization program showed that hospital length of stay was shorter by 3.45 days in the mobilization group [39]. Early mobilization improves functional outcomes and is especially important in older patients; it should be routinely integrated into the ICU care of older adults.

47.3.4 Family Involvement

There is often suboptimal communication between older patients, their families and healthcare providers with regards to care preferences, especially surrounding end-of-life matters [40]. When asked to prioritize health outcomes, the majority of older adults value maintaining independence and quality of life over the prolongation of life [41]. This is frequently not discussed, and when it is, frequently not documented well in the medical record. One recent study found that as few as 13% of older adults had been asked about treatment preferences and willingness to be admitted to the ICU prior to ICU admission [2]. Additionally, family meetings often do not happen even during prolonged ICU stays due to a variety of provider-identified barriers, including time, the presence of multiple specialists, inadequate communication skills training, and lack of dedicated space [42]. A recent large randomized controlled trial (RCT) showed that a multicomponent family-support intervention not only improved surrogates' ratings of communication quality, but also led to shorter ICU lengths of stay [43]. Early and frequent family communication is especially important for older adults and should be routine; the optimal intervention for ensuring this occurs remains to be determined.

47.4 Transitions of Care

Mrs. L requires mechanical ventilator support for three days. On the first day she experiences hyperactive delirium and ventilator dyssynchrony, requiring additional sedation. She is extubated on the third day but remains delirious by CAM-ICU screening. Fortunately, the medical team speaks frequently with her son, and he brings in her hearing aids and glasses, which improves communication and orientation efforts. Her window is open during the day and interruptions are minimized at night, and with improvement in her delirium, she is able to initiate early mobilization. She is ready for transfer to the medical floor on the fifth day of admission.

47.4.1 The Challenge of ICU to Floor Transitions

Transition points are fraught with potential for error. There are lapses in communication, a change in the physical location and daily routine and sometimes suboptimal preparation in terms of discontinuing unnecessary medication, pulling catheters and lines, and in mentally preparing caregivers for the move. A recent qualitative study interviewing patients, families and providers revealed three themes in transition difficulties: resource availability, communication and institutional culture; suggestions for improvement included standardized discharge communication tools and multimodal communication [44].

47.4.2 Early Planning

Early planning for transfer out of the ICU has been shown to be beneficial for older adults. In a 2004 trial, older ICU patients were randomized to an ICU-based nursing intervention of early discharge planning for the transition out of the ICU vs. usual discharge planning. Patients in the ICU early planning intervention felt more ready to be discharged, knew their medications, and knew what warning signs to look for in terms of complications [45]. Similarly, earlier planning for hospital discharge has been shown to be beneficial. A meta-analysis of 1736 hospitalized older adults observed that early discharge planning led to fewer readmissions within 12 months and a lower readmission length of stay if readmitted [46].

47.4.3 Careful Medication Reconciliation and Review

Many medications initiated in the ICU are continued on the floor and at discharge, often inappropriately. Examples include atypical antipsychotics, anticholinergics, hypnotics and opioids. One study of patients age 60 years and older evaluated the inappropriate continuation of dangerous medication as classified by the Beers Criteria; the researchers found over 250 instances of inappropriate medication, most commonly anticholinergics, non-benzodiazepine hypnotics and opioids [47]. Care should be taken to review medications initiated in the ICU prior to transfer to the floor, with a focus on new medication started in the ICU and the Beers Criteria.

47.4.4 Acute Care for Elders Units

In an ideal world, all older adults transferred out of the ICU would be transferred to an Acute Care for Elders unit. Acute Care for Elders units are dedicated geriatrics units based on a patient/family-centered, rehabilitation and function model of care; there is emphasis on frequent medication review, early discharge planning, and thoughtful environmental design. This multidisciplinary team model has been shown to be beneficial in a myriad of ways. A 2012 meta-analysis of 6839 patients showed that Acute Care for Elders units were associated with fewer falls, less delirium, less functional decline, shorter length of stay, fewer discharges to a nursing home and lower costs [48]. Additionally, a retrospective cohort study of 818 patients found that compared with usual care units, there were lower costs per patient on the Acute Care for Elders unit and fewer readmissions within 30 days of discharge (7.9% versus 12.8%) [49].

Because Acute Care for Elders unit beds are a limited resource, studies have also evaluated whether mobile Acute Care for Elders (MACE) teams can improve outcomes for hospitalized older adults [50]. MACE teams include geriatricians, social workers and clinical nurse specialists who rotate throughout the hospital. In this model, the geriatrician may be the attending of record, and there are daily interdisciplinary team meetings and frequent educational meetings with patients and caregivers. The clinical nurse specialist gathers prehospitalization functional and cognitive details and follows up with the patient and family after discharge. The nurse specialist performs a careful medical reconciliation, and the social worker arranges family meetings, provides psychosocial support, and performs discharge planning. In the aforementioned study, the 173 patients receiving MACE care were less likely to experience adverse events (9.5% vs. 17.0%; OR 0.11, 95% CI 0.01–0.88), had shorter lengths of stay, and a lower rate of re-hospitalization at 30-days (OR 0.91, 95% CI 0.39–2.10) when compared with usual care. Although MACE teams have not been studied in the ICU setting, there is great potential for these multidisciplinary teams to help improve the care of older adults in the ICU, on the medical floor, and during the hospital discharge process.

47.5 Conclusion

Mrs. L is transferred to an ACE unit, where planning for post-hospital care begins early. An astute pharmacist discontinues inappropriate medications that were initiated in the ICU and continued on the medical floor. With physical, cognitive, and occupational therapy on the Acute Care for Elders unit, Mrs. L regains a good amount of strength while in the hospital. The unit care coordinator and social worker meet early with family members to ensure they are well-prepared for the transition home. She is discharged home with home nursing and physical therapy services. Immediately after hospital discharge, she is newly disabled in some instrumental activities of daily living (IADLs) including daily meal prep, grocery shopping and finances, but she is able to maintain her independence at home. At her follow-up appointment with her primary care doctor 3 months later, she has recovered independence of her IADLs and has happily resumed her daily walks.

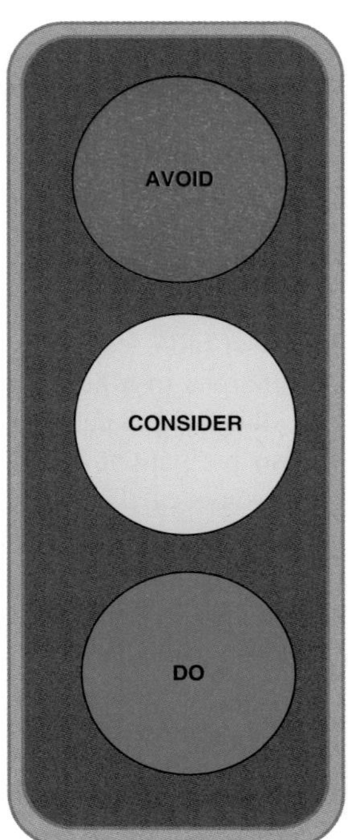

Fig. 47.1 A summary of recommendations for care of older adults in the ICU and upon transfer to the floor

In this chapter, we reviewed principles specific to care of the older ICU patient. Our recommendations, which are summarized in Fig. 47.1, address the phases of inpatient care for critically ill older adults, including triage, the ICU stay and transfer to the hospital floor. Although additional research in ICU triage is warranted, it has become increasingly clear that pre-ICU factors such as functional status are more strongly associated with post-ICU outcomes than age alone. With regard to care in the ICU, the integration of multicomponent interventions, including sensory impairment interventions, holds promise for the future care of critically ill older patients. Progress in delirium research continues, but non-pharmacologic strategies remain the cornerstone of delirium prevention. Early mobilization, family involvement and careful planning are essential to transitions out of the ICU, as is the prompt discontinuation of inappropriate medications. Although Acute Care for Elders units are ideal for the post-ICU care of all older adults, MACE teams are promising alternatives for providing the same benefits on the regular hospital floor. Overall, there have been great strides made in the past decade on how to best care for older adults in the ICU, but this should be an ongoing focus of research, education, and quality improvement efforts in the coming years.

References

1. Wang S, Allen D, Kheir YN, Campbell N, Khan B. Aging and post-intensive care syndrome: a critical need for geriatric psychiatry. Am J Geriatr Psychiatry. 2018;26:212–21.
2. Flaatten H, de Lange DW, Artigas A, et al. The status of intensive care medicine research and a future agenda for very old patients in the ICU. Intensive Care Med. 2017;43:1319–28.
3. Wunsch H, Jones AT, Scales DC. Intensive care for the elderly: current and future concerns. In: Vincent JL, editor. Yearbook of intensive care and emergency medicine. Heidelberg: Springer-Verlag; 2009. p. 935–43.
4. Eymard AS, Douglas DH. Ageism among health care providers and interventions to improve their attitudes toward older adults an integrative review. J Gerontol Nurs. 2012;38:26–34.
5. Garrouste-Orgeas M, Tabah A, Vesin A, et al. The ETHICA study (part II): simulation study of determinants and variability of ICU physician decisions in patients aged 80 or over. Intensive Care Med. 2013;39:1574–83.
6. Garrouste-Orgeas M, Boumendil A, Pateron D, et al. Selection of intensive care unit admission criteria for patients aged 80 years and over and compliance of emergency and intensive care unit physicians with the selected criteria: an observational, multicenter, prospective study. Crit Care Med. 2009;37:2919–28.
7. Sprung CL, Artigas A, Kesecioglu J, et al. The Eldicus prospective, observational study of triage decision making in European intensive care units. Part II: intensive care benefit for the elderly. Crit Care Med. 2012;40:132–8.
8. Guidet B, Leblanc G, Simon T, et al. Effect of systematic intensive care unit triage on long-term mortality among critically ill elderly patients in France: a randomized clinical trial. JAMA. 2017;318:1450–9.
9. Valley TS, Sjoding MW, Ryan AM, Iwashyna TJ, Cooke CR. Association of intensive care unit admission with mortality among older patients with pneumonia. JAMA. 2015;314:1272–9.
10. Ferrante LE, Pisani MA, Murphy TE, Gahbauer EA, Leo-Summers LS, Gill TM. Functional trajectories among older persons before and after critical illness. JAMA Intern Med. 2015;175:523–9.
11. Pietiläinen L, Hästbacka J, Bäcklund M, Parviainen I, Pettilä V, Reinikainen M. Premorbid functional status as a predictor of 1-year mortality and functional status in intensive care patients aged 80 years or older. Intensive Care Med. 2018;44:1221–9.
12. Fried LP, Tangen CM, Walston J, et al. Frailty in older adults: evidence for a phenotype. J Gerontol A Biol Sci Med Sci. 2001;56:M146–56.
13. Ferrante LE, Pisani MA, Murphy TE, Gahbauer EA, Leo-Summers LS, Gill TM. The association of frailty with post-ICU disability, nursing home admission, and mortality: a longitudinal study. Chest. 2018;153:1378–86.
14. Rockwood K, Song X, MacKnight C, et al. A global clinical measure of fitness and frailty in elderly people. CMAJ. 2005;173:489–95.
15. Bagshaw SM, Stelfox HT, Johnson JA, et al. Long-term association between frailty and health-related quality of life among survivors of critical illness: a prospective multicenter cohort study. Crit Care Med. 2015;43:973–82.
16. Muscedere J, Waters B, Varambally A, et al. The impact of frailty on intensive care unit outcomes: a systematic review and meta-analysis. Intensive Care Med. 2017;43:1105–22.
17. Ferrante LE, Murphy TE, Gahbauer EA, Leo-Summers LS, Pisani MA, Gill TM. Pre-intensive care unit cognitive status, subsequent disability, and new nursing home admission among critically ill older adults. Ann Am Thorac Soc. 2018;15:8.
18. Dalton RE, Tripathi RS, Abel EE, et al. Polyneuropathy and myopathy in the elderly. HSR Proc Intensive Care Cardiovasc Anesth. 2012;4:15–9.
19. Brummel NE, Ferrante LE. Integrating geriatric principles into critical care medicine: the time is now. Ann Am Thorac Soc. 2018;15:5.
20. Peterson JF, Pun BT, Dittus RS, et al. Delirium and its motoric subtypes: a study of 614 critically ill patients. J Am Geriatr Soc. 2006;54:479–84.

21. Pisani MA, Kong SYJ, Kasl SV, Murphy TE, Araujo KLB, Van Ness PH. Days of delirium are associated with 1-year mortality in an older intensive care unit population. Am J Respir Crit Care Med. 2009;180:1092–7.
22. Pandharipande PP, Girard TD, Jackson JC, et al. Long-term cognitive impairment after critical illness. N Engl J Med. 2013;369:1306–16.
23. Gusmao-Flores D, Salluh JIF, Chalhub RA, Quarantini LC. The confusion assessment method for the intensive care unit (CAM-ICU) and intensive care delirium screening checklist (ICDSC) for the diagnosis of delirium: a systematic review and meta-analysis of clinical studies. Crit Care. 2012;16:R115.
24. Pisani MA, Murphy TE, Araujo KLB, Slattum P, Van Ness PH, Inouye SK. Benzodiazepine and opioid use and the duration of intensive care unit delirium in an older population. Crit Care Med. 2009;37:177–83.
25. Pandharipande P, Shintani A, Peterson J, et al. Lorazepam is an independent risk factor for transitioning to delirium in intensive care unit patients. Anesthesiology. 2006;104:21–6.
26. van den Boogaard M, Slooter AJC, Bruggemann RJM, et al. Effect of haloperidol on survival among critically ill adults with a high risk of delirium: the REDUCE randomized clinical trial. JAMA. 2018;319:680–90.
27. Devlin JW, Skrobik Y, Gelinas C, et al. Clinical Practice Guidelines for the prevention and management of pain, agitation/sedation, delirium, immobility, and sleep disruption in adult patients in the ICU. Crit Care Med. 2018;46:e825–73.
28. Skrobik Y, Duprey MS, Hill NS, Devlin JW. Low-dose nocturnal dexmedetomidine prevents ICU delirium: a randomized, placebo-controlled trial. Am J Respir Crit Care Med. 2018;197:1147–56.
29. Inouye SK, Bogardus ST, Charpentier PA, et al. A multicomponent intervention to prevent delirium in hospitalized older patients. N Engl J Med. 1999;340:669–76.
30. Barnes-Daly MA, Phillips G, Ely EW. Improving hospital survival and reducing brain dysfunction at seven California community hospitals: implementing PAD Guidelines via the ABCDEF bundle in 6,064 patients. Crit Care Med. 2017;45:171–8.
31. Ferrante LE, Pisani MA, Murphy TE, Gahbauer EA, Leo-Summers LS, Gill TM. Factors associated with functional recovery among older intensive care unit survivors. Am J Respir Crit Care Med. 2016;194:299–307.
32. Vidan MT, Sanchez E, Alonso M, Montero B, Ortiz J, Serra JA. An intervention integrated into daily clinical practice reduces the incidence of delirium during hospitalization in elderly patients. J Am Geriatr Soc. 2009;57:2029–36.
33. Zhou Q, Faure Walker N. Promoting vision and hearing aids use in an intensive care unit. BMJ Qual Improv Rep. 2015;4:u206276.w2702.
34. Gooneratne NS, Vitiello MV. Sleep in older adults: normative changes, sleep disorders, and treatment options. Clin Geriatr Med. 2014;30:591–627.
35. Boyko Y, Jennum P, Toft P. Sleep quality and circadian rhythm disruption in the intensive care unit: a review. Nat Sci Sleep. 2017;9:277–84.
36. Hu RF, Jiang XY, Chen J, et al. Non-pharmacological interventions for sleep promotion in the intensive care unit. Cochrane Database Syst Rev. 2015;2015:CD008808.
37. Ehlenbach WJ, Larson EB, Curtis JR, Hough CL. Physical function and disability after acute care and critical illness hospitalizations in a prospective cohort of older adults. J Am Geriatr Soc. 2015;63:2061–9.
38. Schweickert WD, Pohlman MC, Pohlman AS, et al. Early physical and occupational therapy in mechanically ventilated, critically ill patients: a randomised controlled trial. Lancet. 2009;373:1874–82.
39. Liu B, Moore JE, Almaawiy U, et al. Outcomes of Mobilisation of Vulnerable Elders in Ontario (MOVE ON): a multisite interrupted time series evaluation of an implementation intervention to increase patient mobilisation. Age Ageing. 2018;47:112–9.
40. Heyland DK, Barwich D, Pichora D, et al. Failure to engage hospitalized elderly patients and their families in advance care planning. JAMA Intern Med. 2013;173:778–87.

41. Fried TR, Tinetti ME, Iannone L, O'Leary JR, Towle VR, Van Ness PH. Health outcome prioritization as a tool for decision making among older persons with multiple chronic conditions. Arch Intern Med. 2011;171:1854–6.
42. Gay EB, Pronovost PJ, Bassett RD, Nelson JE. The intensive care unit family meeting: making it happen. J Crit Care. 2009;24:629.e1–12.
43. White DB, Angus DC, Shields AM, et al. A randomized trial of a family-support intervention in intensive care units. N Engl J Med. 2018;378:2365–75.
44. de Grood C, Leigh JP, Bagshaw SM, et al. Patient, family and provider experiences with transfers from intensive care unit to hospital ward: a multicentre qualitative study. CMAJ. 2018;190:E669–76.
45. Kleinpell RM. Randomized trial of an intensive care unit-based early discharge planning intervention for critically ill elderly patients. Am J Crit Care. 2004;13:335–45.
46. Fox MT, Persaud M, Maimets I, Brooks D, O'Brien K, Tregunno D. Effectiveness of early discharge planning in acutely ill or injured hospitalized older adults: a systematic review and meta-analysis. BMC Geriatr. 2013;13:70.
47. Morandi A, Vasilevskis E, Pandharipande PP, et al. Inappropriate medication prescriptions in elderly adults surviving an intensive care unit hospitalization. J Am Geriatr Soc. 2013;61:1128–34.
48. Fox MT, Persaud M, Maimets I, et al. Effectiveness of acute geriatric unit care using acute care for elders components: a systematic review and meta-analysis. J Am Geriatr Soc. 2012;60:2237–45.
49. Flood KL, Maclennan PA, McGrew D, Green D, Dodd C, Brown CJ. Effects of an Acute Care for Elders unit on costs and 30-day readmissions. JAMA Intern Med. 2013;173:981–7.
50. Hung WW, Ross JS, Farber J, Siu AL. Evaluation of the Mobile Acute Care of the Elderly (MACE) service. JAMA Intern Med. 2013;173:990–6.

Part XV

Patient Comfort

Inhaled Sedation and Reflection Systems 48

A. Meiser and H. V. Groesdonk

48.1 Introduction

Volatile anesthetics are increasingly frequently used to sedate intensive care unit (ICU) patients who are receiving invasive mechanical ventilation. The AnaConDa™ (Sedana Medical, Stockholm, Sweden) is the most frequently used administration system. It is intended for use in a single patient for up to 24 h. Up to now, 2.3 million devices have been sold globally [1]. There is a growing body of literature showing advantages of volatile anesthetics over intravenous sedatives [2, 3] and inhaled sedation has been adopted by the German, British and Spanish sedation guidelines [4–6].

However, common anesthesia ventilators are not suitable for use in the ICU. High costs, large space requirements, logistics of soda lime, and limited ability of ventilator modes to augment spontaneous breathing are obstacles to their use. Moreover, because of a different alarm setup, anesthesia ventilators are only approved for use in the presence of specifically instructed and qualified staff. This precondition cannot be met in the ICU.

In recent years, alternative modes for efficient application of volatile anesthetics in patients managed with standard ICU ventilators have become available. In this chapter, these new technical developments will be reviewed as well as some recent clinical studies on inhaled sedation.

A. Meiser (✉) · H. V. Groesdonk
Department of Anaesthesiology, Intensive Care Medicine and Pain Medicine, University Medical Center, University of Saarland, Homburg/Saar, Germany
e-mail: Andreas.meiser@uks.eu

J.-L. Vincent (ed.), *Annual Update in Intensive Care and Emergency Medicine 2019*, Annual Update in Intensive Care and Emergency Medicine,
https://doi.org/10.1007/978-3-030-06067-1_48

48.2 Specific Reflection Versus Total Rebreathing

All new systems to be used with standard ICU ventilators are based on the reflection principle. Instead of rebreathing all expired gases after removal of carbon dioxide, as is the case with circle systems, it is possible to specifically retain volatile anesthetics and re-inhale them with fresh air. Figure 48.1 shows the characteristics of these two principles.

Before entering the circle system, fresh gas passes through a vaporizer to take up volatile anesthetic (Fig. 48.1, left). In the circle, two check valves safeguard the direction of the flow. A bag-in bottle ventilator, a manual ventilation bag, and a carbon dioxide absorber all add considerable compressible volume. An adjustable pressure release valve prevents high pressures and overdistension of the lungs. On the other side, breathing gas leaves the system, washing the anesthetic out again. If the fresh gas flow is less than the minute volume of the patient, consumption of volatile anesthetics is less than in an open system. When the anesthetic concentration needs to be increased, the fresh gas flow is usually also increased to wash the anesthetic in more rapidly. Consequently, anesthetic losses are correspondingly high.

Reflection systems are much simpler (Fig. 48.1, right). Valves or carbon dioxide absorbers are not needed. A small reflector is inserted between the Y piece and the patient. Exhaled anesthetic is retained and re-inhaled during the next inspiration. This process is called anesthetic reflection. The proportion of reflected molecules as part of all molecules exhaled in one breath has been called the reflection efficiency

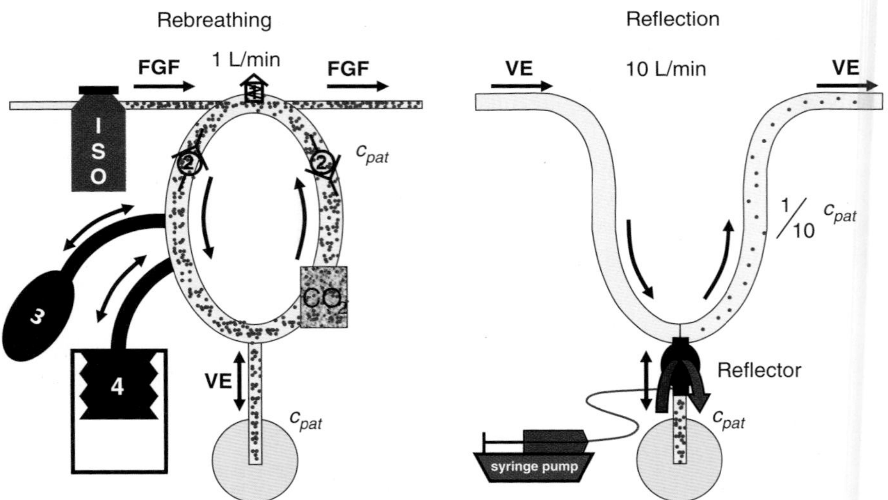

Fig. 48.1 Circle system (left: rebreathing) and reflection system (right) as alternative principles for saving volatile anesthetics. 1 = adjustable pressure release valve, 2 = unidirectional valves, 3 = manual ventilation bag, 4 = bag-in bottle ventilator. *ISO* isoflurane vaporizer; CO_2 carbon dioxide absorber; *FGF* fresh gas flow; *VE* minute volume; C_{pat} patient concentration. Modified from [32] with permission

[7]. Under optimal conditions, reflection efficiency will be about 90%. This means that the savings compared to an open system amount to 90%. The same savings can be achieved with a circle system when the fresh gas flow is reduced to 10% of the minute volume.

48.3 The AnaConDa™

The AnaConDa™ (Fig. 48.2) is the most widely used reflection system. Liquid isoflurane or sevoflurane are delivered by a syringe pump. The end-tidal anesthetic concentration, measured by a separate gas monitor, can be increased rapidly by

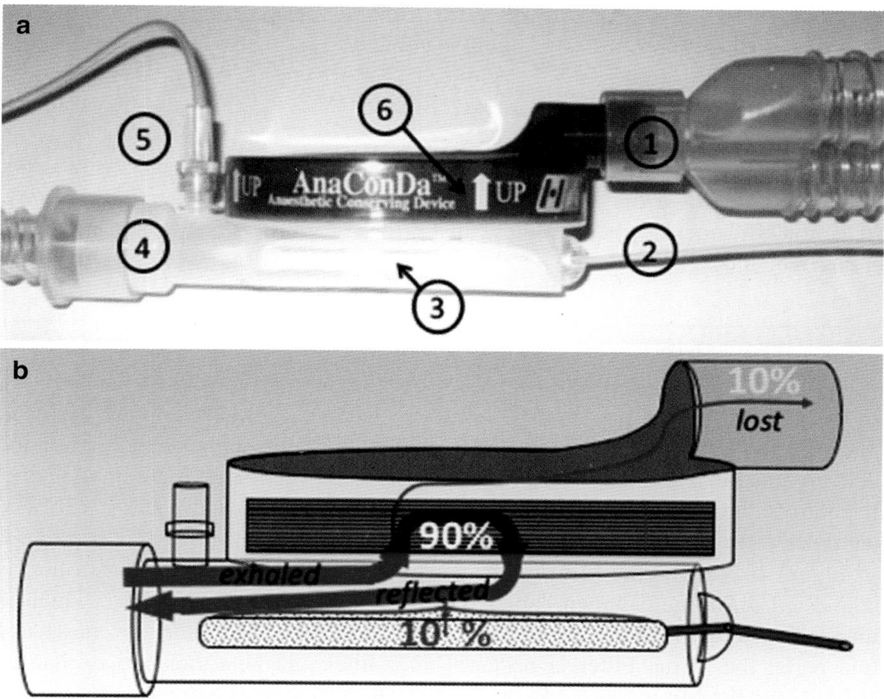

Fig. 48.2 The Anaesthetic Conserving Device (AnaConDa™, Sedana Medical, Stockholm, Sweden). (**a**) Photo. 1 = ventilator side with Y-piece, 2 = anesthetic infusion line, 3 = evaporator (hollow porous rod), 4 = patient side with tube elongation, 5 = port for sampling gas, 6 = anesthetic reflector (felt of black carbon fibers, hidden in black outer case.) (**b**) reflection schematic. With each expiration, about 90% of exhaled anesthetic molecules are absorbed by the reflector and are resupplied during the next inspiration; 10% are lost through the reflector and must be replaced. Liquid volatile anesthetic, either isoflurane or sevoflurane, is infused by a syringe pump through the anesthetic infusion line into the evaporator and evaporates on its surface in the flow of the breathing gas. Modified from [33] with permission

using the bolus function of the syringe pump. When the reflector is taken away, the anesthetic is washed out as quickly as in an open system.

In a bench study, the reflection efficiency of the AnaConDa was determined as 90% for isoflurane and sevoflurane [8]. However, when the volume of anesthetic vapor contained in one expired breath exceeds a certain threshold, the reflection efficiency will decrease. This threshold was determined as 10 mL vapor of isoflurane or sevoflurane. This equals 1 Vol% contained in 1000 mL or 2 Vol% in 500 mL tidal volume. This threshold has been referred to as the reflection capacity [8].

Anesthetic consumption equals uptake by the patient plus losses through the reflector. These losses (V'_{lost} [mL/min]) depend on the respiratory rate (RR, rate per min]), tidal volume (V_T, [mL]), end-tidal anesthetic concentration (C_{pat} [Vol%]), and the reflection efficiency (RE [dimensionless]), and can be calculated according to the following formula:

$$V'_{lost} = RR \times V_T \times C_{Pat} \times (1 - RE)$$

The highlighted part of the equation, $V_T \times C_{Pat}$, describes the anesthetic vapor volume contained in one breath. If this volume exceeds the reflection capacity, reflection efficiency decreases. Below this, in the clinical range, reflection efficiency is constant at 0.9 [8].

48.4 The Mirus

In 2014, a new reflection system became available: the Mirus (TIM Medical, Andernach, Germany). Unlike the AnaConDa, the Mirus comprises an anesthetic delivery unit, an anesthetic reflector, gas monitor, and ventilation monitor all in one. It controls the end-tidal anesthetic concentration to a set value, and it can also administer desflurane [7].

Figure 48.3 shows the Mirus clinical setup. A control unit (Mirus Controller) is connected via a multi-lumen cable to an interface (Mirus Exchanger), which is inserted between the Y-piece and the endotracheal tube. The interface consists of two parts: the Mirus Filter, a bacterial-viral filter and heat-moisture exchanger (HME), and the Mirus Reflector. In the Mirus Reflector, anesthetic is delivered and reflected and, in addition, airway pressure and flow as well as gas concentrations are measured.

As with any side-stream gas measurement, there is a time lag between sampling and measuring. With the Mirus, this time lag is short because of a high sample gas flow rate of 200 mL/h, and it is known and constant, because the sampling line inside the multi-lumen cable is always the same. Taking this time lag into account, the Mirus is able to determine the end-tidal anesthetic concentration according to the airway flow, not according to the carbon dioxide signal.

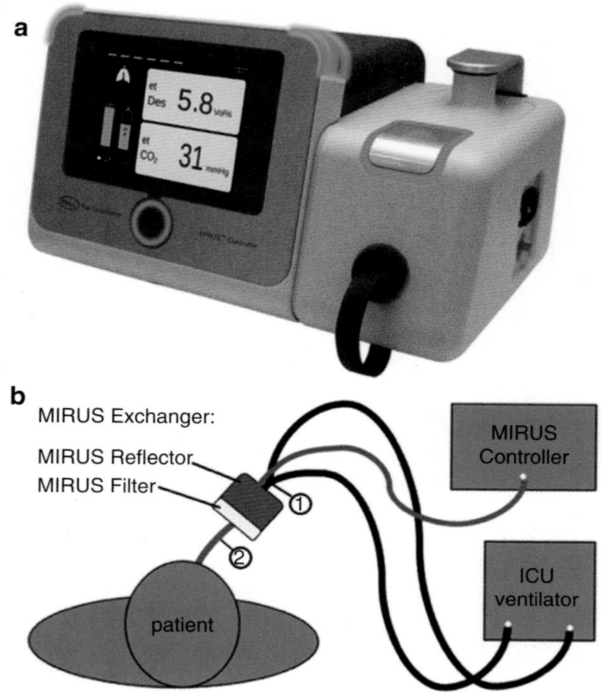

Fig. 48.3 The Mirus system. (**a**) control unit (Mirus Controller); (**b**) setup in a patient. The controller is connected via a multi-lumen cable (blue line) with the cube-like Mirus Exchanger, inserted between the Y-piece (1) and the endotracheal tube (2). The Exchanger comprises two parts: The Mirus Filter constitutes a heat moisture exchanger with a bacterial filter. It can be exchanged separately between patients or when soiled. In the Mirus Reflector, airway pressure as well as flow and gas concentrations are measured; anesthetic is injected as well as reflected. Modified from [7] with permission

Other gas monitors rely on the carbon dioxide signal for determination of the end-tidal concentration. However, when used with a reflection system, such as the AnaConDa, this may lead to falsely high readings [9]. In a bench study, the correct determination of the end-tidal concentration by the Mirus was confirmed by re-measuring with an external gas monitor [7].

To increase the efficiency of anesthetic delivery, saturated vapor is injected at the beginning of inspiration to be carried as far as possible down to the lungs. In a test lung setup with an inspiratory flow time of only 0.5 s, this short time window was always met [7].

The Mirus allows control of the end-tidal concentration by setting a target as a fraction of the age-adjusted minimum alveolar concentration (MAC). Figure 48.4 clarifies the control algorithm. During wash-in, a series of vapor injections takes place with every inspiration. These injections stop when the target is exceeded by

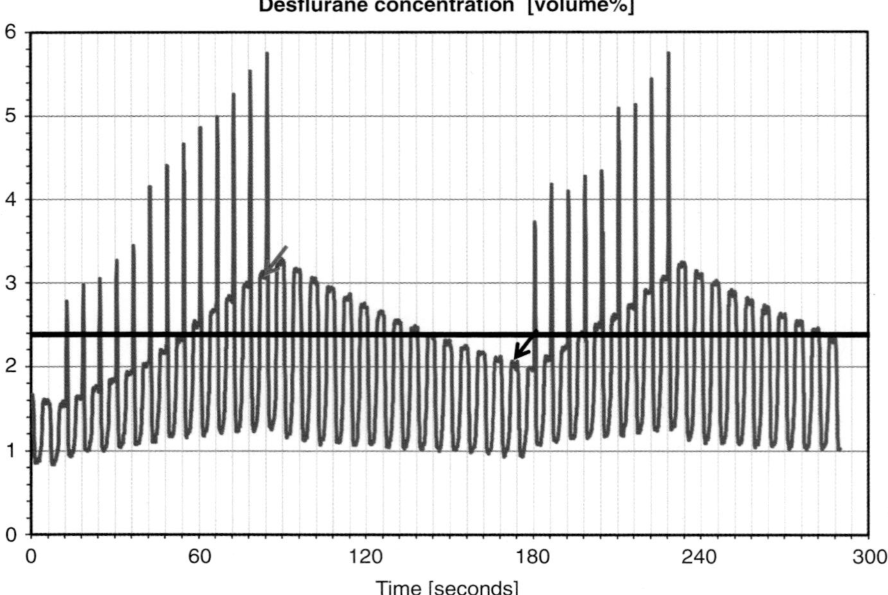

Fig. 48.4 High-resolution recording of the desflurane concentration measured with an external gas monitor over five minutes. The black line represents the target concentration, set at 2.4 Vol%. End-tidal concentrations can easily be identified as plateaus during each breath (arrows). They go up and down swinging around the target. High peak concentrations (spikes) indicate injections of saturated desflurane vapor during the inspiratory flow phases. They stop when the end-tidal concentration is at 130% of the target (red arrow). Then the end-tidal concentration decreases down to 87% of the target (black arrow). Thereafter, another series of injections starts. Trough values show end-inspiratory concentrations. Their dramatic decrease in relation to the end-tidal concentrations indicates the rather low efficiency of the anesthetic reflector. Modified from [7] with permission

about 30%. Thereafter, the end-tidal concentration decreases with every breath. When it reaches 87% of the target, a new series of injections starts. These oscillations around the target may be criticized. However, given the short time interval between two concentration peaks of about 2.5 min, it can be assumed that the amplitude of the oscillations will be attenuated before reaching the brain [7]. In patients, a fluctuating sedation depth has not been noticed using clinical or electrophysiological evaluation [10, 11].

Despite the efficient mode of application described above, consumption of desflurane in this bench study was as high as 40 mL/h when using 6.6 Vol% desflurane. By removing the actual carbon reflector and replacing it with a cut-out of the AnaConDa reflector, consumption was reduced by one third, demonstrating that the efficiency of reflection of the Mirus may still be improved considerably [7].

In the first publication on the clinical use of the Mirus system, a critically ill patient was sedated with desflurane (0.6 MAC) for 24 h; thereafter, isoflurane (0.6 MAC) was used with the AnaConDa system [10]. No significant technical or

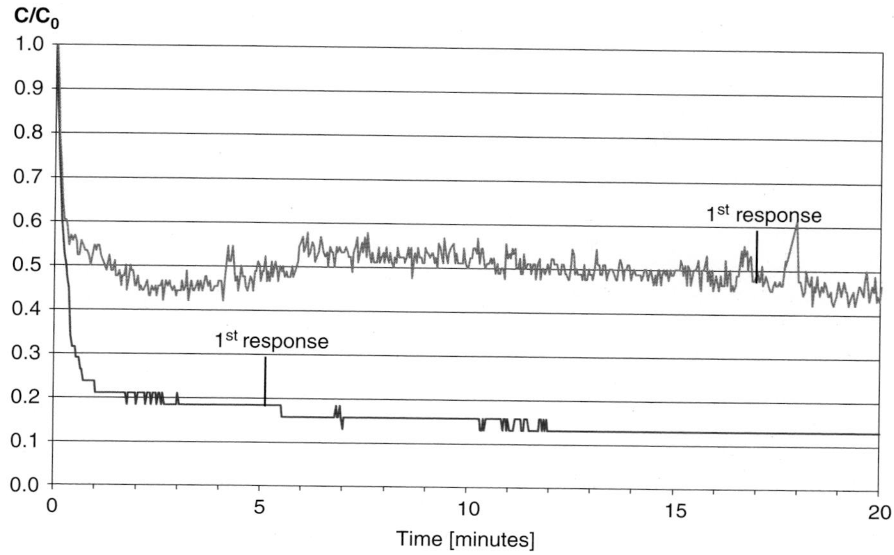

Fig. 48.5 Anesthetic wash-out and awakening after 24-h sedation with desflurane (blue curve) and isoflurane (pink curve) in one patient. The end-tidal desflurane concentration decreases down to 20% of the initial concentration (C_0; 3.8 Vol%) after 1 min; the isoflurane concentration only decreases to 50% of C_0 (0.8 Vol%) during the whole observation period of 20 min. The patient first responded to voice after 5.08 min at 0.7 Vol% desflurane and after 17 min at 0.44 Vol% isoflurane. Modified from [10] with permission

handling problems were reported. Compared to 4 mL isoflurane, 54 mL desflurane were consumed per hour. This high consumption of desflurane may be explained by high minute ventilation (9–12 L/min), frequent suctioning of tracheal secretions, and by use of an earlier version of the Mirus. In two sedation windows, anesthetic wash-out and awakening of this patient were considerably faster after desflurane than after isoflurane (Fig. 48.5).

In a prospective study, 62 patients post-abdominal surgery were ventilated and sedated with sevoflurane using the Mirus in the ICU [11]. On average, end-tidal concentrations were 0.76 Vol% (corresponding to median MAC [interquartile range] values of 0.45 [0.4–0.53]). A total of 7.9 mL sevoflurane were consumed per hour. All patients were breathing spontaneously with pressure support (8–12 cmH_2O); they were deeply sedated (Richmond Agitation and Sedation Scale [RASS] Scores: −4.5 [−3.6 to −5.0]). After 3.3 h (range: 1–19 h) sedation, the time until they were fully cooperative was astonishingly short (4 [2.2–5] min). Room air concentrations of sevoflurane (0.15 ppm) remained well below the recommended thresholds. The authors did not notice any technical failures, handling issues or safety problems. They concluded that the Mirus system is a promising and safe alternative for short-term sedation of ICU patients.

The Mirus was also used in the operating room in patients undergoing knee or hip replacement [12]. Sixty patients were randomized to receive either isoflurane, sevoflurane, or desflurane. Patients were ventilated with an ICU ventilator (Puritan Bennett 840, Medtronic, Dublin, Ireland), for the first hour in volume-controlled mode (tidal volume set at 8 mL/kg); thereafter, spontaneous breathing was facilitated. The times to reach 0.5 MAC (ISO/SEV/DES 1.08/2.42/1.33 min) and to increase the concentration from 0.5 to 1.0 MAC (1.08/2.72/3.40 min) were all very short. Despite the device's dead space of 100 mL, work of breathing, compliance, and resistance measured with the ICU ventilator during spontaneous breathing were not different between groups and were within the normal range in all patients. As expected, times for awakening and recovery were longer after isoflurane compared to sevoflurane and to desflurane. Consumption of desflurane (42 mL/h) was about 4 times that of isoflurane (11 mL/h), and consumption of sevoflurane about twofold higher (24 mL/h). The authors concluded that Mirus was able to reliably deliver and maintain high anesthetic concentrations of 1 MAC in the end-expired gas.

48.5 The AnaConDa-S™

Both the AnaConDa and the Mirus have a dead space of 100 mL that interferes with carbon dioxide elimination. This has been referred to as "volumetric device dead space" [13]. In addition, carbon dioxide is also reflected by the reflectors. Carbon dioxide reflection may be quantified as apparent [14] or "reflective" dead space [13], defined as the increase in tidal volume necessary for its compensation. The reflective dead space of the AnaConDa is large under dry laboratory conditions (almost 200 mL), [13, 14] but small when volatile anesthetics are used under body temperature, pressure, saturated conditions (about 40 mL) [13, 15]. Altogether, this large dead space of 140 mL may interfere with low tidal volume ventilation when lung protective ventilation strategies are indicated.

Therefore, a reduction in dead space has been postulated, even at the cost of a somewhat lower reflection efficiency for anesthetics [8]. Very recently, the AnaConDa-S (Sedana Medical) has become available (Fig. 48.6). This device is very similar to the classical AnaConDa, but its volumetric dead space is only 50 mL and its reflective dead space is also lower by about 15 mL. On the other hand, the reflection efficiency of the AnaConDa-S for isoflurane is still over 80% in the clinical range (0.4 Vol% isoflurane, 500 mL tidal volume) [16].

The AnaConDa-S has been tested in 10 critically ill patients breathing spontaneously with pressure support through endotracheal tubes [17]. In this study, the patients were switched from the classical AnaConDa to the AnaConDa-S. Isoflurane and opioid infusion rates were not changed, and sedation depth, arterial carbon dioxide pressure, and all ventilation parameters remained the same, except that the patients reduced their tidal volumes by 66 mL on average, confirming the data from the bench study of a reduced dead space [16].

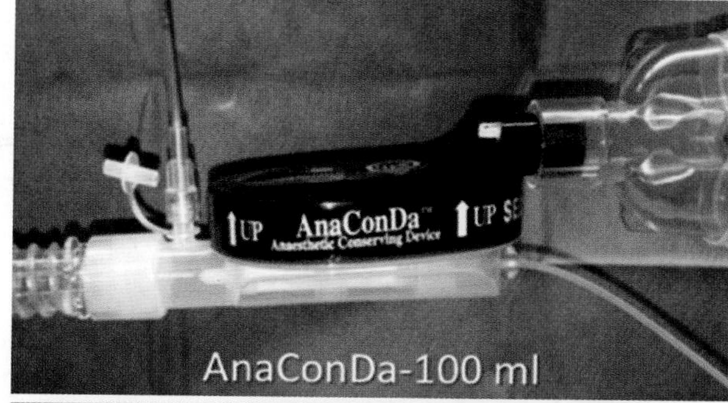

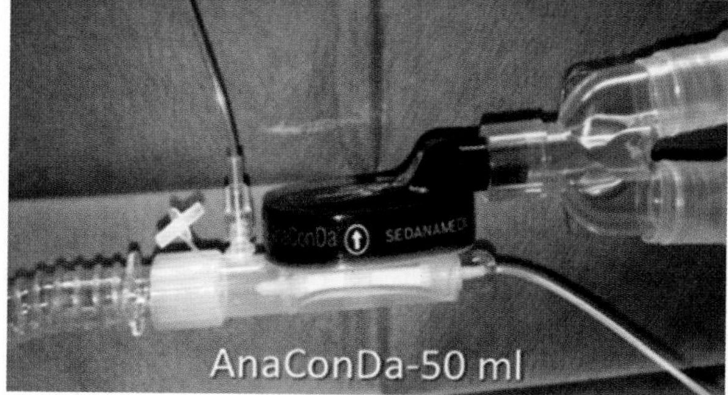

Fig. 48.6 AnaConDa-100 mL (100 mL internal volume) and AnaConDa-50 mL (50 mL internal volume) in the same scale for size comparison. Modified from [16] with permission

48.6 Other Reflection Systems

An anesthetic reflection system has also been used in a different way: interposed between two (!) circle systems (Fig. 48.7) [18]. The primary circle system was part of a common anesthesia ventilator; the secondary contained an in-line vaporizer as well as a second carbon dioxide absorber. As reflector, the active carbon felt from AnaConDa was used. Six small pigs were ventilated with tidal volumes of 200 mL and minute volumes of 3.0–4.0 L/min. The authors compared consumption of sevoflurane with and without the reflector in place: at a fresh gas flow of 1 L/min, the reflector reduced consumption of sevoflurane by 50%. When increasing the fresh gas flow, consumption without the reflector increased drastically, but with the reflector in place, it remained the same. A similar setup had been used by Perhag and colleagues with zeolite as a reflecting material [19]. Ultimately, the reflector, decreasing consumption irrespective of fresh gas flow, could be built into the anesthesia ventilator. Using such a setup, carbon dioxide reflection as well as any additional dead space between Y piece and the patient could be avoided. However, such a system seems too bulky and interposes too much compressible volume between the ventilator and the patient, impairing the ventilator's capabilities to augment spontaneous breathing. No such system is now commercially available.

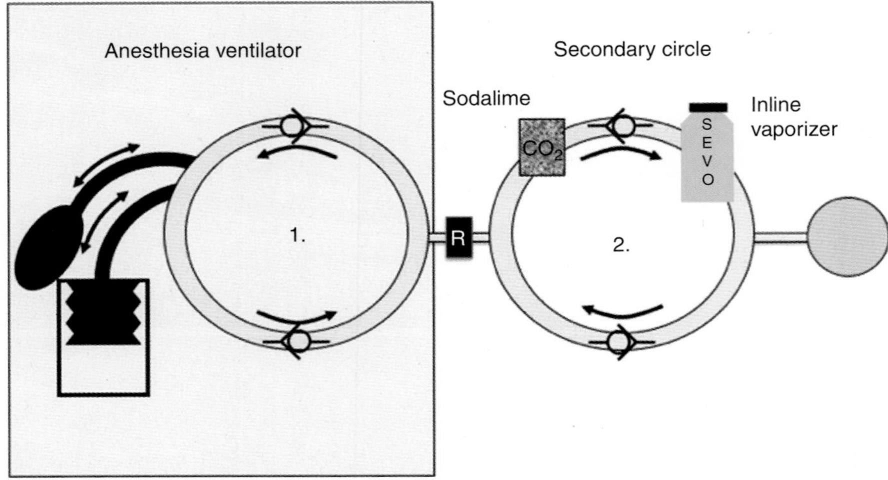

Fig. 48.7 Experimental setup with an anesthetic reflector (R) interposed between two circle systems. Check valves safeguard the unidirectional flow. The secondary circle comprises an inline vaporizer as well as a second carbon dioxide absorber. Modified from [18] with permission

In a test lung study, reflection properties of carbon (charcoal derived from coconut shells) and zeolite granules (ultrastable zeolite Y, US-Y) were evaluated [20]. Glass spheres served as inert controls. The respective granules, 1 mm in diameter, were used to refill the emptied case of an HME. Compared to the glass spheres, consumption of isoflurane was reduced by 70% by carbon and zeolite alike. This rather low reflection efficiency may be explained by several factors: first, 1.5 Vol% isoflurane in a tidal volume of 600 mL, corresponding to 9 mL isoflurane vapor, may have exceeded the reflection capacity of this self-built reflector. Second, the molecular type of charcoal and zeolite may not have been optimal. Third, the size, the shape, and the three-dimensional arrangement of the granules may have limited the surface area exposed to the anesthetics. And finally, the shape and size of the housing may not have been optimal to slow down and disperse the airflow over and through the reflecting material to prolong contact time. Fibers interwoven in a felt instead of loosely packed granules as well as the shape of the AnaConDa housing may have considerable influence on the exposed surface area as well as on contact time, thereby increasing reflection efficiency.

48.7 Clinical Studies

Many clinical studies have shown advantages of inhaled versus intravenous sedation, such as shorter time to extubation [21], more rapid recovery of cognitive functions [22–24], faster mobilization [25], and more rapid discharge [26]. Two recent publications emphasize the possibility of augmented spontaneous breathing despite deep sedation in patients with severe adult respiratory distress syndrome (ARDS) undergoing continuous lateral rotational therapy [27] or veno-venous extracorporeal membrane oxygenation [28].

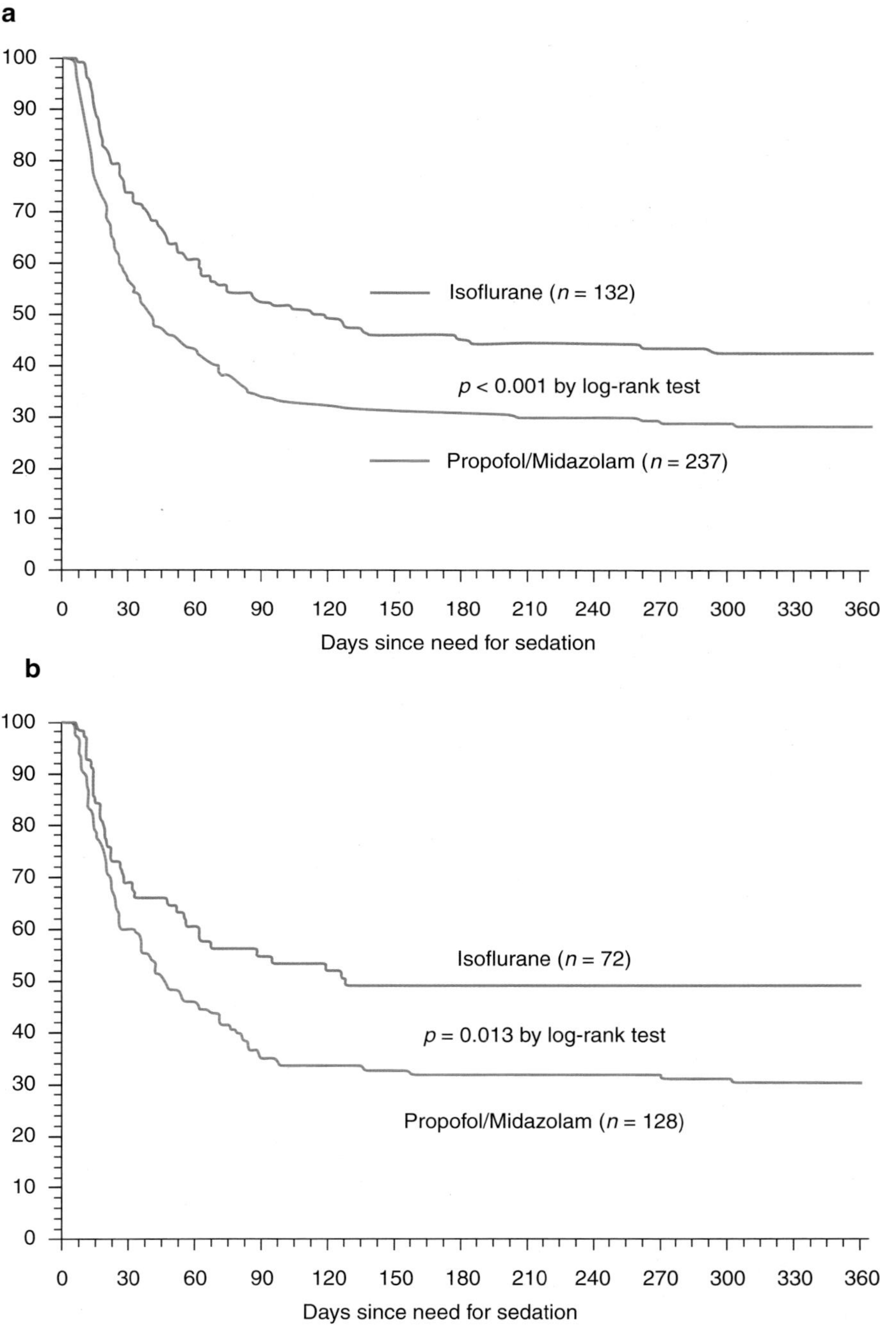

Fig. 48.8 Kaplan-Meier survival curves of a 6-year cohort of critically ill patients ventilated for more than 96 h, sedated with either isoflurane or propofol/midazolam. (**a**) all 369 patients included; (**b**) the selected group of 200 analyzed patients. Modified from [30] with permission

In a randomized controlled multicenter trial involving 50 patients with severe ARDS, patients receiving inhaled sevoflurane showed a significant improvement in oxygenation after 2 days compared to patients receiving intravenous midazolam. This was associated with significantly decreased concentrations of soluble receptor of advanced glycation end-products (sRAGE), a biologic marker of alveolar epithelial injury in plasma as well as in bronchoalveolar lavage fluid [29].

In a retrospective analysis of a 6-year cohort of 369 patients who had received invasive ventilation for more than 96 h, patients that had received inhaled isoflurane showed a significantly reduced hospital (40% versus 63%) as well as 1-year mortality (50% versus 70%) compared to patients sedated with propofol or midazolam (Fig. 48.8). After adjustment for potential confounders, the mortality risk attributable to isoflurane was 0.35 (confidence interval: 0.18–0.68) for hospital mortality and 0.41 (0.21–0.81) for 1-year mortality [30].

Apart from their sedative effect, volatile anesthetics may have widespread effects outside the central nervous system. They possess end-organ protective effects mediated via anti-inflammatory and cytoprotective mechanisms (reviewed in [2]). On the other hand, we know that deep intravenous sedation is associated with increased mortality [31]. The reason for the difference in mortality found in the above cited retrospective analysis [30] may therefore not be a positive effect of inhaled sedation, but simply avoidance of longer lasting, intravenous sedation.

48.8 Outlook

There is not yet explicit approval for ICU sedation with volatile anesthetics. A multicenter study with the title “A randomized controlled open-label study to confirm the efficacy and safety of sedation with isoflurane in invasively ventilated ICU patients using the AnaConDa administration system” (Acronym: Isoconda; Sponsor: Sedana Medical, EudraCT number: 2016-004551-67) is currently under way. Thirty participating hospitals in Germany are going to include 300 patients. A series of substudies will address specific questions, such as the influence of isoflurane on pulmonary artery pressure, monitoring of sedation depth using clinical as well as electrophysiological parameters, delirium, quality of life and neuropsychological outcome, as well as 1-year mortality. With the results of this study, official approval of ICU sedation with isoflurane by the Bundesinstitut für Arzneimittel und Medizinprodukte is expected.

48.9 Conclusion

Inhaled sedation is increasingly used in everyday practice in many ICUs worldwide, with more and more studies showing its benefits. To meet clinical demands, different administration systems have evolved and are now commercially available. These systems can be used with standard ICU ventilators. They are based on the reflection principle: instead of rebreathing all expired gases (after removal of carbon dioxide), savings are achieved by specifically reflecting the volatile anesthetic back to the patient; for the rest, fresh air is inspired. The available systems differ in efficiency, dead space, and technical perfection. Anesthetic wash-in and concentration changes are achieved quickly. When removing the reflectors from the breathing circuit, wash-out is very fast. In terms of anesthetic consumption, reflection systems must compete with circle systems used with low or even minimal fresh gas flow.

Acknowledgments We thank Karen Schneider for critical revision and correction of language.

References

1. Farrell R, Oomen G, Carey P. A technical review of the history, development and performance of the anaesthetic conserving device "AnaConDa" for delivering volatile anaesthetic in intensive and post-operative critical care. J Clin Monit Comput. 2018;32:595–604.
2. Jerath A, Parotto M, Wasowicz M, Ferguson ND. Volatile anesthetics. is a new player emerging in critical care sedation? Am J Respir Crit Care Med. 2016;193:1202–12.
3. Hendrickx J, Poelaert J, De Wolf A. Sedation with inhaled agents in the ICU: what are we waiting for? J Clin Monit Comput. 2018;32:593–4.
4. Baron R, Binder A, Biniek R, et al. Evidence and consensus based guideline for the management of delirium, analgesia, and sedation in intensive care medicine. Revision 2015 (DAS-Guideline 2015) – short version. Ger Med Sci. 2015;13:1–42.
5. Grounds M, Snelson C, Whitehouse A, et al. Intensive care society review of best practice for analgesia and sedation in the critical Care. London: Intensive Care Society; 2014.
6. Celis-Rodríguez E, Birchenall C, de la Cal MÁ, et al. Guía de práctica clínica basada en la evidencia para el manejo de la sedoanalgesia en el paciente adulto críticamente enfermo. Med Intensiva. 2013;37:519–74.
7. Bomberg H, Glas M, Groesdonk HV, et al. A novel device for target controlled administration and reflection of desflurane - The Mirus™. Anaesthesia. 2014;69:1241–50.
8. Meiser A, Bellgardt M, Belda J, Röhm K, Laubenthal H, Sirtl C. Technical performance and reflection capacity of the anaesthetic conserving device - A bench study with isoflurane and sevoflurane. J Clin Monit Comput. 2009;23:11–9.
9. Meiser A, Laubenthal H. Inhalational anaesthetics in the ICU: theory and practice of inhalational sedation in the ICU, economics, risk-benefit. Best Pract Res Clin Anaesthesiol. 2005;19:523–38.
10. Bomberg H, Groesdonk HV, Bellgardt M, Volk T, Meiser A. AnaConDa™ and Mirus™ for intensive care sedation, 24 h desflurane versus isoflurane in one patient. Springerplus. 2016;5:1–5.
11. Romagnoli S, Chelazzi C, Villa G, et al. The new MIRUS system for short-term sedation in postsurgical ICU patients. Crit Care Med. 2017;45:925–31.
12. Bellgardt M, Drees D, Vinnikov V, et al. Use of the MIRUS™ system for general anaesthesia during surgery: a comparison of isoflurane, sevoflurane and desflurane. J Clin Monit Comput. 2018;32:623–7.
13. Bomberg H, Veddeler M, Volk T, Groesdonk HV, Meiser A. Volumetric and reflective device dead space of anaesthetic reflectors under different conditions. J Clin Monit Comput. 2018;32:1073–80.
14. Sturesson LW, Malmkvist G, Bodelsson M, Niklason L, Jonson B. Carbon dioxide rebreathing with the anaesthetic conserving device, AnaConDa®. Br J Anaesth. 2012;109:279–83.
15. Sturesson LW, Bodelsson M, Jonson B, Malmkvist G. Anaesthetic conserving device AnaConDa®: dead space effect and significance for lung protective ventilation. Br J Anaesth. 2014;113:508–14.

16. Bomberg H, Meiser F, Daume P, et al. Halving the volume of AnaConDa: evaluation of a new small-volume anesthetic reflector in a test lung model. Anesth Analg. 2018; https://doi.org/10.1213/ANE.0000000000003452. [Epub ahead of print].
17. Bomberg H, Meiser F, Zimmer S, et al. Halving the volume of AnaConDa: initial clinical experience with a new small-volume anaesthetic reflector in critically ill patients—a quality improvement project. J Clin Monit Comput. 2018;32:639–46.
18. Mashari A, Fedorko L, Fisher JA, Klein M, Wąsowicz M, Meineri M. High volatile anaesthetic conservation with a digital in-line vaporizer and a reflector. Acta Anaesthesiol Scand. 2018;62:177–85.
19. Perhag L, Reinstrup P, Thomasson R, Werner O. The Reflector: a new method for saving anaesthetic vapours. Br J Anaesth. 2000;85:482–6.
20. Sturesson LW, Frennström JO, Ilardi M, Reinstrup P. Comparing charcoal and zeolite reflection filters for volatile anaesthetics. Eur J Anaesthesiol. 2015;32:521–6.
21. Jerath A, Panckhurst J, Parotto M, et al. Safety and efficacy of volatile anesthetic agents compared with standard intravenous midazolam/propofol sedation in ventilated critical care patients: a meta-analysis and systematic review of prospective trials. Anesth Analg. 2017;124:1190–9.
22. Kong KL, Willatts SM, Prys-Roberts C. Isoflurane compared with midazolam for sedation in the intensive care unit. Br Med J. 1989;298:1277–80.
23. Spencer EM, Willatts SM. Isoflurane for prolonged sedation in the intensive care unit; efficacy and safety. Intensive Care Med. 1992;18:415–21.
24. Meiser A, Sirtl C, Bellgardt M, et al. Desflurane compared with propofol for postoperative sedation in the intensive care unit. Br J Anaesth. 2003;90:273–80.
25. Hanafy MA. Clinical evaluation of inhalational sedation following coronary artery bypass grafting. Egypt J Anaesth. 2005;21:237–42.
26. Röhm KD, Wolf MW, Schöllhorn T, Schellhaass A, Boldt J, Piper SN. Short-term sevoflurane sedation using the anaesthetic conserving device after cardiothoracic surgery. Intensive Care Med. 2008;34:1683–9.
27. Meiser A, Groesdonk HV, Bonnekessel S, Volk T, Bomberg H. Inhalation sedation in subjects with ARDS undergoing continuous lateral rotational therapy. Respir Care. 2018;63:441–7.
28. Meiser A, Bomberg H, Lepper PM, Trudzinski FC, Volk T, Groesdonk HV. Inhaled sedation in patients with acute respiratory distress syndrome undergoing extracorporeal membrane oxygenation. Anesth Analg. 2017;125:1235–9.
29. Jabaudon M, Boucher P, Imhoff E, et al. Sevoflurane for sedation in acute respiratory distress syndrome. a randomized controlled pilot study. Am J Respir Crit Care Med. 2017;195:792–800.
30. Bellgardt M, Bomberg H, Herzog-Niescery J, et al. Survival after long-term isoflurane sedation as opposed to intravenous sedation in critically ill surgical patients. Eur J Anaesthesiol. 2016;33:6–13.
31. Shehabi Y, Bellomo R, Reade MC, et al. Early intensive care sedation predicts long-term mortality in ventilated critically ill patients. Am J Respir Crit Care Med. 2012;186:724–31.
32. Bomberg H, Volk T, Groesdonk HV, Meiser A. Efficient application of volatile anaesthetics: total rebreathing or specific reflection? J Clin Monit Comput. 2018;32:615–22.
33. Meiser A, Bomberg H, Volk T, Groesdonk HV. Neue technische Entwicklungen der inhalativen Sedierung. Anaesthesist. 2017;66:274–82.

Intensity Matched Algorithm for Comfort in Intensive Care Patients: I-MAC ICU

49

Y. Shehabi, A. Pakavakis, and W. Al-Bassam

49.1 Introduction

Achieving optimal analgesia and sedation for critically ill patients has been the focus of multiple iterations of guidelines and clinical practice recommendations [1–3]. The common goal has been to deliver adequate analgesia and provide light sedation to reduce patients' dependency on mechanical ventilation and to enhance early physical recovery.

Different algorithms have also been published with the aim of formulating a convenient patient-centered approach that could be implemented in the context of critical illness. The Early Comfort Using Analgesia, Minimal Sedatives and Maximal Humane Care (eCASH) concept focused on early effective pain relief and comfort with light or no sedation to allow earlier mobilization, reduce the risk of agitation and distress and accelerate return to normal routine with improved sleep quality [4]. The level of adoption of eCASH has not been investigated and remains unknown. The evolving "Assessing pain; Both spontaneous awakening and breathing trials; Choice of drugs; Delirium monitoring/management; Early exercise/mobility; and Family empowerment" (ABCDEF) bundle, which has gained popularity in many countries, packages six domains of interventions to be implemented at an organizational level and by bedside care-givers [5, 6]. The bundle emphasizes

Y. Shehabi (✉)
Faculty of Medicine, School of Clinical Sciences, Monash University, Melbourne, VIC, Australia

Clinical School of Medicine, University of New South Wales, Sydney, NSW, Australia
e-mail: yahya.shehabi@monash.edu

A. Pakavakis · W. Al-Bassam
Faculty of Medicine, School of Clinical Sciences, Monash University, Melbourne, VIC, Australia

Department of Intensive Care, Monash Medical Centre, Monash Health, Clayton, VIC, Australia

J.-L. Vincent (ed.), *Annual Update in Intensive Care and Emergency Medicine 2019*, Annual Update in Intensive Care and Emergency Medicine,
https://doi.org/10.1007/978-3-030-06067-1_49

the importance of a change in culture and advocates a multidisciplinary coordinated approach to the assessment and management of pain, ventilator and sedation weaning and delirium.

Despite the increased awareness of these guidelines and bundles, a worldwide survey of the ABCDEF Bundle showed that practice was highly variable around the world [7]. Some strategies, such as the use of pain and sedation scores appear to be widely used, while other elements, such as the use of delirium screening tools, spontaneous breathing trials and sedative interruption and weaning, have been less well implemented.

The Society of Critical Care Medicine's updated 2018 Clinical Practice Guidelines on the management of Pain, Agitation/sedation, Delirium, Immobility and Sleep disruption (PADIS) extended our understanding of current knowledge but identified evidence gaps and research priorities to be addressed, mainly due to limitations associated with previous research in this area [8]. The PADIS included an implementation plan to encourage clinicians and organizations to adopt and/or adapt the PADIS principles [9].

49.2 The Need for a Practical, Personalized, Patient-Centered Approach

Despite the comprehensive nature of Clinical Practice Guidelines and bundles, there are some limitations and barriers to implementation. These Guidelines and bundles were not designed to be prescriptive in nature. They provide general principles and recommendations and leave the details to the clinicians and bedside care givers. Thus, the provision of adequate analgesia and light sedation, two principal recommendations, does not consider individual variability in the intensity of pain, agitation or risk of delirium.

Intensity of pain can be influenced by many variables including patient factors, such as age, ethnicity, prior exposure and acute illness, and procedure-related factors [10]. An individual's perception of pain will vary depending on psychological and physical characteristics. Patient factors, such as young age, non-white ethnicity, sex and a history of anxiety or depression, have been associated with a heightened pain experience [11]. Hospital factors, such as intensive care unit (ICU) length of stay, prolonged time from onset of pain to analgesic administration, the type of procedure and the experience of pre-procedural pain, can also lead to reporting of more intense pain [12]. The importance of understanding the various factors that alter a patient's pain experience become clearer when it is appreciated that moderate to severe pain is an independent risk factor for agitation. Furthermore, the severity of agitation can also be influenced by other factors including sex, prior illness, concurrent medications and the severity of presenting illness [13]. A history of substance abuse, smoking, psychiatric illness and mechanical ventilation also increases the likelihood of a patient becoming agitated. Patients who experience agitation in the ICU have been shown to have fewer ventilation-free days, longer ICU lengths of stay and are more likely to be discharged to a care facility [13].

In addition, risk factors for delirium in the critically ill have been identified. The risk factors can be divided into four domains: patient characteristics, chronic health comorbidities, acute illness factors and environmental factors. Within these groups,

Box 49.1 Factors that increase the risk of delirium in critical illness

Patient factors	Chronic health factors	Acute illness factors	Environmental factors
Age	**Dementia**	**Coma**	No visible daylight
Alcohol use	**Hypertension**	**APACHE II**	Benzodiazepines
Nicotine use	Cardiac disease	**Emergency surgery**	Opiates
	ASA physical status	**Mechanical ventilation**	Epidural analgesia
		Polytrauma	Physical restraints
		Metabolic acidosis	Isolation
		Organ failure	No normal food
		Fever	
		Medical admission	

ASA American Society of Anesthesiologists; higher risk factors in bold font

risk factors should be further considered in terms of ability to modify (Box 49.1) [14]. The individual variability in the intensity of pain, agitation and increasing risk of delirium mandates an approach that takes into account the triggers, drivers and risk factors mentioned.

There is also a need to consider the early phase of critical illness following the initiation of mechanical ventilation. Many reports have suggested that deep sedation in the first 48 h after initiation of mechanical ventilation is a significant risk factor for prolonged mechanical ventilation, increasing risk of delirium and risk of death [15–19]. Therefore, delivery of optimal analgesia and sedation early and consistently to critically ill patients is a clinical imperative.

The scope of illness severity, the multiplicity of intensive care therapeutic interventions and the dynamic nature of critical illness and organ dysfunction influence the metabolism and kinetics of sedative and analgesic agents [20]. All of the above mandate a practical bedside approach, that provides a mixture of pharmacological and non-pharmacological interventions tailored, individualized and personalized to patients' needs.

Based on these principles, we present an Intensity Matched Algorithm for Comfort (I-MAC ICU) that categorizes critically ill adults into three groups according to the severity and complexity of presenting illness including diagnostic category, severity of organ dysfunction and intensity of therapeutic interventions required to support respective organ dysfunction. Patients are divided according to the expected or actual intensity of pain, agitation and risk of delirium into Group 1 (low intensity), Group 2 (intermediate intensity) and Group 3 (high intensity) with correspondingly escalated interventions utilizing the principles outlined in the PADIS guidelines and using multimodal analgesia and sedation (Table 49.1).

49.3 The Perceived Benefits of I-MAC ICU

1. This algorithm provides a standardized, yet personalized, practical approach that can be used in all patients using known and common analgesic and sedative agents that are used in current practice. This can be delivered shortly after

Table 49.1 Intensity-matched escalated interventions and de-escalation algorithm

Group	Escalated interventions	De-escalation[a]
Group 1: low intensity	**Multimodal analgesia** Opioid (e.g., morphine 1–5 mg/h) ± regional analgesia ± low dose ketamine (0.15–0.25 mg/kg/h) Paracetamol injectable or oral Non-steroidal with caution Pregabalin for neuropathic pain	Continue analgesia as needed
	Minimal or no sedation ± propofol[b] (0.5–1 mg/kg//h) or ± dexmedetomidine (0.2–0.5 μg/kg/h)	Cease any sedatives
Group 2: Intermediate intensity	**Multimodal analgesia (as above)** **Minimal sedation** + propofol[b] (1–3 mg/kg/h) ± dexmedetomidine (0.2–1 μg/kg/h)	Continue analgesia as needed Wean sedation as appropriate Add dexmedetomidine if agitated
Group 3: High intensity	**Multimodal analgesia (as above)** **Multimodal sedation:** + propofol[b] (1–3 mg/kg) + intermittent boluses of midazolam (2–5 mg) or continuous midazolam infusion (1–5 mg/h) Recommend suitable neurophysiologic monitoring for sedation depth	Continue analgesia as needed Cease midazolam Low dose propofol[b] (0.5–2 mg/kg) Consider dexmedetomidine (0.7–1 μg/kg/h) Consider quetiapine (12.5 mg –50 mg/day)

[a]De-escalation with frequent assessment of the need for deeper sedation
[b]Propofol dose not to exceed 200 mg/h

admission to intensive care achieving early and targeted delivery of analgesics and sedatives [21].

2. It provides a clinically desirable frequently reviewed sedation target for each group. This can reduce unjustified iatrogenic deep sedation and maintain appropriate target sedation.
3. The use of multimodal analgesia provides the optimal use of pre-emptive and effective pain relief for procedures and therapeutic interventions. The use of opioids, considered the corner stone of pain management, with the N-methyl-d-aspartate antagonist ketamine and local or regional blockade as appropriate provides an effective strategy for pain relief [22–24].
4. It delivers sedative medications to target sedation and allows titration and de-escalation as clinically desirable. It allows the use of multimodal sedation which reduces the side effects and maximizes the benefits of individual agents. It combines the use of propofol, an agent known for fast onset and offset and easy titration to effect, with agents such as dexmedetomidine known for providing conscious light basal sedation, which hastens resolution of agitation and shortens ventilation time [25–27].
5. The de-escalation strategy mandates frequent evaluation of the need for deep sedation. Thus, clinically desirable deeper levels of sedation can be maintained

for the shortest possible time. The use of dexmedetomidine in the de-escalation phase can minimize the risk of emergent delirium [28, 29], which is common following periods of deep sedation in patients with high intensity pain, agitation and increased risk of delirium.

6. Adequate analgesia and light cooperative sedation is an essential pre-requisite to early mobilization and access to physical rehabilitation [19]. I-MAC ICU presents a high degree of individualized titration of analgesics and sedatives that is likely to achieve comfort with effective pain relief and optimal light sedation early in the phase of critical illness. Early access to physical rehabilitation and mobilization is important to earn the desired improvement in clinical outcomes, such as lower delirium and shorter ventilation time and ICU stay [30].
7. The algorithm allows for the early use of non-pharmacological interventions to prevent delirium and sleep disruption at all times in all patients as appropriate and practically feasible [8, 31, 32]. The success of these interventions is enhanced by an improved level of communication and family engagement with comfortable and awake patients, an essential and desired outcome of the I-MAC ICU.

49.4 Key Elements of the I-MAC ICU

We divide critically ill patients into three groups (Fig. 49.1) as follows:

Group 1: Low intensity of pain, agitation and risk of delirium. This is further divided into:

(A) Patients who require ventilation for less than 24 h. This is typically a post-operative patient who remains ventilated following surgery, such as cardiac surgery or complex thoracic or abdominal surgery. It also includes patients who present with a non-operative medical illness that requires short-term ventilation, such as respiratory distress, pulmonary edema or a respiratory infection or sepsis. The target Richmond Agitation Sedation Score (RASS) [33] for these patients should be a RASS of 0, i.e., awake, calm and responsive to voice. The principal I-MAC ICU in this group is multimodal analgesia as described in Table 49.1. The dosages and analgesic medications described present an example of our own practice. In a minority of patients, comfort may be enhanced with the addition of a sedative at the lowest possible dose. Propofol or dexmedetomidine are the agents that we recommend. Consistent with PADIS 2018 Guidelines [8], the use of benzodiazepines in this group of patients should be discouraged.

(B) Patients who require ventilation for more than 24 h and typically for 3–5 days. Typically patients presenting with complicated surgery or medical illness that is associated with more than one organ dysfunction, such as severe intra-abdominal infections, pancreatitis, hospital or community-acquired pneumonia, and cardiogenic shock. The target RASS in this group is 0 to −1, i.e., responsive to voice and able to make eye contact for longer than 10 s. Multimodal analgesia continues to be the principal intervention for comfort in

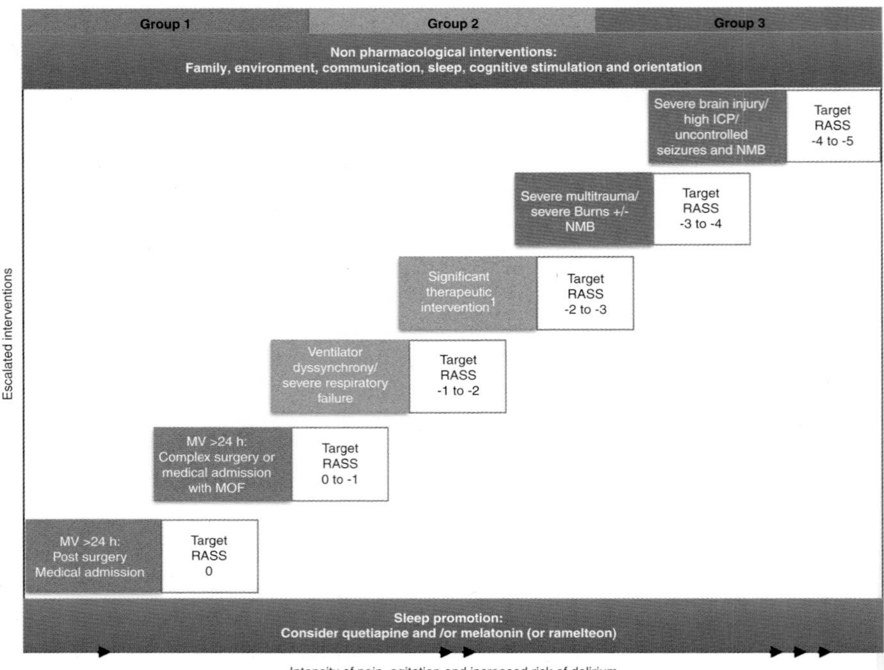

Fig. 49.1 Intensity Matched Algorithm for Comfort (I-MAC) ICU approach. This graph depicts increasing intensity of pain, agitation and risk of delirium on the X-axis according to severity of illness, complexity and diagnostic presentations and therapeutic interventions required. A stepwise algorithm is described with defined Richmond Agitation Sedation Score (RASS) targets, multimodal analgesia and minimal use of sedatives to achieve comfort and clinically desirable sedation targets. Frequent evaluation of sedation targets and titration to effect is an important aspect of the de-escalation process. For detailed doses and agents used, see Table 49.1. [1]Significant therapeutic intervention = extracorporeal life support, therapeutic hypothermia and prone positioning. *MV* mechanical ventilation; *MOF* multiple organ failure; *NMB* neuromuscular blockade

this group of patients, especially following any surgical intervention. Comfort, however, is significantly enhanced by the addition of sedative agents that are short acting and easy to titrate, such as propofol, or agents that allow rousable light sedation, such as dexmedetomidine. The dose of propofol and or dexmedetomidine that may be required in this group of patients is higher than that required for patients needing ventilation for less than 24 h (Fig. 49.1 and Table 49.1).

Group 2: Intermediate intensity of pain, agitation and risk of delirium. This group is further divided into:

(A) Patients with severe respiratory failure requiring high fractional inspired O_2 (FiO_2), high positive end-expiratory pressure (PEEP) with possible ventilator dyssynchrony. The target RASS for these patients is −1 to −2, i.e., responds to voice and makes eye contact. While multimodal analgesia is an essential first component of comfort care, the provision of light sedation using propofol ± dexmedetomidine, at higher doses than prescribed in Group 1 (Table 49.1), will facilitate ventilator therapy and possibly shorten liberation time from mechanical ventilation when compared with using benzodiazepines, such as midazolam [26].

(B) Patients with significant multisystem organ failure who are likely dependent on highly invasive therapeutic interventions, such as extracorporeal life support, targeted temperature management, prone positioning or neuromuscular blockade. The target RASS for these patients is −2 to −3, i.e., patients are responsive to voice but may be unable to make eye contact. In this group of patients, the RASS target should be re-evaluated and reviewed at least twice a day and moved to lighter levels as soon as clinically acceptable. Combination of propofol and dexmedetomidine in appropriate dosages should provide comfort and tolerance for life saving therapeutic interventions.

Group 3: High intensity pain, agitation and risk of delirium. These are the sickest, most critically ill patients in the ICU. This group of patients can be subdivided into:

(A) Those with severe multisystem organ failure, due to severe multi-trauma or burns for example, or severe septic shock or other complicated life-threatening medical conditions. The target RASS for these patients can be typically between −3 to −4, where patients are able to open eyes to tactile stimulation. This is a moderate to deep level of sedation that can be achieved by the addition of intermittent boluses of midazolam in addition to multimodal analgesia and sedation. In principle, the RASS targets should be frequently reviewed and sedation lightened as soon as possible.

(B) Patients with severe traumatic or non-traumatic brain injury with/without raised intracranial pressure (ICP), persistent seizure activity and/or prolonged neuromuscular blockade. These patients need deep levels of sedation to facilitate ICP control and prevent distress and awareness. The target RASS should be −4 to −5. Because of the loss of clinical means of assessing the level of sedation, we recommend using appropriate neurophysiological monitoring to avoid unwarranted extreme levels of deep sedation. The use of midazolam by infusion in these patients may be warranted, however, the dose should be kept to the lowest possible with the use of multimodal analgesia and sedation including propofol, dexmedetomidine and/or suitable enteral agents such as lorazepam or quetiapine. Similar to above, the need for deep sedation must be frequently evaluated and sedative titration, including complete cessation, may be required to achieve lighter sedation targets.

Patients in Group 3 are at high risk of emergent delirium; we suggest the use of a dexmedetomidine infusion during the de-escalation phase to reduce the risk of agitation and delirium [28] and shorten dependency on mechanical support.

49.5 Maximizing Non-pharmacological Interventions

Concomitant non-pharmacological support for critically ill patients represents the humane side of caring for critically ill patients and as such should be a priority in any setting. The I-MAC ICU calls for these interventions to be delivered to all patients as standard. The nature of these interventions, however, is highly institution dependent; it relies on local expertise and the availability of skilled human resources.

Improving communication between patients, families and care-givers is pivotal, this can be facilitated by technology enhancement and the use of visual and hearing aids. The use of music, television, bedside smart phones and e-books and newspapers may maintain a reasonable level of cognitive and intellectual orientation and stimulation. These measures, while common sense interventions, are not simple to deliver consistently and as such have variable success.

49.6 Reducing Sleep Disruption

In addition to the above interventions, day/night orientation, ear plugs, eye masks, noise reduction and implementation of low activity night routine may reduce the risk of sleep disruption, a major issue in the ICU [8]. It is plausible, not proven yet, that adequate sleep may reduce the intensity of pain, agitation and reduce the risk of delirium in critically ill patients. With best intentions, however, non-pharmacological interventions may not be adequate to reduce sleep disruption. Thus, the use of non-benzodiazepine-based medications, such as melatonin, melatonin agonists, such as ramelteon [34] or quetiapine may induce normal sleep architecture and possibly reduce the intensity of pain, agitation and risk of delirium.

49.7 Limitations of I-MAC ICU

The obvious strength of I-MAC ICU is the logical sequence of a stepwise ladder of interventions that utilizes multimodal analgesia and sedation with agents that are commonly used in clinical practice. It is adaptable and practical and can be used in any ICU and for almost all types of patients. The obvious limitation is the lack of a tested hypothesis showing the efficacy of the proposed algorithm. While this is an opinion piece based on the authors' experience, it is consistent with published guidelines and supports the spirit of other bundles, such as the ABCDEF bundle, shown in observational studies to improve patient-specific outcomes, such as ventilation time, delirium and even mortality [35].

49.8 Conclusion

Clinical Practice Guidelines advocate for the provision of effective analgesia and optimal targeted sedation in critically ill adults. The I-MAC ICU is a stepwise escalated, prescriptive, intensity-based algorithm. It provides an individualized practical approach at the bedside to deliver effective multimodal analgesia and targeted optimal multimodal sedation, based on the intensity of pain, agitation and risk of delirium in critically ill patients. It also provides a stepdown de-escalation algorithm designed to reduce unjustified iatrogenic coma and reduce the risk of emergent agitation and delirium. The I-MAC ICU incorporates non-pharmacological strategies and encourages sleep to reduce the need for pharmacological interventions and accelerate the recovery of critically ill patients.

References

1. Jacobi J, Fraser GL, Coursin DB, et al. Clinical practice guidelines for the sustained use of sedatives and analgesics in the critically ill adult. Crit Care Med. 2002;30:119–41.
2. Barr J, Fraser GL, Puntillo K, et al. Clinical practice guidelines for the management of pain, agitation, and delirium in adult patients in the intensive care unit. Crit Care Med. 2013;41:263–306.
3. Girard TD, Alhazzani W, Kress JP, et al. An Official American Thoracic Society/American College of Chest Physicians Clinical Practice Guideline: liberation from mechanical ventilation in critically ill adults. Rehabilitation protocols, ventilator liberation protocols, and cuff leak tests. Am J Respir Crit Care Med. 2017;195:120–33.
4. Vincent J-L, Shehabi Y, Walsh TS, et al. Comfort and patient-centred care without excessive sedation: the eCASH concept. Intensive Care Med. 2016;42:962–71.
5. Pandharipande P, Banerjee A, McGrane S, Ely EW. Liberation and animation for ventilated ICU patients: the ABCDE bundle for the back-end of critical care. Crit Care. 2010;14:1.
6. Marra A, Ely EW, Pandharipande PP, Patel MB. The ABCDEF bundle in critical care. Crit Care Clin. 2017;33:225–43.
7. Morandi A, Piva S, Ely E, et al. Worldwide survey of the "assessing pain, both spontaneous awakening and breathing trials, choice of drugs, delirium monitoring/management, early exercise/mobility, and family empowerment"(ABCDEF) bundle. Crit Care Med. 2017;45:e1111–22.
8. Devlin J, Skrobik Y, Gelinas C, Pandharipande P, Slooter A, Needham D. Clinical practice guidelines for the prevention and management of pain, agitation/sedation, delirium, immobility, and sleep disruption in adult patients in the ICU. Crit Care Med. 2018;46:e825–73.
9. Balas MC, Weinhouse GL, Denehy L, et al. Interpreting and implementing the 2018 pain, agitation/sedation, delirium, immobility, and sleep disruption clinical practice guideline. Crit Care Med. 2018;46:1464–70.
10. Ip HY, Abrishami A, Peng PW, Wong J, Chung F. Predictors of postoperative pain and analgesic consumptiona qualitative systematic review. Anesthesiology. 2009;111:657–77.
11. Devlin JW, Skrobik Y, Gelinas C, et al. Clinical practice guidelines for the prevention and management of pain, agitation/sedation, delirium, immobility, and sleep disruption in adult patients in the ICU. Crit Care Med. 2018;46:e825–73.
12. TMLd A, LCPd A, Nosé PMG, FGRd F, Machado FR. Risk factors for agitation in critically ill patients. Rev Bras Ter Intensiva. 2016;28:413–9.
13. Burk RS, Grap MJ, Munro CL, Schubert CM, Sessler CN. Predictors of agitation in critically ill adults. Am J Crit Care. 2014;23:414–23.
14. Zaal IJ, Devlin JW, Peelen LM, Slooter AJ. A systematic review of risk factors for delirium in the ICU. Crit Care Med. 2015;43:40–7.
15. Shehabi Y, Bellomo R, Reade MC, et al. Early intensive care sedation predicts long-term mortality in ventilated critically ill patients. Am J Respir Crit Care Med. 2012;186:724–31.
16. Shehabi Y, Chan L, Kadiman S, et al. Sedation depth and long-term mortality in mechanically ventilated critically ill adults: a prospective longitudinal multicentre cohort study. Intensive Care Med. 2013;39:910–8.
17. Balzer F, Weiß B, Kumpf O, et al. Early deep sedation is associated with decreased in-hospital and 2-years follow-up survival. Crit Care. 2015;19:197.

18. Stephens RJD, Roberts MR, et al. Practice patterns and outcomes associated with early sedation depth in mechanically ventilated patients: a systematic review and meta-analysis. Crit Care Med. 2018;46:471–9.
19. Shehabi Y, Bellomo R, Kadiman S, et al. Sedation intensity in the first 48 hours of mechanical ventilation and 180-day mortality: a multinational prospective longitudinal cohort study. Crit Care Med. 2018;46:850–9.
20. Devlin JW, Roberts RR. Pharmacology of commonly used analgesics and sedatives in the icu: benzodiazepines, propofol, and opioids. Anesthesiol Clin. 2011;29:13.
21. Shehabi YBR, Reade MC, Bailey M, et al. Early goal directed sedation vs standard care sedation in mechanically ventilated critically ill patients, randomized controlled trial. Crit Care Med. 2013;41:1983–91.
22. Panzer O, Moitra V, Sladen RN. Pharmacology of sedative-analgesic agents: dexmedetomidine, remifentanil, ketamine, volatile anesthetics, and the role of peripheral mu antagonists. Anesthesiol Clin. 2011;29:587–605.
23. Jouguelet-Lacoste J, La Colla L, Schilling D, Chelly JE. The use of intravenous infusion or single dose of low-dose ketamine for postoperative analgesia: a review of the current literature. Pain Med. 2015;16:383–403.
24. Wang L, Johnston B, Kaushal A, Cheng D, Zhu F, Martin J. Ketamine added to morphine or hydromorphone patient-controlled analgesia for acute postoperative pain in adults: a systematic review and meta-analysis of randomized trials. Can J Anesth. 2016;63:311–25.
25. Riker RR, Shehabi Y, Bokesch PM, et al. Dexmedetomidine vs midazolam for sedation of critically ill patients a randomized trial. JAMA. 2009;301:489–99.
26. Jakob SM, Ruokonen E, Grounds RM, et al. Dexmedetomidine vs midazolam or propofol for sedation during prolonged mechanical ventilation: two randomized controlled trials. JAMA. 2012;307:1151–60.
27. Reade MC, Eastwood GM, Bellomo R, et al. Effect of dexmedetomidine added to standard care on ventilator-free time in patients with agitated delirium: a randomized clinical trial. JAMA. 2016;315:1460–8.
28. Skrobik Y, Duprey MS, Hill NS, Devlin JW. Low-dose nocturnal dexmedetomidine prevents icu delirium. a randomized, placebo-controlled trial. Am J Respir Crit Care Med. 2018;197:1147–56.
29. Djaiani G, Silverton N, Fedorko L, et al. Dexmedetomidine versus propofol sedation reduces delirium after cardiac surgery. A randomized controlled trial. Anesthesiology. 2016;124:362–8.
30. Schweickert WD, Pohlman MC, Pohlman AS, et al. Early physical and occupational therapy in mechanically ventilated, critically ill patients: a randomised controlled trial. Lancet. 2009;373:1874–82.
31. Patel J, Baldwin J, Bunting P, Laha S. The effect of a multicomponent multidisciplinary bundle of interventions on sleep and delirium in medical and surgical intensive care patients. Anaesthesia. 2014;69:540–9.
32. Hu RF, Jiang XY, Chen J, et al. Non-pharmacological interventions for sleep promotion in the intensive care unit. Cochrane Database Syst Rev. 2015:CD008808.
33. Sessler CN, Gosnell MS, Grap MJ, et al. The Richmond Agitation–Sedation Scale: validity and reliability in adult intensive care unit patients. Am J Respir Crit Care Med. 2002;166:1338–44.
34. Nichols K, Killian A, Asbury W, Mukhtar A. Ramelteon for the prevention of ICU delirium. Crit Care Med. 2018;46:380. abst 789
35. Barnes-Daly MA, Phillips G, Ely E. Improving hospital survival and reducing brain dysfunction at seven California community hospitals: implementing PAD guidelines via the ABCDEF bundle in 6,064 patients. Crit Care Med. 2017;45:171–8.

Sleep and Circadian Rhythm in Critical Illness

50

I. Telias and M. E. Wilcox

50.1 Introduction

Sleep is controlled by two major regulatory systems: a circadian system that drives 24-h periodicity (Process C), and a homeostatic system (Process S) that ensures adequate amounts of sleep are obtained. Both processes are disturbed in critically ill patients, potentially due to exposure to sleep-altering medications (e.g., propofol), the structure of the intensive care unit (ICU) environment (e.g., workflow), aggravation of a pre-existing sleep disorder, and/or effects of acute illness (e.g., sepsis). As a result, patients may experience delirium, poor respiratory function, and dysregulated immune system reactivity. Several methods of measuring sleep in the ICU exist, although all provide their own challenges. A number of intervention-based therapies to improve ICU sleep and circadian rhythm disturbances have been explored, including noise reduction protocols, music therapy, light treatment, and different modes of mechanical ventilation. These studies have met with limited success.

I. Telias
Interdepartment Division of Critical Care Medicine, University of Toronto, Toronto, ON, Canada

Keenan Research Centre, Li Ka Shing Knowledge Institute, St. Michael's Hospital, Toronto, ON, Canada

Critical Care Medicine, University Health Network and Sinai Health System, Toronto, ON, Canada

M. E. Wilcox (✉)
Interdepartmental Division of Critical Care Medicine, University Health Network, University of Toronto, Toronto, ON, Canada

Division of Respirology, Department of Medicine, Toronto Western Hospital, Toronto, ON, Canada
e-mail: elizabeth.wilcox@mail.utoronto.ca

J.-L. Vincent (ed.), *Annual Update in Intensive Care and Emergency Medicine 2019*, Annual Update in Intensive Care and Emergency Medicine, https://doi.org/10.1007/978-3-030-06067-1_50

50.2 Physiology of Sleep

The brain is active during sleep. Sleep is regulated by several centers in the brainstem, hypothalamus, thalamus and forebrain. Involvement and downregulation of the ascending reticular activating system (ARAS) is important for sleep-wake regulation and involves a number of nuclei in the hypocretinergic, GABAergic, histaminergic, adrenergic, and cholinergic systems. Together, these systems orchestrate sleep into the main phases of rapid eye movement (REM) and non-REM (NREM) sleep, classically described by the Rechtschaffen and Kales Rules (R&K rules) [1]. NREM sleep is further divided into three sleep stages: substages N1, N2 and N3. The N3 substage is known as slow wave sleep (SWS) [1]. Normal sleep architecture consists of stages occurring in cycles of 90–120 min each [1, 2].

Circadian rhythms refer to self-sustained fluctuations with a period of approximately (*cira*) 1 day (*diem*) in various physiological processes. In humans, the circadian system is composed of many individual, tissue-specific clocks with their phase being controlled by the master circadian pacemaker, the suprachiasmatic nucleus (SCN) of the hypothalamus [2]. The most evident circadian rhythm in humans is the sleep-wake cycle. The SCN directly regulates multiple neurotransmitter systems that either drive or modulate sleep, including the hypothalamo-pituitary-adrenal (HPA) axis and melatonin from the pineal gland [2]. Circadian clock genes identified in human peripheral tissues to date include *Period* (*Per-1-3*), *Cryptochrome* (*Cry-1* and *Cry-2*), *Clock*, and *Bmal1*, which coordinate with the master circadian pacer [2]. External factors that are called 'timekeepers' or zeitgebers, such as light/dark cycle, interact with internal clocks by synchronizing their different oscillation phases. Circadian rhythms have a duration of approximately 24 h and can be assessed through chronobiologic analysis of the time series of melatonin, cortisol and temperature [2].

50.3 Altered Sleep in the ICU

Normal sleep architecture varies among individuals [3]. A 'normal' sleep stage in a healthy young adult might be: 2–5% N1, 45–55% N2, 3–15% N3 or SWS and 20–25% REM [3]. Normal transition from wake to sleep onset occurs within 10–20 min, and the first period of REM typically occurs within 90–120 min [2]. Although the total sleep time within a 24-h period in the ICU is similar to that of a non-hospitalized individual, marked differences exist in sleep architecture. As much as half of a critically ill patient's sleep occurs during daytime hours with N1 and N2 representing a larger percentage of the total sleep time. The duration and frequency of both SWS and REM sleep are reduced, and frequent arousals lead to high sleep fragmentation. Altered patterns of sleep during an ICU stay take days to normalize and in certain cases may persist after transfer to the general floor/ward. In a recent study by Wilcox et al. characterizing the quality and quantity of sleep in ICU survivors within 7 days of discharge to the ward, approximately two-thirds (61%) of patients had persistent sleep disturbances. Further, patients continued to experience little or no SWS and/or REM sleep, independent of external factors (e.g., frequency of vital sign measurement or number of beds in the room) [4].

Critically ill patients experience circadian rhythm disruption likely secondary to the absence of effective zeitgebers in the ICU environment. In addition, systemic inflammation may also disrupt circadian rhythmicity of chronobiologic markers. In a study by Haimovich et al., the administration of intravenous endotoxin in human volunteers dramatically altered circadian clock gene expression in peripheral blood leukocytes, suggesting a misalignment of central and peripheral clocks in the modulation of the inflammatory response [5]. Mundigler et al. assessed circadian disruption in 17 septic patients, 7 non-septic patients and 21 controls admitted to an ICU [6]. Urinary 6-sulfatoxymelatonin (6-SMT) exhibited loss of circadian rhythmicity with no daytime decline in septic patients [6]. Recently, Li et al. measured plasma levels of melatonin, tumor necrosis factor (TNF)-α, interleukin (IL)-6 and messenger RNA of the circadian genes *Cry-1* and *Per-2* for 24-h in septic and non-septic ICU patients (n = 22) [7]. Altered circadian rhythm of melatonin secretion, reduced expression of *Cry-1* and *Per-2*, and elevated levels of TNF-α and IL-6 were seen in patients with sepsis [7]. Further, peripheral circadian gene expression was suppressed independent of the melatonin rhythmicity, confirming that, at least in the acute phase of sepsis, there is an uncoupling of the central master clock and peripheral tissue-specific clock genes.

50.4 Mechanisms and Physiological Consequences of Sleep Disturbances in the ICU

50.4.1 Light-Dark Cycle

Light is measured in units of lux. On a sunny day in early spring, light levels range from 32,000 to 60,000 lux. In the ICU, reported daytime light levels range from mean illumination levels of 30–165 lux; nocturnal light levels vary from 2.4 to 145 lux; and during procedures (e.g., central line insertion) light devices can deliver up to 10,000 lux [8, 9], which definitely can alter a patient's circadian rhythm. Different studies modulating light exposure, have been shown to decrease incident delirium, possibly through a mechanistic link with modulation of sleep. For example, nocturnal light exposure decreases the secretion of melatonin, a hormone secreted by the pineal gland in response to darkness, which can ultimately result in sleep disruption [2]; the disruption of the circadian rhythm seen in patients with severe sepsis (n = 7) was reflected in the first 48 h of ICU admission by disordered diurnal variation of urinary 6-SMT excretion [10]. In animal models, circadian rhythm disruption due to constant light exposure led to reduced expression of *Per-2* in the SCN and subsequent behavioral symptoms of delirium (i.e., executive dysfunction and memory impairment) [11]. Clinical symptoms were reversed with nobiletin, a known enhancer of Per-2 function [11]. Findings of diurnal disruption have been reported in traumatic brain injury (TBI), trauma and medical patient populations [12]; any association between diurnal disruption and resultant outcome (e.g., sedative use, incidence delirium or length of stay) in these patient populations has yet to be demonstrated.

50.4.2 Noise in the ICU

Noise has been reported as an important contributing factor to sleep disturbance in the ICU. The most common contributing sources of sound disruption are staff conversation, alarms, and patient care interventions [13]. As per the World Health Organization, sound levels should not exceed 30 A-weighted decibels (dBA). Sound levels in numerous ICU studies have reported levels of noise at mean values of 53–59 dBA with peak noise levels of 67–86 dBA [13, 14]. ICU noise levels during daytime and nighttime hours have been found to be similar. ICU noise contributes to patients' lack of REM sleep [13].

50.4.3 Sensorimotor Experience

50.4.3.1 Sedation

Unlike natural sleep that serves an essential biological function, sedation frequently leads to atypical electroencephalogram (EEG) patterns that are not commonly observed in normal sleep. Benzodiazepines and propofol, both GABA agonists, are frequently used for sedation in critically ill patients, propofol being recommended as a first-line agent by current guidelines [15]. Benzodiazepine administration results in decreased sleep latency but adversely effects sleep architecture, decreasing SWS and REM stages of sleep [16]. Propofol is also a potent suppressor of SWS and at high doses can induce EEG burst suppression. Opioids, commonly administered in conjunction with sedatives in critically ill patients, bind the μ-receptors of the ponto-thalamic arousal pathway, a key pathway in REM generation [17]. In a dose-dependent manner, opioids can suppress both SWS and REM [17]. In an observational study ($n = 21$) of mechanically ventilated medical ICU patients on intravenous sedation and analgesia, pronounced temporal disorganization and a paucity of normal sleep EEG findings were seen [18]. Although circadian rhythm was preserved in this study, patients exhibited a phase delay in their excretion of urinary 6-SMT, suggesting that their circadian pacemakers were free-running [18].

Dexmedetomidine is one of the most recently introduced agents for sedation in the ICU. It is a potent and highly selective α-2-adrenergic agonist, with the action of dose-dependent sedation, anti-anxiolysis, and analgesia adjunct. Dexmedetomidine has been shown to more closely create natural sleep than other GABA agonist agents. In two small pilot studies, one study showed improved sleep efficiency and sleep time at night with dexmedetomidine [19] and another study also demonstrated improved sleep efficiency and stage 2 sleep as well as a modification of sleep pattern, shifting sleep (i.e., more than 75% total sleep time) to evening hours [20]. Recently, low-dose nocturnal dexmedetomidine was found to reduce the incidence of delirium in the ICU, without having an effect on patient-reported sleep quality [21]. Numerous outstanding questions remain in investigating the interplay of sleep, circadian rhythm and sedatives in the ICU. Efforts to date have focused on minimizing administration of these agents whilst mechanistic investigations are ongoing.

50.4.3.2 Restraint Use

Conditions encountered by a patient in the ICU could resemble those deliberately created for experiments of sensory and perceptual deprivation. The use of physical restraints deprives patients of a normal sensory interaction with their environment. Short-term arm immobilization was shown in healthy volunteers to reduce local synaptic activity in sensorimotor areas, suggesting that cortical plasticity may be linked to local sleep regulation [22]. A study exploring the impact of physical restraints on sleep quantity and quality would help in informing care recommendations.

50.4.4 Organ Function

50.4.4.1 Mechanical Ventilation

Sleep disturbances in patients under mechanical ventilation are key; however, the interaction between sleep and mechanical ventilation is complex. There is a pathophysiological link between patient-ventilator interaction and sleep disturbances directly or through a necessity for higher doses of sedative drugs. In addition, sleep disturbances in and of themselves, and incident delirium, possibly due to a need for more sedation may all lead to prolonged weaning course and lengthier durations of mechanical ventilation.

Over assistance during pressure-support ventilation (PSV) leads to sleep disruption. During sleep, ventilatory demand, respiratory drive and inspiratory effort decrease. Therefore, it is not uncommon for ventilatory support during PSV to become excessive in relatively normal lungs. This results in hyperventilation and $PaCO_2$ decreasing below the apnea threshold. Asynchronies, related to a high respiratory drive, such as flow starvation, short cycling, and double triggering might theoretically contribute to sleep disturbances and delirium in the context of air hunger necessitating greater sedative exposure [23]. On the other hand, patient-ventilator asynchronies are associated with longer duration of mechanical ventilation that might be associated, at least in part with disturbances of sleep. Thille et al. recently demonstrated that the weaning process was longer in patients who, after failing the first spontaneous breathing trial (SBT), had atypical sleep and an absence of REM as compared to those exhibiting a normal sleep pattern [24]. Preliminary data from a physiological study assessing the relationship between quantity and quality of sleep and weaning outcome shows that patients who passed an SBT and were successfully extubated had a polysomnography (PSG) trace compatible with being more awake (assessed by the odds ratio product [25]) compared to those who failed an SBT or passed but were not extubated (Martin Dres, personal communication). This complex interaction might be mediated by higher use of sedatives, as described by Mehta et al. [26], where patients receiving higher doses of sedatives and opioids at night were more likely to fail readiness-to-wean criteria, fail a SBT, or not be extubated despite having passed an SBT after clinical assessment. Again, in the preliminary data by Dres et al. (personal communication), patients who failed the SBT were shown to have had lesser degrees of interhemispheric correlation during sleep. This is consistent with a study of delirious patients (n = 70), where reductions in peak, mean, and total amplitude of urinary 6-SMT was associated with inability to wean [27]. Although circadian rhythm may influence one's ability to wean, how this effect is mediated through incident delirium or on the weaning process directly is unknown.

50.4.4.2 Immune System

Melatonin, in addition to mediating the effects of the photoperiod, also plays an important role in the adaptive response of an organism. Experimental studies have shown that binding of melatonin to specific receptors in antigen-activated Type 1 T-helper cells (Th-1) upregulates pro-inflammatory cytokine production as well as enhancing phagocytosis and antigen presentation [28]. Animal models have demonstrated a protective effect of melatonin against lethal viral encephalitis, infectious hepatitis, and hemorrhagic or septic shock; it has been shown to inhibit TNF-α, and to reduce post-shock levels of IL-6, superoxide production in the aorta, and inducible nitric oxide synthase (iNOS) in the liver preventing endotoxin induced circulatory shock [28]. Altered patterns of illumination in the ICU have been found to abolish the physiological regulation of melatonin secretion in response to darkness and light [29]; this pathway is directly linked to the inflammatory response and possibly mortality. For a complete review of circadian aspects of the immune response see Papaioanno et al. [28].

50.4.4.3 Nutrition

Although guidelines advise that enteral nutrition be initiated within 24–48 h in the critically ill patient [30] there is no specific recommendation around the timing of nutrition delivery (e.g., daytime hours versus continuous 24-h feeds). Peripheral circadian oscillators are sensitive to stimuli associated with food intake, enabling animals to uncouple rhythms of behavior and physiology from light-dark cycles and instead align them with predictable mealtimes. In our experience, the current practice in the ICU is to administer feeds, as tolerated, over a 24-h period with multiple interruptions during the day for procedures (e.g., bronchoscopy), medication administration (e.g., levothyroxine) or radiographic tests. It may be reasonable to consider the restriction of feeds to daytime hours to assist in the re-entrainment of the SCN. The literature is currently primed for a survey of ICU practices around the timing of feeds (e.g., daytime, 24-h) as this information may help to inform how to best study the impact of nutrition delivery on circadian rhythm disruption in the ICU.

50.4.4.4 Delirium and Other Neuropsychological Sequelae

Studies have found a correlation between sleep deprivation and mental status changes in the ICU. Delirium is characterized by inattention, fluctuating mental status, disorganized thinking and an altered level of consciousness, findings which are also characteristics of sleep deprivation. Sleep disturbances are common in delirious patients. While sleep deprivation is regarded as a potentially modifiable risk factor for the development of delirium, it is also possible that delirium itself may contribute to experienced sleep disturbances. Studies conducted mainly in cardiac surgical patients indicate that sleep deprivation can cause [31], be a result of [32], or simply lower the threshold for transitioning to delirium. Decreased SWS and REM sleep have been hypothesized to contribute to developing delirium. A recent study of ICU patients demonstrated an association between delirium and severe REM sleep reduction (<6% of total sleep time), however a causal relationship was not clearly established [33]. The association between sleep disturbance and delirium remains unclear, but it is possible that their relationship shares a common pathophysiologic pathway.

There is considerable evidence linking sleep-related breathing disorders and poor sleep quality with cognitive impairment in many patient populations. Cognitive domains particularly associated with sleep disruption include working memory, semantic memory, processing speed, and visuospatial abilities [34]. Experimental studies support a number of potential neurobiological mechanisms including accumulation of beta-amyloid pathology, abnormalities of tau, synaptic abnormalities, changes in hippocampal long-term potentiation, impaired hippocampal neurogenesis, and gene expression changes. Few studies have rigorously evaluated the prevalence of sleep disruption after critical illness and its potential role in potentiating cognitive impairment. A recent systematic review by Altman and colleagues reported on 22 studies examining sleep after hospital discharge in survivors of critical illness; however, none of these studies reported on cognitive outcomes [35]. Despite sleep disturbances improving over time, up to two-thirds (61%) of patients reported persistently poor sleep at 6 months follow-up [35]. Analyses of risk factors for sleep disturbances have had conflicting results, but persistent sleep disturbances were consistently associated with post-discharge psychological comorbidities and impaired quality of life.

The risk of developing psychological morbidity after discharge from intensive care is as high as 60% [36]; psychological morbidity includes depression, anxiety and post-traumatic stress disorder. Numerous follow-up studies have demonstrated an association between depressive symptoms and increased levels of fatigue, stress, and anxiety in healthy participants subject to sleep restriction. The underlying mechanism between sleep, circadian rhythm disruption and depression is not well understood; it is theorized that generation of sleep and mental health disorders share overlapping neural mechanisms such that defects in these endogenous pathways result in pathologies to both behaviors. Sleep and circadian rhythm disruption after critical illness may contribute to post-ICU psychological disorders, such as depression; associated risks may be challenging to understand given the complexities of pre-existing comorbid conditions and ICU exposures (e.g., sedation).

50.5 Sleep Measurement in the ICU

Sleep can be measured using a variety of objective and subjective techniques. The gold standard for the objective measurement of sleep is laboratory-based PSG. PSG is a multi-parametric test that monitors brain activity by EEG, eye muscles (electrooculography), muscle activity or skeletal muscle activation (electromyography) and heart rhythm. It is the only method of sleep measurement capable of identifying individual sleep stages following the R&K rules; these stages are scored epoch-by-epoch in accordance with the American Association of Sleep Medicine criteria [1]. The application of conventional classification criteria is challenging in the ICU as alteration in cerebral metabolism, electrolyte disorders, intoxications, and medications influence sleep patterns. Alternative or supplementary criteria for PSG scoring have been proposed by Drouot et al. separating EEG recordings into states of either pathological wakefulness or atypical sleep. Devised and validated on non-sedated patients in the ICU, this method of scoring predicted atypical sleep with a sensitivity of 100% and a specificity of 97% [37].

As classical R&K sleep stages are discrete, they are unable to describe the continuum between wakefulness and sleep. Recently, an automated algorithm named odds ratio product was developed that enables continuous measurement of sleep state ranging from full wakefulness (2.5) to deep sleep (0) [25]. EEG is assessed by rating epochs based on the relative power spectrum of each frequency band (delta, theta, alpha-sigma and beta). In a validation dataset of outpatient PSG recordings, an odds ratio product <1 predicted sleep and odds ratio product >2 wakefulness, with 95% accuracy. Additionally, correlation ($r^2 = 0.98$) was high between the odds ratio product and the probability of arousals and awakenings. Formal validation in a cohort of ICU patients has yet to be performed.

Bispectral index (BIS), an EEG-derived method for assessing the depth of sedation, mainly used during general anesthesia in the operating room, has been proposed as an alternative means of sleep assessment. Unfortunately, BIS is sensitive to technique and its interpretation is difficult. Further, its use for sleep assessment is poorly documented. Spectral edge frequency has been evaluated to assess sleep states as well as circadian rhythmicity [18], but suffers from inconsistency in selecting which epochs to include. In addition, further studies are needed to determine its validity in an ICU population.

Actigraphy, which continuously measures an individual's movement using a wristwatch-like device on the wrist or ankle, is another alternative to PSG. The presence of movement indicates wakefulness, and its absence indicates sleep. This widely-used method has been validated in several populations for measurement of total sleep time and sleep fragmentation [38]. Actigraphy has been validated against biochemical markers of circadian rhythmicity [39]. A recent systematic review of actigraphy in the ICU showed that when compared to PSG, nurse assessment and patient questionnaires, actigraphy tended to consistently overestimate total sleep time and sleep efficiency [40]. When compared to PSG, actigraphy under-reported nocturnal awakenings. Overall awakenings were more frequently reported by nurse assessment and patient questionnaires compared to actigraphic recordings in the ICU.

The use of subjective measures of sleep assessment, such as patient or nurse questionnaires, is simple, easy and relatively inexpensive compared to other objective measures of sleep. Patients may keep daily sleep diaries or a sleep log. The Richards-Campbell Sleep Questionnaire (RCSQ), the Sleep in the Intensive Care Unit Questionnaire, and the Verran/Snyder Halpern Sleep Scale have all been tested in ICU patient populations [41]. Incident delirium and the frequent use of sedatives limit the use of instruments. Further, they typically report only on nighttime sleep, whereas sleep in the ICU is distributed over a 24-h period. Nursing assessment using the Echols Sleep Behavior Observation Tool, Nurses' Observation Checklist and the RCSQ can be used to estimate sleep [41]. Nursing-derived assessments however tend to overestimate total sleep time and sleep efficiency but underestimate awakenings when compared to PSG. Subjective assessments of sleep are variably reliable and provide no information on experienced sleep stages or circadian rhythmicity, limiting their utility in assessing sleep outcomes the ICU.

50.6 Efforts to Improve Sleep in the ICU

A number of studies have evaluated interventions targeting sleep optimization in the ICU, including non-pharmacologic sleep bundles, bright light therapy, earplugs, pharmacologic therapy, relaxation techniques and differing modes of mechanical ventilation, with mixed results. While it is likely that a successful sleep improvement program will need to address both internal and external factors disturbing ICU sleep, no single study has strongly proven its efficacy as an intervention (Fig. 50.1). The widespread use of an ICU specific sleep protocol would require a substantial commitment on the part of the individual center for its implementation. Precipitating such a culture change would likely require the demonstration of a substantial outcome benefit justifying a change to long-held workflow and care provision habits.

50.6.1 Reducing Environmental Impact on Sleep

As the duration, intensity, and wavelength of a light stimulus modulates circadian rhythm via the central circadian clock, it makes intuitive sense to try to restore temporal disorganization of circadian pacemakers by modulating light exposure in the ICU. A single center randomized interventional study (n = 11) evaluating two different light exposures in postoperative patients with esophageal cancer, showed that subjects provided with more intense light had lower incident delirium [42]. Further, in a multicenter, prospective study of 523 non-intubated patients, delirium incidence was reduced in those exposed to visible sunlight in their hospital room [43]. In contrast, however, a large study of medical ICU patients (n = 3577) exposed to differing ambient light levels, with an approximately threefold difference in mean light levels due to different room orientations (south facing 399.2 ± 146 lux as compared to east facing rooms 30.6 ± 1.3 lux), there were no associated differences in sedative, analgesic or neuroleptic use, suggesting no impact on delirium incidence [9]. Conversely, in a small single center prospective study of elderly patients admitted for acute cardiac, respiratory or renal diseases (n = 10), decreases in nocturnal lighting thresholds led to progressive resynchronization of circadian rhythm; circadian rhythms were severely altered during the first 24 h but progressively resynchronized by day 5 [44].

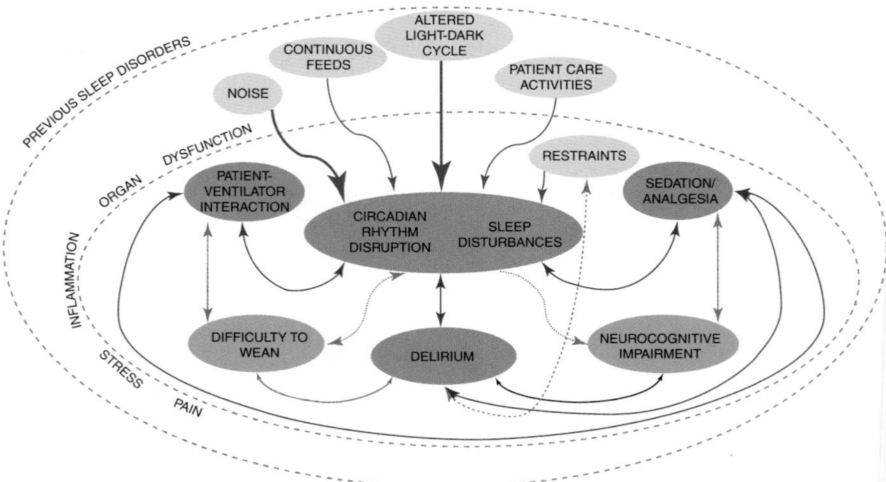

Fig. 50.1 Determinants and physiological consequences of sleep and circadian rhythm disruptions in the intensive care unit (ICU). Interaction between determinants (light blue) and possible consequences (light green) of sleep and circadian rhythm disruptions are shown. Interestingly, most interactions are bidirectional, meaning that the determinants might predispose the patient to such disturbances and be a consequence of them. An intimate relationship between sleep, circadian rhythm disruption and delirium is shown (purple). Main interactions are represented by thicker and continuous arrows. More complex and less proven interactions have dashed arrows. Most of the determinants are modified by factors related to the disease process such as pain, inflammation and end-organ dysfunction. Additionally, many patients admitted to the ICU have previous sleep disturbances, which will probably increase the risk of having them in the ICU

The effects of noise reduction strategies on sleep in the ICU remain controversial. Demoule et al. found that in non-sedated ICU patients, adding earplugs and eye masks to standard care reduced anxiety and improved sleep quality, specifically reducing long awakenings and increasing the duration of SWS [45]. Beneficial effects of noise reduction may be limited to the early stage of ICU admission [43]. Limitations of these studies include small sample sizes, lack of standard measures, and before-after study design. Well-designed trials of environmental interventions with adequate sample sizes are needed.

50.6.2 Pharmacological Considerations

Pharmacological therapy for sleep and circadian rhythm disruption includes a careful review of existing pharmacological treatments, including the omission of chronic medications that may lead to withdrawal symptomatology. As many of the medications administered in the ICU have effects on normal sleep physiology, if medications such as opioids or sedatives cannot be discontinued then their administration should be limited to a minimal effective dose. Medications specifically used for acute sleep disturbances should be used for short periods with ongoing reassessment of necessity. Further, any medication prescribed for sleep should be accompanied by non-pharmacologic interventions (e.g., daytime mobilization and attempts at maintaining daytime wakefulness). Although medications for acute sleep disturbances may increase total sleep time they may not improve sleep quality. As an example, a small randomized controlled trial was able to show that patients who received 10 mg of oral melatonin as compared to placebo demonstrated improved nocturnal sleep efficiency as measured using BIS [46]. Pharmacokinetic analyses suggested that 10 mg dosing was too high, and that 1–2 mg of melatonin could be used in future studies. Studies of melatonin, sleep and delirium are ongoing.

50.6.3 Mechanical Ventilation

Mechanical ventilation represents another important potential cause of sleep disruption. Reducing patient-ventilator asynchrony by optimizing ventilatory settings has been shown to mitigate the impact of mechanical ventilation on sleep [47]. Improved sleep efficiency has been achieved either by limiting the amount of ventilatory support [48, 49] or by altering ventilatory modes (e.g., proportional assist ventilation or neutrally-adjusted ventilatory assist modes). Surprisingly, few studies have examined the effect of time of day on minute ventilation. Recently, difficult to wean tracheostomized patients were reconnected to the ventilator at night to improve sleep efficiency [50]. Airway caliber is known to vary in healthy human beings across a 24-h period. In asthmatics, airflow obstruction tends to worsen in the early morning, corresponding to circadian changes in pulmonary function and abundance of immune cells in the airway. Little is known about how the molecular clock controls lung physiological function and how its disruption might influence respiratory mechanics during ventilation or weaning processes.

50.7 Conclusion

There are complex interactions between physiological, behavioral and environmental factors that contribute to sleep and circadian rhythm disturbances in ICU patients. Little is known about the exact mechanisms leading to these disruptions or the importance of each factor individually on the experienced sleep disturbance. The relationship between sleep, circadian rhythm and outcome after critical illness requires further study. Moreover, measurement of sleep quantity and quality is technically difficult, creating further challenges in delineating relationships. Efforts to date have been focused on non-pharmacologic and pharmacological strategies to improve sleep, with some promising results; however, for broader implementation a change in culture needs to occur. Less attention has been directed towards understanding underlying biological mechanisms of disturbed sleep and circadian disruption. Designing interventions grounded in basic biological principles might prove more effective in improving sleep in the ICU. Without strong evidence of benefit to facilitate changes in practice, the implementation of sleep-specific improvement bundles will be challenging.

References

1. American Academy of Sleep Medicine. The AASM manual for the scoring of sleep and associated events: rules, terminology and technical specifications, version 2.5. Westchester: American Academy of Sleep Medicine; 2018.
2. Collop NA, Salas RE, Delayo M, Gamaldo C. Normal sleep and circadian processes. Crit Care Clin. 2008;24:449–60.
3. Hirshkowitz M, Whiton K, Albert SM, et al. National Sleep Foundation's sleep time duration recommendations: methodology and results summary. Sleep Health. 2015;1:40–3.
4. Wilcox ME, Lim AS, Pinto R, Black SE, McAndrews MP, Rubenfeld GD. Sleep on the ward in intensive care unit survivors: a case series of polysomnography. Intern Med J. 2018;48:795–802.
5. Haimovich B, Calvano J, Haimovich AD, Calvano SE, Coyle SM, Lowry SF. In vivo endotoxin synchronizes and suppresses clock gene expression in human peripheral blood leukocytes. Crit Care Med. 2010;38:751–8.
6. Mundigler G, Delle-Karth G, Koreny M, et al. Impaired circadian rhythm of melatonin secretion in sedated critically ill patients with severe sepsis. Crit Care Med. 2002;30:536–40.
7. Li CX, Liang DD, Xie GH, et al. Altered melatonin secretion and circadian gene expression with increased proinflammatory cytokine expression in early-stage sepsis patients. Mol Med Rep. 2013;7:1117–22.
8. Dennis CM, Lee R, Woodard EK, Szalaj JJ, Walker CA. Benefits of quiet time for neuro-intensive care patients. J Neurosci Nurs. 2010;42:217–24.
9. Verceles AC, Liu X, Terrin ML, et al. Ambient light levels and critical care outcomes. J Crit Care. 2013;28:110 e111–8.
10. Verceles AC, Silhan L, Terrin M, Netzer G, Shanholtz C, Scharf SM. Circadian rhythm disruption in severe sepsis: the effect of ambient light on urinary 6-sulfatoxymelatonin secretion. Intensive Care Med. 2012;38:804–10.
11. Gile J, Scott B, Eckle T. The Period 2 enhancer nobiletin as novel therapy in murine models of circadian disruption resembling delirium. Crit Care Med. 2018;46:e600–8.
12. Seifman MA, Gomes K, Nguyen PN, et al. Measurement of serum melatonin in intensive care unit patients: changes in traumatic brain injury, trauma, and medical conditions. Front Neurol. 2014;5:237.
13. Freedman NS, Gazendam J, Levan L, Pack AI, Schwab RJ. Abnormal sleep/wake cycles and the effect of environmental noise on sleep disruption in the intensive care unit. Am J Respir Crit Care Med. 2001;163:451–7.
14. Freedman NS, Kotzer N, Schwab RJ. Patient perception of sleep quality and etiology of sleep disruption in the intensive care unit. Am J Respir Crit Care Med. 1999;159:1155–62.
15. Barr J, Fraser GL, Puntillo K, et al. Clinical practice guidelines for the management of pain, agitation, and delirium in adult patients in the intensive care unit. Crit Care Med. 2013;41:263–306.
16. Plante DT, Goldstein MR, Cook JD, et al. Effects of oral temazepam on sleep spindles during non-rapid eye movement sleep: a high-density EEG investigation. Eur Neuropsychopharmacol. 2015;25:1600–10.
17. Dimsdale JE, Norman D, DeJardin D, Wallace MS. The effect of opioids on sleep architecture. J Clin Sleep Med. 2007;3:33–6.
18. Gehlbach BK, Chapotot F, Leproult R, et al. Temporal disorganization of circadian rhythmicity and sleep-wake regulation in mechanically ventilated patients receiving continuous intravenous sedation. Sleep. 2012;35:1105–14.
19. Lu W, Fu Q, Luo X, Fu S, Hu K. Effects of dexmedetomidine on sleep quality of patients after surgery without mechanical ventilation in ICU. Medicine (Baltimore). 2017;96:e7081.
20. Alexopoulou C, Kondili E, Diamantaki E, et al. Effects of dexmedetomidine on sleep quality in critically ill patients: a pilot study. Anesthesiology. 2014;121:801–7.

21. Skrobik Y, Duprey MS, Hill NS, Devlin JW. Low-dose nocturnal dexmedetomidine prevents icu delirium. a randomized, placebo-controlled trial. Am J Respir Crit Care Med. 2018;197:1147–56.
22. Huber R, Ghilardi MF, Massimini M, et al. Arm immobilization causes cortical plastic changes and locally decreases sleep slow wave activity. Nat Neurosci. 2006;9:1169–76.
23. Pham T, Telias I, Piraino T, Yoshida T, Brochard LJ. Asynchrony consequences and management. Crit Care Clin. 2018;34:325–41.
24. Thille AW, Reynaud F, Marie D, et al. Impact of sleep alterations on weaning duration in mechanically ventilated patients: a prospective study. Eur Respir J. 2018;51:1702465.
25. Younes M, Ostrowski M, Soiferman M, et al. Odds ratio product of sleep EEG as a continuous measure of sleep state. Sleep. 2015;38:641–54.
26. Mehta S, Meade M, Burry L, et al. Variation in diurnal sedation in mechanically ventilated patients who are managed with a sedation protocol alone or a sedation protocol and daily interruption. Crit Care. 2016;20:233.
27. Dessap AM, Roche-Campo F, Launay JM, et al. Delirium and circadian rhythm of melatonin during weaning from mechanical ventilation: an ancillary study of a weaning trial. Chest. 2015;148:1231–41.
28. Papaioannou V, Mebazaa A, Plaud B, Legrand M. 'Chronomics' in ICU: circadian aspects of immune response and therapeutic perspectives in the critically ill. Intensive Care Med Exp. 2014;2:18.
29. Perras B, Meier M, Dodt C. Light and darkness fail to regulate melatonin release in critically ill humans. Intensive Care Med. 2007;33:1954–8.
30. McClave SA, Taylor BE, Martindale RG, et al. Guidelines for the provision and assessment of nutrition support therapy in the adult critically ill patient: society of critical care medicine (SCCM) and American Society for Parenteral and Enteral Nutrition (A.S.P.E.N.). J Parenter Enter Nutr. 2016;40:159–211.
31. Sveinsson IS. Postoperative psychosis after heart surgery. J Thorac Cardiovasc Surg. 1975;70:717–26.
32. Harrell RG, Othmer E. Postcardiotomy confusion and sleep loss. J Clin Psychiatry. 1987;48:445–6.
33. Trompeo AC, Vidi Y, Locane MD, et al. Sleep disturbances in the critically ill patients: role of delirium and sedative agents. Minerva Anestesiol. 2011;77:604–12.
34. Lim AS, Yu L, Costa MD, Leurgans SE, Buchman AS, Bennett DA, Saper CB. Increased fragmentation of rest-activity patterns is associated with a characteristic pattern of cognitive impairment in older individuals. Sleep. 2012;35:633–40.
35. Altman MT, Knauert MP, Pisani MA. Sleep disturbances after hospitalization and critical illness: a systematic review. Ann Am Thorac Soc. 2017;14:1457–68.
36. Davydow DS, Gifford JM, Desai SV, Bienvenu OJ, Needham DM. Depression in general intensive care unit survivors: a systematic review. Intensive Care Med. 2009;35:796–809.
37. Drouot X, Roche-Campo F, Thille AW, et al. A new classification for sleep analysis in critically ill patients. Sleep Med. 2012;13:7–14.
38. Lim AS, Yu L, Kowgier M, Buchman AS, Bennett DA. Modification of the relationship of the apolipoprotein E ε4 allele to the risk of Alzheimer disease and neurofibrillary tangle density by sleep. JAMA Neurol. 2013;70:1544–51.
39. Lim AS, Chang AM, Shulman JM, et al. A common polymorphism near PER1 and the timing of human behavioral rhythms. Ann Neurol. 2012;72:324–34.
40. Schwab KE, Ronish B, Needham DM, To AQ, Martin JL, Kamdar BB. Actigraphy to evaluate sleep in the intensive care unit. a systematic review. Ann Am Thorac Soc. 2018;15:1075–82.
41. Matthews EE. Sleep disturbances and fatigue in critically ill patients. AACN Adv Crit Care. 2011;22:204–24.
42. Taguchi T, Yano M, Kido Y. Influence of bright light therapy on postoperative patients: a pilot study. Intensive Crit Care Nurs. 2007;23:289–97.

43. Van Rompaey B, Elseviers MM, Schuurmans MJ, Shortridge-Baggett LM, Truijen S, Bossaert L. Risk factors for delirium in intensive care patients: a prospective cohort study. Crit Care. 2009;13:R77.
44. Vinzio S, Ruellan A, Perrin AE, Schlienger JL, Goichot B. Actigraphic assessment of the circadian rest-activity rhythm in elderly patients hospitalized in an acute care unit. Psychiatry Clin Neurosci. 2003;57:53–8.
45. Demoule A, Carreira S, Lavault S, et al. Impact of earplugs and eye mask on sleep in critically ill patients: a prospective randomized study. Crit Care. 2017;21:284.
46. Bourne RS, Mills GH, Minelli C. Melatonin therapy to improve nocturnal sleep in critically ill patients: encouraging results from a small randomised controlled trial. Crit Care. 2008;12:R52.
47. Fanfulla F, Delmastro M, Berardinelli A, Lupo ND, Nava S. Effects of different ventilator settings on sleep and inspiratory effort in patients with neuromuscular disease. Am J Respir Crit Care Med. 2005;172:619–24.
48. Cabello B, Thille AW, Drouot X, et al. Sleep quality in mechanically ventilated patients: comparison of three ventilatory modes. Crit Care Med. 2008;36:1749–55.
49. Parthasarathy S, Tobin MJ. Effect of ventilator mode on sleep quality in critically ill patients. Am J Respir Crit Care Med. 2002;166:1423–9.
50. Roche-Campo F, Thille AW, Drouot X, et al. Comparison of sleep quality with mechanical versus spontaneous ventilation during weaning of critically ill tracheostomized patients. Crit Care Med. 2013;41:1637–44.

Part XVI

Medical Education

Social Media in Critical Care: Entering an Exciting New Era

51

J. N. Wilkinson, A. V. K. Wong, and M. L. N. G. Malbrain

51.1 Introduction

The way we communicate and learn has been revolutionized by technology such that we are never more than a phone call, message or text away from family, friends and colleagues. Mirroring this, social media is beginning to change the way that medicine is taught and practiced. It has the power to engage both healthcare professionals and members of the public with regards to health and policy discussions, networking and facilitating access to health information and services. In this chapter, we will discuss the way social media and free open access medical education impacts on the way we learn, teach and keep up to date with medicine.

51.2 Social Media and Free Open Access Medical Education

'Social media' describes the myriad of cloud- and web-based applications that enable people to create and exchange content. The UK's General Medical Council guidance uses the term to include blogs and microblogs (such as Twitter), internet

J. N. Wilkinson (✉)
Department of Intensive Care Medicine and Anaesthesia, Northampton General Hospital, Northampton, UK
e-mail: jonathan.wilkinson@ngh.nhs.uk

A. V. K. Wong
Department of Intensive Care Medicine and Anaesthesia, King's College Hospital, London, UK

M. L. N. G. Malbrain
Department of Critical Care Medicine, Brussels University Hospital (UZB), Brussels, Belgium

Faculty of Medicine and Pharmacology, Vrije Universiteit Brussel (VUB), Brussels, Belgium

J.-L. Vincent (ed.), *Annual Update in Intensive Care and Emergency Medicine 2019*, Annual Update in Intensive Care and Emergency Medicine,
https://doi.org/10.1007/978-3-030-06067-1_51

forums (such as doctors.net), content communities (such as YouTube and Flickr), and social networking sites (such as Facebook and LinkedIn) [1].

Closely related to social media is the concept or principle of free open access medical education, with which online resources are shared freely and openly to the wider audience [2]. The free open access medical education community spontaneously emerged from the collection of constantly evolving, collaborative and interactive open access medical education resources being distributed on the web. It is independent of platform or media and includes blogs, podcasts, tweets, Google hangouts, online videos, text documents, photographs, Facebook groups, and a whole lot more [3, 4]. Some examples of free open access medical education sites are shown in Box 51.1.

There are inherent differences between traditional printed media and those resources available on social media. First, the quality of traditional media is mediated by publishers, with peer reviewers selected from a pool of 'experts'. Publishing via this route is expensive and access is limited to those paying the necessary subscription fees (paywalls). Another aspect regularly debated and often objected to, is the time taken for information to reach readers.

Box 51.1 List of recommended free open access medical education sites (list is not exhaustive and in no specific order)

Site Name	Web Address	Content
Critical Care Northampton	www.criticalcarenorthampton.com	Critical care, point-of-care ultrasound and anesthesia resources, including regular free open access medical education trawl, blogs, videos, infographics and podcasts
Critical Care Reviews	www.criticalcarereviews.com	Critical care newsletters, symposia, resources and peer reviewing
EMcrit	www.emcrit.org	Emergency medicine resources, including critical care as well as emergency medicine. Blogs included.
International Fluid Academy	www.fluidacademy.org	Critical care resources, includes symposia, blogs, podcasts, vodcasts, videos, powerpoint slides and free open access medical education publications.
Propofology	www.propofology.com	Critical care and anesthesia infographics, resources and podcasts
Life in the Fast Lane	www.lifeinthefastlane.com	Critical care and anesthesia resources including regular free open access medical education trawl, blog and 'best of' sections from other sites
The Bottom Line	www.thebottomline.org.uk	Critical care 'Big Trial' peer review site and resources
Thinking Critical Care	www.thinkingcriticalcare.com	Critical care, point-of-care ultrasound, symposia and blogs
RebelEM	www.rebelem.com	Emergency medicine resources. Includes blogs, podcasts and videocasts.

Modified from [14]

Social media on the other hand has many sources (multiple receivers) and differs in that the quality of the information is mediated by participants, many of whom will not have had training in the peer review process or have no previous scientific publication record. It is, however, cheaper or free to publish, providing easy, unlimited access. Publication is immediate, and information is flexible, even after publication (which can also be seen as a weakness).

In a move supporting the spirit of improving accessibility to new scientific publication and research, research funders from France, the United Kingdom, the Netherlands and eight other European nations have unveiled a radical initiative [4]. The 11 agencies, who together spend €7.6 billion in research grants annually, will mandate by the year 2020 that the scientists they fund must make resulting papers free to read immediately on publication. Currently more than a third of journals publish articles behind a paywall limiting their access. The challenge is how to adapt to this ever-changing environment, whilst still training the next generation of healthcare professionals to deliver the high-quality care expected by society. It is also apparent that the general public is becoming increasingly aware of the availability of this easily accessible information. As their medical practitioners, some may expect us to engage with it.

51.3 Assessing Impact

It is very difficult to quantify the impact of social media using the techniques that we are familiar with using for traditional learning resources. Twitter attracts a high number of 'followers' and retweets that are difficult to compare with traditional impact factors. However, many web blogs are used to host daily summaries of conferences and have demonstrated, via web analytics, an increase in the visitor traffic over the duration of a conference, indicating the presence of a significant audience over a longer period of time (even before or after the actual conference) who make use of the social media resources.

Similarly, online resources providing peer-reviewed summaries of relevant publications have steadily gained momentum and readership through re-tweets by readers, generating publicity to capture interested readers [5]. Such resources have also been used to interview authors of trials, enabling a wide audience to engage in critical discussion of their results just days (and in some case hours) after publication [6]. This may provoke earlier changes in practice than we had previously seen with more traditional methods of information dissemination. But this carries also a potential danger.

The question therefore arises whether free open access medical education could possibly replace peer review? The answer is, perhaps: free open access medical education ignores traditional hierarchy, it is free and has equitable access 24/7, it crosses professional boundaries, it is multinational, transparent, robust and apolitical. Due to the increasing use and awareness of free open access medical education, measures such as the Social Media Index (SMI) [7] and the so-called Kardashian index (KI) [8] have been proposed. The SMI enables assessment of the impact and quality of free open access medical education resources, enables educators to receive scholarly credit and permits learners to identify respected resources.

The KI measures the discrepancy between a scientist's social media profile and publication record, based on the direct comparison of numbers of citations and Twitter followers.

Altmetric (https://www.altmetric.com/) also offers a potentially valuable analysis of the extent to which any given publication has gained attention on social media beyond the classic citations in peer-reviewed journals. It is a system that tracks the attention that research outputs such as scholarly articles and datasets receive online. It pulls data from social media like Twitter, Facebook, and Google+, and traditional media — both mainstream (e.g., The Guardian, New York Times) and field specific (e.g., New Scientist, Bird Watching). Many non-English language titles are covered, blogs (both major organizations (e.g., Cancer Research UK) and individual researchers), and online reference managers (e.g., Mendeley and CiteULike). While Altmetrics has been criticized as a poor surrogate for scientific validity, research quality, and future citation potential, such data can highlight publications that are shared via social media or may otherwise come to the attention of the public via mainstream media outlets.

In addition to Altmetric, PlumX Metrics (https://plumanalytics.com/) also provides insight into the ways people interact with individual pieces of research output (articles, conference proceedings, book chapters, and much more) in the online environment. Examples include when research is mentioned in the news or is tweeted about. These PlumX metrics are divided into five categories to help make sense of the huge amounts of data involved and to enable analysis by comparing like with like: usage, capture, mentions, citations, and social media exposure. As of today, there is no scientific publication looking at the correlation between Altmetric or PlumXmetric scores against the more traditional citation index or impact factor.

Possible dangers of free open access medical education relate to the reliability and correctness of the information provided. Recently, a quality label for medical websites has been launched, the so called HONcode by the Health on the Net foundation [9]. Another danger related to social media and free open access medical education is reductive education and information: first we read the textbook, then we just read the chapter, then just the paper, then just the abstract and now we just read the Tweet.

Not everyone is active on social media and, indeed, opinion on its perceived benefits have divided the scientific community. Those who are active on social media in medicine can often find themselves immersed in a world governed by like-minded individuals and, as a result, can fall securely and often naively into their own closed bubble. Ultimately though, it is up to the individual learner as to how much they engage with social media at conferences/meetings or during the normal working day.

51.4 Keeping Up to Date

The sheer volume of new medical knowledge and publications makes it nearly impossible to keep up to date with everything. With the rapid expansion of digital media worldwide, it is unsurprising that the medical literature has followed this trend.

Box 51.2 Some relevant online medical education hashtags and their descriptors

Hashtag term	Specialty or subject
#FOAMed	Anything medical
#FOAMcc	Critical care
#FOAMem	Emergency medicine
#FOAMim	Internal medicine
#FOAMped	Pediatrics
#FOAMres	Resuscitation
#FOAMsim	Simulation
#FOAMtox	Toxicology
#FOAMus	Ultrasound
#FOANed	Nursing
#MedEdFOAM	Medical education
#POCUS	Point-of-care ultrasound

An estimated 6000 papers are published every day at present, thus keeping up with recent and relevant advances in medicine is an enormous challenge. Social media, when used correctly, can be an effective way of optimizing opportunities for self-directed learning, holding discussions with other healthcare professionals (commonly including the principal authors of landmark studies) and reflecting on newly-acquired knowledge. It is possible to document these learning experiences for your personal record and as evidence for appraisals and revalidation.

Filtering and compiling relevant articles of interest is clearly more efficient digitally. All social media platforms vary but each has its own mechanism to aid the user to search for relevant material. For example, placing a hashtag (#) symbol before an item being described allows every Twitter user rapid access to anything associated with it (Box 51.2).

51.5 Personal Learning Networks, Remote Learning and Early Access

Social media and free open access medical education have the power to facilitate global conversations about the latest medical practice and literature. They allow anyone to follow conferences remotely (but in real-time), help users develop professional networks and friendships and can consolidate information with colleagues at home and abroad. Following attendees using meeting hashtags on Twitter permits in real-time remote access to the meeting, viewed through their interest/opinion spectrum.

New and unpublished innovations, upcoming trial ideas and recruitment to studies are often showcased. Innovative safety ideas and discussions thereon can often open doors to new and exciting practices, many promoting patient safety.

51.6 Appraisals, Records and Continuing Medical Education

With many of us now increasingly learning from blogs and podcasts, it is important to reference these resources for the purpose of appraisals. The problem is how best to record this activity. Some methods include the use of IFTTT or "If This, Then That". This is a web service that aggregates many other web apps into one place and can perform actions given a certain set of criteria. All you need to do is create your recipe and let it store all of your social media activity on Twitter and Facebook for you. Other more specific resources include an online zone for members of the Association of Anaesthetists of Great Britain and Ireland (AAGBI) that hosts a wealth of educational, learning and continuing professional development (CPD) resources [10]. Here you can learn in your own time and keep a record of your completed CPD for use in appraisals and revalidation.

51.7 Policing, Etiquette and Caution

The Royal College of Anaesthetists (RCOA) in the UK encourages the use of social media and in its guidance states that social media use by doctors can benefit patient care, enhance learning and strengthen professional relationships [11]. Social media can facilitate networking by linking like-minded people through tweets at conferences and meetings, and has enhanced communication between and within trainee research groups. As an educational resource, it encourages the use of open access journals and time-limited free access to articles in subscribed journals to further distribute new information.

Like any tool, there are risks and consequences of using social media. Communication and rapid dissemination of new information allows almost instantaneous access to the results of new trials, and allows for critical discussion when the information is fresh and without any traditional peer review process. Clearly, we need to be mindful that any information can be misinterpreted or distorted, especially when subjected to multiple layers of filtering through the social media channels (a broken telephone effect) and the unchecked dissemination of distorted information (gray evidence). Often, it can take some time to sift the so called, 'wheat from the chaff' and learn the patterns of 'the good, the bad and the ugly'.

The General Medical Council UK (GMC) has issued specific guidance relating to the use of social media by doctors, stating that "the standards expected of doctors do not change because they are communicating through social media rather than face to face or through other traditional media" [1]. It must be considered that if one is to place a message out into the vapor of social media, it should be done with exactly the same degree of caution, candor and humility one would exercise when orating it in person from a conference stage to friends, patients and strangers in the crowd. Disappearing behind a username should not be an excuse to abuse the privileged of freedom of speech, or indeed the privileged position of a medical professional.

More detailed guidance has been written as a collaborative publication of Australasian groups of doctors in training, illustrating the application of professional standards with examples both fictional and based on previous cases [12]. Other guidance has been issued by medical defense/indemnity and professional organizations [13].

51.8 Conclusion

There is little doubt about the reach and immense potential that social media and free open access medical education have within critical care. They influence how we access information and how we spread important messages to millions of like-minded clinicians. They may indeed be one of the most effective and efficient platforms for publishers, researchers and clinicians alike. They allow us to rapidly disseminate ground-breaking results, new therapies and trial methodologies. Of course, the information must be used with due care, as peer review processes are not the same as those involved in major journals. One can become influenced by gray information, as well as by the biases of others. In our opinion, with due care and attention, this is one of the most exciting and promising areas to become involved in within critical care.

References

1. General Medical Council UK. Doctors' use of social media. 2013. Available at: https://www.gmc-uk.org/ethical-guidance/ethical-guidance-for-doctors/doctors-use-of-social-media/doctors-use-of-social-media. Accessed 19 Nov 2018.
2. Nickson C. Life in the Fast Lane: FOAM. 2017. Available at: https://lifeinthefastlane.com/foam/. Accessed 19 Nov 2018.
3. Cadogan M, Thoma B, Chan TM, et al. Free open access meducation (FOAM): the rise of emergency medicine and critical care blogs and podcasts. Emerg Med J. 2014;31:e76–7.
4. Holly E. Radical open-access plan could spell end to journal subscriptions. Nature. 2018;561:17–8.
5. The Bottom Line website. Available at: http://www.thebottomline.org.uk. Accessed 19 Nov 2018.
6. Bastian H, Glasziou P, Chalmers I. Seventy-five trials and eleven systematic reviews a day: how will we ever keep up? PLoS Med. 2010;7:e1000326.
7. Thoma BS, Lin JL, Paterson M, et al. The social media index: measuring the impact of emergency medicine and critical care websites. West J Emerg Med. 2015;16:242–9.
8. Hall N. The Kardashian index: a measure of discrepant social media profile for scientists. Genome Biol. 2014;15:424.
9. Health on the Net Foundation Code of Conduct. Available at: https://www.healthonnet.org/HONcode/Conduct.html. Accessed 19 Nov 2018.
10. Association of anaesthetists of great britain and ireland: lifelong learning in anaesthesia. Available at: https://learnataagbi.org. Accessed 19 Nov 2018.
11. Royal College of Anaesthetists UK: What to expect from the RCoA on Social Media. Available at: https://www.rcoa.ac.uk/system/files/Guidelines-WhatExpect.pdf. Accessed 19 Nov 2018.

12. Australian Medical Association Council of Doctors-in-Training, the New Zealand Medical Association Doctors-in-Training Council, the New Zealand Medical Students' Association and the Australian Medical Students' Association. Social media and the medical profession. A guide to online professionalism for medical practitioners and medical students. 2010. Available at. http://www.amawa.com.au/wp-content/uploads/2013/03/Social-Media-and-the-Medical-Profession_FINAL-with-links.pdf. Accessed 19 Nov 2018.
13. Medical Defence Union. Guide to social media. 2017. Available at https://www.themdu.com/guidance-and-advice/guides/consultant-pack/guide-to-social-media. Accessed 19 Nov 2018.
14. Nickson CP. Free open-access medical education and critical care. ICU Management and Practice. 2017. Available at https://healthmanagement.org/c/icu/issuearticle/free-open-access-medical-education-foam-and-critical-care. Accessed August 2018.

Index

J.-L. Vincent (ed.), *Annual Update in Intensive Care and Emergency Medicine 2019,* Annual Update in Intensive Care and Emergency Medicine,
https://doi.org/10.1007/978-3-030-06067-1